School Violence and Primary Prevention

Thomas W. Miller

Editor

School Violence and Primary Prevention

Second Edition

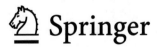 Springer

Editor
Thomas W. Miller
Department of Psychiatry, College of Medicine
Department of Gerontology, College of Public Health
University of Kentucky
Lexington, KY, USA

ISBN 978-3-031-13136-3   ISBN 978-3-031-13134-9   (eBook)
https://doi.org/10.1007/978-3-031-13134-9

This Springer imprint is published by the registered company Springer Nature Switzerland AG
The registered company address is: Gewerbestrasse 11, 6330 Cham, Switzerland

"Dr. Thomas Miller has once again made a major contribution to the scientific literature on one of the most pressing issues of our times: school violence. School Violence and Primary Prevention covers the expansive landscape, ranging across the conceptualization of this psychosocial problem, including neurobiology's contributions – but also explores scholarship concerning cultural, developmental, intergenerational, racial, and gender aspects of school violence, as well as proposed approaches and solutions. Dr. Miller's approach in his previous and extremely influential volumes contributing to stress, health psychology, and adult development are always grounded in historical, theoretical, and conceptual terms that set the framework for empirical studies. He has replicated this sophisticated approach in this volume.

A representative list of topics includes school bullying; sexual exploitation; abuse; trafficking; dating violence; traumatic factors; school shootings; boundary violations; harassment on campus; and the impacts of COVID-19. These contributions reflect the hundreds of compelling questions that galvanize this research and practice domain, and Dr. Miller ably steers the reader through the complexities.

In sum, Dr. Miller has organized complex information for practitioners, teachers, researchers, and policymakers. As a forensic behavioral health researcher, educator, clinician, and policy consultant, I find it an extremely important book that sets forth the state-of-the science for this important field. And it appears at a crucial time in our nation's history."

—James J. Clark, LCSW, PhD, Provost & Executive Vice President, *Florida State University, Tallahassee, FL, USA*

"In this second volume of School Violence and Primary Prevention, Thomas W. Miller has yet again assembled a clear and comprehensive guide to this tragically timely topic. Chapters range from the conceptual to the practical, detailing the many forms of violence, prevention, assessment, and treatment. Issues related to key figures involved in addressing violence in our schools—school superintendents, law enforcement, educators, psychiatrists—are discussed as well. Teachers, administrators, parents, health professionals, and other readers will be enormously grateful to Miller, and the many esteemed authors in this important work, for helping us to understand how we can create the safer learning environments our children need and deserve."

—Madelaine Claire Weiss, LICSW, MBA, BCC, Licensed Psychotherapist, Mindset Expert, and Board-Certified Executive, *Career, and Life Coach, Private Practice, Washington, DC, USA*

"In the new School Violence and Primary Prevention, Dr. Tom Miller addresses the anguish and horror of emerging school violence and the public and academic community's urgent need to fathom and respond. Framing the scope, developmental and neurobiological underpinnings afford a concrete foundation guiding inquiry. The chapters exploring the myriad forms and formats in urban schools will be eye-opening for many: sexual and gender harassment and abuse, boundary violations, bullying, shootings, and trafficking, in relation to cohort perpetrator and victim age, cultural and socialization variables. The roles and options for prevention and responding among education, mental health law enforcement professionals and parents is a comprehensive plan for cogent action for my patients and colleagues as well as the general public and media. I strongly endorse and recommend this resource."

—Steven Nisenbaum, PhD, JD, *Department of Psychiatry, Massachusetts General Hospital, Boston, MA, USA*; *Department of Public Health and Community Medicine, Tufts University School of Medicine, Boston, MA, USA*

"Thomas Miller has created, just at the right time for us all, a second volume, to prevent school violence. For the COVID pandemic not only causes illness and death but, likewise, COVID secondarily is associated with violence and victimization increasing in schools. Schools, as children grow up, are essential for promoting physical and mental well-being. Changes in schooling—such as suspending education, shifting to remote and virtual learning—now require that parents, teachers, school administrators, clinicians, health specialists, many others, learn how to cope and to prevent school violence that once again is increasing as surge upon surge by pandemics increase violence and victimization. And Thomas Miller has done just that, assembled the most knowledgeable experts to teach us all how to conceptualize school violence in our 'new normal', including new factors and forms of school violence, for key personnel learning to master and to deliver prevention interventions. Thomas Miller, himself, has written several excellent chapters on prevention of school violence, as he brings together the most experienced researchers and teachers to train us all on both how to conceptualize new forms of school violence and to deliver new techniques to prevent violence and victimization."

—Walter Penk, PhD, ABPP, Consultant; *Department of Veterans Affairs*; *Department of Defense*; *Texas A&M College of Medicine*; *New Braunfels, TX, USA*

This volume is a collaborative effort to address the changes that we have come to witness in this first quarter of the twenty-first century among our school-age population. From preschool through college, significant shifts have occurred in the way we relate socially to one another that has impacted our lives. It is for the children, parents, teachers, administrators, legislators, and the general public that this volume is intended. May it be a resource that aids in our awareness of the issues and directions that need to be taken to address the safety and well-being of school-aged children. May this compendium of the latest in evidence-based perspectives provide that steppingstone. Finally, it is for my children David and Jeanine as parents, my grandchildren Colin, Francis, Hillarie, Derek, and Heidie as students, and their children that this volume is dedicated.

Foreword

About a month after I was invited to contribute to a foreword to the book entitled *School Violence and Primary Prevention*, edited by Dr. Thomas W. Miller, I remember hearing about mass school shootings that occurred in Oxford High School, which claimed the lives of four innocent students with very promising futures. The shootings also left six students and one teacher critically injured and a community in Oxford Township emotionally scarred. Prior to the incident, I had been aware that the number of people victimized in school shootings was higher this year compared to the previous years and like the general public, I gradually became inured to the school shootings that make the news. I conceded that school shootings are inevitable phenomena in American school districts.

The shootings at Oxford High School, however, hit close to home given my proximity to the school as a faculty at Wayne State University, which is located a little less than one hour away from the school. I have also taught many students who had graduated from Oxford High. Indeed, a week after the incident, one of my students had informed me that the shootings at Oxford High left her quite distressed, and she was unable to concentrate on her assignments. Even though I did what I can to comfort her and all my students, I had frankly stated that "Despite my years of research [on bullying and school violence], I really have no answers."

The good news is, however, that all is not lost. In the aftermath of the Columbine shootings, there has been a burgeoning of research on school violence and school safety conducted by notable researchers in the United States. A quick search by Dr. Dorothy L. Espelage yielded over 4000 published articles on school bullying from 1995 to today (Peguero & Hong, 2020). My own research findings within the past 14 years have uncovered multitudes of factors, such as parent-adolescent relationship quality, number of close friends, presence of caring teachers, and poverty status, which school practitioners need to seriously consider in their assessments and treatment plans. Even more importantly, several anti-bullying programs and policies have been developed and implemented in school districts, and today, public schools in all 50 states are mandated to have an anti-bullying program or policy in place. Despite numerous efforts made to tackle school violence, school shootings remain to be a serious public health concern today. According to *The Washington Post*, since the Columbine High School shootings in 1999, which were followed by other infamous shootings, such as the West Nickle Mines Amish School shootings in 2006, Virginia Tech shootings in 2007, Sandy Hook Elementary School shootings in 2012, and Marjory Stoneman Douglas High School shootings in 2018, more than 278,000 US students had experienced gun violence at their school (Cox et al., 2021).

This book is a highly important contribution to research and practice concerning school violence. Researchers over the years have recognized the significance of primary prevention, defined as "intervening *before* [italics added] health effects occur" by the Centers for Disease Control and Prevention (2017), in addressing school violence. A recent study by Ngo and colleagues (2019) also underscores a critical need for an effective primary prevention approach that aims to increase safe storage of firearms by caregivers and decrease firearms carriage/use by youth, which can significantly reduce firearm-related deaths, such as those at the Oxford High School. Firearms-related injury is the second leading cause of death among adolescents in the United States, and it is paramount that school personnel, researchers, practitioners, and policy makers find ways to prevent shootings from happening. Many thanks to Dr. Miller and the book contributors for this outstanding and highly relevant contribution to the field of school safety.

School of Social Work, Wayne State University   Jun Sung Hong
Detroit, MI, USA

References

Centers for Disease Control and Prevention. (2017). *Picture of America: Prevention*. https://www.cdc.gov/pictureofamerica/

Cox, J. W., Rich, S., Chiu, A., Muyskens, J., & Ulmanu, M. (2021, December 2). More than 278,000 students have experienced gun violence at school since Columbine. *The Washington Post*. https://www.washingtonpost.com/graphics/2018/local/school-shootings-database/

Ngo, Q. M., Sigel, E., Moon, A., Stein, S. F., Massey, L. S., Rivara, F., King, C., Ilgen, M., Cunningham, R., & Walton, M. A. For the FACTS Consortium (2019). State of the science: A scoping review of primary prevention of firearm injuries among children and adolescents. *Journal of Behavioral Medicine, 42*, 811–829. https://doi.org/10.1007/s10865-019-00043-2

Peguero, A. A., & Hong, J. S. (2020). *School bullying: Youth vulnerability, marginalization, and victimization* (Springer Series on Child and Family Studies). Springer.

Acknowledgments

Special appreciation is expressed to the expertise reflected by the contributors and the breadth of knowledge that they have brought to this volume. Appreciation is extended to Springer and to Janet Kim, MPH, Senior Editor, Subhalakshmi, Project Manager and their staff for their guidance and support. For their support and encouragement, special appreciation is extended to my family and to Seth Himelhock, MD; Jeffrey Fisher, PhD; Deborah Corman, PhD; Lane J. Veltkamp, MSW, ACSW, BCD; Walter Penk, PhD; Skip Lowe, PhD; Joanna Hawthorne; Alla Moeller; Howard Coleman; Steve Campbell, MSW; Steve Nisenbaum, PhD, JD; James McCormick, MD; James Holsinger, MD; Neil Carey, MSW; James Clark, PhD, Kathleen Banas, MLS; Tag Heister, MLS.; Deborah Kessler, MLS; Katrina Scott, MLS; and Jill Livingston, MLS. Library Services are acknowledged for their support and assistance in the completion of this volume.

Contents

About the Editor

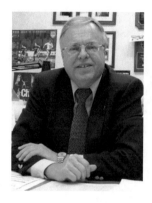

Thomas W. Miller, PhD, ABPP, is a professor emeritus at the University of Connecticut in Storrs and a professor in the Department of Psychiatry, College of Medicine, and the Department of Gerontology, College of Public Health, at the University of Kentucky in Lexington. Dr. Miller is boarded in clinical psychology, a licensed psychologist, and certified in school psychology. He is certified by the American College of Forensic Examiners. He received his doctorate from the State University of New York at Buffalo, is a Diplomate of the American Board of Professional Psychology in Clinical Psychology, and is a Fellow of the American Psychological Association, the American Psychology Society, and the Royal Society of Medicine. Dr. Miller has published several books, chapters, and numerous articles in professional refereed journals, and has presented at a number of national and international symposia and conferences. Dr. Miller is the recipient of the Master Teacher Award at the University of Kentucky College of Medicine, the prestigious RHR International Award for Excellence in Consulting Psychology from the American Psychological Association (APA), the Distinguished Researchers Award from the APA, the Distinguished Psychologist Award of the Kentucky Psychological Association, the Distinguished Contribution to the Science of Psychology by the Connecticut Psychological Association, Hall of Fame at St. John Fisher College, the Distinguished Service Award of the APA, and the Outstanding Alumnus Award of the State University of New York.

Contributors

Jean M. Alberti, PhD Alberti Psychological Services, Glen Ellyn, NY, USA

Mark Barden Sandy Hook Promise, Newtown, CT, USA

Christopher S. Barrier Montgomery County Schools, Mount Sterling, KY, USA

Allan Beane, PhD Bully Free Systems, Denton, TX, USA

Elissa P. Benedek, MD Department of Psychiatry, University of Michigan, Ann Arbor, MI, USA

Sharla D. Biefeld, PhD (candidate) Department of Psychology, University of Kentucky, Lexington, KY, USA

Paul Boxer, PhD Department of Psychology, Rutgers University, Newark, NJ, USA

Shaniqua Bradley, PhD Department of Social Work and Child Advocacy, Montclair State University, Montclair, NJ, USA

Amanda Breese, BS Alberti Center for Bullying Abuse Prevention, University at Buffalo, The State University of New York, Buffalo, NY, USA

Carol T. Brown, EdD Equipping Minds™, Frankfort, KY, USA

Christia Spears Brown, PhD Department of Psychology, University of Kentucky, Lexington, KY, USA

Barbara Burcham, PhD Georgetown College, Lexington, KY, USA

R. Davis Dixon, PhD Department of Psychology, Hampton University, Hampton, VA, USA

Dorothy L. Espelage, PhD School of Education, University of North Carolina at Chapel Hill, Chapel Hill, NC, USA

Annie Farmer, PhD Private Practice, Austin, TX, USA

William P. French, MD Department of Psychiatry and Behavioral Sciences, University of Washington, Seattle, WA, USA

Division of Child and Adolescent Psychiatry, Seattle Children's Hospital, Seattle, WA, USA

Sara E. Goldstein, PhD Department of Family Science and Human Development, Montclair State University, Montclair, NJ, USA

Maedah Golshirazi, PhD (candidate) Graduate School of Education, University of California, Berkeley, Berkeley, CA, USA

Jenna E. Greenstein, PhD (candidate) Graduate School of Education, University of California, Berkeley, Berkeley, CA, USA

Nicole Hockley Sandy Hook Promise, Newtown, CT, USA

Praveen R. Kambam, MD Court-Based Mental Health Programs, Division of Forensic Psychiatry, Los Angeles County Department of Mental Health, Los Angeles, CA, USA

Department of Psychiatry and Biobehavioral Sciences, The David Geffen School of Medicine at UCLA, UCLA Semel Institute for Neuroscience and Human Behavior, Los Angeles, CA, USA

Mackenzie Leachman, PhD Fayette County Public Schools, Lexington, KY, USA

Susan Logan, MS, MPH Injury and Violence Surveillance Unit, Community, Family Health, and Prevention Section, Connecticut Department of Public Health, Hartford, CT, USA

Virginia Luftman, PhD Department of Psychiatry, University of Kentucky, Lexington, KY, USA

Linda Malone-Colon, PhD Department of Psychology, Hampton University, Hampton, VA, USA

Sarah Manchanda, PhD (candidate) Graduate School of Education, University of California, Berkeley, Berkeley, CA, USA

Zina T. McGee, PhD Department of Social Sciences, Hampton University, Hampton, VA, USA

Thomas W. Miller, PhD, ABPP Department of Psychiatry, College of Medicine, Department of Gerontology, College of Public Health, University of Kentucky, Lexington, KY, USA

Institute for Collaboration on Health, Intervention, and Policy, University of Connecticut, Storrs, CT, USA

Amy L. Murphy, PhD Department of Curriculum and Instruction, Angelo State University, San Angelo, TX, USA

Amanda B. Nickerson, PhD Alberti Center for Bullying Abuse Prevention, University at Buffalo, The State University of New York, Buffalo, NY, USA

Jeanie Park, MA Department of Family Science and Human Development, Montclair State University, Montclair, NJ, USA

Susan K. Reuter, RPh Step-by-Step, Louisville, KY, USA

Sarah C. Savoy, PhD Department of Psychology, Stephen F. Austin State University, Nacogdoches, TX, USA

Brian Simmons New York Insight Meditation Center, New York, NY, USA

Food and Finance High School (Manhattan) NYC DOE, Astoria, NY, USA

Ginny Sprang, PhD Department of Psychiatry, College of Medicine, University of Kentucky, Lexington, KY, USA

Center on Trauma and Children, Department of Psychiatry, College of Medicine, University of Kentucky, Lexington, KY, USA

Susan M. Swearer, PhD, LP College of Education and Human Sciences, University of Nebraska – Lincoln, Lincoln, NE, USA

Michelle J. Tam, PhD (candidate) Department of Psychology, University of Kentucky, Lexington, KY, USA

Marie L. Tanaka, PhD (candidate) College of Education, University of Arizona, Tucson, AZ, USA

Andrew M. Terranova, PhD Department of Psychology, Gupta College of Science, Coastal Carolina University, Conway, SC, USA

Matthew D. Thompson, EdD Montgomery County Schools, Mt. Sterling, KY, USA

Brian Van Brunt, EdD Author, New Orleans, LA, USA

Candice M. Wallace, PhD Department of Psychological Science, Central Connecticut State University, New Britain, CT, USA

Dai Williams, MSc., C.Psychol. Eos Career Services, Surrey, UK

Tammy Yabiku, BA Graduate School of Education, University of California, Berkeley, Berkeley, CA, USA

Chunyan Yang, PhD Graduate School of Education, University of California, Berkeley, Berkeley, CA, USA

Jina Yoon, PhD Department of Disability and Psychoeducational Studies, College of Education, University of Arizona, Tucson, AZ, USA

Part I
Conceptualizing School Violence

Chapter 1
School-Related Violence: Definition, Scope, and Prevention Goals

Thomas W. Miller

Introduction

The purpose of this volume is to provide a compendium of theory, research, and applied models addressing school violence and the critical ingredients in prevention interventions that contribute to reducing and/or eliminating various forms of violence in the school setting. The United Nations International Children's Fund (2020) has been an international leader in addressing children who are at heightened risk of abuse, neglect, exploitation, and violence in search of prevention interventions that reduce the potential for victimization (UNICEF, 2020). Researchers have been instrumental in developing assessment strategies when it comes to understanding the issues and problems encountered with school violence (Vossekuil et al., 2015). The US Department of Justice and the Center for the Study and Prevention of Violence (1999) developed a research-based definition of "school violence." The definition, which emerged from a detailed microanalysis, suggests that school violence is any behavior that violates a school's educational mission or climate of respect or jeopardizes the intent of the school to be free of aggression against persons or property, drugs, weapons, disruptions, and disorder (US Department of Justice and the Center for Study and Prevention of Violence, 1999). School violence involves a spectrum of crimes taking place within the spectrum of educational institutions.

Twentieth-century monitoring of disease fell on the Centers for Disease Control and Prevention (CDC) and continues to do so with collaboration among several

T. W. Miller (✉)
Department of Psychiatry, College of Medicine, Department of Gerontology, College of Public Health, University of Kentucky, Lexington, KY, USA

Institute for Collaboration on Health, Intervention, and Policy, University of Connecticut, Storrs, CT, USA
e-mail: tom.miller@uconn.edu

© The Author(s), under exclusive license to Springer Nature Switzerland AG 2023
T. W. Miller (ed.), *School Violence and Primary Prevention*,
https://doi.org/10.1007/978-3-031-13134-9_1

other organizations nationally and globally. According to the CDC (2016), within the conceptualization of school *violence is the understanding that school violence involves children in the school setting and mostly occurs on school property or on the way to or from school, or at school-sponsored events. Children exposed to school violence can be viewed as a victim, a perpetrator, or a witness of school violence. School violence may also involve or impact adults (CDC, 2016). Youth violence includes various behaviors that may include but are not limited to bullying, pushing, and shoving. When such behaviors occur, they may cause emotional and/ or physical harm. Other forms of violence, such as gang violence and assault with or without weapons, can lead to serious injury or even death according to the* CDC *(2016).*

In examining the breadth and dimensions of school-related violence, the *School Survey on Crime and Safety* (SSOCS) (Irwin et al., 2021) is the primary source of school-level data on crime and safety for the U.S. Department of Education. The National Center for Education Statistics (NCES) has crafted the definition and scope of violence in our schools. The *School Survey on Crime and Safety* is a nationally representative cross-sectional survey of about 4800 public elementary and secondary schools. This is a collaborative effort involving the National Center for Education Statistics and the Bureau of Justice Statistics to address school violence.

Resources provided through this annual report examine crime occurring in schools and colleges nationally along with data on crime at schools from the perspectives of students, teachers, principals, and the general population from an array of sources. Sources include research from the National Crime Victimization Survey, the School Crime Supplement to the National Crime Victimization Survey, the Youth Risk Behavior Survey, the School Survey on Crime and Safety, the Schools and Staffing Survey, and the Campus Safety and Security Survey. Within the annual report are topics such as victimization, bullying, school conditions, fights, weapons, the presence of security staff at school, availability and student use of drugs and alcohol, student perceptions of personal safety at school, and criminal incidents at postsecondary institutions (Irwin et al., 2021).

In examining the incidence, for example, of cyberbullying abuse among tweens (defined as youth between the ages of 9 and 12 years) in the school setting, the research generated by the Cyberbullying Research Center (Patchin & Hinduja, 2020) found one in five or 20% of students experienced cyberbullying of some form (as victim, perpetrator, or witness) during their school experience. These findings are consistent with findings reported by the National Center for Education Statistics and the Bureau of Justice Statistics in the annual *School Survey on Crime and Safety – Report on Indicators of School Crime and Safety: 2020* (Irwin et al., 2021).

There are some educational specialists, along with legislators, who have recognized that bullying behavior is a form of "discriminatory harassment" when it is found to be based on race, national origin, color, and sex (including sexual orientation, gender identity, age, disability, or religion). There are numerous considerations when discriminatory harassment may be recognized as occurring and is found to be motivated by the presence of bias against the victim due to race, color, religion, national origin, sexual orientation, gender, gender identity, or disability of the victim. There is consistency across several sources that identify the forms that bullying can take in the school setting: (1) verbal, (2) physical, (3) relational/social, and (4) damage to a person or property related to the person (CDC, 2021). Modecki et al. (2014) performed a meta-analysis examining a comparison between traditional and newer forms of bullying behavior involving cyberbullying which provided the needed research platform for further investigation in this arena. Factors such as these should be applied for consideration of bullying as a form of discriminatory harassment. Ensuring safer schools requires establishing valid and reliable indicators of the current state of school crime and safety across the nation and periodically monitoring and updating such indicators. More than two decades ago, the term "school violence" itself was widely used to describe violent and aggressive acts on school campuses. Today, the definition is much broader in scope.

Definition

Since the first edition of this volume, the realm of bullying has been more thoroughly examined by the scientific community in more detail and provided a more comprehensive definition. The Centers for Disease Control and Prevention recognizes two primary modes of bullying and four types of bullying (Gladden et al., 2014). A mode of bullying involves the form it takes such as direct or indirect. More specifically, it is how the aggressive behavior is experienced by the victim. Direct bullying is then viewed as aggressive behavior that occurs in the presence of the victim (Gladden et al., 2014; Allanson et al., 2015), while indirect bullying is aggressive behavior that is not directly communicated to the victim (Gladden et al., 2014). There are several types of bullying identified by the Centers for Disease Control and Prevention (2021) that include physical, verbal, relational/social, and damage to property. Physical bullying is defined as the use of physical force by the perpetrator against the target which includes hitting, kicking, and punching (Gladden et al., 2014). Verbal bullying is oral or written communication that causes harm like taunting and inappropriate sexual comments (Gladden et al., 2014). With advances in media technology, Hinduja and Patchin (2014) have provided a definition of cyberbullying as "the willful and repeated harm inflicted through the use of computers, cell phones, and other electronic devices." With the broadening conceptualization of bullying, there have been numerous bullying prevention programs available to the community and educational units, and school-created bullying prevention programs have emerged over the past two decades producing several meta-analyses and systematic reviews to assess the effectiveness of these bullying prevention programs, as summarized by Huang et al., 2019; Gaffney et al., 2019; and Nickerson and Parks (2021). Several researchers (Gaffney et al., 2019; Ttofi & Farrington, 2011) have examined more studies and revealed encouraging results with several prevention intervention programs that suggest a 19–23% reduction in bullying perpetration and a 15–20% reduction in victimization. Characteristics of the more effective programs are marked by multiple components such as intense training, higher dosage, and comprehensive monitoring of intervention integrity and include a parental component that demonstrates greater effectiveness in reducing bullying victimization and perpetration (Huang et al., 2019).

When we come to an understanding of school violence, we find that it includes but is not limited to such behaviors as child and teacher victimization, child and/or teacher perpetration, physical and psychological exploitation, cyber victimization, cyber threats and bullying, fights, bullying, classroom disorder, physical and psychological injury to teacher and student, cult-related behavior and activities, sexual and other boundary violations, and use of weapons in the school environment. Social media has played a prominent role in so many aspects of school-related violence and has become a driving force in the lives of our children. At the very least, it has influenced so many aspects of their relationships that have developed within the school setting.

In considering the number of resources available for understanding school-related violence, there are several state and federal agencies that may be beneficial in expanding one's understanding of the complexities of violence experienced in the school or college environment. It is suggested that some that are very helpful for this topic include but are not limited to the U.S. Department of Education, the National School Safety Center, the US Department of Health and Human Services, the National Center for Education Statistics (NCES), the Federal Bureau of Investigation (FBI), the Centers for Disease Control and Prevention (CDC), the Office of the U.S. Surgeon General (2001), the U.S. Secret Service National Threat Assessment Center (NTAC) (2018), the Office of Juvenile Justice and Violence Prevention, the U.S. Preventive Services Task Force, and the National Consortium of School Violence Prevention Researchers and Practitioners that provide important data in monitoring school-related violence and greater specificity to the definition of violence in schools.

Since the first edition of *School Violence and Primary Prevention* (2008), the interest in school-related violence and strategies for primary prevention have generated new directions and guidelines for school administrators, teachers, educators, and violence-focused researchers in addressing the arena of school violence and primary prevention.

Over the first two decades of the twenty-first century, there have been several important initiatives to address school-related violence. The Alliance for Child Protection in Humanitarian Action (2020), the United Nations Children's Fund (UNICEF, 2020), the New Zealand Family Violence Clearinghouse (NZFVC) (2020), and CDC's Division of Violence Prevention (2016) have provided new directions in safety and child protection.

Educators and researchers internationally (Barlow et al., 2016; Cicchetti et al., 2000; Espelage, 2014; Cornell et al., 2012; Goodrum et al., 2018) have emphasized that it is essential to assess the threat, monitor the presence of school-related violence, and develop creative intervention initiatives that focus on prevention in the school violence domain.

Scope of the Problem

In addressing the scope of school-related violence, it is important to understand the incidence and prevalence factors that have been the focus of monitoring from the US Department of Education along with the Centers for Disease Control and Prevention (CDC). An important source in addressing the scope of school-related violence is the *Youth Risk Behavior Survey*. The school-based *Youth Risk Behavior Survey*, a division of the Youth Risk Behavior Surveillance System (YRBSS), conducts their survey biennially on health-risk behavior. This survey analyzes the data collected that address student characteristics such as gender, race and ethnicity, grade level, and urbanicity of the school. These researchers evaluated children based on age and grade level and found that 19.0% of children in grades 9–12 were bullied on school property and 14.9% of children in grades 9–12 were electronically bullied (Kann et al., 2018). Findings suggest that prevention intervention strategies that utilize "social learning theory and established client-centered, community-based, and experiential methods have been shown to be [among the more] successful" prevention intervention strategies with children who have experienced bullying (Feather & Bordonada, 2019).

Violence in American society generally, and concerning children and adolescents specifically, who are the victims of more crimes than any other age group in the United States (Steinberg, 2000; Rennison, 2000), has become an increasingly difficult factor to control. When we speak of the scope of the problem, we realize that this problem is not uniquely our own but crosses national and international boundaries. Globalization and technology and its availability to students and adults have influenced the growth of such behavior in the school environment. Suicide and homicide in the school setting are responsible for about 25% of deaths among persons aged 10–24 years in the United States (Arias et al., 2003).

Epidemiological data on forms of violence come from multiple primary sources that include health-related information such as records from hospitals, emergency medical services, and medical examiners. Other primary sources of such data include public law enforcement records such as police reports and arrest records and reports of child abuse from child protective services and other agencies. An additional source is data that has been collected through self-report surveys and interviews (Greene, 2002). University-based data collection and studies that address several forms of violence in schools and on college campuses have proven to be very helpful in understanding the scope of violence in our society.

In considering the scope of lethal violence in the school setting, it is essential to examine the problem of homicide and gun-related violence or firearm homicides overall. The National Center for Health Statistics (2020) reports 1.2 million emergency room visits for assaults with 19,384 deaths and a rate of 5.9 deaths per 100,000 of the population reported. Globally, the United Nations Office on Drugs and Crime (2019) reports that 464,000 people were estimated to have been victims of intentional homicide in 2017 with an average global homicide rate of 6.1 victims per 100,000 population for that year. The report further notes that about 90% of all homicides recorded worldwide were committed by male perpetrators and that males make up almost 80% of all homicide victims recorded worldwide.

"Our World in Data" is another excellent resource for assessing the scope of the problem, which includes those affected by school-related shootings and school-related lethal violence. According to the Global Burden of Disease study, a component of the "Our World in Data" source, just over 415,000 individuals died from homicide in 2019, which is consistent with other sources. This was around three times the number of those killed in armed conflict and terrorism combined for that year (Roser & Ritchie, 2019). An earlier report of the World Health Organization (2015) reported that an estimated 470,000 individuals worldwide were victims of homicide, with a global rate of 6.4 deaths per 100,000.

School shootings and fatalities from such shootings broaden the scope of the numerous forms of school violence. Greene (2002) reported the global homicide rate in 1998 was 12.5 per 100,000, significantly higher than that of the United States, which was 6.2 per 100,000. At that time, the United States owned the third highest homicide rate among some 40 countries, making homicide a factor in understanding the scope of school violence which is substantiated by several researchers (Thornton et al., 2000; Blum et al., 2000; Brener et al., 2004).

Everytown for Gun Safety (2022) is a viable resource for data on incidents of gun violence at US schools, as is World Population Review (2022). The latter provides both incidence and prevalence data that are current along with rankings of school shootings by country globally. School shooting by country found that the United States has led the world in the number of school shootings. Noted in their report is the definition of a school shooting, which is an event that occurs when firearms are used. Specifically emphasized is that perpetrators who resort to the use of such violence desire attention, have been bullied, and may have been victims themselves of various forms of exploitation, abuse, and violence in their lives.

Data analyzed from the Gun Violence Archive (2020), a nonprofit organization that tracks school shootings, report that for many youths growing up in at-risk neighborhoods with high firearm access, the role of social media has played a significant role in influencing youth behavior resulting in school shootings. In considering the sources for such acts of violence in the school setting, one cannot rule out the influence of video games, movies, or online media sources. Prevention interventions are necessary to address this burgeoning problem in our country and worldwide.

Furthermore, school shootings have occurred at several levels of education including preschool and kindergarten, elementary such as the Sandy Hook Elementary School shooting in Connecticut in 2012; special education school units such as South Education Center in Richfield, Minnesota in February 2022; high schools that include Heath High School shooting in Paducah, Kentucky in 1997, Columbine High School shooting in Colorado in 1999, and the Marjory Stoneman Douglas High School shooting in Florida in 2018. Similarly, there have been reported incidents at the college and university levels, such as the University of Texas Tower shooting in 1966 and the Virginia Tech shooting in 2007. The Youth Participatory Action Research (2022) (YPAR) is viewed as a needed approach for developing effective developmentally appropriate youth engagement as a preventative intervention. School-related violence has continued to be an unwanted presence at all levels of education in this country.

Risk Factors in Violence

Howell (2000) and Murphy (2000) are credited with researching indicators also referred to as risk factors that, if present, may indicate that a child who possesses these characteristics is more likely to subsequently engage in violent thinking and behaviors. The reader is encouraged to review these publications to gain a more complete understanding of these risk factors. As we have come to understand the role of risk factors in diagnosing the likelihood of a child developing violent thoughts and/or behaviors, patterns of development indicate that they may be addictive and increase with age. Furthermore, the presence and the severity of risk factors are likely to increase or decrease proportionately (Howell, 2000; Murphy, 2000). Risk factors begin to show themselves in smaller ways during the childhood years, while becoming a more prominent part of the personality of the individual during adolescence. Adolescence requires peer involvement and peer acceptance. The individual's need for peer acceptance and belonging, as well as the need for enhanced social status, particularly for unpopular youth and for those youth who feel socially powerless, lend itself to attention-getting acts of bullying and other forms of violence. Prevention interventions that focus on community-based outreach efforts in association with community policing operations are required. Such efforts need to address the individual's social, psychological, interpersonal, and economic needs (Howell, 2000; Murphy, 2000).

Goals for School-Based Prevention

Violence in our society and communities has increased dramatically over the past decade. *Healthy People 2030* continues in the tradition of *Healthy People 2000, Healthy People 2010, and Healthy People 2020* with an ambitious 10-year agenda for improving the nation's health, including community-related violence among our school-aged population. *Healthy People 2030*, which focuses on reducing different types of violence, is the result of a multiyear process that reflects input from a diverse group of individuals and organizations that have, through a national health-care policy agenda, set the goal of reducing the prevalence of violence in our communities and our schools (U.S. Department of Health and Human Services, Office of Disease Prevention and Health Promotion, n.d.). Many people in the United States experience physical assaults, sexual violence, and gun-related injuries. According to *Healthy People 2030*, adolescents are especially at risk for experiencing violence. Interventions to reduce violence are needed to keep people safe in their homes, schools, workplaces, and communities. Children who experience violence are at risk for long-term physical, behavioral, and mental health problems. Strategies to protect these children from violence can help improve their health and well-being later in life (U.S. Department of Health and Human Services, Office of Disease Prevention and Health Promotion, n.d.).

Schools and communities must continue efforts to establish physical and social environments that prevent violence and promote actual and perceived safety in schools. While the decline in school violence-related behaviors is encouraging, prevention efforts must be sustained if the nation is to achieve its 2030 national health objectives. To further reduce violence-related behaviors among young persons and to have an impact on behaviors that are more resistant to change, continued efforts are needed to monitor these behaviors and to develop, evaluate, and disseminate effective prevention strategies.

School personnel including school and college administrators, teachers, clinicians, researchers, educators, legislators, and justice department personnel must continue efforts to reduce the incidence and prevalence of violence. It has generally gone unnoticed that the use and meaning of the term school violence have evolved over the past 10 years. School violence is conceptualized as a multifaceted construct that involves both criminal acts and aggression in schools, which inhibits development and learning as well as harms the school's climate.

School climate is important as the role of schools as a culture and as an organization has not always received attention because of different disciplinary approaches to studying the problem. Researchers have brought divergent orientations to their work, and these interests have not always been well coordinated with the primary educational mission of schools. An understanding of the multidisciplinary basis of school violence research is necessary in order to critically evaluate the potential use of programs that purport to reduce "school" violence.

Prevention research scientists and practitioners hold a unique responsibility in the realm of school-based violence. Contained in this volume are a series of chapters that address the spectrum of issues related to preventing the perpetration of school-related violence. Their role is to offer an understanding of theory, incidence, and prevalence and provide a forum for discussion of the need of understanding the multiple variables that must be considered in addressing prevention-based approaches to school violence as we approach the second quarter of the twenty-first century.

School Violence as a Public Health Issue

School violence as a public health issue has been the focus of parents such as Nicole Hockley, Tim Makris, and Mark Barden who cultivated the Sandy Hook Promise to address gun control after the school shooting at Sandy Hook Elementary School in Newtown, Connecticut in 2012 (also see Chap. 28).

In approaching the prevention of violence in our schools and our communities, the Centers for Disease Control and Prevention (2022) provides a "social-ecological"

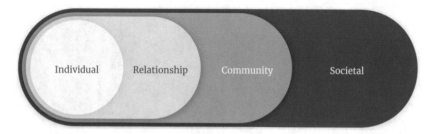

Fig. 1.1 The social-ecological model (CDC, 2022b)

public health approach to prevention interventions that address the interaction between the person, the community, and society (Fig. 1.1).

The social-ecological model provides an integrated, multidisciplinary public health approach to addressing violence that is adaptable to school-related violence. The multidisciplinary integration is nested in diverse disciplines represented by health, justice, education, social services, and the private sector. It employs a four-stage approach outlined in Fig. 1.2 that requires in the first stage, defining and monitoring violence-related activities. The second stage searches for both risk and protective factors present to aid in identifying where prevention efforts need to be focused. The third stage is one of identifying and testing the effectiveness of evidence-based prevention strategies reported in the literature. The fourth stage involves implementation that assures the adoption of the evidence-based strategies and plans for use in schools and is viewed as a critical part of the social-ecology of the community (CDC, 2022a).

Understanding the Stages of Prevention

There have been changes to the understanding of the various levels or stages of prevention within the healthcare arena. Prevention is recognized as involving three distinct stages: primary, secondary, and tertiary. The US Preventive Services Task Force's (USPSTF) *Guide to Clinical Preventive Services, 2nd Edition* (1996), defines primary prevention measures as those that are taken in anticipation of an event or events that intervene before any risk behavior occurs for the victim. Since successful primary prevention intervention strategies tend to reduce the chances of a negative event or abusive issue occurring, it is typically considered the most cost-effective form of health care.

The USPSTF (1996) describes secondary prevention measures as those that "identify and treat asymptomatic persons who have already developed risk factors or preclinical disease but in whom the condition is not clinically apparent." These activities are focused on early case finding of asymptomatic conditions that occur commonly and have a significant risk of negative outcomes without treatment or some form of intervention. Screening tests are examples of secondary prevention

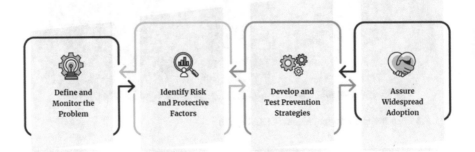

Fig. 1.2 The public health approach to violence prevention (CDC, 2022a)

activities, as these are done on those without clinical presentation of condition that has a significant latency period such as hypertension, prostate, and breast cancer conditions.

With early case findings, the natural history of disease or condition, or how the course of an illness or condition unfolds over time without treatment, can often be altered by maximizing the well-being of an individual and in this case, the child, and therefore minimizing the severity of the condition. Tertiary prevention involves the care of established disease or condition such as fear or apprehension by the child when bullying or another form of school-related violence occurs. Primary prevention is the first line of intervention before any issues or problems exist, while secondary intervention is valued once some signs or symptoms occur for the child. Finally, tertiary intervention is needed to reduce or minimize the negative effects of the abuse or violence experienced by the child. When tertiary interventions are successful, the child impacted by various forms of violence usually begins to show some degree to adaptation or recover to improved functioning and coping with the traumatic target experienced.

Major Goals and Approaches to Prevention

There are three key goals of prevention-oriented programs at schools. The goals that follow are specific to the student population at all levels. These include that (1) students understand their own peer culture; (2) students provide a typically untapped human resource; (3) the program is a network of involved youth; and (4) the involvement of students in implementing such programs provides an alternative for antisocial, violent, and delinquent behavior. School-based peer mediation, in which a trained student mediates a dispute between two other students with the goal of establishing a mutually agreed-upon peaceful solution, is considered to be an essential ingredient (Thompson & Kyle, 2005; Miller et al., 2005; McCord et al., 2001; Herrenkohl et al., 2000). An extremely important factor involves school bonding.

The reader is encouraged to review the discussion in Chap. 24 that focuses on character education as a prevention intervention strategy for school-related violence.

The use of evidence-based scientific models of study has been recognized as critical in assessing the effectiveness of prevention intervention programs. Such scientific evaluations are costly and only a small proportion of programs now in use at schools and in communities have been evaluated using such scientific models. Those programs that have been evaluated are generally highly structured, implemented by professionals, and developed at academic institutions. While this body of research has revealed that some programs do indeed reduce rates of aggression and violence in the schools, several programs have not been studied but have realized some observable positive changes in students' behavior. The reader is cautioned that some programs that have been shown to be effective in research studies may not necessarily work equally well in other or in all school settings, with both genders and in other contexts. There remains the need for further evidence-based research programs that continually monitor and evaluate both existing and new prevention intervention programs.

In Search of School-Related Violence Prevention

During the last quarter of the twentieth century, several approaches on prevention toward school violence have been documented (Edwards et al., 2005; Afkinich & Klumpner, 2018; Gaffney et al., 2019; Huang et al., 2019). Results of the most effective models for violence prevention programs utilize social skills training. Social skills training programs generally utilize structured and interactive curricula (e.g., role-playing) and are usually classroom-based. In addition to social skills training, these programs focus on parent training, family interaction, and family dynamics. A third component involves teacher–student bonding and healthy interaction with peers in the school environment. Critical components to social skills training models nationally include humanistic education also known as emotional literacy, self-control with respect to one's emotional and behavioral reactions to another, social competence to adopt and carry out a response pattern that results in positive peer relations, and effective interpersonal problem-solving skills. Other models have created applied psychoeducational strategies to reduce the likelihood of a person engaging in violent types of behavior. Some well-established community-based training and mentoring programs have been shown to be effective violence prevention strategies.

The significant contributions of Daniel Olweus, a Swedish-Norwegian Professor of Psychology at the University of Bergen, and his associates must be recognized for framing the foundation for violence prevention in the school setting. Their research led to a "hybrid" model entitled the Olweus Bullying-Prevention Program (Olweus, 1993). This program has several key features, including skills-based classroom training, parent involvement, policy development, "hot spot" analysis, and counseling. Evaluations of this program suggest that it is effective in reducing levels of bullying and harassment. Indeed, multicomponent programs are generally viewed as preferable, particularly for high-risk school-aged youth.

Safer Schools Through Primary Prevention

Prevention educators along with research scientists can be very helpful in consulting with school administrators, teachers, psychologists, nurses, social workers, and counselors in playing an effective role in limiting and mitigating the influence of problematic behavior, including violence in the school setting. Programs that incorporate the use of mindfulness (Simmons, Chap. 22), cognitive training with the Equipping Minds Cognitive Development Curriculum (Brown, Chap. 23), and empathy with the Step-by-Step Student Stewardship © program (Reuter, Chap. 25) are described in this volume. With empathy comes acknowledging a student's issues and laying the foundation for improving the management of a strategy that will result in improved thinking and behavior on the part of the student. Also examined are clinical issues and case analyses involving violence in the classroom and school setting.

Concluding Thought

An effort toward gaining some understanding as to why victims and perpetrators seek various forms of violence in the school setting may be explained by the work of psychologist Roy Baumeister and his research addressing the concept of escape theory (Baumeister, 1990). The escape theory model suggests that peer victimization is driven by the desire of the perpetrator to escape a state of painful self-awareness characterized by inadequacy, negative affect, and low self-esteem. And so, in this volume, the reader will find chapters that will address critical issues and essential components of the task of preventing school-related violence and a potential pathway to safer schools.

Furlong et al. (2000, as cited in Overstreet & Mazza, 2003) noted that the social problem of community violence has created a critical need for: (1) prevention programs to foster resilience in the face of various forms of violence; (2) the development of research-based intervention programs to help children who are challenged to cope with these forms of violence; and (3) prevention and intervention programs aimed at reducing the occurrence of community violence. Meeting these needs will require researchers to move beyond a focus on narrow definitions and single outcomes. An integrated and multidimensional approach to this challenge is required.

The focus of *Healthy People 2030* is on reducing different types of community-based violence. It targets bullying, all forms of abuse, exploitation, physical assaults, sexual violence, and gun-related incident in the school setting and beyond. *Healthy People 2030* recognizes that children and adolescents are especially at risk for experiencing violence. According to *Healthy People 2030*, prevention interventions that address strategies that reduce all forms of violence provide the essential agenda to assure safety for children, adolescents, adults, and the elderly in their homes, schools, workplaces, and their communities. When it comes to our children who experience any form of violence, they are identified as at-risk for long-term emotional, physical, behavioral, and mental health concerns. Strategies to protect children from violence can contribute to improving their health and well-being throughout their lives (U.S. Department of Health and Human Services, Office of Disease Prevention and Health Promotion, n.d.).

Several strategies have been addressed in response to the need for more effective intervention in addressing violence and safety in our schools by Afkinich and Klumpner (2018). Among the strategies identified are programs that address the needs of at-risk youth. Programs focusing on peer and adult mentoring aimed at conflict resolution and peer mediation intervention strategies provide the basis for team-building, problem-solving, and self-confidence. To reduce and prevent youth violence, the authors encourage educators to provide full-service schools which are designed to offer a safe place for youth to meet and participate in meaningful school activities including the arts and academics.

Meeting the needs to address school violence and safety will require educators, administrators, legislators, clinicians, the public, clinical practitioners, and researchers to seek a comprehensive theoretical model that facilitates the integration of information across subdisciplines in psychology, sociology, public health, social work, nursing, criminology, education, law, and medicine to increase our understanding of the developmental impact of exposure to community violence. More specifically, clinical symptoms associated with posttraumatic stress disorder have been linked to exposure to community violence in community-based research (Overstreet & Chafouleas, 2016). As a result of such exposure to various forms of violence, school-aged children and adolescents have a greater probability of developing over time the clinical consequences which may result in the need for more professional clinical services in the future.

References

Afkinich, J. L., & Klumpner, S. (2018). Violence prevention strategies and school safety. *Journal of the Society for Social Work and Research, 9*(4), 637–650.

Allanson, P. B., Lester, R. R., & Notar, C. E. (2015). A history of bullying. *International Journal of Education and Social Science, 2*, 31–36. http://www.ijessnet.com/uploads/volumes/1576145463.pdf

Alliance for Child Protection in Humanitarian Action. (2020). *Technical note: Protection of children during the coronavirus pandemic*. Available at: https://alliancecpha.org/en/COVD19

Arias, E., Anderson, R. N., Kung, H. C., Murphy, S. L., & Kochanek, K. S. (2003). Deaths: Final data. *National Vital Statistics Reports, 52*, 1–100.

Barlow, D. H., Allen, L. B., & Choate, M. L. (2016). Toward a unified treatment for emotional disorders—Republished article. *Behavior Therapy, 47*, 838–853. https://doi.org/10.1016/j.beth.2016.11.005

Baumeister, R. F. (1990). Suicide as escape from self. *Psychological Review, 97*, 90–113. Available at:. https://doi.org/10.1037/0033-295X.97.1.90

Blum, R. W., Beuhring, T., & Rinehart, P. M. (2000). *Protecting teens: Beyond race, income and family structure*. Center for Adolescent Health, University of Minnesota.

Brener, N. D., Simon, T. R., Anderson, M., Barrios, L. C., & Small, M. L. (2004). Effect of the incident at Columbine on students' violence- and suicide-related behaviors. *American Journal of Preventive Medicine, 22*, 146–150.

Centers for Disease Control and Prevention. (2021). *Violence prevention – Fast fact: Preventing bullying.* https://www.cdc.gov/violenceprevention/youthviolence/bullyingresearch/fast-fact.html

Centers for Disease Control and Prevention. (2022a). *The public health approach to violence prevention.* Available at: https://www.cdc.gov/violenceprevention/about/publichealthap-proach.html

Centers for Disease Control and Prevention. (2022b). *The social-ecological model: A frame-work for prevention.* Available at: https://www.cdc.gov/violenceprevention/about/social-ecologicalmodel.html

Centers for Disease Control and Prevention, Division of Violence Prevention. (2016). *Understanding school violence: Fact sheet.* Atlanta. Available at: http://www.cdc.gov/violen-ceprevention/pdf/school_violence_fact_sheet-a.pdf

Cicchetti, D., Toth, S. L., & Maughan, A. (2000). An ecological–transactional model of child maltreatment. In A. Sameroff, M. Lewis, & S. Miller (Eds.), *Handbook of developmental psy-chopathology* (2nd ed., pp. 689–722). Kluwer Academic Publishers. Available at: https://doi.org/10.1007/978-1-4615-4163-9_37

Cornell, D. G., Allen, K., & Fan, X. (2012). A randomized controlled study of the Virginia Student Threat Assessment Guidelines in kindergarten through grade 12. *School Psychology Review, 41*(1), 100–115.

Edwards, D., Hunt, M., Meyers, J., Grogg, K., & Jarrett, O. (2005). Acceptability and student outcomes of a violence prevention curriculum. *The Journal of Primary Prevention, 26*(5), 401–418.

Espelage, D. L. (2014). Ecological theory: Preventing youth bullying, aggression, and victimiza-tion. *Theory Into Practice, 53*(4), 257–264. https://doi.org/10.1080/00405841.2014.947216

Everytown for Gun Safety. (2022). *Everytown research & policy: Gunfire on school grounds in the United States* [Internet]. Available at: https://everytownresearch.org/maps/gunfire-on-school-grounds/

Feather, K. A., & Bordonada, T. M. (2019). Leading an anti-bullying intervention for students with disabilities. *Counseling Today.* https://ct.counseling.org/2019/01/leading-an-anti-bullying-intervention-for-students-with-disabilities/

Furlong, M., Morrison, G., & Pavelski, R. (2000). Trends in school psychology for the 21st cen-tury: Influences of school violence on professional change. *Psychology in the Schools, 37*, 81–90. https://doi.org/10.1002/(SICI)1520-6807(200001)37:1<81::AID-PITS9>3.0.CO;2-O

Gaffney, H., Ttofi, M. M., & Farrington, D. P. (2019). Evaluating the effectiveness of school-bullying prevention programs: An updated meta-analytical review. *Aggression and Violent Behavior, 45*, 111–133. https://doi.org/10.1016/j.avb.2018.07.001

Gladden, R. M., Vivolo-Kantor, A. M., Hamburger, M. E., & Lumpki, C. D. (2014). *Bullying surveillance among youths: Uniform definitions for public health and recommended data ele-ments, version 1.0.* National Center for Injury Prevention and Control, Centers for Disease Control and Prevention and U.S. Department of Education. Available at: https://www.cdc.gov/violenceprevention/pdf/bullying-definitions-final-a.pdf

Goodrum, S., Thompson, A. J., Ward, K. C., & Woodward, W. (2018). A case study on threat assessment: Learning critical lessons to prevent school violence. *Journal of Threat Assessment and Management, 5*(3), 121–136. https://doi.org/10.1037/tam0000104

Greene, M. B. (2002). Violence. In L. Breslow (Ed.), *Encyclopedia of public health* (pp. 1284–1293). Macmillan Reference USA.

Gun Violence Archive. (2020). *Evidence based data summary*. Available at: https://www.gunvio-lencearchive.org/

Herrenkohl, T. I., Magiun, E., Hill, K. G., Hawkins, J. D., Abbott, R. D., & Catalano, R. F. (2000). Developmental risk factors for youth violence. *Journal of Adolescent Health, 26*, 176–186.

Hinduja, S., & Patchin, J. W. (2014). *Bullying beyond the schoolyard: Preventing and responding to cyberbullying*. Corwin.

Howell, J. C. (2000). *Youth gang programs and strategies*. Department of Justice. Office of Justice Programs, Office of Juvenile Justice and Delinquency Prevention. Available at: https://www.ojp.gov/pdffiles1/ojjdp/171154.pdf

Huang, Y., Espelage, D. L., Polanin, J. R., & Hong, J. S. (2019). A meta-analytic review of school-based anti-bullying programs with a parent component. *International Journal of Bullying Prevention, 1*, 32–44. https://doi.org/10.1007/s42380-018-0002-1

Irwin, V., Wang, K., Cui, J., Zhang, J., & Thompson, A. (2021). *Report on indicators of school crime and safety: 2020 (NCES 2021-092/NCJ 300772)*. National Center for Education Statistics, U.S. Department of Education, and Bureau of Justice Statistics, Office of Justice Programs, U.S. Department of Justice. Available at: https://nces.ed.gov/pubsearch/pubsinfo.asp?pubid=2021092

Kann, L., McManus, T., Harris, W. A., Shanklin, S. L., Flint, K. H., Queen, B., Lowry, R., Chyen, D., Whittle, L., Thornton, J., Lim, C., Bradford, D., Yamakawa, Y., Leon, M., Brener, N., & Ethier, K. A. (2018). Youth risk behavior surveillance – United States, 2017. *MMWR Surveillance Summaries, 67*(SS-8), 1–114. https://doi.org/10.15585/mmwr.ss6708a1

McCord, J., Widom, C. S., & Crowell, N. A. (Eds.). (2001). *Juvenile crime, juvenile justice*. National Academy Press.

Miller, T. W., Veltkamp, L. J., & Kraus, R. F. (2005). Character education as a prevention strategy in school related violence. *The Journal of Primary Prevention, 26*(5), 455–467.

Modecki, K. L., Minchin, J., Harbaugh, A. G., Guerra, N. G., & Runions, K. C. (2014). Bullying prevalence across contexts: A meta-analysis measuring cyber and traditional bullying. *The Journal of Adolescent Health: Official Publication of the Society for Adolescent Medicine., 55*(5), 602–611. https://doi.org/10.1016/j.jadohealth.2014.06.007

Murphy, S. L. (2000). Deaths: Final Data for 1998. *National vital statistics reports*; 48(11). Atlanta: National Center for Health Statistics (U.S.). Division of Vital Statistics. https://stacks.cdc.gov/view/cdc/22289

National Center for Health Statistics. (2020). *National vital statistics system – Mortality data (2020) via CDC WONDER* [Internet]. Available at: https://www.cdc.gov/nchs/fastats/homicide.htm

New Zealand Family Violence Clearinghouse. (2020). *National Centre for family and whanau violence research and information*. Available at: https://nzfvc.org.nz/

Nickerson, A. B., & Parks, T. (2021). Preventing bullying in schools. In P. J. Lazarus, S. Suldo, & B. Doll (Eds.), *Fostering the emotional well-being of our youth: A school-based approach* (pp. 338–354). Oxford University Press. https://doi.org/10.1093/medpsych/9780190918873.003.0017

Office of the Surgeon General (US), National Center for Injury Prevention and Control (US), National Institute of Mental Health (US), & Center for Mental Health Services (US). (2001). *Youth violence: A report of the surgeon general*. Office of the Surgeon General (US). https://www.ncbi.nlm.nih.gov/books/NBK44294/

Olweus, D. (1993). *Bullying at school*. Blackwell Publishers.

Overstreet, S., & Chafouleas, S. M. (2016). Trauma-informed schools: Introduction to the special issue. *School Mental Health, 8*, 1–6. https://doi.org/10.1007/s12310-016-9184-1

Overstreet, S., & Mazza, J. (2003). An ecological-transactional understanding of community violence: Theoretical perspectives. *School Psychology Quarterly, 18*(1), 66–87. https://doi.org/10.1521/scpq.18.1.66.20874

Patchin, J. W., & Hinduja, S. (2020). *Tween Cyberbullying in 2020. Cyberbullying Research Center in partnership with Cartoon Network*. Available at: https://cyberbullying.org/tween-cyberbullying-in-the-united-states

Prevention (2004), OJJDP Statistical Briefing Book. Available at: https://ojjdp.ojp.gov/statistics.

Rennison, C. M. (2000). *Criminal victimization 1999: Changes 1998–99 with trends 1993–99.* U.S. Department of Justice.

Roser, M., & Ritchie, H. (2019). *Homicides* [Internet]. OurWorldInData.org. Available at: https://ourworldindata.org/homicides

Steinberg, L. (2000). Youth violence: Do parents and families make a difference? *National Institute of Justice Journal, 243,* 30–38.

Thompson, S., & Kyle, K. (2005). Understanding mass shootings: Links between personhood and power in the competitive school environment. Developmental issues in school based aggression prevention. *The Journal of Primary Prevention, 26*(5), 419–438.

Thornton, T. N., Craft, C. A., Dahlberg, L. L., Lynch, B. S., & Baer, K. (2000). *Best practices of youth violence: A sourcebook for community action.* Centers for Disease Control and Prevention, National Center for Injury Prevention and Control.

Ttofi, M. M., & Farrington, D. (2011). Effectiveness of School-Based Programs to Reduce Bullying: A Systematic and Meta-Analytic Review. *Journal of Experimental Criminology, 7,* 27–56.

U.S. Department of Health and Human Services, Office of Disease Prevention and Health Promotion. (n.d.). *Healthy people 2030: Violence prevention* [Internet]. Washington, DC. Available from: https://health.gov/healthypeople/objectives-and-data/browse-objectives/violence-prevention. Accessed on: 28 Mar 2022.

U.S. Preventive Services Task Force. (1996). *Guide to clinical preventive services, 2nd edition: Report of the U.S. preventive services task force.* Williams & Wilkins. Available from: https://www.ncbi.nlm.nih.gov/books/NBK15435/

U.S. Secret Service National Threat Assessment Center (NTAC), U.S. Department of Homeland Security. (2018). *Enhancing school safety using a threat assessment model: An operational guide for preventing targeted school violence.* https://www.cisa.gov/enhancing-school-safety-using-threat-assessment-model

UNICEF. (2020). *COVID-19: Children at heightened risk of abuse, neglect, exploitation and violence amidst intensifying containment measures.* Available at: https://www.unicef.org/press-releases/covid-19-children-heightened-risk-abuse-neglect-exploitation-and-violence-amidst

United Nations Office on Drugs and Crime. (2019). *Global study on homicide, 2019 edition.* Available at: https://www.unodc.org/unodc/en/data-and-analysis/global-study-on-homicide.html

United States Department of Justice and the Center for the Study and Prevention of Violence. (1999). *Blueprints: A violence prevention initiative.* OJJPD Fact Sheet. Available at: https://www.ojp.gov/pdffiles1/fs99110.pdf

Vossekuil, B., Fein, R. A., & Berglund, J. M. (2015). Threat assessment: Assessing the risk of targeted violence. *Journal of Threat Assessment and Management, 2,* 243–254. https://doi.org/10.1037/tam0000055

World Health Organization. (2015). *Homicides: WHO Global Health estimates (2015 update).* Available at: https://apps.who.int/violence-info/homicide/

World Population Review. (2022). *School shootings by country 2022* [Internet]. Available at: https://worldpopulationreview.com/country-rankings/school-shootings-by-country

Youth Participatory Action Research. (2022). *Learn about youth participatory action research (YPAR).* Available at: http://yparhub.berkeley.edu/learn-about-ypar/

Chapter 2
The Neurobiology of Violence and Victimization: Etiology, Biological Substrates, Clinical Implications, and Preventive Strategies

William P. French

Introduction

The primary purpose of this chapter is to provide a theoretical framework for understanding the neurobiology of violence and victimization, especially as it relates to school violence. In recent years, progress in neurobiological study designs, imaging techniques, and animal models has led to an expansion in our knowledge and understanding of the neurobiological structures, chemicals, circuits, and systems that regulate the expression of violence and victimization. However, more than simply describing the nature and function of these biological substrates, it is important to examine how environmental factors, especially early childhood experiences, influence (and are influenced by) the formation and function of these neurobiological systems. The expression of violence and victimization is best viewed within a developmental context beginning with gene expression in the embryo and continuing throughout the lifespan (Conner, 2002; Mash & Dozois, 1996). Compared to the 2008 first publication of this chapter, this revision incorporates findings about racial disparities and provides additional guidance about how neuroscience findings can inform educational policies designed to decrease the prevalence of violence in school settings.

Key in understanding the current discussion is to keep in mind, that while individuals begin the developmental process with certain innate propensities, based mainly on inherited genetic factors, the expression and direction of these propensities depends in large part on the interactions between these factors and the individual's environment. To understand the impact of these interactions, the individual's

W. P. French (✉)
Department of Psychiatry and Behavioral Sciences, University of Washington, Seattle, WA, USA

Division of Child and Adolescent Psychiatry, Seattle Children's Hospital, Seattle, WA, USA
e-mail: william.french@seattlechildrens.org

© The Author(s), under exclusive license to Springer Nature
Switzerland AG 2023
T. W. Miller (ed.), *School Violence and Primary Prevention*,
https://doi.org/10.1007/978-3-031-13134-9_2

environment needs to be defined broadly enough to include the totality of environmental interactions that shape the destiny of the individual. Examples of such interactions include but are not limited to gene–protein (e.g., growth factor) interactions, gene–environment interactions, embryo–intrauterine interactions (e.g., the presence or absence of neurotoxic substances such as alcohol during gestation), infant–caregiver interactions (e.g., the quality of their attachment), adolescent–peer group interactions, and individual–community interactions. It is also important to emphasize the bidirectional nature of this process. For example, although it is true that males with high levels of testosterone have been found to display increased aggression (biology acting on the environment), it has also been found that males placed in situations of social dominance experience increases in their testosterone levels (environment acting on biology) (Conner, 2002; Rutter et al., 1997).

Note In the remainder of this chapter, aggression and violence will be used interchangeably. Technically, aggression can only be exerted by an animate agent, while violence can be produced by both animate and inanimate forces. Furthermore, the words aggression and aggressive both have potential positive meanings, while the words violence and violent do not. Therefore, it is important to note that adaptive aggression in animals and humans, if displayed in the right environmental context, is an adaptive trait. For example, a teenager, who fights off an intruder at home, may be aggressive, but this does not mean that he or she suffers from psychopathology. On the other hand, maladaptive aggression implies that the aggressive action being displayed is inappropriate to the context, ultimately harmful to the organism in its consequences, and represents a dysfunction of the organism, i.e., it is psychopathological. Therefore, while the word "aggression" will be frequently used in the rest of the chapter, the implication is that the "aggression" being discussed is maladaptive unless otherwise noted (Conner, 2002). Additionally, when discussing victims and victimization, often it will be more convenient to discuss the topic using words such as maltreatment, trauma, and traumatized.

Gene–Environment Interactions in Violence and Victimization

From a biological-oriented perspective, the study of the root causes of violence and victimization in school and in society involves attempting to understand how human biology interacts with the environment in ways that lead to maladaptive behavior. This approach inevitably brings us to discuss current concepts in the long-standing historical, philosophical, and scientific debates over the role of "nature" versus "nurture" in determining human behavior. Since the rise of the biological sciences, there have been several significant swings of the pendulum from extremes of biological determinism on one hand to extreme behavioralism on the other (Niehoff, 1999). In recent years, however, this either/or dichotomy has been transcended (at least in certain fields such as developmental biology and neurobiology) to be replaced by a growing appreciation of the interdependent bidirectional role of *gene–environment interactions* in directing the development of organisms.

Gene–environment interactions play a role in all aspects of an organism's development from conception to death. The following example, examining the relationship between developing neural cells and certain proteins called growth factors that regulate their development, illustrates the basic model of *gene–environment interactions*. Growth factors, also known as trophic factors (meaning, "to nourish"), are essential in guiding and nurturing neurons during nervous system development. By binding to receptors on the cell surfaces of young, differentiating neurons, trophic factors initiate biochemical changes that lead to selective gene expression. This process ultimately produces specialized neurons that are able to carry out the specific functions that are required in their local environments. For example, under the influence of nerve growth factor (NGF), precursor neural crest cells migrate out of the neural tube to become sympathetic neurons, which function in the autonomic nervous system (ANS). These same precursor cells, when they migrate to the adrenal gland, however, come under the influence of a different trophic factor glucocorticoid and do not develop into sympathetic neurons but into a different class of cells called Chromaffin cells, which have similar but distinct function compared to the sympathetic neurons (Niehoff, 1999). Trophic factors, thus, serve as environmental elements that interact with genetic elements to influence genetic expression. Dysregulation of trophic factors has been found in trauma victims with posttraumatic stress disorder (PTSD) and in animal and human subjects with aggression, which highlights the potential multilevel (micro to macro) influence of *gene–environment interactions* in selecting, regulating, and controlling neurobiological development. The study of *gene–environment interactions* has been able to progress beyond describing how local factors such as proteins are able to modify genetic expression. Through the work of leaders in the field of developmental psychopathology (such as Michael Rutter, Terrie Moffitt, and Avshalom Caspi), studies have been conducted to show how environmental influences, as far removed from direct contact with the genome as parental treatment of children, can modulate gene expression in ways that influence the expression of behaviors such as aggression and the development of depression (see Rutter et al., 2006 for an overview of the field).

An Example of the Role Gene–Environment Interactions That Play in Modulating Aggression and Violence

A number of studies have been undertaken over the last several decades to explore how genes interact with the environment to modify the expression of aggression and violence. One of the most interesting lines of inquiry in this regard has been into the role a class of neurochemicals called monoamines plays in mediating aspects of violence. An influential study on violence in maltreated children reported by Caspi et al. (2002) highlights some of the important research findings in this area. Their study draws on a large cohort of 1037 children born in 1972 who are part of the Dunedin Multidisciplinary Health and Development Study. The researchers looked at gene–environment interactions in children who either had or had not been exposed to maltreatment between the ages of 3 and 11 years. They were interested in determining the effect maltreatment would have in these children in predicting antisocial behavior across development, depending on whether the children had one of two types of polymorphisms (different versions of the same gene) for the gene monoamine oxidase A (MAOA) located on the X chromosome.

The gene product MAOA enzyme is a protein that metabolizes monoamines such as dopamine, norepinephrine, and serotonin. Thirty-seven percent of a subsample of 442 males in the study had a version of the MAOA gene, which produces a low-activity enzyme. Sixty-three percent of the males had a version of this gene, which produces a high-activity enzyme. Additionally, they categorized the children according to whether they had been exposed to severe maltreatment (8%), probable maltreatment (28%), or no maltreatment (64%). When they looked at the gene–environment interactions, they found that the 55 males who had both probable or severe maltreatment and *low* MAOA activity were twice as likely to have received a diagnosis of conduct disorder in their teens, and three times as likely to have been convicted of violent crime by age 26, compared to the 99 males with maltreatment **and** *high* MAOA activity. This subgroup of 55 boys, which was only 12% of the sample, was responsible for 44% of the violent convictions.

One conclusion which can be drawn from this study is that neither maltreatment nor genetic risk alone was associated with an appreciable level of antisocial behavior. It was only the interaction of a high-risk gene with a susceptible environment (a specific *gene–environment interaction*) that (presumably) produced a change in gene expression, which then contributed to a higher incidence of antisocial behavior.

A later study by Manuck (2006) investigating 531 white healthy males from the general population produced findings consistent with Caspi's original study. In this study, men with the low-activity MAOA allele were more likely to report a history of emotional reactivity, impulsive aggression, and antagonistic and confrontational behavior than those with the high-activity allele but only if they *also* had poorly educated fathers and were perceived as being cynical and hostile by others.

Other investigations in this area have examined the effect these polymorphisms of the MAOA gene may have on brain structure and function, especially during neurodevelopment. Meyer-Lindenberg et al. (2006), using fMRI to measure brain volume and activity differences, reported that compared to individuals with the high-activity allele, individuals with the low-activity allele (and thus presumably with higher serotonin levels during neurodevelopment) had reduced brain volumes in several neural structures known to crucial roles in emotional and behavioral regulation, including the anterior cingulate, bilateral amygdala, and the hypothalamus. Their results also showed increased activity in the left amygdala and decreased activity in the cingulate cortex and orbital frontal cortex (OFC), as well as decreased OFC-amygdala connectivity in males in response to emotionally provocative stimuli. These findings underscore what are thought to be the respective roles of these structures in modulating aggressive, impulsive behavior—namely, that an overly reactive amygdala, with dysfunctional inhibitory modulation by important neural structures involved in its regulation (OFC and cingulate cortex), may be playing a significant role in contributing to the pathology seen in emotionally disturbed children with impulsive, reactive aggression. While some subsequent studies examining how maltreatment affects the expression of the MAOA gene (including attempts to replicate Caspi's original finding) have had mixed results, meta-analyses by Kim-Cohen et al. (2006) and Byrd and Manuck (2014) concluded that the essential findings remain valid, though the latter meta-analysis, which included female subjects, found that the interaction between the low-activity MAOA allele and exposure to early maltreatment was significant only in male cohorts.

Of course, neither the aforementioned authors nor other researchers investigating the role of the MAOA gene in impulsive aggression are claiming that violence in youths and adults is caused solely by the low-activity version of the MAOA gene. In contrast, most recent research in behavioral genetics stresses the probable influence of multiple genes in the etiology of any given pathological condition. Moreover, as it is being suggested in this section, environmental interactions at multiple levels (biological, psychological, and social) probably impact how multiple genes contribute to the manifestation of aggression and violence (and most likely for victimization as well, though no data supporting this will be presented here).

Clinical Considerations

As the previous study suggests, understanding human maladaptive behavior (in this case impulsive aggression) requires consideration of biology, the environment, and the interaction between them.

While the use of knowledge of the allelic variation of genes is consistently expanding as a method to guide treatment for a number of psychiatric disorders (see de Leon et al., 2006; van Schaik et al., 2020), it is currently not widely utilized, or unequivocally considered to be beneficial, to identify or guide clinical treatment for youth at risk or engaged in aggression and violence and/or those youth with histories of victimization. Unfortunately, the widespread application of behavioral genetics to societal problems like violence and mental illness has a tainted past in the form of the eugenics movement of the early 1900s (Niehoff, 1999). In the future, though, as data on the importance genes–environment interactions in determining behavior continues to accumulate, efforts to identify youth at risk for aggression (based on genetic polymorphisms or other genetic information) may be critical in efforts to initiate early interventions to decrease the risk of environmental exposure to potential pathological influences, such as parental maltreatment. The following discussion of two studies investigating gene–environment interactions in toddlers illustrates this potential.

While not at the level of single-gene polymorphism analysis, both studies investigated the role of gene–environmental interactions in the development and persistence of callous-unemotional (CU) behaviors in children less than 3 years of age. (For further description of callous-unemotional behaviors, see below.) In the first study (Hyde et al., 2016), researchers studied a cohort of 561 adopted children who were removed from their biological parents at a mean age of 2 days. To investigate both heritable and non-heritable pathways to the development of CU behaviors, in addition to examining the role that adoptive mothers' parenting had in modifying their children's inherited risks for developing CU behaviors, they also quantified the severity of antisocial behaviors in their biological mothers. Their results indicated that high levels of antisocial behaviors in biological mothers predicted corresponding high levels of CU behaviors in their adopted children at 27 months. Importantly, they were also able to demonstrate that high, but not low, levels of positive adoptive parenting (e.g., warm praise given for prosocial child behaviors during a task demand) observed at 18 months acted to buffer this heritable risk, leading to lower levels of CU behaviors at 27 months for the children who received high levels of positive praise from their adoptive parents.

The earlier example demonstrates the influence of parent-driven effects on the development of CU behaviors in young children; the other study (Flom et al., 2020) investigated the role of child-driven effects in the development of CU behaviors. In this study, researchers examined a community sample of 314 same-sex twin pairs (roughly ½ of whom were monozygotic and ½ dizygotic) at age 2 and then again at age 3. By using a twin-sample cohort design, the researchers were able to parse out the relative genetic and shared environmental contributions to behavior. Their results indicated that genetically mediated childhood CU behaviors at age 2 predicted negative parenting behaviors at age three. Interestingly, this study did not find that negative parenting (parent-driven effect) at age 2 contributed to CU behaviors at age 3. Only when broader conduct problems were included as a co-variable in the analyses (not just strictly defined CU behaviors) did they find evidence of negative (vs. positive parenting) increasing the risk for worsening maladaptive behaviors at the later timepoint. While the authors acknowledge the likely bidirectionality of child and parental factors playing a role in subsequent behavioral problems, this study highlights the negative effects that genetically mediated CU behaviors in children have on parenting.

Additional research on the early emergence of CU behaviors identifies heritable temperamental risks for both *fearlessness* and *low interpersonal emotional sensitivity* (which can be identified in research settings in the first 2 years of life or earlier) as contributing to the formation and persistence of CU traits across the lifespan. Impairments in interpersonal emotional sensitivity are thought to lead to deficits in developing affective empathy characterized by diminished concerned for others' distress and low levels of positively expressed emotions. Fearlessness, a manifestation of low physiological arousal in face of threat, on the other hand, can undermine a child's ability to learn to avoid behaviors that lead to negative consequences, including parental limit setting, and may reinforce the development of patterns of dominance and high reward seeking, even when such behaviors transgress social norms. Importantly, these inherited temperamental patterns interact with parenting practices with research indicating that harsh, low warmth parenting serves to amplify the risks for further crystallization of CU behaviors, while high warmth, positive parenting can serve to buffer to some degree the risks that these temperamental patterns will ultimately lead to the emergence of persistent CU characteristics during the course of development (Waller & Hyde, 2018).

Callous and unemotional behaviors (e.g., lack of remorse and guilt, fearlessness, low empathy, lack of response to negative consequences) are seen in a subset of youth with conduct disorder. Conduct disorder is associated with the violation of the rights of others (including acts of aggression) and often precedes the development of antisocial, and in extreme cases, psychopathic traits in older individuals. One approach to decrease the likelihood of societal aggression (e.g., school violence) is to intervene early enough in development, so that maladaptive, but possibly modifiable, behaviors (e.g., CU behaviors) do not crystalize over time into becoming recidivistic behavioral or personality traits.

While several steps removed from the level of genetic analysis (however, see an animal model in the next paragraph), the work of Jerome Kagan (Kagan, 1989) is an example of how understanding nature–nurture interactions can lead to changes in developmental trajectory through first identifying unique biological traits in children and then applying targeted environmental interventions in an attempt to modify these traits. In his work on childhood temperament, Kagan has been able to show that shy children, whose parents encouraged them to be more curious in novel situations, developed more outgoing behaviors than children whose parents did not offer this encouragement. Shy children have been shown to have larger corticosteroid responses to stress than uninhibited children. By carefully attempting to modify inhibited children's behavioral responses through graduated, supported exposure to novel environments, these parents may be helping their children to alter corticosteroid response to stress leading to altered gene expression in the brain, which ultimately may further influence behavior change. Victimized children, such as those who suffer from PTSD, often also show exaggerated hormonal responses to subsequent stressors, which can lead to physiological symptoms that serve to maintain their hyper-responsive behavior (Siegel, 2001).

One example of an animal model: Cross-fostering studies in rats where high pup licking and grooming mothers raise offspring of low pup licking and grooming parents have shown that gene expression changes, in response to the cross-fostering, promote changes in the function of the HPA axis that leads these pups to have more modest hormonal responses to stress and be less fearful as adults than those low licking and grooming pups that were not cross-fostered (Kramer, 2005).

If we accept the premise that early intervention is one of the key factors in preventing the later emergence of maladaptive behaviors, such as aggression, at what age should those interventions begin? Research in the field of maternal–fetal health suggests that one critical opportunity for intervention begins with prenatal and perinatal care, given what is known about the relationship between poor maternal mental health (e.g., a history of maternal child maltreatment) being associated with an increased risk for negative mental health outcomes in mothers' offspring. Such intergenerational transmission of adverse mental health risks and outcomes is related not only to genetic and postnatal caregiving environment risk factors but also to maternal–intrauterine–fetal environment vulnerabilities. Though the mechanisms that underlie the role of the intrauterine environment in mediating these risks are yet to be fully elucidated, it is hypothesized that negative events (e.g., history of maternal maltreatment) lead to deleterious alterations in the fetal gestational biology (involving endocrine, immune/inflammatory, and metabolic processes) that, in turn, contribute to later negative healthcare outcomes in children (Buss et al., 2017). Given the emerging research findings in this area, it is not surprising that the field of child mental health is progressively moving upstream (e.g., perinatal psychiatry) in an effort to positively shape developmental trajectories.

One reason to include this information is to highlight the scope of the problem, as it relates to school violence and aggression from a neurobiological perspective. As William Wordsworth wrote, "The Child is the father of the Man." If we are not able to identify ways to change the conditions (e.g., maternal maltreatment) that lead to an increased risk for a mother's child to experience aberrant fetal brain development (and eventually possible behavioral challenges), then our efforts to create safer school environments will unlikely succeed to the degree we hope.

Youth Trauma, Abuse, and Neglect

Adverse Childhood Experiences

Since the publication of *The Adverse Childhood Experiences (ACE) Study* (Felitti et al., 1998), our understanding of the long-term negative health and developmental outcomes associated with early adverse childhood experiences (ACEs) has grown exponentially. Oftentimes discussed in terms of exposure to toxic stress, the ACE literature has documented the cumulative negative effects that exposure to maltreatment (e.g., sexual and physical abuse, neglect) and household dysfunction (e.g., substance abuse, domestic violence) have on individuals throughout their lifespan in terms of increased risks for developing unhealthy coping behaviors in response to childhood adversity and higher susceptibility to developing chronic diseases, such as asthma, heart disease, substance use disorders, and a range of mental health disorders. Research in this area has identified that exposure to ACEs leads to the disruption of multiple developmental processes involving the nervous, immune, and endocrine systems, among others (Jonson-Reid & Wideman, 2017). Most worrisome is the fact that multiple exposures to trauma lead to a graded dose–response relationship wherein a higher number of ACEs are correlated with a concomitant worsening of health outcomes over the lifespan.

Another rapidly expanding body of research related to the previous discussion on ACEs is building on evidence that early life adversity (ELA) accelerates biological aging at genomic, molecular, and cellular levels. In a recent systematic review and meta-analysis, Colich et al. (2020) found that ELA involving threat (e.g., violence exposure), but not deprivation (e.g., neglect) or low-socioeconomic status, was associated with accelerated timing of puberty, cellular aging (as measured by DNA methylation age and telomere length), and cortical thinning in the ventromedial prefrontal cortex. Accelerated aging, like ACEs, is linked to a wide range of negative health outcomes across multiple biological systems including cardiovascular, reproductive, neurobiological, and is associated with increases in all-cause mortality, unhealthy lifestyle decision-making, and numerous health disorders.

While it is easy to understand the burden of suffering ACEs exact on the individuals who experience them, research also finds that early childhood adversity can also increase the likelihood of future perpetration of aggression and violence against others. For example, in a study that compared adult convicted offenders (of child abuse, domestic violence, sexual assault, and stalking) to a normative sample, rates of adverse childhood experiences in the offender sample were nearly four times higher than the normative sample (Reavis et al., 2013). It is also important to note here that racial inequities in the US criminal justice system contribute to significant disparities in the rate of incarceration for blacks, especially black males, compared to whites. For example, a 2016 publication using cohort data ($n = 5189$) from the National Survey of American Life found that, compared to respondents who had never experienced trauma, black Americans experiencing 4 or more traumas were 5 times more likely to have been jailed. The authors note black children experience maltreatment at twice the rate of white children and that incarceration rates for adult black males are up to six times greater compared to their white counterparts (Jäggi et al., 2016).

Even more salient to the topic of prevention of school violence, a study published in *Pediatrics* in 2010, involving nearly 140,000 Minnesota 6th, 9th, and 12th grade student survey responses, found that those students who had experienced one or more of 6 ACE categories investigated were significantly more likely to have engaged in interpersonal acts of violence perpetration, such as bullying, delinquency, physical fighting, bringing a weapon on school grounds, intimate partner violence, and self-directed violence (e.g., suicide attempts). For females, having experienced any ACE was associated with a 1.7- to 5-fold increased risk for violence perpetration; for males, the risk increase was 1.7- to 44-fold. In terms of added risk per each increase in ACE score, violence perpetration risk increased from 30% to 88% for females and 35% to 88% for males (Duke et al., 2010). These examples of the relationship between violence and victimization highlight a central theme of this chapter, which is that maltreatment sows the seeds for future maltreatment both for the initial victim and for others who the victim may later encounter. The neurobiological underpinnings of this reciprocal relationship will be covered later in this chapter.

Trauma Through the Lens of the DSM-5

In America, childhood and adolescent psychiatric disorders are usually diagnosed and categorized utilizing the American Psychiatric Association's *Diagnostic and Statistical Manual of Mental Disorders* (DSM-5) (American Psychiatric Association, 2013). The DSM uses categorical descriptions of observable or reported signs and symptoms to define disorders. With this system, to be diagnosed with a particular psychiatric disorder, for example, PTSD, a person must meet the discreet criteria for the disorder and be experiencing impairment in daily functioning as a consequence. With the DSM, a person either has a disorder or does not. While this chapter will discuss several DSM disorders, it focuses on understanding the neurobiological substrates associated with violence and victimization, which are not considered in the DSM. Furthermore, the approach utilized here, in addition to the categorical approach in the DSM, also utilizes a dimensional approach and assumes that behavior, if viewed as a reflection of neurobiology interacting with the environment, exists on a continuum from adaptive to maladaptive. (For diagnostic criteria of the various DSM disorders discussed, please refer to the DSM-5.)

As for the previous discussion regarding ACEs, our understanding of the effects of childhood trauma, abuse, and neglect has evolved over the last four-and-a-half decades since Fraiberg's 1975 seminal work *Ghosts in the Nursery* (Fraiberg et al., 1987) described the multigenerational deleterious effects that occur in impaired mother–infant relationships. One of the main features of current research-driven formulations of childhood trauma is that multiple variables influence the generation and severity of psychopathology. Depending on frequency, severity, the degree to which caregivers are involved, the age of the child, and factors related to individual vulnerability and resilience, the consequences of maltreatment can range from little or no effect to profound disruptions of multiple aspects of normal development lasting across the lifespan (van der Kolk, 2003).

In current US psychiatric and psychological practice, diagnoses of PTSD and Acute Stress Disorder (ASD), under the broader category of Trauma-and Stress-Related Disorders, are commonly employed in attempting to categorize the consequences of childhood maltreatment. However, the range and degree of potential disruption to normal development that occurs as a result of childhood trauma (especially when severe) fail to be captured in these diagnoses (Cook et al., 2005). It is not surprising, therefore, that child victims of trauma and neglect often meet criteria for multiple disorders other than PTSD and ASD, including but not limited to, anxiety disorders, mood disorders, attentional disorders such as ADHD, disruptive behavior disorders, sensory integration disorder, and reactive attachment disorder (Cook et al., 2005). In severe and chronic maltreatment cases, symptoms of PTSD may not even be prominent and may be obscured by other behavioral, affective, and cognitive concerns (van der Kolk, 2003). Child trauma experts often use terms such as *complex trauma* and *developmental trauma* to better capture the significance of maltreatment and neglect in the young. Early trauma causes pervasive and lasting impact on the developing mind and brain leading to disruption of developing neurobiological systems, which in turn manifests in the development of complex behavioral and psychological symptoms. In order to facilitate a more informed clinical approach to children whose experiences of violence, fear, and neglect play a significant role in their early development, van der Kolk has argued for new diagnostic criteria *Developmental Trauma Disorder* to guide the assessment and treatment of children with complex trauma histories (van der Kolk, 2005). Alexandra Cook et al. (2005) list seven domains affected by complex trauma, some of which are incorporated in the following discussion.

Domains of Trauma

Attachment

Mary Ainsworth and Mary Main expanding on John Bowlby's formulation of caregiver-infant attachment theory have described four patterns of relating that infants and young children use to organize their cognitive, affective, and behavioral approaches to their environments: secure, insecure-avoidant, insecure-ambivalent, and insecure-disorganized (Davies, 1999). Newborns are born with immature nervous systems that are unable to self-regulate in the face of internal and environmental stressors. Children with secure attachment receive assistance in self-regulation from attentive caregivers, who by responding caringly to their infants' needs and signals of distress, help them modulate their stress responses. By responding to children with a balance of soothing and stimulation, caregivers serve as "hidden regulators" of infant physiological states of arousal and relaxation. This capacity to provide comfort and security acts bidirectionally creating a state of "affect attunement" that reinforces the attachment process. At the same time, it creates the stable conditions necessary for the healthy maturation of the nervous system and ultimately enables the child to independently and flexibly modulate his or her stress responses (van der Kolk, 2003; Ainsworth, 1985). Caregiver–infant interactions, by contributing to the maturation of the nervous system, are one example of how interpersonal relationships influence neurobiology in the formation and function of the developing mind and brain (Siegel, 2001).

Childhood trauma, violence, and neglect often disrupt the normal attachment process; this is especially likely if the caregiver is the source of the trauma, suffers from the trauma as well, or responds to the trauma in a disorganized, chaotic fashion (van der Kolk, 2003; McFarlane, 1988). While all the insecure attachment patterns are less than optimal, a study by Carlson found that 80% of traumatized children show the unhealthiest pattern—insecure-disorganized attachment (Carlson et al., 1989). A high percentage of parents with children who show disorganized attachment have histories themselves of abuse, neglect, and unresolved trauma. These parents are often anxious and fearful and commonly display intense emotions in the present related to unresolved traumas in the past. In interactions with their parents, children with disorganized attachment often show signs of alarm and may appear frightened by their parents' intense expression of negative emotions, inconsistent parenting, and potentially violent behavior.

Disorganized children are at high risk for the development of psychopathology for several reasons: (1) they are exposed (perhaps chronically) to frightening experiences, which produce large physiological stress responses that overcome their underdeveloped coping capacities; (2) though they are unable to cope with their stress, their caregivers not only do not serve as "hidden regulators" of physiological arousal, but they often are the source of the distress; and (3) although they may feel intense anger and other negative emotions toward their attachment figures, they may be filled with conflicting feelings because they also still must rely on these caregivers as sources of security and belonging. Studies of traumatized children with disorganized styles of attachment show that they often respond to stress and perceived threat with fear-driven fight-flight-freeze reactions that: (1) lead to withdrawing, self-destructive, or aggressive behaviors and (2) prevent them from developing (and learning to use) skills such as affect regulation and cognitive inhibition of impulses that enable healthy children to flexibly respond and manage stress.

While disorganized attachment increases the risks for later pathology, there is evidence that having attachment security buffers some of the potential negative consequences of early pre- and post-natal adverse experiences. In a 2018 study examining the relationship of infant attachment style at 36 months and (a) measures of cognitive and behavioral development and (b) genomic DNA methylation, researchers were able to demonstrate that in a large cohort of infants recruited from the Maternal Adversity Vulnerability and Neurodevelopment study, securely attached infants showed distinct methylation patterns compared to those infants without secure attachments, with the differences being most evident when comparing secure versus disorganized attachment styles. Compared to infants without secure attachment styles, the securely attached infants showed relative advantage in cognitive and behavioral development. Many of these identified variations in methylation patterns occurred in genes known to encode for proteins involved in neuronal development (e.g., ephrin signaling pathway) and the biological stress response system (e.g., glucocorticoid signaling). The authors suggest their study and others, which demonstrate the biological embedding of early life experiences (biological response to adversity being moderated by attachment style), provide molecular evidence that early interventions aimed at improving the quality of parent–child attachment may be able to mitigate some of the downstream negative consequences of early adversity (Garg et al., 2018).

One such intervention is the Nurse-Family Partnership (NFP), which provides interventions to promote maternal health and improve mother–child relationships for pregnant women with identified risks (e.g., young age, low socioeconomic status) for poor parenting outcomes including abuse and neglect. Utilizing data from the original NFP cohort, diagnostic interviews, and DNA methylation analyses, researchers conducted a study comparing psychosocial outcomes and methylation patterns in the adult offspring (mean age 27.4 years) of the intervention (NFP intervention group) and control groups hypothesizing that differences in adult DNA methylation patterns would be evident for: (1) adult offspring in either group who were exposed to childhood abuse and neglect (from birth to age 15) and (2) between those offspring assigned to the NFP (versus the control group). Both intervention and control groups were assessed for evidence of depression, anxiety, PTSD, substance abuse, and conduct disorder/antisocial personality disorder. Blood samples were drawn to conduct DNA methylation pattern analyses. Results showed clear evidence that participant exposure to childhood abuse and neglect was associated with significant changes to the methylation patterns compared to those without exposure. There was also evidence of significant (albeit, small) differences in genome-wide methylation patterns in those offspring of mothers who received the NFP intervention indicating that the NFP intervention had lasting impact on the epigenome (DNA methylation) that regulates genomic function from infancy into adulthood (O'Donnell et al., 2018).

The Role of Biology, Trauma, and Working Models in the Development of Psychopathology

Trauma affects multiple neurotransmitter systems, disrupts the normal development of important neural structures such as the hippocampus, impairs the connectivity and information flow between neural structures, and is implicated in producing persistent functional alterations in important stress regulating systems such as the autonomic nervous system (ANS) and the hypothalamic-pituitary-adrenal (HPA) axis (van der Kolk, 2003).

As a child grows, modifications (as from trauma) to the biological systems that regulate functions, such as arousal, behavior, affect and cognition will, in turn, affect the way the child relates to organizes, interprets, and responds to his or her environment. Perry and Pollard describe this process in terms of bidirectional interactions between children's brains and their early experiences, whether typical or filled with trauma, as shaping (in a use-dependent manner) how they will ultimately come to interpret reality (Perry & Pollard, 1998; van der Kolk, 2003). Bowlby believed this process begins during the attachment period and used the term *internal working model* to describe the process in which children develop inner maps or representations of themselves, their relationships, and their environments that help them organize and regulate their responses to situations and people. Working models contribute to the development of a sense of self and play a role in a child's ability to regulate states of arousal and respond flexibly to stress. By the third year, internal working models are relatively enduring and thus tend to become stable filters through which subsequent events and relationships are experienced (Davies, 1999).

Fear conditioning in animals provides a model for understanding how childhood trauma affects internal working models, nervous system development, and t development of psychopathology. Animals exposed to aversive unconditioned stimuli (i.e., an electrical shock) paired with a neutral conditioned stimulus (e.g., a light) will develop an enduring conditioned fear response to the conditioned stimulus even in the absence of a shock. This conditioning is difficult to extinguish, and depending on laboratory conditions, can produce chronic alterations in biological systems involved in fear conditioning and the stress response such as the ANS and HPA-axis (Conner, 2002).

Children undergoing nervous system development are especially vulnerable to developing enduring conditioned fear responses in the face of trauma. If they occur during the early attachment period, traumatic fear responses may be one of the earliest (and therefore most impactful) organizing experiences of their developing nervous system (Perry & Pollard, 1998). If trauma is ongoing, the nervous system may undergo lasting changes that "hard-wire" these fear-conditioned biological changes in a use-dependent manner producing children who are chronically hyper-aroused, fearful, and insecure and who show evidence of lasting alterations in CNS function. Heim et al. (2000) report that adult women sexually or physically abused as children show abnormal HPA axis and ANS responses to mild stress, while Bremmer et al. (1997) using MRI have documented hippocampal atrophy in adult patients with PTSD who had been abused as children.

Along with changes in neurobiological function, trauma produces alterations in the working models that children use to make sense of their world and organize their experiences. The working models of many severely traumatized children show a pattern of lack of self-confidence, mistrust of others, and experiencing the world as threatening. As mentioned earlier, working models are relatively stable after the third year, and since they are unconsciously formed, are unconsciously projected onto future relationships and situations leading to additional dysfunctional experiences even in the absence of continuing sources of trauma. Such adaptations to a traumatic experience, which then serves as a template for processing future experiences, may also occur in older children, adolescents, and adults exposed to trauma as part of a trauma accommodation syndrome (Miller & Veltkamp, 1996). Previously physically abused children, who behave in ways that invite aggressive responses from otherwise well-intentioned foster parents, and child sexual assault victims, who, as adults, become involved in relationships with abusive partners, or otherwise demonstrate behaviors that put them at risk for re-assault, are examples of how past trauma acts in the present to recreate past patterns of behavior (Davies, 1999; Porter et al., 2015).

While neurobiological underpinnings of these types of behaviors are complex, animal models can provide insight. For example, researchers utilizing an odor-shock conditioning model in rat pups demonstrated that when a specific odor (peppermint) was paired with a shock during a significant developmental window for attachment learning, the rats, as adults, developed a strong preference for the odor. Furthermore, presentation of this trauma-associated odor acted to reverse depressive symptoms (i.e., have an antidepressant effect), repair amygdala dysfunction, and reduce stress-related cortisol levels through mechanisms involving amygdala serotonin and the glucocorticoid system (Rincón-Cortés et al., 2015). Such findings provide a provocative, and disturbing, model as to why a child, who experiences caregiver trauma during a critical period of attachment formation, would be attracted to trauma-related cues in later life.

Cognition, Affect Regulation, and Behavioral Control—The Role of the Amygdala in the Threat Response

As discussed earlier, neurobiological systems that regulate arousal and stress responses, though functional, are immature at birth and therefore require caregiver intervention to modulate their activities. As development continues, however, securely attached children gain greater control in their abilities to self-soothe and control their response to stress. Part of this control is due to the gradual development of functional competencies in biological systems that regulate cognition and affect. Unlike many structures more directly involved with survival that are fully functional from birth, structures such as the hippocampus (involved in memory and emotion processing) and the prefrontal cortex (PFC) (involved in executive functioning, impulse control, and affect regulation) develop their functional capacities more slowly. As these affective and cognitive (executive) capacities come "on-line" during normal development, they provide additional layers of regulatory capacity enabling children and adolescents to fine-tune their behavioral responses to situations and people. The following discussion highlighting the role of the prefrontal cortex and hippocampus in regulating the fear pathway provides an example of how cognitive and affective input contributes to overall stress regulation.

The amygdala is a key neural structure in the limbic system that registers threats. When activated, it produces fear. It functions by assigning emotional valency (or intensity) to incoming stimuli. (For example, for humans, a snake usually has more emotional valency than a stick.) When activated by a threat, the amygdala sends signals to the hypothalamus, which activates stress responses via the HPA-axis and autonomic nervous system thus preparing a person for defensive action. The hippocampus only begins to develop from approximately 3 years. As it matures, it provides a child with the capacity to form context-dependent autobiographical memories, which include the ability to organize and place sources of threat in a spatial context. It has inhibitory inputs to the hypothalamus, which serve to inhibit the activation of the stress response. This in turn leads to inhibition of the amygdala through feedback mechanisms involving cortisol. In fear-provoking situations, the hippocampus, through its role in memory, is able to provide greater flexibility of response and behavioral control by helping a child better interpret the emotional significance of incoming stimuli through connecting the current threatening experience to similar past emotional experiences and responses (LeDoux, 2002; Conner, 2002; van der Kolk, 2003).

The prefrontal cortex also plays an inhibitory role in relation to the amygdala and thus is able to provide additional regulatory control to the fear pathway. In situations of immediate threat, sensory information reaches the thalamus, which then directs it on two separate pathways: one to the amygdala and one to the prefrontal area (via sensory association areas), which then continues on to the amygdala. The short pathway allows for rapid responses to threats by direct amygdala activation of the fear pathway, while the long pathway permits frontal areas of the brain to gather more detailed information about the threat, which then can be used to modulate the initial response. When you come upon an object resembling a snake, the short pathway allows you to quickly move out of the way, while the long pathway, though it takes more time, allows you to gather more detailed visual information to determine if the object is really a snake or just a stick. While slower than the pathway directly to the amygdala, the long pathway, via pathways through the PFC to the amygdala, permits cortical areas of the brain capable of reasoning, planning, problem solving, and representational memory to modulate emotional, physiological, and behavioral responses to threats and stress (LeDoux, 1996).

In normal development, neurobiological structures and processes involving cognition, emotion, behavior, and physiology all work together in producing an integrated, functional, and flexible nervous system that enables developing children to successfully respond to their environments. As discussed in the introduction to this section, trauma potentially produces deficits in multiple aspects of nervous system function including those that involve affect regulation, cognition, and behavioral control.

Affect

In studies involving affect regulation, maltreated children show deficits in their ability to identify and label emotional states in themselves and others, which may impair their own ability to understand, regulate, and respond appropriately to their feelings and the feelings of others (Beeghly & Cicchetti, 1996). Such deficits in important social skills often lead to social withdrawal or bullying of other children (van der Kolk, 2003). Damage to the hippocampus, as seen in sufferers of PTSD, may lead to impairments in autobiographical memory impacting the ability of traumatized children to use past experiences to regulate current affective states. Studies of the long-term consequences of maltreatment on affect regulation indicate that past trauma is the third most common predictor of adult depression aside from heredity and current stress (Harvard Mental Health Letter, 2005). Perhaps the most common association between childhood trauma and later problems with affect regulation, however, occurs in borderline personality disorder where a history of previous maltreatment, especially sexual abuse, is the norm rather than the exception. Such individuals commonly exhibit dysregulation of nervous system function across multiple domains including instability of emotional affect manifesting in intense mood swings, irritability, anxiety, periodic dysphoria often associated with suicidal ideation or attempts, and severe problems with anger and interpersonal relationships.

Cognition

Victimized children and adolescents also display deficits in multiple areas of cognition. Studies of maltreated children have shown decreased overall IQ; deficits in receptive and expressive language abilities; problems in learning and memory; deficits in executive functioning leading to problems in attention, impulse control, and abstract reasoning; decreased creativity, flexibility, and sustained interest in problem solving; greater need for special education services; and dropout rates three times that of the general population (Culp et al., 1991; Beers & De Bellis, 2002; Shonk & Cicchetti, 2001). Longstanding, stable deficits to executive functioning (EF), and more broadly downstream increased risks for general psychopathology (P), have been demonstrated in ongoing studies of institutionally raised children participating in the Bucharest Early Intervention Project. Severe, early neglect is associated with global deficits in EF, which appears to serve as a transdiagnostic mediator cutting across both internalizing and externalizing disorders leading to an increased risk for the development (measured at age 8, 12, and 16) of discrete psychiatric disorders in both externalizing and internalizing domains (Wade et al., 2020).

Problems with autonomic hyperarousal and affect regulation may contribute to short-term cognitive difficulties by creating physiological, emotional, social, and environmental conditions that interfere with immediate cognitive tasks; over time, these dysfunctional patterns of arousal and affect, however, can lead to permanent alterations in cognitive systems through their deleterious effects on important neural structures and circuits. Short-term impairment of cognitive capacity may occur when excessive subcortical "noise" from the brain stem, autonomic, and limbic systems overwhelms cortical functioning. Hyperarousal, partly mediated by elevated epinephrine, has been associated with decreased executive functioning capacity in areas involved in working memory, attention, and impulse inhibition (Crittenden, 1997). Mezzacappa et al. (1998) showed that traumatized boys have decreased vagal modulation in parasympathetic branches of the ANS that are involved in executive control. Additional sources of cognition dysfunction in traumatized children involve: (1) deficits in language due to underdevelopment of the left cortex (responsible for language function in most humans) and (2) impairments in learning and memory involving the hippocampus brought on by excess secretion of cortisol and impaired secretion of BDNF, a trophic factor that supports hippocampal development (Bremner, 2006).

Behavior

Childhood and adolescent trauma is associated with both overcontrolled (i.e., rigid, compulsive) and under-controlled (i.e., impulsive, aggressive) behavior patterns. Some commonly seen behaviors patterns include re-enactment of the trauma (i.e., sexualized behaviors in sexually abused youth); heightened sensitivity to threat (i.e., aggressive behaviors); attempts to gain control (i.e., eating disorders); avoidance (i.e., social withdrawal); and maladaptive efforts to self-soothe (i.e., cutting) (Cook et al., 2005). Except for discussions involving the neurobiology of fear and fear-based aggression, the neurobiology involved in these complex behaviors is beyond the scope of this chapter.

Risk and Resiliency

Not everyone exposed to trauma develops PTSD or some other psychopathology. In fact, some clinicians and researchers believe that an overemphasis on the potential pathological responses to negative events places trauma victims at risk for developing maladaptive outcomes by pathologizing these experiences. In their view, such catastrophizing engenders a negative expectation concerning future outcomes that can actually serve to undermine a healthy adaptive response. These researchers focus on the concept of resiliency and emphasize that stress is common, successful adaptation to stress is the norm, and overcoming stress actually can promote resiliency against future stress (Levin, Psychiatric News, August, 2006). Research in resiliency attempts to identify the biological, psychological, and environmental characteristics of individuals who experience stressful events and adversity but are able to recover quickly without developing maladaptive responses or dysfunction.

Animal research in rats has provided evidence as to how resiliency might occur at the neurobiological level. Amat and colleagues exposed rats to two sets of experimental conditions. In the first condition, they first exposed rats to a controllable stressor and then to an uncontrollable one; in the second condition, they first exposed rats to an uncontrollable stressor and then to an additional stressor. They were able to show that rats exposed to the controllable stressor were resistant to the development of depression-like behavior when exposed to future stressors, while the rats first exposed to the uncontrollable stressor were susceptible to the development depression-like behaviors when faced with future stressors. Further experimental work showed that the ventral medial prefrontal cortex (vmPFC) and the dorsal raphe nucleus in the brainstem were both involved in this process in a way that suggests that when the rats "sense" control over stressful situations the vmPFC is able to inhibit the release of serotonin from the dorsal raphe nucleus. The clinical implication here is that perceived control is able to buffer against the deleterious effects of stress through the action of prefrontal structures inhibiting stress-responsive structures in lower brain areas such as the brainstem. This competency in the face of stress may promote resiliency by "inoculating" the organism against maladaptive responses to future stressors (Amat et al., 2006). Additional work in stress inoculation done by Parker et al. (2006) demonstrated that early stress can have beneficial in primates as well by showing that in male squirrel monkeys early, intermittent stress in infancy, such as increasing foraging demands on mothers, leads to a reduced HPA-axis response in face of stress as adults.

In humans, Laura Campbell–Sills and coworkers (Campbell-Sills et al., 2006) report that individuals with childhood neglect, who also scored high on tests of resiliency, showed fewer psychiatric symptoms as adults than other individuals with high resiliency but who did not experience childhood neglect. While the neurobiological mechanism for this finding was not studied, these results echo those of the aforementioned studies in non-human animals and suggest that the combination of resiliency and exposure to stress creates conditions for mental health in the face of challenge (Arehart-Treichel, Psychiatric News, September, 2005).

Clinical Considerations

Paul MacLean, former director of the NIH's Laboratory of Brain Evolution and Behavior, is best known as the originator of the concept of *the triune brain* (Ploog, 2003). Introduced in 1970, the theory of the triune brain uses concepts and research findings in evolutionary theory, comparative neuroanatomy, and neurochemistry to describe how modern human brains are the result of three successive, hierarchically organized stages of animal evolution that in humans (and other closely related mammals) has led to the formation of three-brains-in-one. MacLean termed these three distinct "brains" *reptilian* (sensorimotor and autonomic systems), *paleomammalian* (limbic system), and *neomammalian* (executive system). He believed, that though connected and organized to operate in an integrated fashion, because each "brain" evolved separately, each has separate distinct functions mediated through its unique anatomy and phylogeny (LeDoux, 1996).

MacLean's model provides a useful heuristic for discussing how human cognitive (executive), emotional (limbic), and behavioral (sensorimotor, endocrine, and autonomic) systems operate hierarchically to produce both adaptive and maladaptive responses to victimization. Moreover, conceiving of the brain as a triune system can be useful in assessing and devising treatment strategies, not only for victims of trauma but also for other categories of psychopathology (including maladaptive aggression) by helping clinicians analyze and breakdown complex clinical presentations into more manageable cognitive, emotional, and behavioral components. For example, in the treatment of PTSD, such a strategy can aid in selecting appropriate medications by helping categorize target symptoms (arising from a background of neurobiological malfunction) into cognitive, affective, and behavioral (including autonomic) components in order to better align medication's mechanisms of action with intended treatment outcomes.

Another application of the triune model is to use its hierarchical structure to separate therapeutic approaches to victimization and trauma into "top-down" or "bottom-up" interventions (Ogden et al., 2006). As discussed earlier, the human brain develops through the emergence of inborn potentialities that are realized in a time-dependent developmental sequence that involves interaction with caregivers and other environmental inputs. While a child is born able to breathe and regulate many physiological processes without caregiver support, higher order capacities such as behavioral control, affect regulation, and cognitive function only develop over time through interactions with the environment.

In young people, the impact of trauma is thought to especially affect subcortical neurobiological systems, such as the limbic system and brainstem, which are critical for stress regulation and innate and learned responses to threats (van der Kolk, 2003). While top-down interventions (e.g., talk therapy) may attempt to enlist a patient's cognitive capacities in order to understand, process, or make sense of past trauma, such attempts may be misguided if the child's cognitive capacities are not yet sufficiently developed or he or she remains "stuck" in a dysregulated physiological and emotional state that blocks effective cognitive processing of potentially curative information (Ogden et al., 2006). As such, one approach clinicians may choose to take is a bottom-up intervention using pharmaceuticals (such as a beta-adrenergic blocker or alpha 2-adrenergic agonist) to treat physiological hyperarousal through manipulating the autonomic nervous system. While this approach may ameliorate some of the physiological symptoms that are contributing to suffering, it does not address the cause of the continued hyperarousal and activation of the stress response system in the absence of persisting threat.

Van der Kolk suggests a key cause of a persistent state of conditioned fear and chronic stress in a child following trauma is the loss of a sense of safety and security, created in part by the subcortical systems responsible for responding to stress and danger having been overwhelmed and/or caregivers having been unable to intervene in their role as "hidden regulators." What needs to occur ultimately then is a restoration of a sense of security in the environment but often the child remains biologically "stuck" following the trauma in a state of chronic fear, stress, and hyperarousal and is unable to experience safe environments as unthreatening. By creating safe, predictable environments free from past trauma triggers, however, parents, caregivers, and therapists can intervene from the bottom-up by creating conditions for controllable stress responses and thus help the child to begin to modulate his or her limbic and brainstem responses to novel situations in more flexible, less frozen ways (van der Kolk, 2003). Another aspect of involvement at the bottom-up level may involve addressing, not hyperarousal, but the numbing, hypo-arousal, and dissociative states of mind that often occur as a result of trauma. Here the task is to help the child begin to feel his or her body again, possibly through play or other body-focused therapies (Ogden et al., 2006).

As progress occurs and bodily sensations and feelings associated with trauma are better tolerated without creating hyper or hypo-aroused physiological states or disorganized behaviors or states of mind, top-down approaches may become more effective. At this point, therapies and interventions, such as talk therapy, that call on the children's cognitive capacities to process their traumatic experiences (and their limbic and brainstem responses reactions to them) can be better utilized to help children begin to understand and process memories and reactions to past trauma. Through being able to put feelings and sensations into words, or other symbolic representations such as drawings, children acquire the ability to objectify past experiences, understand factors outside their control that contributed to them, and gain a sense of mastery and control, which permits adaptive responses to future environmental encounters. Importantly, a child's aptitude and preference for cognitive processing of trauma need to be monitored carefully as children who seem out of touch with their emotions and rely heavily on cognitive approaches in dealing with stress have as many problems as children who primarily rely on their emotions (van der Kolk, 2003; Crittenden, 1992).

Youth Violence and Aggression

Aggression Subtypes—"Hot" and "Cold" Aggression

Adolescent males make up 8% of the total United States population but are responsible for 50% of violent crimes (Fox, 1995). Research into the neurobiology and phenomenology of violence and aggression has revealed discrete patterns of aggression that arise from different neurobiological pathways and sources of pathology. Efforts to understand these different patterns have led to the segregation of aggression into different subtypes. Two important subtype groupings that have emerged are the distinctions between proactive and reactive aggression (Dodge, 1991; Dodge & Coie, 1987) and between predatory and affective aggression (Eichelman, 1987; Moyer, 1976). These two subtype groupings, though sharing different conceptual origins, overlap sufficiently to be combined for our discussion (following Steiner) into "hot" and "cold" subtypes of aggression. What follows is a brief introduction to research into the phenomenology and clinical utility of this area of aggression research (Soller et al., 2006). Note, earlier in this chapter, there was a discussion of callous and unemotional behaviors in very young children. While not entirely synonymous concepts, CU behaviors can be viewed as an example of what is meant by "cold" aggression.

"Hot" aggression comprises impulsive, aggressive, and defensive behaviors that arise in the face of actual or perceived attack or provocation. This type of aggression is best conceptualized as a defensive fear-driven response to threat and frustration often with the expectation of a negative situational outcome. There is high CNS autonomic arousal and irritability due to activation of the fight, flight, and freeze response, while behaviorally there is an uncoordinated, poorly modulated response to the threat with a high risk of self-harm and low probability of successful outcome or reward. Children and adolescents with "hot" aggression often display biases that, in the setting of socially provocative or ambiguous situations, lead them to make inappropriate, exaggerated, and aggressive responses to peers and adults, who they believe have hostile intentions toward them (Conner, 2002; Dodge, 1991; Crick & Dodge, 1996). Compared to "cold" aggression, "hot" aggression has an earlier age of onset and is more commonly associated with early developmental disturbances, such as physical abuse or social instability, and neuropsychiatric problems, such as inattention and impulsivity (Conner, 2002). Despite this seemingly greater burden of pathology, studies by Vitaro et al. (1998) and Pulkkinen (1996) showed children with "hot" aggression to be less likely than those with "cold" aggression to continue to exhibit disruptive and antisocial behaviors in adolescence and adulthood. Finally, "hot" aggression is correlated with lower IQ, greater likelihood of treatment with psychotropics, and greater likelihood of favorable response to psychotropics.

"Cold" aggression combines aspects of the proactive and predatory aggression formulations to describe a pattern of behavior and physiological arousal quite distinct from "hot" aggression. Children and adolescents with "cold" aggression typically have little CNS autonomic arousal or visible signs of fear, irritability, and anger when engaged in aggressive acts (Conner, 2002). This type of aggression is pursued in order to obtain desired goal or favorable outcome whether for food, property, or social status. Unlike "hot" aggression, the execution of "cold" aggressive acts occurs in an organized, patterned, goal-directed, and controlled manner, which increases the likelihood of a successful outcome. "Cold" aggression models in humans postulate that this behavior is often learned and practiced in the context of social environments that provide social role modeling and external reinforcements for such behavior (Bandura, 1973).

In the latest iteration of the DSM (DSM-5), a specifier has been added to the diagnosis of conduct disorder to identify those youth diagnosed with conduct disorder who display evidence of "cold" aggression. While essentially describing youth who display evidence of CU behaviors, DSM task force members chose to specify these youth as: *With limited prosocial emotions* (LPE), as evidenced by exhibiting a lack of remorse or guilt, being callous/lacking empathy, being unconcerned about their performance (e.g., does not seem concerned about poor academic functioning), or displaying a shallow, insincere, or superficial affect. For the remaining of this chapter, LPE, CU, and "cold" aggression will be used interchangeably.

Psychopathy—A Lack of Conscience and Moral Sense

Current research in the neurobiology of aggression, in delineating between "cold" and "hot" aggression, seeks to identify unique neural circuitry that leads to the separate motivational, behavioral, and physiological manifestations of each pattern. In addition, this distinction between the two patterns of aggression may aid in identifying common maladaptive pathways operating in both perpetrators and victims of violence insofar as both victims and perpetrators often show evidence of pathological adaptations to perceived or actual threats in the environment.

The concept of psychopathy, while not currently recognized in the DSM-5, is an important construct in the study of aggression and violence that further clarifies the distinction between "cold" and "hot" aggression and aids in elucidating the relationship between violence and victimization. Defined in multiple ways across different fields, the definition to be used here follows from Cleckley and Hare. Hare describes psychopaths as "intraspecies predators who use charm, manipulation, intimidation, and violence to control others and to satisfy their own selfish needs. Lacking in conscience and in feeling for others, they take what they want and do as they please violating social norms and expectations without guilt or remorse" (Hare, 1995). Research in psychopathy identifies, unlike in oppositional defiant disorder (ODD), conduct disorder (CD), and antisocial personality disorder (ASPD) populations, a fairly *homogenous* group of individuals with *stable* symptoms across childhood into adulthood. Psychopaths present with excessive use of instrumental, proactive, predatory (i.e., "cold") behaviors and have been hypothesized as having deficits in neural structures and circuitry responsible for the development of empathy and socialization (Blair, 1995; Blair et al., 1997). As a result of these deficits, individuals with psychopathy are at increased risk of learning antisocial behaviors that lead to criminal activity and to DSM diagnoses such as ODD, CD, and ASPD (Blair et al., 2006). However, as suggested earlier, ODD, CD, and ASPD represent a heterogeneous population and most individuals diagnosed with these disorders do not have psychopathy. Distinguishing youth who present with psychopathy versus other types of aggression has important implications for prevention and intervention strategies and for understanding the relationship between exposure to trauma and the development of aggression. Research in the neurobiology of psychopathy hypothesizes that at the core of the development of the disorder are genetic/molecular/neural circuit alterations that lead to emotional dysfunction, which impairs socialization and the development of empathy. This impairment, while increasing the risk for learning antisocial behaviors, does not necessarily mean that a such a child will develop persistent antisocial behaviors, as long as other more socially acceptable means to obtain goals are available (Blair et al., 2006). However, individuals with high levels of CU traits, even those who manage to play by society's rules, potentially pose harm to others through self-centered, emotionally shallow interactions with people and their environment (see Babiak and Hare, 2006, *Snakes in Suits: When Psychopaths Go to Work*).

The Role to the Amygdala in Psychopathy, "Cold" Aggression, and Deficit Empathy

Some theories on the origins of psychopathy have speculated that early childhood maltreatment could lead to the development of psychopathy by disruption of the basic threat response system leading to heightened autonomic arousal thereby increasing the risks of maladaptive, fear-driven responses to stress and threat. As discussed earlier, the amygdala plays a key role in activating endocrine and ANS responses to threat and is found to be overresponsive in many individuals previously exposed to trauma. Blair and others, however, argue that in individuals who present with primarily "cold" aggression, the amygdala is *not overactive* but shows *reduced activation*.

The amygdala plays a central role in both conditioned and learned responses to aversive and appetitive cues in the environment. Individuals with amygdala damage and those with psychopathic instrumental aggression show similar levels of dysfunction on a number of laboratory tests designed to elicit amygdala integrity. Individuals with psychopathy show reduced autonomic responses to other individuals' sadness—which in normal subjects typically will elicit empathy (Aniskiewicz, 1979; Blair et al., 1997; House & Milligan, 1976), reduced recognition of the fearful expressions in others (Blair et al., 2001, 2015), impairment in aversive conditioning (Lykken, 1957; Blair et al., 2015), reduced augmentation of the startle reflex by threat primes (Levenston et al., 2000), deficits in passive avoidance (Newman & Kosson, 1986) and instrumental learning, and decreased amygdala volume as measured by volumetric MRI (Tiihonen et al., 2000).

Blair has suggested that amygdala dysfunction in the areas described above contributes to the formation of psychopathy by impairing normal moral development and induction of empathy. During normal development, caregivers reinforce desired behaviors and punish undesired ones. During a transgression, a victim's distress, pain, or sadness (unconditioned stimuli) results in activation (unconditioned response) of an aggressor's threat response system, which leads to autonomic arousal (and usually) postural freezing. This association of unpleasant, unconditioned cues in the victim with unpleasant, unconditioned responses in the aggressor leads (especially when intentionally paired by caregivers) a normally developing child to experience the distress of others as aversive to them as well (aversive conditioning). Caregivers then, by focusing the aggressor's attention on the victim and connecting the cause of his or her suffering (and the autonomic arousal being experienced by the aggressor) to the action committed by the aggressor, are able (through instrumental conditioning) to promote the development of conscientiousness, socialization, and the induction of empathy. As indicated earlier, amygdala dysfunction disrupts this process and leads to impairments in socialization (Blair, 2004, 2005). In fact, deficits in autonomic fear conditioning (mediated by amygdala dysfunction) at age 3, measured by electrodermal responses to aversive and non-aversive tones, predicted criminal behaviors at age 23 by showing higher levels of criminal behavior in the subjects who exhibited abnormal fear conditioning in the face of an aversive unpleasant tone (Gao et al., 2010). Thus, the amygdala, when normally developed, through its central role in the "fear" circuit, promotes a healthy "fearfulness," while dysfunction leads to under activation of the threat circuitry and an inability to recognize or properly respond to fear in others, leading to the potential for development of psychopathic traits and behaviors later in life.

Heightened Threat Sensitivity—The Role of the Prefrontal Cortex and Amygdala in Reactive, "Hot" Aggression

While instrumental "cold" aggression and deficit empathy appear to be core pathologies in youth with CU traits and psychopathy, individuals with internalizing disorders (e.g., anxiety) and externalizing disorders (e.g., ODD) can also present with "hot," or reactive, aggression. While the display of "cold" aggression is unique to psychopathy, many other individuals with psychopathology also display reactive aggression, including children with intermittent explosive disorder, borderline personality disorder, disruptive mood dysregulation disorder, pediatric bipolar disorder, and anxiety disorders (Leibenluft et al., 2003), ODD, CD, *and victims of maltreatment and violence*. The prefrontal cortex, specifically the OFC, (and portions of the ventrolateral cortex), has been identified as an area that is dysfunctional both in individuals with histories of trauma and in those who display reactive aggression. As discussed earlier, the OFC is a key regulating component of the threat response system, which includes the amygdala, HPA-axis, and other areas such as the dorsal periaqueductal gray (PAG), brain stem, and association cortex (Gregg & Siegel, 2001; Panksepp, 1998; Blair et al., 2015). Specifically, in both humans and other animals, a brain circuit involving the amygdala, PAG, and hypothalamus mediates graded response to threats prompting a sequence of behavioral freezing, fleeing, and if faced with the inability of escape, reactive aggression, depending upon the proximity the threat. Heightened sensitivity and over-reactivity in this threat response circuit, including a tendency to display a hostile attributional bias, are seen both in both youths with conduct disorder without CU traits and in individuals with elevated rates of anxiety, including those who have suffered trauma. Cortical input from the OFC to the amygdala is critical in accurately assessing and responding to environmental threats. Severe trauma, which leads to overactivation of catecholamines, has been associated with the impairment of the OFC's ability to inhibit amygdala activity (Arnsten, 1998). Failure of the OFC to properly inhibit amygdala activity in the face of threatening or ambiguous environmental situations can lead to uncontrolled, maladaptive behavioral responses, including reactive aggression.

Deficient Decision-Making—The Role of the OFC, Ventromedial PFC, and Striatum in Impulse Control Problems, Frustration, and Reactive Aggression

Note: the following discussion assumes that the OFC and vmPFC are anatomically related with the OFC designating a specific region in the anatomically broader vmPFC area.

Research has targeted frontal lobe dysfunction as a potential mediator of aggressive behavior in psychopathic individuals. Damage to prefrontal areas, specifically the OFC/vmPFC, is associated with an increased likelihood of violence and aggression and is often seen in individuals following traumatic brain injury. This association has led to speculation that OFC/vmPFC dysfunction or damage may play a major role in the pathology of psychopathy (Damasio, 1994). However, patients with OFC/vmPFC damage only show increases in "hot," reactive aggressive, not the "cold," instrumental aggression which is considered the defining characteristic of the disorder (Blair, 2005).

Neurocognitive research has shed light on additional neural circuitry connected to the OFC/vmPFC, which may help clarify unresolved questions related to the conflicting hypotheses regarding the source of reactive aggression in CD youth presenting with a predominance of CU characteristics. The circuitry involves connections between the OFC/vmPFC and a subcortical region of the brain—the ventral portion of the striatum (which includes the nucleus accumbens). The ventral striatum, particularly the nucleus accumbens, has important functions in reward processing, reinforcement of behaviors, punishment processing, and avoidance learning. Taken together, impairments in this circuit (and neurocognitive tasks which utilize these neural substrates) lead to *deficit decision-making* when faced with tasks that require flexible responses to changing circumstances or contingencies (Blair et al., 2015). CD youth with CU characteristics show evidence of deficit decision-making on neurocognitive tasks designed to engage this neural pathway, which, at least in experimental paradigms, increases the risk for frustration-based reactive aggression (Fairchild et al., 2019). However, deficits in decision-making, which clinically are more often encountered than deficits in empathy and heightened threat sensitivity, are seen in many youth with conduct problems, not just youth who have CU traits, including those with CD without CU characteristics, ODD, and in youth diagnosed with other impulse control disorders, such as ADHD and substance use disorder. Nonetheless, this neural circuitry, and its association with deficit decision-making, while being less specifically linked to youth with CU traits, may be an important pathway to understand the source of reactive aggression in CD youth with CU traits and help distinguish them from other youth who display reactive aggression as a result of having higher threat sensitivity but do not show CU traits.

Individuals prone to frustration and reactive aggression show impairments in OFC/vmPFC and striatum circuitry, especially during *response reversal tasks* that require cognitive flexibility in the face of changing task contingencies. In response reversal tasks, individuals with conduct disorder have more difficulty than controls in changing patterns of goal-seeking behavior when contingencies arise that require alterations of behavior in order to obtain reward or avoid punishment. This impairment in the ability to modify stimulus-response associations in the face of contingency change leads to frustration-based reactive aggression, as the individuals are less able to respond flexibly to environmental demands. Patients with OFC/vmPFC lesions also have been shown to have impairment in a related test known as social response reversal. This task is employed as an index of OFC/vmPFC capacity to modify behavioral responses when confronted with actions that are in violation of societal norms or rules. Compared to controls, individuals with OFC/vmPFC damage show impairments in multiple parameters involving social response reversal, including the capacity to recognize facial expressions, especially anger.

Neurocognitive tasks, such as response reversal tasks, essentially serve as an index for an individual's ability to tolerate frustration and flexibly respond to changing contingencies. Frustration here is defined as resulting when an individual attempts a behavior with the expectation of obtaining a goal but then having that goal go unmet (Blair et al., 2006). Frustration is associated with reactive aggression (Berkowitz, 1993). Individuals with dysfunction in OFC/vmPFC areas show impairments in their ability to achieve goals and rewards, especially during situations involving contingency change (response reversal). Due to impairments in prefrontal function, subcortical systems mediating reactive aggression may be underregulated putting these individuals at heightened risk for displaying reactive aggression as a result of experiencing frustration in their interactions with others and their environment.

The Connection Between Victimization and Violence

Toward an Integrated Model of Neurobiological Function in Violence and Victimization

When one brings together the neurocognitive research findings discussed earlier regarding (1) youth who display deficits in empathy (CU traits); (2) youth with heightened threat sensitivity (who may respond to perceived threat with reactive aggression); and (3) youth who experience neurocognitive deficits in flexible decision making and reward processing, which increases the likelihood of reactive aggression (due to frustrative non-reward), we begin to see the contours of three different endophenotypes, or intermediate phenotypes, which connect unique impairments in genetic and neurobiological substrates and circuitries to observable behaviors (phenotypes). From a clinical standpoint, while youth with impulse control and conduct problems may, from a superficial perspective, look similar in their behaviors, youth with CD and other impulse control and behavioral issues (many of whom have histories of significant trauma) form a very heterogeneous group. It is only when we start to be able to parse out and describe the different types of impairments in the neural circuitry driving individuals' behaviors that we can properly characterize the source and nature of their impairments and develop treatment interventions that are specifically tailored to their needs.

Key Neurobiological Substrates Underlying Victimization and Violence and Their Interaction: Summary

Though incomplete and speculative, the previous discussion of neurobiological correlates of trauma and subtypes of aggression suggests the following generalizations:

1. *Fear-driven victimization*—neurobiological description: *Heightened threat sensitivity* trauma and maltreatment produce heightened fear responses mediated partly by a dysregulated fear circuit involving an over-responsive amygdala; one source of amygdala over-reactivity may be impaired prefrontal cortex inhibition of the amygdala. "Hot," reactive aggression is one of the possible maladaptive behavioral responses that can result from dysfunction of the threat response system.

2. *Fearless-driven "cold" aggression*—neurobiological description: *Deficient empathy* "cold" aggression involves instrumental, predatory, goal-directed aggressive behavior with little autonomic arousal; it is mediated partly through amygdala dysfunction and can be identified, for example, in experimental conditions by impairments in typical responses to the expression of fear and sadness in others. Behavioral manifestations include impaired empathy, disregard for social norms, and proactive aggression.

3. *Frustration-driven, impulsive, reactive "hot" aggression*—neurobiological description: *Deficient decision-making.*

   Deficits in this circuitry involving prefrontal and striatal brain areas implicated in reward processing create challenges for affected youth to be able to flexibly respond to changes in environmental contingencies, which increases the likelihood of them failing to obtain rewards and/or avoid punishment, which in turn, produces feelings of frustrative non-reward and increases their risks of responding in these situations with impulsive, reactive aggression. While youth with CD youth with CU traits have been shown to have deficits in this circuitry, so do many other youth with reactive aggression, including youth diagnosed with CD without CU, and other youth with impulse-control disorders, a certain portion of whom have trauma-exposed histories.

As is clear from the multiple mass shootings that have occurred on American soil since the deaths of 14 students and one teacher at Columbine High School in 1999, school violence is a national problem of critical importance and concern for ordinary citizens and professionals alike. One of the main challenges that arise in an integrative perspective that takes a developmental, longitudinal approach to behavior and emphasizes the impact of genetic-neurobiological-environmental interactions on the expression of this behavior is that it becomes difficult to attribute differences in behavior to simple, isolated, non-dynamic linear cause and effect relationships. This is especially problematic in discussing the topic of violence and victimization because, while society would prefer to separate victims and perpetrators into distinct groups based on clear differences in biology, environment, and behavior (and assign the causes of these differences in behavior to mutually exclusive etiologic factors), the situation is much more complex than that on many levels, one of which is that there is much behavioral overlap (and interaction) between the two groups in that victims of trauma often act aggressively (both to themselves and others) while perpetrators often themselves are victims of past maltreatment and traumatization.

While there is no reliable psychological profile that can be used to identify those at risk for committing school violence, the vast majority of youth who have engaged in school shootings have been male. Many perpetrators have histories of growing up in unstable families, were exposed to violence in the home, and experienced maltreatment and neglect. Oftentimes there is a history of significant loss as well, such as the Parkland, Florida defendant who lost his adopted mother several months before months prior to his attack on Marjory Stoneman Douglas High School. For many perpetrators, there is also a history of being bullied, harassed, and socially excluded in school settings. Such experiences can lead to social isolation, feelings of hopelessness, and unfortunately can also breed anger, resentment, a sense of being persecuted, feelings of rage, and a desire to kill oneself and to seek retribution on others. Investigation of many school shootings reveals that the actions of the perpetrator were not done impulsively but appear to have been carefully planned and executed. In this aspect, the violence perpetrated appears to display characteristics of the "cold" aggression pattern of planned goal-directed behavior, perhaps accompanied by low physiological arousal. On the other hand, to the degree that the perpetrator's action is a response to perceived or past actual threats from others, the planned violence may be preceded by prior feelings of victimization, accompanied by heightened physiological arousal, negative self-appraisal, and a sense of threat from and mistrust of his or her environment. While presenting no evidence here, in some youth who commit such violence against others, the type of impairments in neurocognitive decision-making described by Blair et al. (2015) may have had a role in creating an ongoing sense of frustration in their efforts to create rewarding relationships with others and feel their lives are fulfilling and meaningful. Thus, for at least a percentage of school shootings, the perpetrator may exhibit aspects of all three impairments in neurocognitive functioning described earlier—impairments in empathy, threat detection, and decision-making.

Clinical Studies Investigating the Connection Between Violence and Victimization

Numerous clinical studies have documented associations between trauma exposure, victimization, violence perpetration, and their interrelation. Research on the association between being exposed to traumatic events (e.g., abuse, sexual molestation, witnessing violence, unsafe communities, etc.) and the development of psychopathology and delinquency is well-documented (Foy et al., 1996). In such environments, it is not surprising that exposure to trauma sets up a "cycle of violence" of victim later becoming perpetrator (Ryan et al., 1996). Previous sexual molestation of male youth (often by females) leading to later sexual victimization by these males of women is one specific example (Rubinstein et al., 1993). Steiner et al. (1997) investigated 85 adolescents incarcerated by the California Youth Authority for a range of offenses from first-degree murder to auto theft. The study found that 32% of the youth had PTSD and 20% had PTSD symptoms but did not meet full criteria, which is significantly higher than estimates of approximately 9% lifetime prevalence in young adults. Fifty percent of these youth had witnessed interpersonal violence. The individuals diagnosed with PTSD had increased levels of distress, depression, and anxiety, poor impulse control, and increased levels of aggression. Another study by Ford et al. (2000) found trauma in general, but more specifically physical and sexual maltreatment, to be associated with ODD (and ADHD). In their sample, 48–73% of children diagnosed with ODD had been exposed to physical maltreatment, while 18–31% had been exposed to sexual maltreatment. Investigations into the underlying biological mechanisms involved in the development of ODD reveal dysregulation of emotional and information processing (Lahey et al., 1999; Pennington & Ozonof, 1996) leading youth with ODD to (1) have negative biases toward themselves, peers, and relationships; (2) more likely experience social inter-actions as hostile; (3) possess rigid and limited problem-solving skills; and (4) often express frustration, rage, and aggression (Dodge et al., 1997; Matthys et al., 1999). These impairments parallel findings from victimization research and are consistent with the data above linking traumatization to the development of "hot" aggression.

Baskin-Sommers and Baskin (2016) published a study that is particularly rele-vant to the role of psychopathy in mediating the development of aggressive behav-iors following exposure to violence. Using data from the Pathways to Desistance study (n = 1170) of serious juvenile defenders, they explored potential links between exposure to violence (ETV) and juvenile offending. They were particularly inter-ested in whether psychopathic traits played a role in mediating ETV exposure and later offending behaviors. Using the Youth Psychopathic Traits Inventory (YPI), their results indicated that while ETV predicted later involvement in violent offend-ing, results from the YPI showed the presence or absence of identified psychopathic traits was the primary mediator of whether ETV led to later violent offending. They speculated that, especially for youth with psychopathic traits who experienced high or ascending ETV, engagement in violence may become normative and to be seen as a pragmatic response to chronic exposure to interpersonal or community vio-lence. As such, these individuals, when initially identified, should be offered prompt and specifically tailored interventions to address their maladaptive response to ETV, including more robust case management, cognitive remediation treatment, and juve-nile diversion strategies in order to prevent further ingraining of these maladaptive behaviors and ultimate legal system involvement. The authors also acknowledge that identification of psychopathic traits in youth is not without controversy, as such identification can lead to labeling and stigmatization of such youth as deserving punishment versus care.

Given the well-documented relationship between exposure to trauma and subse-quent engagement in disruptive and delinquent behavior, including violence perpe-tration, what factors or interventions can decrease the likelihood of these downstream deleterious outcomes, including involvement with the criminal justice system. A 2019 publication investigating the association of childhood trauma with subsequent criminal justice involvement (CJI) offers one clue. The study involved analyzing data (n = 12,288) from the National Longitudinal Study of Adolescent to Adult Health investigated the impact that having a mentor (i.e., having at least one support from outside of the family system) at age 14 or older had on adolescents' later CJI. In addition to documenting a dose-dependent relationship between cumulative trauma exposure to CJI (e.g., having 5 or more traumas increased the odds of being incarcerated before age 18 by 26 times), the authors also found that, indeed, having at least one *close* mentor during adolescence significantly decreased the association between past trauma and CJI, both before and after the age of 18, compared to those adolescents reporting no mentor or having only a *non-close* mentor, with the biggest mitigating impact of having a *close* mentor seen in those youth with more than one childhood traumatic event (Scanlon et al., 2019).

Social Media—A New World, New Risks for Victimization and Perpetration

A 2005 study involving video games highlights changes that occur in the amygdala and prefrontal regions in youths exposed to video game violence. Forty-four healthy adolescents previously exposed to a violent video game called "Medal of Honor" showed increased activation in the right amygdala and decreased activation in prefrontal areas compared to a comparison group of adolescents shown a nonviolent game called "Need for Speed" during functional MRI imaging obtained during two Stroop tasks. The individuals who played the nonviolent game showed more activation in the prefrontal areas, especially the anterior cingulate and the dorsolateral prefrontal cortex. These results (decreased prefrontal and increased amygdala activation in violent video game players), while not *proving* that watching violent media causes violence, parallel findings above that implicate exposure to previous violence in biasing the threat response system to maladaptive behavioral responses such as displays of "hot" aggression (Mathews et al., 2005).

A 2017 abstract published in *Pediatrics* summarizes the current scientific consensus related to the relation between violent video game exposure and youth aggression, which is quoted in part here: "The Workgroup on Media Violence and Violent Video Games reviewed numerous meta-analyses and other relevant research from the past 60 years, with an emphasis on violent video game research. Consistent with every major science organization review, the Workgroup found compelling evidence of short-term harmful effects, as well as evidence of long-term harmful effects. The vast majority of laboratory based experimental studies have revealed that violent media exposure causes increased aggressive thoughts, angry feelings, physiologic arousal, hostile appraisals, aggressive behavior, and desensitization to violence and decreases prosocial behavior (e.g., helping others) and empathy" (Anderson et al., 2017).

Jeffrey Gray's Biobehavioral Model of Brain Functioning— An Additional Endophenotype Model to Consider

Jeffrey Gray has developed a comprehensive theory of how separate but interrelated neurobiological systems function in the brain to control a variety of human qualities and characteristics such as temperament, emotions, and behaviors. His theory can be used to create a relatively simple but plausible framework to facilitate an understanding of the neurobiological systems involved in controlling violence and victimization, including aspects of hot and cold aggression (Gray, 1982, 1987; Conner, 2002).

Gray's model consists of three major branches: a behavioral activation system (BAS), a behavioral inhibition system (BIS), and a fight, flight, freeze system (FFFS). By aligning these components of brain function to neurobiological findings in trauma and aggression research, the following associations are hypothesized: "Cold" aggression results when an organism displays a relative excess of behavioral activation versus inhibition. "Hot" aggression, on the other hand, is likely to arise in the context of an overactive, dysregulated FFFS, possibly from prior trauma, which is biased toward exaggerated responses to threat. Finally, in children exposed to trauma, who go on to develop the symptomatology of victimization, there is not only the risk of dysregulation of the FFFS but also the possibility of dysregulation of the BAS and BIS, leading to the development of multiple psychiatric symptoms. While trauma is not explicitly discussed in Gray's model, Gray's colleague Neil McNaughton does briefly discuss PTSD. He states that PTSD is not included in the model because, more than a single disease entity, it should be viewed as a trauma-related phenomenon that predisposes affected individuals to the development of multiple disorders, echoing conclusions presented earlier on the numerous possible sequelae of complex trauma (McNaughton & Corr, 2004).

The BAS is the primary system in animals that promotes behavioral approach when conditions exist such that conditioned stimuli for reward are present and conditioned stimuli for punishment are absent (McNaughton & Corr, 2004). This system is critical in producing predatory and instrumental aggression (i.e., "cold" aggression). Evidence suggests that dopamine (DA) and dopaminergic pathways are critical in the functioning of this system (Lara & Akiskal, 2006). This pathway begins in brainstem nuclei in fibers that ascend from the substantia nigra and the ventral tegmental area and project via the medial forebrain bundle to many areas in the midbrain and forebrain. The nucleus accumbens and the ventral striatum of the midbrain receive dopaminergic fibers that release DA, the main neurotransmitter responsible for appetitive, reward-influenced behavior.

The BIS provides a brake to the acceleration of the BAS. It works to inhibit behavioral approach in situations where conditions are present that could lead to possible danger, punishment, or frustration of non-reward. Like the BAS, it functions in response to learned conditioned stimuli; but in this case, it becomes activated, not by the promise of reward, but by conditions that limit reward and predict punishment. A key concept of the BIS is that while it balances the BAS, it is still a system of approach, albeit a defensive approach. That is, in conditions where both reward and punishment are present, the BIS serves as a tool for risk assessment and conflict resolution to analyze environmental circumstances and past learning in order to guide behavior. The primary emotion or felt neurophysiological experience associated with the BIS is anxiety. McNaughton not only identifies the septo-hippocampal system and the amygdala as being critical in the function of the BIS but also includes other important structures such as the PAG, the hypothalamus, and the prefrontal cortex. Norepinephrine (NE) and serotonin (5-HT) are the neurotransmitters most active in this system.

The FFFS, unlike the BAS and BIS, is an innate (not learned) system that mediates animal responses to unconditioned stimuli such as pain, punishment, and frustration. In Gray's model, the FFFS is responsible for the generation of the emotion of fear and mobilizes an animal to attempt escape, or if that option is not available, to engage in defensive aggression. It, therefore, provides direction in situations where animals, confronted with threats to survival and livelihood, act defensively to avoid the source of danger. For example, cat–naïve rats when confronted with a cat respond either by freezing, fleeing, or fighting according to options available to them. While there is much overlap between the FFFS and the BIS, a key difference between them is that the FFFS involves moving away (defensive avoidance) from a negative stimulus, whereas the BIS involves a defensive approach toward the stimulus (or cues related to the stimulus). Thus, if a rat exposed to a cat is placed in the same environment but without the cat, the rat may initially remain still (but with a different posture than is seen in fear-related freezing) and then begin to cautiously explore its environment (behavioral inhibition) in a manner that has been characterized as risk assessment (Gray & McNaughton, 2000; Blanchard & Blanchard, 1990). As mentioned earlier, the FFFS may be overactive in some people who display reactive or affective ("hot") aggression. Such people may be subject to autonomic over-arousal and biases toward feeling threatened and fearful in situations that others find non-threatening. The neuroanatomical substrates of the FFFS are very similar to that of the BIS. Key structures include the prefrontal cortex, the amygdala, and the PAG. Mobilization of the fear response involves the elaboration of many neurochemicals including NE, 5-HT, DA, endorphins, and cortisol.

Gray's model predicts that different forms of psychopathology can result from relative deficiencies or excesses of the function of any of the aforementioned three interrelated systems. In terms of different forms of aggressive behavior, the model predicts that individuals with excessive BAS activity and deficient BIS activity will be especially prone not only to aggression, as they will be highly driven to seek rewards, but also be unresponsive to cues discouraging reward, such as warnings of punishment. These individuals should have low ANS arousal even in potentially aversive environments and therefore should not be easily inhibited by anxiety. Furthermore, due to their reward-dominant behavior, such individuals will be less able to learn from punishment and therefore are likely to persist in maladaptive reward-seeking behavior despite negative consequences (Conner, 2002). Evidence for this type of aggression is present in studies of CD children and adolescents where youth with and without CD play computerized card games in which money is either rewarded or taken away from the participants based on whether they make correct or incorrect responses. The game is set up to decrease the probability of choosing a correct response as the game proceeds. Compared to youth without CD, children and adolescents with CD are more likely to persist playing the game (and therefore lose more money) despite being able to pass on trials (Daugherty & Quay, 1991; Shapiro et al., 1988).

Gray's theory also predicts that in youth with CD and strong BIS (and therefore more prone to anxiety), the active BIS should inhibit antisocial behavior compared to CD youth with an active BAS and weaker BIS. In fact, several studies have provided this kind of evidence by showing that anxious boys with CD are less likely to become involved with the police than boys with CD without anxiety (Walker et al., 1991). Additional studies looking at chemical markers of the BAS and BIS have generally supported Gray's theory with some exceptions. For example, several studies have shown decreased NE and 5-HT function to be associated with increased antisocial behavior and aggressiveness, while there is yet no data available that show increased DA to be associated with increased antisocial behavior (Rogeness et al., 1992). Another marker used to assess BIS function is EDA, a chemical released during sweat production. In studies that measure sweating, increased EDA is used as a marker for increased peripheral sympathetic ANS arousal, which in turn is used as a marker for BIS activation. Gray's theory predicts that youth with CD should exhibit lower EDA production compared to controls when presented with stimuli suggestive of impending punishment or non-reward. According to Conner, seven of seven studies in youth with CD that have tested this hypothesis have results consistent with this prediction.

Clinical Considerations

While there is significant evidence to support the external and internal validity of the two distinct subtypes of aggression discussed earlier, there is also substantial overlap found in experimental studies. For example, in a study by Vitiello et al. of 73 aggressive child and adolescent psychiatric patients, a scale describing fully predatory (+5) and fully affective (−5) patterns had bimodal peaks of −3 (predominately affective) and 1 (mixed) (Vitiello et al., 1990). One conclusion drawn from this study is that purely predatory children are less likely to receive psychiatric treatment (Vitiello & Stoff, 1997). Furthermore, both in animals and humans, the same subject at different times can display aggression more predominately in one of the two subtypes according to the circumstances that the subject is involved in (Vitiello & Stoff, 1997). Thus, clinical utility in the "cold" and "hot" formulation will likely involve a dimensional approach that respects the difficulty of identifying patients and formulating treatments purely on a clear-cut categorical basis (Vitiello & Stoff, 1997).

As discussed earlier, Blair argues that the developmental pathology associated with psychopathy is the result of genetic influences that impair the function of the amygdala resulting in deficits in moral development, empathy induction, and socialization. While neglectful and/or harsh (coercive) parenting has been identified as a risk factor for the development of conduct problems in previously healthy children, this association is weaker for children who show CU/psychopathic tendencies (Blair et al., 2006; Oxford et al., 2003; Wootton et al., 1997). In fact, no studies to date have linked *any* causal environmental factor to the reduced amygdala functioning thought to be at the core of psychopathy. While the study findings (Hyde et al., 2016) presented at the beginning of this chapter showing decreases in children's CU behaviors with higher levels of adoptive parental warmth and positive praise are promising in terms of identifying a potential mechanism to change CU trajectory, it may be prudent to assume that a child or adolescent with CU traits, even in a supportive and warm caregiving environment, is going to carry an increased genetic and neurobiological risk for using antisocial means for obtaining goals. Conversely, with children and adolescents primarily at risk of "hot" aggression due to prior exposure to trauma, environmental factors are implicated in both the etiology and the continuation of their maladaptive responses to their environment.

Psychometric tools designed to aid in identifying "cold" aggression have been developed (e.g., the Psychopathy Checklist—Revised, the Hare Psychopathy Checklist—Youth Version, and the Inventory of Callous-Unemotional Traits (developed by Paul J. Frick, Ph.D.) but are primarily used in research settings (Conner, 2002). More recently, Frick and colleagues have developed the Clinical Assessment of Prosocial Emotions (CAPE 1.1), which is designed as a screening instrument for clinical use in identifying youth with CU traits. However, at this time, it is still undergoing clinical validation (available at https://faculty.lsu.edu/pfricklab/). The implementation of these and other psychometric tools into clinical practice may aid in developing tailored treatment strategies that respect the discreet developmental etiologies and developmental pathways, of different subtypes of aggression. The identification of CU/psychopathic tendencies in youth is beginning to inform the development of interventions that clinicians undertake with aggressive youth. In general, until the last 10 years or so, youth (and adults) with CU traits have been viewed as largely treatment-resistant, and for those in the criminal system, at high risk of recidivism. White et al. (2013), however, have shown that youth with CU traits enrolled in a comprehensive program utilizing Functional Family Therapy displayed significant improvement in overall functioning following treatment. The caveat is that compared to conduct-disordered youth without CU traits, CU youth entered treatment with much greater impairment, so even with significant improvement as a result of treatment, they still had significant behavioral issues. The take-home message from this study is that evidence-based treatments (EBT) for youth with CU traits can be effective to reduce impairments but need to be improved/enhanced (better tailored to the unique needs of these youth) to be optimally effective. A colleague of Frick, Eva Kimonis, has undertaken just such an enhancement to a widely available EBT for disruptive children called Parent–Child Interaction Therapy (PCIT). In addition to applying the standard interventions of PCIT, she enhanced the treatment by (1) teaching parents to be more warm and emotionally responsive to their children; (2) increasing the use of rewards (compared to punishment) as a way to shape desired behaviors; and (3) adding a module called CARES (Coaching and Rewarding Emotional Skills) to target the children's impairments in empathy. An uncontrolled trial of this program in children ages 3–6 published in 2019 (Kimonis et al., 2019) showed robust decreases in conduct problems and CU traits and improved displays of child empathy. At 3 months after treatment, 75% of participants remained free of clinically significant conduct problems.

While studies demonstrating the clinical utility of developing individualized treatment strategies based on different aggression subtypes are still few in number (but growing, as discussed earlier), research does support several additional general guidelines. One is that, since children and adolescents with predominately "cold" aggression are at risk for using instrumental aggression to achieve goals, it is important to minimize exposure to environments where such behavior is typically modeled and rewarded (e.g., gangs) while maximizing exposure to environments where guidelines of expected behavior (to achieve rewards and avoid punishments) are clearly outlined. Treatment paradigms for this type of aggression support the use of behavioral therapy and parent education strategies that create environments where expectations for behavior are clearly outlined and consequences enforced consistently in a non-aggressive manner. Commitment to and successful implication of these strategies are especially critical in light of evidence that suggests psychopharmacological interventions in this subtype of youth aggression have somewhat limited efficacy.

The other general guideline relates to children and adolescents who predominantly display pure "hot" or mixed aggression. Because these youth tend to be easily aroused physiologically and are biased to mistrust their environment, they are likely to react impulsively and defensively in response to threat or provocation. Such children tend to escalate as a response to coercive, harsh, or authoritarian parenting but respond more favorably to interventions that create safe and predictable environments, teach social problem-solving skills and the management of negative emotions, and, if indicated, utilize medications capable of modulating mood, anxiety, physiological arousal, and the level of attention (Conner, 2002; Vitiello & Stoff, 1997). Helping parents learn to modulate their own emotions more skillfully when interacting with their children is also an important component to many of EBTs designed to promote better emotional and behavioral regulation in youth.

Finally, studies examining psychiatric comorbidities associated with aggression, for example, those looking at the separate emotional and behavioral components of psychopathy, have found anxiety and depression to be inversely correlated with the emotional component (lack of empathy) and positively correlated with the antisocial behavioral component, especially the expression of reactive aggression. In other words, greater levels of anxiety are associated with greater levels of "hot" reactive aggression and decreased levels of "cold" aggression. One interpretation of the significance of this data is that psychopathy, to the degree that it is associated with "cold" aggression and low autonomic arousal and response to threat, while putting an individual at higher risk of expression for amoral, instrumental, goal-directed aggression, may actually protect against the development of psychiatric sequelae, which can result from environmental insults such as trauma and maltreatment. As such, *their* pathology will be experienced more through their ability to achieve goal-directed goals at the expense of *others* than through the development of emotional problems in *them* from exposure to childhood maltreatment or trauma (Blair et al., 2006; Frick et al., 1999).

Appendix: Additional Interventions

Adolescence as a Critical Period

The adolescent developmental period is not only a time of rapid growth in multiple areas of brain development (e.g., reasoning abilities, physical capacity) but also a time of increased health risks with a twofold increase in disability and mortality (e.g., suicide, violence perpetration) compared to younger children. From a psychiatric perspective, it is also a period of emergence of a wide range of mental disorders with an estimated 50% of all mental illnesses emerging by age 14 (Kessler et al., 2005). Likely hypotheses to explain this mismatch between emerging strengths coupled with increased risks point to differential rates of maturity in key regions of the brain regulating reward-seeking behavior (nucleus accumbens/NA), emotional regulation (amygdala), and cognitive control (PFC) as contributing to a mismatch between adolescents' experiencing strong emotions (accelerator) without yet being able to apply adaptive cognitive control (brakes). For example, during this high-risk period, due to lack of PFC inhibition of the amygdala, many normally developing teens may display "hot" emotional reactions or misinterpret facial expressions of neutrality or curious inquiry from parents or teachers as intrusive or threatening. At around the age of 16, amygdala volume growth begins to decelerate and form stronger connections to PFC areas involved in emotional regulation (Giedd, 2015).

Developmental neuroscience-informed educators working with such youth may be in a better position to help youth experiencing these "hot" emotions to understand their source and learn to "take it down a notch" to decrease the likelihood that their "hot" emotions coupled with high motivation for action (NA) will lead to a potentially dangerous behavioral outcome. Additionally, educators should be aware that until the cortical areas of the brain (PFC) catch up to subcortical areas (NA and amygdala) that their adolescent students will have tendencies to emotionally over-value the potential reward, while undervaluing their potential negative consequences of their actions, be more likely to engage in sensation seeking (and risky) behaviors when in the presence of peers, and will be more susceptible to behaving impulsively when under stress (Chung & Hudziak, 2017).

Ludvik (2017) offers these additional recommendations for educators in *Leveraging Neuroscience and Education to Prevent Youth Aggression and Violence.*

- Introduce mindfulness (for both students and educators) to promote attentional regulation training and improved emotional regulation.
- Consider helping youth regulate their sensory input (e.g., allowing headphones), especially for youth with traumatic backgrounds.
- Couple heightened sensation/novelty/reward seeking to long-term versus immediate gains.
- Promote exercise for healthy brain regulation and growth, including increases in neurotrophic factors, such as BDNF.

- Introduce emotional regulation-related training to help youth learn to identify their emotions (e.g., distinguish between feelings of fear, anger, sadness, and irritability).
- Introduce compassion training to students, which can decrease implicit biases.
- Introduce activities to promote strengthening of executive functioning.
- While not de-valuing adolescents' strong emotional drive (their "hot" emotions) help them couple these "bottom-up" brain processes with "cooler" "top-down" brain functions, such as mindfulness, self-reflection, executive functioning, and goal setting in order to help them be less emotionally reactive and more thoughtful with their behavioral choices.

Additional Recommended Interventions for Youth of Various Ages

There are numerous interventions—preventative, clinic-based, home-based, school-based, criminal justice system-based, etc.—that are available for families and youth, which can promote resilience, change mental health trajectories, offer individual and family supports, and in general, help youth at risk for, or who have had negative outcomes, due to trauma and violence perpetration. The following are just a sampling of available interventions and programs. Please check web resources in the next section for descriptions, age ranges, and strength of evidence base.

For the very young Home Health Visiting Programs for Prevention of Child Abuse and Neglect, such as the Nurse-Family Partnership; Early Start; Head Start; Attachment, Regulation, and Competency (ARC); Promoting First Relationships (PRF); Attachment and Biobehavioral Catch-up (ABC); Triple P (Positive Parenting Program; Parent–Child Interaction Therapy (PCIT); Child–Parent Psychotherapy.

For school-age children, including school-based programs The Good Behavior Game; Families & Schools Together (FAST).

For middle and high school youth Multisystemic Therapy (MST); Multidimensional Treatment Foster Care (MTFC) for court-involved youth; Adolescent Diversion Project; Aggression Replacement Therapy (ART) for youth in state institutions; Functional Family Therapy for Youth Post-release.

For youth of various ages School-Based Health Alliance (https://www.sbh4all.org/), which supports nationwide School-Based Health Centers; Trauma-Focused Cognitive Behavior Therapy (TF-CBT); RULER: Recognizing Understanding, Labeling, Expressing, and Regulating Emotions (Yale Center for Emotional Intelligence, https://www.ycei.org/); Intensive Family Preservation Services and Intensive Family Reunification Services, such as HOMEBUILDERS®; Full-Fidelity Wraparound.

Programs/Interventions without a strong evidence base Boot Camps; Drug Court; Restorative Justice Conferencing.

Websites Providing Evidence-Based Resources

The National Registry of Evidence-Based Programs and Practices (NREPP): https://www.samhsa.gov/ebp-resource-center

U.S. Federal website created by the Interagency Working Group on Youth Programs: https://youth.gov/

U.S. Federal Bullying Prevention: https://www.stopbullying.gov/

Washington State Institute for Public Policy: http://www.wsipp.wa.gov/

The California Evidence-Based Clearinghouse for Child Welfare https://www.cebc4cw.org/

References

Ainsworth, M. (1985). Patterns of infant-mother attachment: Antecedents and effects on development. *Bulletin of the New York Academy of Medicine, 61*, 771–791.

Amat, J., Paul, E., Zarza, C., Watkins, L. R., & Maier, S. F. (2006). Previous experience with behavioral control over stress blocks the behavioral and dorsal raphe nucleus activating effects of later uncontrollable stress: Role of the ventral medial prefrontal cortex. *The Journal of Neuroscience, 26*(51), 13264–13272.

American Psychiatric Association. (2013). *Diagnostic and statistical manual of mental disorders* (5th ed.). American Psychiatric Association.

Anderson, C. A., Bushman, B. J., Bartholow, B. D., Cantor, J., Christakis, D., Coyne, S. M., Donnerstein, E., Brockmyer, J. F., Gentile, D. A., Green, C. S., Huesmann, R., Hummer, T., Krahé, B., Strasburger, V. C., Warburton, W., Wilson, B. J., & Ybarra, M. (2017). Screen violence and youth behavior. *Pediatrics, 140*(Suppl 2), S142–S147.

Aniskiewicz, A. S. (1979). Autonomic components of vicarious conditioning and psychopathy. *Journal of Clinical Psychology, 35*, 60–67.

Arehart-Treichel, (2005). Psychiatric News. Resilence shown in youth protects against adult stress, Joan Arehart-Treichel. Published Online 2 Sep 2005. https://doi.org/10.1176/pn.40.17.00400014.

Arnsten, A. (1998). Catecholamine modulation of prefrontal cortical cognitive function. *Trends in Cognitive Science, 2*, 336–447.

Babiak, P., & Hare, R. D. (2006). *Snakes in suits: When psychopaths go to work*. Collins.

Bandura, A. (1973). *Aggression: A social learning analysis*. Prentice-Hall.

Baskin-Sommers, A. R., & Baskin, D. (2016). Psychopathic traits mediate the relationship between exposure to violence and violent juvenile offending. *Journal of Psychopathology and Behavioral Assessment, 38*, 341–349.

Beeghly, M., & Cicchetti, D. (1996). Child maltreatment, attachment, and the self system: Emergence of an internal state lexicon in toddlers at high social risk. In M. Hertzig & E. Farber (Eds.), *Annual progress in child psychiatry and child development* (pp. 127–166). Brunner/Mazel.

Beers, S. R., & De Bellis, M. D. (2002). Neuropsychological function in children with maltreatment-related posttraumatic stress disorder. *American Journal of Psychiatry, 159*(3), 483–486.

Berkowitz, L. (1993). *Aggression: Its causes, consequences, and control.* Temple University Press.

Blair, R. J. R. (1995). A cognitive developmental approach to morality: Investigating the psychopath. *Cognition, 57*, 1–29.

Blair, R. J. R. (2004). The roles of orbital frontal cortex in the modulation of antisocial behavior. *Brain and Cognition, 55*, 198–208.

Blair, R. J. R. (2005). Applying a cognitive neuroscience perspective to the disorder of psychopathy. *Development and Psychopathology, 17*, 865–891.

Blair, R. J. R., Jones, L., Clark, F., & Smith, M. (1997). The psychopathic individual: A lack of responsiveness to distress cues? *Psychophysiology, 34*, 192–198.

Blair, R. J. R., Colledge, E., Murray, L., & Mitchell, D. G. (2001). A selective impairment in the processing of sad and fearful expressions in children with psychopathic tendencies. *Journal of Abnormal Child Psychology, 29*, 491–498.

Blair, R. J. R., Peschardt, K. S., Budhani, S., Mitchell, D. G. V., & Pine, D. S. (2006). The development of psychopathy. *Journal of Child Psychology and Psychiatry, 47*(3/4), 262–275.

Blair, R. J., Leibenluft, E., & Pine, D. S. (2015). Conduct disorder and callous-unemotional traits in youth. *The New England Journal of Medicine, 371*(23), 2207–2216.

Blanchard, R. J., & Blanchard, D. C. (1990). Anti-predator defense as models of animal fear and anxiety. In P. F. Brain, S. Parmigiani, R. J. Blanchard, & D. Mainardi (Eds.), *Fear and defense* (pp. 89–108). Harwood Academic.

Bowlby, J. (1973). *Attachment and loss: Vol. II. Separation.* Basic Books.

Bremmer, J. D., Randall, P., Vermetten, E., Staib, L., Bronen, R. A., Mazure, C., Capelli, S., McCarthy, G., Innis, R. B., & Charney, D. S. (1997). Magnetic resonance imaging-based measurement of hippocampal volume in posttraumatic stress disorder related to childhood physical and sexual abuse: A preliminary report. *Biological Psychiatry, 41*, 23–32.

Bremner, J. D. (2006). Traumatic stress: Effects on the brain. *Dialogues in Clinical Neuroscience, 8*(4), 445–461.

Buss, C., Entringer, S., Moog, N. K., Toepfer, P., Fair, D. A., Simhan, H. N., Heim, C. M., & Wadhwa, P. D. (2017). Intergenerational transmission of maternal childhood maltreatment exposure: Implications for fetal brain development. *Journal of the American Academy of Child and Adolescent Psychiatry, 56*(5), 373–382.

Byrd, A. L., & Manuck, S. B. (2014). MAOA, childhood maltreatment, and antisocial behavior: Meta-analysis of a gene- environment interaction. *Biological Psychiatry, 75*(1), 9–17.

Campbell-Sills, L., Cohan, S. L., & Stein, M. B. (2006). Relationship of resilience to personality, coping, and psychiatric symptoms in young adults. *Behavior Research and Therapy, 44*(4), 585–599.

Carlson, V., Barnett, D., Cicchetti, D., & Braunwald, K. (1989). Disorganized/disoriented attachment relationships in maltreated infants. *Developmental Psychology, 25*(4), 525–531.

Caspi, A., McClay, J., Moffitt, T. E., Mill, J., Martin, J., Craig, I. W., Taylor, A., & Poulton, R. (2002). Role of genotype in the cycle of violence in maltreated children. *Science, 297*, 851–854.

Chung, W. W., & Hudziak, J. J. (2017). The transitional age brain: "The best of times and the worst of times". *Child and Adolescent Psychiatric Clinics of North America, 26*(2), 157–175.

Colich, N. L., Rosen, M. L., Williams, E. S., & McLaughlin, K. A. (2020). Biological aging in childhood and adolescence following experiences of threat and deprivation: A systematic review and meta-analysis. *Psychological Bulletin, 146*(9), 721–764.

Conner, D. F. (2002). *Aggression and antisocial behavior in children & adolescents.* Guilford Press.

Cook, A., Spinazzola, J., Ford, J., Lanktree, C., Blaustein, M., Cloitre, M., DeRosa, R., Hubbard, R., Kagan, R., Liautaud, J., Mallah, K., Olafson, E., & van der Kolk, B. (2005). Complex trauma in children and adolescents. *Psychiatric Annals, 35*(5), 390–398.

Crick, N. R., & Dodge, K. A. (1996). Social information-processing mechanisms in reactive and proactive aggression. *Child Development, 67*(3), 993–1002.

Crittenden, P. (1992). Treatment of anxious attachment in infancy and early childhood. *Development and Psychopathology, 4*, 575–602.

Crittenden, P. (1997). Truth, error, omission, distortion, and deception: The application of attachment theory to the assessment and treatment of psychological disorder. In S. Dollinger & L. F. DiLalla (Eds.), *Assessment and intervention issues across the life span* (pp. 35–76). Erlbaum.

Culp, R., Watkins, R., Lawrence, H., et al. (1991). Maltreated children's language and speech development: Abused, neglected, and abused and neglected. *First Language, 11*(33 Pt. 3), 377–389.

Damasio, A. R. (1994). *Descartes' error: Emotion, rationality and the human brain*. Putnam (Grosset Books).

Daugherty, T. K., & Quay, H. C. (1991). Response perseveration and delayed responding in childhood behavior disorders. *Journal of Child Psychology and Psychiatry, 32*, 453–461.

Davies, D. (1999). *Child development*. Guilford Press.

de Leon, J., Susce, M. T., & Murray-Carmichael, E. (2006). The AmpliChip CYP450 genotyping test: Integrating a new clinical tool. *Molecular Diagnosis & Therapy, 10*, 135–351.

Dodge, K. A. (1991). The structure and function of reactive and proactive aggression. In D. J. Pepler & K. H. Rubin (Eds.), *The development and treatment of childhood aggression* (pp. 210–218). Lawrence Erlbaum.

Dodge, K. A., & Coie, J. D. (1987). Social-information-processing factors in reactive and proactive aggression in children's peer groups. *Journal of Personality and Social Psychology, 53*(5), 1289–1309.

Dodge, K., Lochman, J., Harnish, J., Bates, J., & Pettit, G. (1997). Reactive and proactive aggression in school children and psychiatrically impaired chronically assaultive youth. *Journal of Abnormal Psychology, 106*, 37–51.

Duke, N. N., Pettingell, S. L., McMorris, B. J., & Borowsky, I. W. (2010). Adolescent violence perpetration: Associations with multiple types of adverse childhood experiences. *Pediatrics, 125*(4), e778–e786.

Eichelman, B. (1987). Neurochemical and psychopharmacologic aspects of aggressive behavior. In H. Y. Meltzer (Ed.), *Psychopharmacology: The third generation of progress* (pp. 697–704). Raven Press.

Fairchild, G., Hawes, D. J., Frick, P. J., Copeland, W. E., Odgers, C. L., Franke, B., Freitag, C. M., & De Brito, S. A. (2019). Conduct disorder. *Nature Reviews. Disease Primers, 5*(1), 43.

Felitti, V. J., Anda, R. F., Nordenberg, D., Williamson, D. F., Spitz, A. M., Edwards, V., Koss, M. P., & Marks, J. S. (1998). Relationship of childhood abuse and household dysfunction to many of the leading causes of death in adults. The Adverse Childhood Experiences (ACE) Study. *American Journal of Preventive Medicine, 14*(4), 245–258.

Flom, M., White, D., Ganiban, J., & Saudino, K. J. (2020). Longitudinal links between callous-unemotional behaviors and parenting in early childhood: A genetically informed design. *Journal of the American Academy of Child and Adolescent Psychiatry, 59*(3), 401–409.e2.

Ford, J. D., Racusin, R., Ellis, C. G., Daviss, W. B., Reiser, J., Fleischer, A., & Thomas, J. (2000). Child maltreatment, other trauma exposure, and posttraumatic symptomatology among children with oppositional defiant and attention deficit hyperactivity disorders. *Child Maltreatment, 5*(3), 205–217.

Fox, J. A. (1995). Homicide offending patterns: A grim look ahead (abstract). In: *Scientific proceedings of the annual meeting of the American Academy for the Advancement of Science.*

Foy, D., Guevara, M., & Camilleri, A. (1996). Community violence. In D. J. Miller (Ed.), *Handbook of posttraumatic stress disorders* (pp. 2–25). Basic Books.

Fraiberg, S., Adelson, E., & Shapiro, V. (1987). Ghosts in the nursery: A psychoanalytic approach to the problems of impaired infant-mother relationships. In *Selected writings of Selma Fraiberg* (pp. 101–136). Ohio State University Press.

Frick, P. J., Lilienfeld, S. O., Ellis, M., Loney, B., & Silverthorn, P. (1999). The association between anxiety and psychopathy dimensions in children. *Journal of Abnormal Child Psychology, 27,* 383–392.

Gao, Y., Raine, A., Venables, P. H., Dawson, M. E., & Mednick, S. A. (2010). Association of poor childhood fear conditioning and adult crime. *The American Journal of Psychiatry, 167*(1), 56–60.

Garg, E., Chen, L., Nguyen, T., Pokhvisneva, I., Chen, L. M., Unternaehrer, E., MacIsaac, J. L., McEwen, L. M., Mah, S. M., Gaudreau, H., Levitan, R., Moss, E., Sokolowski, M. B., Kennedy, J. L., Steiner, M. S., Meaney, M. J., Holbrook, J. D., Silveira, P. P., Karnani, N., Kobor, M. S., et al. (2018). The early care environment and DNA methylome variation in childhood. *Development and Psychopathology, 30*(3), 891–903.

Giedd, J. N. (2015). The amazing teen brain. *Scientific American, 312*(6), 32–37.

Gray, J. A. (1982). *The neuropsychology of anxiety: An enquiry into the functions of the septohippocampal system.* Oxford University Press.

Gray, J. A. (1987). *The psychology of fear and stress* (2nd ed.). Cambridge University Press.

Gray, J. A., & McNaughton, N. (2000). *The neuropsychology of anxiety: An enquiry into the functions of the septo-hippocampal system* (2nd ed.). Oxford University Press.

Gregg, T. R., & Siegel, A. (2001). Brain structures and neurotransmitters regulating aggression in cats: Implications for human aggression. *Progress in Neuropsychopharmacology and Biological Psychiatry, 25,* 91–140.

Hare, R. D. (1995). Psychopaths: New trends in research. *The Harvard Mental Health Letter, 12,* 4–5.

Harvard Mental Health Letter. (2005). The biology of child maltreatment, *21*(12), 1–3.

Heim, C., Newport, D. J., Miller, A. H., & Nemeroff, C. B. (2000). Long-term neuroendocrine effects of childhood maltreatment. *Journal of the American Medical Association, 284*(18), 2321.

House, T. H., & Milligan, W. L. (1976). Autonomic responses to modeled distress in prison psychopaths. *Journal of Personality and Social Psychology, 34,* 556–560.

Hyde, L. W., Waller, R., Trentacosta, C. J., Shaw, D. S., Neiderhiser, J. M., Ganiban, J. M., Reiss, D., & Leve, L. D. (2016). Heritable and nonheritable pathways to early callous-unemotional behaviors. *The American Journal of Psychiatry, 173*(9), 903–910.

Jäggi, L. J., Mezuk, B., Watkins, D. C., & Jackson, J. S. (2016). The relationship between trauma, arrest, and incarceration history among black Americans: Findings from the National Survey of American Life. *Society and Mental Health, 6*(3), 187–206.

Jonson-Reid, M., & Wideman, E. (2017). Trauma and very young children. *Child and Adolescent Psychiatric Clinics of North America, 26*(3), 477–490.

Kagan, J. (1989). Temperamental contributions to social behavior. *American Psychologist, 44,* 668–674.

Kessler, R. C., Berglund, P., Demler, O., Jin, R., Merikangas, K. R., & Walters, E. E. (2005). Lifetime prevalence and age-of- onset distributions of DSM-IV disorders in the National Comorbidity Survey Replication. *Archives of General Psychiatry, 62*(6), 593–602.

Kim-Cohen, J., Caspi, A., Taylor, A., Williams, B., Newcombe, R., Craig, I. W., & Moffitt, T. E. (2006). MAOA, maltreatment, and gene-environment interaction predicting children's mental health: New evidence and a meta-analysis. *Molecular Psychiatry, 10,* 603–913.

Kimonis, E. R., Fleming, G., Briggs, N., Brouwer-French, L., Frick, P. J., Hawes, D. J., Bagner, D. M., Thomas, R., & Dadds, M. (2019). Parent-child interaction therapy adapted for preschoolers with callous-unemotional traits: An open trial pilot study. *Journal of Clinical Child and Adolescent Psychology: The Official Journal for the Society of Clinical Child and Adolescent Psychology, American Psychological Association, Division 53, 48*(sup1), S347–S361.

Kramer, D. A. (2005). Commentary: Gene-environment interplay in the context of genetics, epigenetics, and gene expression. *Journal of the American Academy of Child and Adolescent Psychiatry, 44*(1), 19–27.

Lahey, B., Waldman, I., & McBurnett, K. (1999). Annotation: The development of antisocial behavior. *Journal of Child Psychology and Psychiatry, 29,* 669–682.

Lara, D., & Akiskal, H. S. (2006). Toward and integrative model of the spectrum of mood, behavioral, and personality disorders based on fear and anger traits: II. Implications for neurobiology, genetics, and psychopharmacological treatment. *Journal of Affective Disorders, 94*(1–3), 89–103.

LeDoux, J. (1996). *The emotional brain.* Simon & Schuster.

LeDoux, J. (2002). *The synaptic self.* Penguin Books.

Leibenluft, E., Blair, R. J. R., Charney, D. S., & Pine, D. S. (2003). Irritability in pediatric mania and other childhood psychopathology. *Annals of the New York Academy of Sciences, 10008,* 201–218.

Levenston, G. K., Patrick, C. J., Bradley, M. M., & Lang, P. J. (2000). The psychopath as observer: Emotion and attention in picture processing. *Journal of Abnormal Psychology, 109,* 373–386.

Levin, A. (2006). PTSD not sufficient to explain response to trauma. *Psychiatric News, 41*(16), 20.

Ludvik, M. B. (2017). Leveraging neuroscience and education to prevent youth aggression and violence. *US-China Education Review Bulletin, 7*(9), 401–433.

Lykken, D. T. (1957). A study of anxiety in the sociopathic personality. *Journal of Abnormal and Social Psychology, 55,* 6–10.

Manuck, S. (2006). 6th International Congress of Neuroendocrinology (ICN 2006).

Mash, E. J., & Dozois, D. J. A. (1996). Child psychopathology: A developmental-systems perspective. In E. J. Mash & R. A. Barkley (Eds.), *Child psychopathology* (pp. 3–60). Guilford Press.

Mathews, V. P., Kronenberger, W. G., Wang, Y., Lurito, J. T., Lowe, M. J., & Dunn, D. W. (2005). Media violence exposure and frontal lobe activation measured by functional magnetic resonance imaging in aggressive and non-aggressive adolescents. *Journal of Computer Assisted Tomography, 29*(3), 287–292.

Matthys, W., Cuperus, J. M., & Van Engeland, H. (1999). Deficient social problem-solving in boys with ODD/CD, with ADHD, and with both disorders. *Journal of the American Academy of Child & Adolescent Psychiatry, 38*(3), 311–321.

McFarlane, A. (1988). The phenomenology of posttraumatic stress disorders following a natural disaster. *Journal of Nervous and Mental Disorders, 176,* 22–29.

McNaughton, N., & Corr, P. J. (2004). A two-dimensional neuropsychology of defense: Fear/ anxiety and defensive distance. *Neuroscience and Biobehavioral Reviews, 28,* 285–305.

Meyer-Lindenberg, A., Buckholtz, J., Kolachana, B. S., Pezawas, L., Blasi, G., Wabnitz, A., Honea, R., Hariri, A. R., Verchinski, B., Callicott, J., Egan, M. F., Mattay, V. S., & Weinberger, D. R. (2006). Neural mechanisms of genetic risk f or impulsivity and violence in humans. *Proceedings of the National Academy of Sciences, 103*(16), 6269–6274.

Mezzacappa, E., Earls, A., & Kindlon, D. (1998). Executive and motivational control of performance task behavior, and autonomic heart-rate regulation in children: Physiologic validation of two-factor solution inhibitory control. *Journal of Child Psychology and Psychiatry, 39,* 525–531.

Miller, T. W., & Veltkamp, L. J. (1996). Trauma accommodation syndrome. In T. W. Miller (Ed.), *Theory and assessment of stressful life events* (pp. 95–98). International Universities Press.

Moyer, K. E. (1976). *The psychobiology of aggression.* Harper & Row.

Newman, J. P., & Kosson, D. S. (1986). Passive avoidance learning in psychopathic and non-psychopathic offenders. *Journal of Abnormal Psychology, 95,* 252–256.

Niehoff, D. (1999). *The biology of violence.* Free Press.

O'Donnell, K. J., Chen, L., MacIsaac, J. L., McEwen, L. M., Nguyen, T., Beckmann, K., Zhu, Y., Chen, L. M., Brooks-Gunn, J., Goldman, D., Grigorenko, E. L., Leckman, J. F., Diorio, J., Karnani, N., Olds, D. L., Holbrook, J. D., Kobor, M. S., & Meaney, M. J. (2018). DNA methylome variation in a perinatal nurse-visitation program that reduces child maltreatment: a 27-year follow-up. *Translational psychiatry, 8*(1), 15. https://doi.org/10.1038/s41398-017-0063-9

Ogden, P., Minton, K., & Pain, C. (2006). *Trauma and the body.* Norton Series on Interpersonal Neurobiology.

Oxford, M., Cavell, T. A., & Hughes, J. N. (2003). Callous-unemotional traits moderate the relation between ineffective parenting and child externalizing problems: A partial replication and extension. *Journal of Clinical Child and Adolescent Psychology, 32*, 577–585.

Panksepp, J. (1998). *Affective neuroscience: The foundations of human and animal emotions.* Oxford University Press.

Parker, K. J., Buckmaster, C. L., Sundlass, K., Schatzber, A. F., & Lyons, D. M. (2006). Maternal mediation, stress inoculation, and the development of neuroendocrine stress resistance in primates. *Proceedings of the National Academy of Sciences, 103*(8), 3000–3005.

Pennington, B., & Ozonof, S. (1996). Executive functions and developmental psychopathology. *Journal of Child Psychology and Psychiatry, 37*, 51–87.

Perry, B., & Pollard, R. (1998). Homeostasis, stress, trauma and adaptation. *Child and Adolescent Psychiatric Clinics of North America, 7*, 33–51.

Ploog, D. W. (2003). The place of the triune brain in psychiatry. *Physiology & Behavior, 79*, 487–493.

Porter, K. E., Koch, E. I., & Saules, K. (2015). The impact of sexual assault history on perceived consequences of risky dating Scenarios. *Acta Psychopathologica, 1*, 1.

Pulkkinen, L. (1996). Proactive and reactive aggression in early adolescence as precursors to anti- and prosocial behaviors in young adults. *Aggressive Behavior, 22*, 241–257.

Reavis, J. A., Looman, J., Franco, K. A., & Rojas, B. (2013). Adverse childhood experiences and adult criminality: How long must we live before we possess our own lives? *The Permanente Journal, 17*(2), 44–48.

Rincón-Cortés, M., Barr, G. A., Mouly, A. M., Shionoya, K., Nuñez, B. S., & Sullivan, R. M. (2015). Enduring good memories of infant trauma: Rescue of adult neurobehavioral deficits via amygdala serotonin and corticosterone interaction. *Proceedings of the National Academy of Sciences of the United States of America, 112*(3), 881–886.

Rogeness, G. A., Javors, M. A., & Pliszka, S. R. (1992). Neurochemistry and child and adolescent psychiatry. *Journal of the American Academy of Child and Adolescent Psychiatry, 31*, 765–781.

Rubinstein, M., Yeager, C. A., Goodstein, C., & Lewis, D. O. (1993). Sexually assaultive male juveniles: A follow-up. *The American Journal of Psychiatry, 150*(2), 262–265.

Rutter, M., Dunn, J., Plomin, R., Simonoff, E., Pickles, A., Maughan, B., Ormel, J., Meyer, J., & Eaves, L. (1997). Integrating nature and nurture: Implications of person-environment correlations and interactions for developmental psychopathology. *Development and Psychopathology, 9*, 335–364.

Rutter, M., Moffitt, T. E., & Caspi, A. (2006). Gene-environment interplay and psychopathology: Multiple varieties but real effects. *Journal of Child Psychology and Psychiatry, 47*(3/4), 226–261.

Ryan, G., Miyoshi, T., Metzner, J., Krugman, R., & Fryer, G. (1996). Trends in a national sample of sexually abusive youths. *Journal of the American Academy of Child & Adolescent Psychiatry, 35*, 17–54.

Scanlon, F., Schatz, D., Scheidell, J. D., Cuddeback, G. S., Frueh, B. C., & Khan, M. R. (2019). National study of childhood traumatic events and adolescent and adult criminal justice involvement risk: Evaluating the protective role of social support from mentors during adolescence. *The Journal of Clinical Psychiatry, 80*(5), 18m12347.

Shapiro, S. K., Quay, H. C., Hogan, A. E., & Schwarz, K. P. (1988). Response perseveration and delayed responding in undersocialized aggressive conduct disorder. *Journal of Abnormal Psychology, 97*, 371–373.

Shonk, S. M., & Cicchetti, D. (2001). Maltreatment, competency deficits, and risk for academic and behavioral maladjustment. *Developmental Psychology, 37*(1), 3–17.

Siegel, D. (2001). *The developing mind: How relationships and the brain interact to shape who we are.* Guilford Press.

Soller, M. V., Karnik, N. S., & Steiner, H. (2006). Psychopharmacologic treatment in juvenile offenders. *Child and Adolescent Psychiatric Clinics of North America, 15*(2), 477–499.

Steiner, H., Garcia, I. G., & Matthews, Z. (1997). Posttraumatic stress disorder in incarcerated juvenile delinquents. *Journal of the American Academy of Child & Adolescent Psychiatry, 36*(3), 357–363.

Tiihonen, J., Hodgins, S., & Vaurio, O. (2000). Amygdaloid volume loss in psychopathy. *Society for Neuroscience Abstracts,* 2017.

van der Kolk, B. A. (2003). The neurobiology of childhood trauma and abuse. *Child and Adolescent Psychiatric Clinics of North America, 12,* 293–317.

van der Kolk, B. A. (2005). Developmental trauma disorder: Toward a rational diagnosis for children with complex trauma. *Psychiatric Annals, 35*(5), 401–408.

van Schaik, R., Müller, D. J., Serretti, A., & Ingelman-Sundberg, M. (2020). Pharmacogenetics in psychiatry: An update on clinical usability. *Frontiers in Pharmacology, 11,* 575540.

Vitaro, F., Gendreau, P. L., Tremblay, R. E., & Oligny, P. (1998). Reactive and proactive aggression differentially predict later conduct problems. *Journal of Child Psychology and Psychiatry, and Allied Disciplines, 39*(3), 377–385.

Vitiello, B., & Stoff, D. M. (1997). Subtypes of aggression and their relevance to child psychiatry. *Journal of the American Academy of Child & Adolescent Psychiatry, 36*(3), 307–315.

Vitiello, B., Behar, D., Hunt, J., Stoff, D., & Ricciuti, A. (1990). Subtyping aggression in children and adolescents. *The Journal of Neuropsychiatry and Clinical Neurosciences, Spring, 2*(2), 189–192.

Wade, M., Zeanah, C. H., Fox, N. A., & Nelson, C. A. (2020). Global deficits in executive functioning are transdiagnostic mediators between severe childhood neglect and psychopathology in adolescence. *Psychological Medicine, 50*(10), 1687–1694.

Walker, J. L., Lahey, B. B., Russo, M. F., Frick, P. J., Christ, M. A. G., McBurnett, K., Loeber, R., Stouthamer-Loeber, M., & Green, S. M. (1991). Anxiety, inhibition, and conduct disorder in children: I. Relations to social impairment. *Journal of the American Academy of Child and Adolescent Psychiatry, 30,* 187–191.

Waller, R., & Hyde, L. W. (2018). Callous-unemotional behaviors in early childhood: The development of empathy and prosociality gone awry. *Current Opinion in Psychology, 20,* 11–16.

White, S. F., Frick, P. J., Lawing, K., & Bauer, D. (2013). Callous-unemotional traits and response to functional family therapy in adolescent offenders. *Behavioral Sciences & the Law, 31*(2), 271–285.

Wootton, J. M., Frick, P. J., Shelton, K. K., & Silverthorn, P. (1997). Ineffective parenting and childhood conduct problems: The moderating role of callous-unemotional traits. *Journal of Consulting and Clinical Psychology, 65,* 292–300.

Chapter 3
Developmental Issues in the Prevention of Aggression and Violence in School

Sara E. Goldstein, Andrew M. Terranova, Sarah C. Savoy, Shaniqua Bradley, Jeanie Park, and Paul Boxer

Results from the National Crime Victimization Survey indicated that during the 2016–2017 school year, 20.2% of students in grades 6–12 reported being bullied in school and 15.3% reported being bullied online or by text (Seldin & Yanez, 2019). According to 2017 Youth Risk Behavior Surveillance System data, on at least one day during the 30 days before the survey, 3.8% of students in grades 9–12 had carried a weapon on school property (e.g., gun, knife, or club; Kann et al., 2018). In the 12 months before the survey, 8.5% of students had been in a physical fight on school property and 6% had been threatened with a weapon on school property. Offering hope to students who are targets, it is the norm for the frequency and prevalence of victimization to decline across grades K-12 (Ladd et al., 2017). Some data even suggest that the total victimization rate in schools has declined; this progress has occurred alongside a shift in school security standards and anti-violence efforts in recent decades (Waasdorp et al., 2017; Wang et al., 2020). Concerns regarding safety remain, however, among students, educators, and parents (e.g., Kann et al.,

S. E. Goldstein (✉) · J. Park
Department of Human Development and Family Sciences, University of Delaware, Newark, DE, USA
e-mail: sgolds@udel.edu

A. M. Terranova
Department of Psychology, Gupta College of Science, Coastal Carolina University, Conway, SC, USA

S. C. Savoy
Department of Psychology, Stephen F. Austin State University, Nacogdoches, TX, USA

S. Bradley
Department of Social Work and Child Advocacy, Montclair State University, Montclair, NJ, USA

P. Boxer
Department of Psychology, Rutgers University, Newark, NJ, USA

© The Author(s), under exclusive license to Springer Nature Switzerland AG 2023
T. W. Miller (ed.), *School Violence and Primary Prevention*, https://doi.org/10.1007/978-3-031-13134-9_3

2018; Mowen & Freng, 2019; Waasdorp et al., 2017; Wang et al., 2020). Moreover, rare incidents of extreme school violence can have serious consequences. A total of 66 school shootings were documented at U.S. public and private elementary and secondary schools during the 2018–2019 school year, 37 involving injuries only and 29 involving deaths (Wang et al., 2020).

Aggressors and victims alike are at increased risk for negative psychosocial ramifications when involved with aggressive behavior and violence. For example, youth who have been victimized are more likely than their peers to have challenges with depression, anxiety, and self-concept (Brunstein Klomek et al., 2015; Guerra et al., 2011; Tiiri et al., 2020; Turner et al., 2017) and they are also at an increased risk for suicidal ideation and behavior (Gunn III & Goldstein, 2017). Perpetrators are at higher risk for mental health challenges as well (Kozasa et al., 2017; LeBrun-Harris et al., 2019; Ttofi et al., 2011; Wolke et al., 2014) and also may get involved in the justice system depending on the specifics of their aggressive behavior (Matlasz et al., 2020; Ttofi et al., 2011). Clearly, it behooves educators and mental health professionals to identify and utilize the most effective and reliable methods to prevent aggressive behavior at school. As is the case with other types of educational material and psychosocial interventions, it is imperative that aggression prevention efforts are developmentally sound and that they consider aspects of social, cognitive, and psychological development in their design and implementation. Prevention efforts are most effective when they are easily understood by the targeted population, and when they are culturally, socially, and developmentally relevant (Chan et al., 2016; Hahn et al., 2007).

Given these issues, the current chapter will focus on developmental issues in the primary prevention of aggressive behavior among children, adolescents, and emerging adults. First, we will define and introduce the concept of primary prevention. Next, we will discuss the need to consider aspects of social, cognitive, and psychological development when designing and implementing primary prevention programs. We will then review ways in which the topography of aggression changes with age and the associated age-related factors of social goals and social context. This will move into a general discussion of different forms and functions of aggressive behavior, where we will discuss variations in severity as well as relational/overt and reactive/proactive distinctions. We will also review research regarding sexual harassment and harassment based on gender, sexual orientation, and race. Due to the increasing likelihood of online schooling due to the COVID-19 pandemic at the time of this chapter writing, we will also include a discussion of cyberbullying and online aggression.

In the final sections of the chapter, we will review the relevant theories of the development of aggressive behavior, focusing on social learning/social cognitive information processing (SCIP) theory (e.g., Anderson & Huesmann, 2003; Anderson & Bushman, 2002; Boxer et al., 2005; Huesmann, 1998) and aspects of the bioecological theory (Bronfenbrenner, 2005; Bronfenbrenner & Evans, 2000; Bronfenbrenner & Morris, 2006). We will conclude the chapter by specifically discussing what we know about the mediating mechanisms of aggression specifically from a SCIP perspective and how these can be linked to developmentally sensitive prevention programs. We will also include suggestions for future directions for research and practice, including ideas that discuss the potential for online or socially distanced programming in the future that has become important to consider as a result of COVID-19 or another future crisis.

Primary Prevention

Primary prevention programming typically refers to a type of programming that is provided to children as early as possible in their development, intended to prevent the development of some type of problem or pathological behavior. Primary prevention programming should ideally be implemented as soon as possible in human development. The exact timing would vary by type of behavior, but universally this should occur as soon as youth have reached the necessary social, emotional, and cognitive capacities to address in an effort to prevent the particular undesired behavior (McGorry et al., 2011). Primary prevention is a cost-and resource-effective way of promoting positive, healthy human development (Roberts & Peterson, 1984; Serna et al., 2000; Weissberg et al., 1991). Without prevention programming, the cost of later intervening in the undesirable behaviors can be enormous, far exceeding the initial cost of primary prevention (National Research Council and Institute of Medicine, 2009).

With regard to aggressive behavior, evidence suggests that an early start for primary prevention programming is warranted. Aggressive behavior occurs relatively early in human development (Tremblay, 2000), with toddlers and preschoolers engaging in well-documented and sometimes frequent acts of school-based aggressive behavior (Goldstein et al., 2002; Ostrov et al., 2014). Although the aggressive behavior of young children often starts out modestly (e.g., a small pushing incident over a toy dispute), it can escalate and modify over time leading to much larger acts, and socially and financially costly outcomes during adolescence and adulthood (Huesmann et al., 2002; Jones et al., 2002). Psychologically and educationally, the impact of aggression and bullying in school can be devastating from a young age, with victims showing decreased school motivation and belonging and an increase in mental health problems as early as the early elementary years and potentially lasting through college and beyond (Goldstein et al., 2008; Woods & Wolke, 2004; Young-Jones et al., 2015). Thus, it is imperative that aggression and violence prevention programs should target children at as young of an age as possible and should target all relevant forms of aggression (discussed in detail later in this chapter) for the particular age range.

Even though starting primary prevention programming to prevent aggression as early as possible is critical, there is a clear need for continued approaches beyond early and middle childhood. Aggressive behavior aggression shows moderate continuity from childhood to adolescence and into adulthood (Huesmann et al., 2006, 1984; Kokko & Pulkkinen, 2005). Children who exhibit high levels of aggression at a young age are also more likely to be more aggressive than their peers into adulthood. Second, the impact of aggressive behavior on school experiences is evident from elementary school through post-secondary experiences, with frequency of school-based aggression peaking in middle school but continuing to evolve and morph (Pellegrini & Long, 2007; Pepler et al., 2008). Relatedly, other challenges with mental health associated with bullying and aggression also begin to increase during early adolescence, including depression, anxiety, and behaviors and cognitions associated with suicide (Arseneault et al., 2010; Gunn III & Goldstein, 2017; Hinduja & Patchin, 2010; Kowalski & Limber, 2013; Litwiller & Brausch, 2013). Further compounding things, as youth age aggressive behavior may become increasingly difficult to detect. As youth gain in social sophistication and insight about the potential legal or educational consequences of their behavior (e.g., Goldstein, 2016; Goldstein et al., 2008), the topography of aggression evolves. Aggression in younger children typically involves low-impact physical and acquisitive behaviors such as pushing, shoving, or taking a classmate's toy/other possessions, or disobeying authority. In contrast, aggression among older children and adolescents includes more varied behaviors such as an increase in the frequency of relational/social aggression (e.g., ostracizing, spreading defamatory gossip) cyberbullying and aggression, sexual harassment, and interpersonal violence (dating violence and sexual aggression). At different ages, varying social, emotional, and cognitive factors may be more impactful for understanding the development and maintenance of particular forms of aggressive behavior. For example, programs targeting emotional reactivity and regulation may be especially important for working with young children (e.g., Eisenberg et al., 2001), whereas aggressive older youth might benefit more from an approach that emphasizes social-cognitive processing (e.g., Huesmann, 1998).

Developmental Considerations in Designing Primary Prevention Programming

There are numerous factors to consider when establishing a developmentally sensitive primary prevention program. Primary or universal approaches to preventing aggression among youth must be sensitive to these factors to be effective. Social goals and interpersonal needs change over time, and developmental tasks evolve as well (cf. Boxer et al., 2006). The most effective programming will take these factors into consideration, and the approaches that will work best on young children will vary greatly from what will work best with older youth.

First, the age of program implementation needs to be carefully reviewed. How old should children be when they first begin programming targeted at preventing the specific type of unwanted behavior? Ideally, it is best to target the behavior before it starts, but after one is developmentally ready to handle the programming about the specific type of behavior (e.g., Durlak & Wells, 1997). For example, very young children have experience with physical and relational aggression (e.g., Ostrov et al.,

2014, 2015) so these forms of aggression are appropriate (and important) to begin targeting early.

One important reason to start targeting various types of behavior as soon as they become relevant is so that prevention can be the focus rather than changing pre-existing, engrained behavioral patterns – this would be considered intervention, which presents additional challenges. For example, parents and teachers begin to differentially socialize physically versus relationally aggressive behavior during the preschool years, with increased sanctions and punishments being given for physical aggression versus relational aggression (Goldstein & Boxer, 2013). This type of messaging becomes internalized and facilitates the belief that relational aggression is less harmful than physical aggression, which can lead to increases in relationally aggressive behavior. This is a well-established belief among older children and adolescents (e.g., Goldstein & Tisak, 2010), and is held despite the fact of the myriad negative consequences associated with relational aggression in school and beyond (Kawabata et al., 2013; Marshall et al., 2015; Merrell et al., 2006). Thus, targeting relational aggression early and often in school-based prevention programming can help to prevent these harmful behaviors from occurring in the first place, and can help by spreading a consistent message that *all* forms of harmful behavior are not acceptable (even those forms that do not leave physical bumps and bruises).

Second, cognitive characteristics of specific age groups need to be attended to when establishing developmentally sensitive programs. There are several aspects of cognitive development that should be carefully considered here, including attentional limitations, perspective-taking ability, and ability to use various cognitive strategies to calm down or distract oneself in an emotionally arousing moment. An important first consideration has to do with youth attention span; that is, their ability to remain focused on a stimulus (in this case aggression prevention programming) in the face of various distractions (internal or external). How long can the child or adolescent be expected to remain interested and engaged with the type of programming delivered? In the preschool years, the answer to this question is "not too long," although there can be a good deal of variability (e.g., McClelland et al., 2013). For universal prevention programming, however, it is important to keep the program at levels that most children in the grade could be expected to focus on and attend to, rather than to get side tracked and focus on an unrelated stimulus. Very young pre-school children will have difficulty focusing on prevention programming for too long if other, more attractive stimuli are available. However, by the early elementary school years, children can be expected to remain focused on a selected task for longer periods of time (e.g., Diamond et al., 2002; Sabbagh et al., 2006). Selective attention also improves over the course of the early elementary school years (e.g., DeMarie-Dreblow & Miller, 1988), making programming easier in the face of tempting classroom distractions. Older elementary school-aged youth and adolescents can be expected to remain focused for longer periods of time (e.g., a typical "academic period" of 45 minutes or so in school should be fine), although some disruptions still may occur and should be addressed constructively (e.g., Bundge & Zelazo, 2006; Munakata et al., 2012).

Although older elementary-school aged youth and adolescents are able to sustain attention for longer periods of time, they also need more autonomy and peer engagement and participation. Without peer interaction, adolescents are at risk of losing focus quite quickly and may shift their attention elsewhere (Makara & Madjar, 2015). Thus, activities with older elementary-aged children and adolescents should rely heavily on opportunities for peer engagement and social interaction (Hwang et al., 2017). It is also important to note here that when opportunities for in-person instruction and interaction are put on hold due to the 2020 Coronavirus pandemic or other highly unprecedented circumstances, these relationship needs are still incredibly salient for youth. Programmers are urged to find creative and safe mechanisms for program delivery that still honors the developmentally relevant relational needs of youth.

Similar to attention span, perspective-taking ability changes over time from childhood through adolescence. During the preschool years, young children still have difficulty taking others' perspectives during an argument or a fight without scaffolding (Dominguez & Trawick-Smith, 2018), although data suggest that this is a skill that can be encouraged and taught in children from a young age (Kirova & Jamison, 2018). Given the developmental challenges, though, associated with perspective taking during the preschool and even early elementary school years, it behooves prevention programs to focus on this component of cognition as part of the developing programming. As youth get older and more socially sophisticated, programmers can assume the ability to take others' perspectives in a conflict or a fight but should also acknowledge that this skill may be impaired by high levels of emotional arousal (Arsenio & Lemerise, 2004). Programming targeting (and practicing) perspective-taking abilities can help to make these skills more automatic and thus more likely to be enacted during a stressful peer conflict that could result in aggression or bullying. This type of emphasis may be especially useful in younger children where these skills are starting to develop.

Emotion regulation capacities are another important factor to consider when designing prevention programming. The ability to regulate emotional expression changes over time, as does the ability to do this on one's own initiative versus counting on others to assist with this challenge (Harden et al., 2017). As reviewed by Rademacher and Koglin (2019), it is typical for preschool-aged children to struggle with self-initiated soothing and calming down activities, although there can be variability. Their ability to recognize basic emotions is newly emerging (Widen & Russell, 2008), and in order to calm down from a state of emotional arousal that may lead to aggression, one has to identify the feeling of anger/frustration first. Thus, programming targeting this age group should keep in mind that these strategies for identifying basic feelings and emotions are important building blocks for later regulatory capacities. At older ages, children's and adolescents' ability to regulate their own emotions remains questionable when faced with potential highly arousing/salient perceived threats or insults (Hessler & Fainsilber Katz, 2007). Thus, as discussed later in this chapter in detail, research demonstrates the efficacy of providing youth with social-cognitive programming that targets perceptional biases that can negatively impact emotion regulation capabilities (Hudley &

Graham, 1993). As youth move into adolescence, emotion regulation may be especially compromised in peer situations (which is where aggression and bullying are most likely) thus programming should target strategies for youth to "do the right thing" even when they are confronted with potential peer pressure or negative peer influence. This challenge is likely heightened during early adolescence when susceptibility to peer influence is at its peak (Goldstein et al., 2020).

Along with the cognitive development considerations of attention span, perspective-taking ability, and emotion regulatory capacities, the role of relational context needs to be considered. In other words, which relationships are most salient and frequent in youths' lives during a particular point of development? Which relationships are most important to youth, and which are they less invested in over time? Early in development, the family of origin is prioritized in terms of meeting relational needs (Bowlby, 1969), although as the youth moves toward adolescence the peer world expands to take an increasing emphasis in terms of companionship and emotional support. School is a critical context for establishing these peer relationships and learning how to maintain them, and thus it is a key context for establishing healthy and safe conflict resolution strategies. By early adolescence, peers first "catch up to" then replace family as most frequent companions and confidants (e.g., Levitt et al., 1993). As adolescence continues, romantic relationships also take on increased importance as there is a continued shift in intimacy and companionship from family to peers, friends, and intimate partners during the emerging adult years (Arnett, 2015; Eshbaugh, 2010). Thus, programming for high school-aged youth and college students should include a variety of relational contexts including the family of origin but most certainly also peers and romantic partners.

A final developmental consideration that we will mention here is the increasing need for personal autonomy, especially as youth move into middle school and beyond. The middle school years are a unique developmental period within adolescence. Rapid changes in social, cognitive, and physical development occur during this time. Young adolescents desire increased autonomy from their parents during this period (Smetana, 1995, 2000; Smetana & Asquith, 1994). They believe that an increasing number of behaviors are outside of parental or authority jurisdiction to regulate, especially with regard to behaviors that they believe to be "personal" or under their individual jurisdiction (Smetana & Bitz, 1996; Tisak & Tisak, 1990). Usually, this does not include aggressive behavior which is acknowledged as being harmful to others (Tisak et al., 2006), although there is some variation in the way that youth believe certain acts fall in the personal-moral continuum such as relational aggression (Goldstein & Tisak, 2010) or cyberbullying (Goldstein, 2016). This shift co-occurs with other social transitions including puberty, romantic interest, rapid neurological and cognitive growth, and the new social and academic structure of secondary school (Eccles et al., 1996, 2003; Kloep et al., 2016). Early adolescents are especially vulnerable to peer influence, often struggling to find a balance between fitting in with their peer group and making healthy, positive choices (Dawes, 2017; Goldstein et al., 2015, 2020). These simultaneously occurring transitions increase early adolescents' risk for impulsive and short-sighted behaviors (Shulman et al., 2016; Steinberg, 2008), such as aggressive behavior. The middle school years, therefore, are especially critical for prevention programming from the perspective of addressing aggression and bullying when it is most salient and potentially impactful for social and academic trajectories.

Types and Trajectories of Aggressive Behavior During Childhood, Adolescence, and Emerging Adulthood

All aggressive behavior shares the commonality of being a behavior intended to "injure or irritate" the victim (Eron, 1987), and research has clearly indicated that some individuals consistently engage in more aggressive behaviors than their peers across development (Olweus, 1979; Huesmann et al., 2009). That said, decades of research on aggressive behavior indicate a broad topography of behavior. Aggression ranges from relatively mild behaviors (e.g., a light shove between two preschoolers), to moderately severe behaviors like spreading a defamatory rumor about a friend around middle school, to very serious behaviors such as assault with a knife in adolescence or spousal abuse in adulthood (cf. Huesmann et al., 1984). This has led some to try to better understand aggressive behaviors by reclassifying the behaviors into more homogenous categories (Björkqvist et al., 1992). Moreover, the topography of the aggressive behaviors in which people engage changes as they develop, with some evidencing escalation in the severity of their aggressive behaviors (Tolan et al., 2000). Thus, it is imperative to identify the different manifestations of aggression and how these manifestations change with development.

Classifying Aggressive Behaviors

In an effort to better understand these varying forms of aggression, researchers have found it useful to distinguish aggression based on its severity, its *form* (i.e., the concrete characteristics of the behavior), and its *function* (i.e., the motivation behind the behavior). These distinctions have been shown to be useful in terms of developing targeted and effective prevention and intervention strategies (e.g., Barker et al., 2010; Dambacher et al., 2015; Leff et al., 2010).

Some have asserted that the severity of the impact of aggressive behaviors is important to consider when creating a classification system for aggression. Some aggressive behaviors are relatively mild in terms of the implications that they have for the victim, for example, a single light shove or an eye roll that the victim does not notice. In sharp contrast, other aggressive behaviors have devastating and long-lasting consequences for the victim, such as is the case regarding assault with a deadly weapon or rape. Still, the severity of many other aggressive acts is somewhere between the two extremes (e.g., pushing and kicking a classmate to obtain lunch money, or telling a group of friends to exclude another child). Loeber and colleagues have categorized aggressive behaviors into three categories based on degree of severity: minor aggression, fighting, and violence. According to this classification scheme, minor aggression involves bullying and annoying behaviors. Fighting involves physical altercations such as fighting with fists, and finally, violence includes more harmful aggression such as attacking someone, forced sex, and similar types of behavior (Tolan et al., 2000).

Alternatively, others have focused on the topological characteristics of the behaviors when making the distinction between indirect and direct aggression. The contrast between these two forms of aggression rests on whether the identity of the perpetrator is known. For direct aggression, it is clear who has perpetrated the behavior whereas, for indirect aggression, the identity of the perpetrator remains unknown (Björkqvist et al., 1992). When this original formulation was conceptualized, it was possible to have indirect physical behavior (e.g., covertly sticking gum on a classmate's seat) and direct socially aggressive behavior (e.g., openly excluding a victim from a birthday party where the whole class was invited except for them).

A similar typological distinction of more general covert versus overt antisocial behavior has also been proposed, with a focus on whether the harmful behavior is committed with others present (overt) or in secret/private. Over time, the original distinction between indirect and direct aggression has come to be understood as the difference between aggression that relies on social/relationship manipulation to cause harm (indirect) versus behaviors that involve overt physically or verbally harmful behaviors to cause harm. Others have further elaborated on this distinction by referring to most indirectly aggressive behaviors as social aggression (Galen & Underwood, 1997). Cairns, Underwood, and colleagues also emphasize the functional aspect of social aggression as damaging the victim's social status and/or self-esteem. Thus, social aggression can also include behaviors such as negative facial or body language (e.g., eye rolling) and direct verbal social rejection ("you can't play with us"), in addition to the more covert/indirect socially aggressive behaviors such as spreading a defamatory rumor (Galen & Underwood, 1997).

Crick and colleagues have employed a similar distinction between relational and overt aggression. Relational aggression harms others through the manipulation of social relationships. Thus relational aggression can too be direct (e.g., threatening to end a friendship) or indirect (starting an anonymous slanderous social media account about somebody). In contrast to relational aggression, Crick and colleague refer to overt aggression as behaviors that use physical aggression or verbal attacks. Similar to relational aggression, overt aggression can be direct (one child punches another child) or indirect (a child secretly puts a thumbtack on a classmate's chair). Other researchers have also included verbal aggression (direct verbal threats and insults), and cyber aggression/cyberbullying as unique forms of aggression. Cyberbullying/ aggression typically refers to harm inflicted through electronic means such as text messaging, emails, or online social network attacks), although especially in the case of cyberbullying, there is often an overlap between the forms in a single incident (e.g., a socially/relationally aggressive incident that occurs in social media, or a physical threat expressed through a text message; Goldstein, 2016).

It is important to note that the field has not come to a unanimous consensus regarding this terminology and that the interested applied researcher or program developer should review all of these terms when searching for evidence to support programming material for development. Further, as articulated in greater detail below, other researchers have emphasized the importance of including additional types of harmful behaviors – such as sexual harassment (Goldstein et al., 2007, 2020) or other types of aggression targeting race, gender, or sexual orientation (e.g., Sugarman et al., 2018) in research on aggressive behavior and prevention and intervention programming.

Another well-established way of classifying aggression has been to distinguish between reactive and proactive functions of aggression. These behaviors are distinguishable based on the antecedents of the aggressive incident (the motivation behind the incident), rather than on the form of aggression enacted (e.g., relational versus overt aggression). In general, reactive aggression is enacted in response to a perceived provocation (e.g., one teen hears that another teen has been spreading lies about them). In contrast, proactive aggression is typically operationalized as being unprovoked and unemotional. Proactive aggression is generally enacted to achieve some types of instrumental goals, such as to obtain a personal gain or reward or to demonstrate social dominance.

It is also important to note that although a rather large body of research has identified subgroups of youth who are either primarily reactively aggressive or proactively aggressive, the correlation is relatively high between these behaviors (e.g., Dodge & Coie, 1987). In fact, these have led some researchers to suggest that this line of inquiry is of little further need. Despite these concerns, developmental research has produced evidence supporting the validity of the distinction (see Merk et al., 2005 for review). For instance, children and youth who are proactive, as opposed to solely reactively aggressive, have been shown to exhibit unique cognitive, social, and affective characteristics (e.g., Hubbard et al., 2010). While attentional biases toward aggressive cues are associated with higher levels of reactive aggression, weaker attentional biases toward aggressive cues are associated with higher levels of proactive aggression (Brugman et al., 2015). Additionally, researchers have examined social conditions that are associated with higher levels of proactive or reactive aggression common. These data suggest that although bullies and victims are relatively likely to be reactively aggressive, only bullies are at an increased risk for proactive aggression. Regarding the affective characteristics that are differentially associated with proactive and reactive aggression, proactive aggression is characteristic of callous-unemotional youth who feel little remorse or empathy for victims of aggression or other antisocial acts. Likewise, Euler et al. (2017) found that cognitive and affective empathy was associated with lower levels of proactive aggression, but not reactive aggression. With regard to preventive programming, then, it is important to target varied forms and functions of aggressive behavior, being mindful that information may not be generalized from one form of aggression to another in terms of students' internalization of programming material.

Trajectories of Aggressive Behaviors Throughout Development

A large body of research has made it clear that engagement in high levels of aggression, relative to one's similar aged peers, early in development, is a risk factor for elevated levels of aggression (Olweus, 1979; Huesmann et al., 2009) and other adjustment difficulties (e.g., Campbell et al., 2006; Tremblay, 2000) throughout the first few decades of life. There are several prominent explanations for why young, aggressive children follow this development trajectory. In one of these explanations, researchers have proposed a developmental pathway model to describe progressions over time in aggression, based on escalating severity. As described by these authors, there are three pathways: covert, authority conflict, and overt. The covert pathway involves a progression from relatively minor, secretive behaviors in early adolescence (e.g., shoplifting) to increasingly serious property-focused crimes in mid-adolescence (e.g., vandalism, fire setting), and then to even more serious property-focused crimes through the transition to adulthood such as fraud and burglary. With regard to the authority conflict pathway, younger children engage in a variety of oppositional and defiant behaviors (e.g., not listening to teachers) and transition into more serious disobedience and truancy in adolescence. Youth who follow the overt pathway, however, escalate from provoking and bullying peers as children, to physical fighting in early adolescence, and then move to serious violence during later adolescence and the transition to adulthood – including assault and rape. It is important to note that these pathways are not conceptualized as being mutually exclusive. Thus, an individual can escalate through more than one of these pathways at the same time.

Focusing more on the overt pathway, as its focus on the development of aggression is of most relevance to the current review, research indicates that the overt pathway is associated with an increased risk of later violence (e.g., Gorman-Smith & Loeber, 2005). Factors that predicted whether youth would escalate along this overt pathway and later commit violent offenses in young adulthood included psychopathic traits (Jolliffe et al., 2016; Pardini et al., 2014), physical abuse, parental stress, association with deviant friends, and low school motivation (Ahonen et al., 2015). Factors predicting which youth managed to exit the overt pathways have also started to be identified and include better self-regulation skills, supportive friendships, parental warmth, positive relationships with teachers, and a stronger sense of personal responsibility. While self-regulation skills and personal responsibility seemed to serve as protective factors across large periods of development, the importance of many other protective factors has been found to vary with development. For example, parental warmth in early adolescence, but not late adolescence, reduces the likelihood of engaging in violence in young adulthood. Additionally, although having supportive friends in early adolescence increases the likelihood of violence in young adulthood, having supportive friends in late adolescence decreases the likelihood of violence perpetration in young adulthood. Many of the factors associated with "exiting" this overt pathway can be targeted in prevention programming (e.g., self-regulation skills, a sense of personal responsibility) and thus should be highlighted in prevention curriculum in various age groups in developmentally sensitive manners.

In another potential explanation, when subtle neurological deficits (e.g., low verbal intelligence, difficult temperament) and family adversity co-occur in early development, these factors increase the risk of life-course persistent antisocial and aggressive behaviors. Alternatively, Patterson et al. (1989) have proposed that children on what is called the "early-starter pathway" to antisocial and aggressive behaviors are inadvertently trained to engage in coercive behaviors through faulty parenting practices, and later in development, through interactions with deviant peers. These early parenting practices in early childhood and deviant peer associations in adolescence are both thought to reinforce persistent problematic behaviors. Both of these explanations have since received extensive support (see Moffitt, 2007; Reid et al., 2002 for reviews). Thus, it is worth considering that primary prevention in the younger grades includes parents and guardians as well, at least in part, to begin to address some of these challenging parenting practices associated with persistent and increasing aggressive behavior. For example, parents could be offered free parenting seminars on bullying or on coping with challenging child behaviors.

Changes in the Forms and Functions of Aggressive Behaviors with Development

Recent research has also begun to establish that the distinction between the forms and functions of aggression seems to emerge relatively early in development and might point to more developmentally nuanced factors that could be considered by intervention efforts. More specifically, the distinctions between reactive and proactive (e.g., Jia et al., 2014) and relational and physical aggression (e.g., Ostrov et al., 2006) have been established in children as young as aged 3–6 years old. Just as age-specific developmental tasks and relationship context variations are important to consider with regard to the development of prevention programs, they are also important to consider when understanding the manifestation of aggressive behavior (cf. Boxer et al., 2005).

For example, during the preschool years, it appears that physical aggression precedes and is replaced by the use of relational aggression, as many forms of relational aggression require better verbal abilities and closer relationships. Having an older sibling who engages in relational aggression is also associated with an increased likelihood of younger siblings engaging in relational aggression (Ostrov et al., 2006). In the preschool and early elementary school years, friendships also are typically formed over shared activities and proximity, and conflicts tend to be focused on objects such as toys. Conflict among friends is theorized to be an important social and cognitive learning experience (Chen et al., 2001; Keltner et al., 2001; Mills & Carwile, 2009), and it is common among friends throughout childhood (Barnett et al., 2004). That said, children who engage in a high frequency of conflict with their friends may be at an increased risk for later challenges with aggression. To illustrate, Salvas et al. (2014) found that the frequency of conflicts during early elementary school predicts later involvement in some forms of aggressive behavior (physical aggression for boys), if certain other characteristics of friendship support are not also present.

As children transition into and through middle childhood (approximately 8 through 12 years of age), friendship not only continues to be based on shared activities and proximity but also expands to include a focus on the affective quality of the relationship and to perceptions of loyalty and commitment. During this time, the focus of peer conflicts shifts from conflicts over objects to conflicts over control of other's behaviors (Murphy & Eisenberg, 2002).

Overall, more direct forms of physical aggression continue to decrease or remain infrequent for most children during middle childhood (Dodge et al., 2006), in part, because of a developing awareness that this form of aggressive behavior is associated with relationship difficulties with peers, (e.g., Kawabata et al., 2014). However, there also remains a small group of children, primarily boys, who continue to exhibit high levels of physical aggression, which is predictive of long-term antisocial behaviors (Broidy et al., 2003). While it was once thought that declines in direct physical aggression during middle childhood were replaced by more covert and relational forms of aggressive behavior at this developmental period (Björkqvist et al., 1992), when examining physical and relational forms of aggression within individuals, it appears this is not the case. Though there are decreasing rates of one form of aggression, and not the other in some youth, the two types of aggression remain highly correlated. Further, changes in rates of one form of aggression during this period in development tend to mirror changes in rates of other forms of aggression in most (Côté et al., 2007; Orpinas et al., 2015; Underwood et al., 2009). Thus, there seems to be more homotypic continuity in the use of specific forms of aggression during middle childhood than once thought at this developmental stage.

Still, the use of relational aggression increases across time in many children. This is likely due to several factors. For example, throughout early and middle childhood, teachers (Bauman & Del Rio, 2006; Swit et al., 2018; Yoon & Kerber, 2003; Yoon et al., 2016) and parents (e.g., Goldstein & Boxer, 2013; Swit et al., 2018) differentially punish physical versus relational aggression, laying down much harsher punishments for physical aggression. Children internalize these messages, and by early adolescence believe that relational aggression is less wrong than physical aggression and less under the authority of adults (Goldstein & Tisak, 2006). Additionally, relational aggression has been associated with some positive aspects of peer status such as acceptance and mutual friendships (Kawabata et al., 2014; Tseng et al., 2013), even if this aggression also has some social costs or negative consequences (e.g., Grills & Ollendick, 2010; Gunn III & Goldstein, 2017; Klomek et al., 2008).

In recent decades, electronic devices with internet access have increasingly become a more central context for social interactions for children during middle childhood and adolescence, and like any other context in which youth interact, aggression can be problematic. Though research on cyber aggression is just emerging, it seems that cyberbullying, a form of cyber aggression, is associated more strongly with proactive, rather than reactive, aggression, but some aspects of cyber aggression, such as aggressive messaging and posting embarrassing photos, have been linked to more traditional aspects of reactive aggression (Law et al., 2012). It has also been discussed that reactive aggression may manifest differently as cyber aggression because of the opportunity to revisit the offending comments/threats multiple times online (e.g., revisiting a defamatory social media page; see Goldstein, 2016 for a discussion).

As youth move into adolescence, friendships become more intimate and emotionally supportive, and take up an increasing amount of time and focus. Gender differences in friendship maintenance become fairly striking during adolescence. For example, whereas girls may tend to focus on conversation and discourse (often about other people and relationships), boys' friendships have a greater emphasis on shared activities. Interestingly, youth who are relatively high in proactive aggression seem to also have increased peer influence and dominance, and maybe even be viewed as more attractive (Pellegrini & Long, 2007). Similarly, during adolescence, youth who are perceived as being popular by their peers are also relatively likely to be relationally aggressive, highlighting the potentially socially instrumental implications of aggression (Kawabata et al., 2014; Smith et al., 2009). Thus, programming efforts should be mindful of this challenge, in that some youth may be reluctant to desist from a behavior that is socially rewarding or that is *perceived to be* socially rewarding in others.

Additionally, youth begin to be interested in developing and maintaining romantic relationships during adolescence, even though these early relationships are typically transient and fluid (e.g., Meier & Allen, 2009). The move toward finding other peers physically and romantically attractive may occur well before appropriate romantic approach behavior has been learned and may co-occur at a time of increased susceptibility to peer influence, thus setting the stage for engagement in sexually harassing behaviors. Goldstein et al. (2020) found that early adolescents who were relatively high in susceptibility to peer influence were also more likely to sexually harass their peers. Relational aggression remains a common strategy in romantic relationships throughout adolescence and young adulthood (Goldstein et al., 2008), and is associated with lower levels of relationship satisfaction and security (Linder et al., 2002).

With the increased interest in romantic relationships dating violence also becomes a concern during adolescence and young adulthood. For example, dating violence has been recorded in youth as young as 13 years of age (Wolitzky-Taylor et al., 2008), and an earlier sexual debut is one of the more consistent risk factors for dating violence (Halpern et al., 2009). The risk of dating violence increases with age into young adulthood (Howard et al., 2007; Wolitzky-Taylor et al., 2008), especially as the number of sexual partners increases (Halpern et al., 2009). While engaging in antisocial behaviors (Howard et al., 2007) and prior associations with violent and antisocial peers (Gagne et al., 2005) are both associated with a greater likelihood of dating violence, having better quality relationships with peers and better conflict resolution skills are associated with a lower likelihood of being involved in dating violence (Linder & Collins, 2005). As noted previously, this evidence suggests that school-based programs targeting older teens and college students must also include a focus on romantic relationships.

Implications for Primary Prevention

The above-discussed research highlights the importance of attending to the fairly complex interweaving of form, function, and youth developmental status for the prevention program developer. One approach has been to select children for prevention programming if they show any early signs of potentially challenging aggressive behavior (e.g., kindergarten). Starting in preschool, school-based programs have been developed to help young children develop social and emotional skills that have been shown to reduce the likelihood of aggression (Bierman et al., 2008; Domitrovich et al., 2007). Other programs, in turn, have been revised to include parenting components (Webster-Stratton & Reid, 2010). Other approaches target relatively mild forms of aggression which can be fairly common at a variety of ages across development (e.g., name calling, peer exclusion), and more recently, there has been a movement toward developing interventions that are more sensitive to the different types of aggression. For example, in addition to addressing risk factors for physical aggression, the friend-to-friend intervention includes material designed to address relationally aggressive behaviors among girls, and it has shown some success (Leff et al., 2015, 2016).

The critical call for primary prevention program developers is to consider carefully what forms and functions of aggression are most relevant for youth in their current stage of development. To illustrate, programming aimed at preschoolers should focus on concrete, easily observable social and physical behaviors that are developmentally relevant (e.g., for this age group, it is relevant to discuss sharing, social inclusion, identifying and regulating big emotions like anger and frustration). Likewise, focusing on targeted behaviors such as resolving conflicts about sharing would be well below the zone of proximal development for high-school students. In this age group, it would be appropriate to discuss more covert and circuitous behaviors such as rumor spreading and displaying romantic interest in a socially appropriate and respective manner and how to take "no" for an answer.

Sexual Harassment and Harassment Based on Gender, Race, or Sexual Orientation

Youth begin to feel physically attracted to others approximately 2 years before the pubertal process begins (McClintock & Herdt, 1996). Over the course of the next several years, leading up to the early teen years, youth must learn to address these new and strange feelings in a way that is emotionally and physically safe for themselves and others. Fledgling romantic relationships can begin as early as the middle school years, although early intense romantic relationships are linked to other forms of risky behavior such as substance use and problem behavior (Neemann et al., 1995). Most relevant to the current chapter, though, are the unrequited crushes and desires that may be expressed in inappropriate and harassing ways. Sexual harassment, defined here as unwelcome and unwanted sexual or romantic attention (see Goldstein et al., 2007), becomes a challenge when young teens have not been educated and socialized in terms of how to approach a potential romantic interest in a respectful manner where "no" is clearly understood, acknowledged, and acted upon. Sexual harassment has been associated with an array of negative psychosocial consequences disproportionately impacting girls. Girls, as compared to boys, are relatively more likely to be victimized by sexual harassment (Goldstein et al., 2007; Gruber & Fineran, 2016; Schnoll et al., 2015). Additionally, girls are at particular risk for negative implications including substance use, objectified body consciousness, lowered self-esteem, and self-injury (e.g., Goldstein et al., 2007; Lindberg et al., 2007). Boys are not immune to the negative consequences of sexual harassment, rather; they are just less likely to be victims and if they are at lower risk for associated challenges. Given this pattern of evidence, it is clear that prevention programming aimed at middle school-aged youth and older should incorporate psychoeducational resources regarding appropriate displays of romantic interest. Youth may have been socialized to assertively pursue their romantic interests – this has been embedded in media depictions of romance stories, depicting male dominance and persuasion (e.g., Ybarra et al., 2014). Thus, especially with younger adolescents, sexual harassment may be enacted when the intent is not actually to harm the victim but rather to get them to change their minds about romantic interests. Young teens may also succumb to peer pressure to assertively pursue their intended romantic interest; data suggest that those early adolescents who are most susceptible to peer influence are also the most likely to sexually harass (Goldstein et al., 2020). Unfortunately, the implications for the victim are likely quite similar, whether the intent was to harm or to acquire a relationship. Victimization by sexual harassment is tied to an array of mental health challenges as well as declines in academic motivation (Chiodo et al., 2009; Goldstein et al., 2007). When one is worried about getting catcalled while walking to one's locker, it is challenging to focus on schoolwork. Thus, addressing sexual harassment and working to prevent it are clearly indicated as important parts of school-based aggression prevention programming. It is also important to not wait until high school to address this issue –programmers and school districts should address it early and often from middle school age on up.

In addition to including sexual harassment prevention programming in school-based programs, it is important to address other issues of diversity and tolerance as well. For example, sexual minority youth (youth who identify as having same-sex attraction) or gender-questioning or transitioning youth are at an increased risk for peer victimization, as compared to their peers (Berlan et al., 2010; LeVasseur et al., 2013; Russell & Joyner, 2001). This increased likelihood of victimization, compounded by other social stressors including the stress of minority status (Meyer, 2015) and potential challenges with social support (Safren & Pantalone, 2006), are linked to an increased risk for mental health challenges in this group, including an increased risk of suicidal thoughts and behavior (Gunn III & Goldstein, 2017).

In addition to victimization based on sexual orientation or gender identity, race or class may serve as a target for peer-based aggression and harassment (Fisher et al., 2000; Russell et al., 2012). Like other forms of bullying and aggression, race-based incidences are associated with increased mental health challenges and increased academic and social risks (Wong et al., 2003). Positive racial socialization messages might help mitigate some of these negative experiences with peer aggression and institutionalized discrimination (Mallett & Swim, 2009), but it is clearly preferable to have these negative experiences not happen in the first place. The recent increase in the visibility of the Black Lives Matter Movement (Kershner, 2020) might yield an increased focus on race-based discrimination and bullying in the media and in various mental health promotion projects. We would urge that this attention be sustained and that these factors stay central in prevention and intervention programs. These experiences may be especially salient during adolescence when peers take on increased prominence in youths' day-to-day activities and in the development of self-concept and self-competence (Feiring & Lewis, 1991). Moreover, it is during adolescence when youth start to link aspects of their identity to their prospects for future success (Eccles, 2009). Thus, it is especially urgent that prevention programming during adolescence targets not only traditional aggression and bullying, but also the critical topics of institutionalized racism, tolerance, diversity, and civil rights. It is important that these efforts are undertaken regardless of the ethnic/racial composition of the school, as lessons about diversity and tolerance as a part of comprehensive violence prevention programs can serve to promote positive outcomes throughout development.

Cyberbullying and Internet-Based Harassment

With the rise in the availability of electronic devices and online spaces, there are many new avenues through which youth can act aggressively (Cassidy et al., 2013). Features of cyber aggression can contribute to a sense of desperation among victims who are limited in their ability to escape, defend themselves, or seek help. Many victims of cyberbullying also experience other forms of bullying (Waasdorp & Bradshaw, 2015). Cyberbullies can use expertise in technology to exert power over and publically humiliate their victims (Perren et al., 2012). Incidents of cyber aggression can occur any time and any place that a person can be online, both on and off school grounds, and even anonymously (Juvonen & Gross, 2008; Tokunaga, 2010). Via reposts, forwarding, and "likes" of damaging messages or pictures, cyber aggression can quickly spread and be reinforced throughout a school community, allowing repeated trauma for the victim (Dooley et al., 2009; Kowalski et al., 2014; Machackova & Pfetsch, 2016). Because it is rare for bystanders of cyber aggression to intervene by comforting the victim, confronting the bully, or reporting the incident to an authority figure or adult (Dillon & Bushman, 2015; Huang & Chou, 2010), an impression of tacit peer approval can be formed (Bastiaensens et al., 2014). Unfortunately, many of these same features have the potential to make cyber aggression difficult for schools and the legal system to identify and control (Patchin & Hinduja, 2012).

Prior research has identified characteristics that are common among those involved in cyber aggression. Adolescents who are involved in cyber aggression (i.e., as perpetrators, victims, or both) report more time online, more online game use, and more exposure to violent media compared to adolescents who are not involved (Baldry et al., 2015; Chang et al., 2015; Chen et al., 2017). Sharing personal information or photos and "friending" online strangers have been identified as risky online behaviors that are more common among victims of cyberbullying (Kwan & Skoric, 2013). As is the case with other methods of aggression, cyber aggression is also predicted by peer norms (Ang et al., 2017; Dang & Liu, 2020) and moral disengagement (Meter & Bauman, 2018). Cyberbullying victimization is associated with a variety of negative psychosocial and academic outcomes (e.g., low self-esteem, depression, anxiety, academic underachievement, absenteeism, and suicidal ideation) even after controlling for offline victimization (Giumetti & Kowalski, 2016; Kowalski et al., 2019).

More research is needed to identify risk and protective factors for cyberbullying within the school context; however, preliminary evidence suggests that cyberbullying is more common in schools without clear rules to address it and in schools that are perceived by students as unsafe or having a negative climate and little teacher support (Álvarez-García et al., 2015; Baldry et al., 2015; Bottino et al., 2015; Kowalski et al., 2014; Lee et al., 2018). Because offline bullying is associated with cyberbullying victimization, researchers have recommended that prevention efforts for cyberbullying begin with improving school climate to reduce offline bullying. There also have been calls for educating students and parents about risky online behaviors, internet safety, and guidelines for ethical and prosocial online behaviors (Lee et al., 2018; Perren et al., 2012; Sabella et al., 2013). Youth begin to engage regularly with technology as early as 3–4 years of age and report perpetration of and victimization by cyberbullying as early as 6–7 years of age, yet prevention and intervention programs for students under the age of 11 are not common (Kowalski et al., 2019; Tanrikulu, 2018). Prevention efforts may therefore need to be expanded and tailored to address the developmental needs of younger children.

Theories of Aggressive Behavior and Violence

Any primary prevention effort targeting aggression should be grounded in a strong developmental theoretical framework that allows for a clear specification of risk factors, quantifiable indicators of behavioral outcomes, and well-elaborated internal mediating mechanisms that account for changes in behavior over time (Boxer & Dubow, 2001; Hunter et al., 2001). Many school-based prevention programs target individual behaviors and social functioning but it is important to acknowledge that aggressive behavior develops in a broad social-ecological context (e.g., Smith et al., 2005). Contemporary theorizing on the development of aggressive behavior has focused extensively on internal cognitive and emotional mechanisms in the stimulation and expression of aggressive behavioral responses. For example, the social-cognitive information-processing (SCIP) view (Boxer et al., 2005; Dodge, 2006; Huesmann, 1998) asserts broadly that the way youth process social information plays a central role in the emergence and subsequent persistence of aggressive behavior. According to SCIP, in any social conflict situation, the process by which a youth initially attends to and interprets environmental cues, searches for and evaluates potential behavioral responses, and then evaluates the consequences of the chosen responses is central to explaining whether the specific behavior enacted will become an enduring style of behavioral response. According to the emotion regulatory (ER) framework, the critical determinant of behavioral styles over time is the extent to which children appropriately manage and express their emotional arousal (Eisenberg et al., 2001; Eisenberg & Morris, 2002; also see Frick & Morris, 2004). In particular, the ER view emphasizes the importance of effortful control over emotional arousal in accounting for habitual behavior. Children unable to regulate appropriately their negative arousal, and especially their angry arousal, are more prone to developing aggressive behavioral styles. Whereas both of these perspectives suggest that critical targets for prevention services – teaching better social problem-solving or training effective arousal management, for example – neither draw into full consideration the broader context in which prevention programming might occur.

Recently, Boxer and colleagues (Boxer et al., 2020) showed that violent crimes occurring in neighborhoods around school buildings (coded geospatially from police reports) were significantly linked to aggregate academic outcomes (based on proficiency rates in English and Math learning) in those buildings, even after controlling for the economic disadvantage of the school community. This effect is consistent with other theory-driven research that has shown the consistent impact of the larger ecological context in shaping children's individual outcomes related to aggressive behavior (Boxer et al., 2013), even at the level of internal mediating mechanisms such as social cognition (Guerra et al., 2003) and emotion regulation (Niwa et al., 2016). All of this work is aligned with a general ecological perspective on human development (Bronfenbrenner, 1979, 2005). Indeed, aggression is a learned behavior, which therefore can be unlearned (Eron, 1987), and it is imperative for prevention practitioners to take into account all the possible sources of observational and direct learning of aggression that could be brought to bear on children. A complete and current theoretical framing of aggressive behavior integrates both personal, individual social and psychological process with contextual conditions and circumstances (Guerra & Huesmann, 2004; Anderson & Bushman, 2002). Importantly, contemporary best-practice recommendations related to the prevention of aggression (at all levels – primary and universal, secondary and selected, and tertiary and indicated prevention) incorporate school-communitywide programming along with classroom or individual programming. These might include whole-school approaches (Olweus & Limber, 2010) or whole-community approaches that include schools (David-Ferdon et al., 2016).

Future Research and Evidence-Based Applications of Research to Practice

School intervention efforts must take a comprehensive approach to effectively implement school violence prevention programs. One such aspect to this approach is to consider the makeup of the student population and ensure that the prevention efforts align with the cultural, social, and developmental characteristics of the population of focus (Cawood, 2012). For example, implementing technological strategies such as computer programs may be effective for younger elementary aged children (Scheckner & Rollin, 2003), whereas intervention efforts for adolescents should incorporate self-awareness, managing negative emotions, effect problem-solving skills, and self-care strategies (Kongsuwan et al., 2012). It is also important to take into account school size, school location, and the grade level(s) present within the school building (Nickerson & Spears, 2007). Another aspect to the comprehensive approach involves assessing internal school factors such as the relationship between students and their school environment (Johnson et al., 2011), as the makeup of the school environment plays a role in deterring school aggression and violence (Cobbina et al., 2019). As such, it is essential to assess the relationship between students and staff.

School violence prevention teams should include a multidisciplinary team of professionals who can effectively collaborate and utilize their unique expertise to effectively aid in prevention efforts (Eklund et al., 2017). It is important to consider which stakeholders are integral in program development and implementation prior to the actual intervention (Kongsuwan et al., 2012). Teachers are an integral part and often the first to encounter violent and aggressive acts among students (Cobbina et al., 2019; Sela-Shayovitz, 2009). As such, they should actively participate in school violence prevention training programs (Sela-Shayovitz, 2009). Additionally, the presence of Student Resource Officers (SROs) and School Security Guards are the important aspects for school safety and prevention efforts (Cobbina et al., 2019). However, it should be noted that it is not enough to just have Security Guards and SROs present, they need to build and establish rapport that is founded on genuine care and concern for the safety and well-being of the students (Johnson et al., 2011). It is also important that those who are leading and facilitating the school violence prevention efforts are able to relate to the students and establish a collaborative environment where the students are included as part of the change process (Fawson et al., 2016; Nickerson & Spears, 2007). Establishing a collaborative setting where students feel valued and respected and have input is vital for program success (Fawson et al., 2016).

School social workers, school psychologist, and school counselors should be at the forefront of these intervention efforts as they play a vital role in shaping the social-emotional development of youth (Cawood, 2012; Nickerson & Spears, 2007). Unfortunately, school mental health professionals are often bombarded with large caseloads of students making it difficult to manage some of the intricate details necessary for effective school violence prevention efforts (Cawood, 2012). As such, school systems need to increase the number of school mental health professionals that are available to service the students (Cawood, 2012; Nickerson & Spears, 2007). School systems should also provide staff with regular professional development focused on school violence prevention efforts (McAdams et al., 2011; McKellar & Sherwin, 2003; Sela-Shayovitz, 2009).

It should be noted that institutions that prepare school mental health professionals need to ensure that their curricula are effective in preparing these professionals to intervene and provide support with regard to school violence prevention (Cawood, 2012; McAdams et al., 2011; McKellar & Sherwin, 2003). It is also equally important that teacher preparation programs have components of their curricula that focus on the teacher's role in school violence prevention programs (Sela-Shayovitz, 2009). Curricula should focus on (1) providing education around school violence prevention and (2) providing opportunities to engage in fieldwork or practicum experiences where hands-on training can be acquired (McAdams et al., 2011; McKellar & Sherwin, 2003).

In addition to the aforementioned factors, the external school factors of parental and community involvement (Cuellar, 2016) are equally important. Parental and community involvement is critical to effective school violence prevention efforts (Cuellar, 2016; Nickerson & Spears, 2007; Song et al., 2018). Parental involvement is instrumental in promoting positive behaviors and assisting in school violence prevention efforts (Cuellar, 2016; Nickerson & Spears, 2007; Song et al., 2018). While community involvement is important, the types of community involvement, as well as the role of community stakeholders' involvements are equally important (Song et al., 2018). For example, having law enforcement officials visit the school only in response to a negative behavior or situation is not beneficial and can actually increase school violence (Song et al., 2018). However, collaborations with colleges and universities may help to aid in school violence and aggressive behavior intervention efforts (Haymes et al., 2003). Additionally, school systems that collaborate with professional evaluators that assist in assessing the effectiveness of the school violence prevention program (Cawood, 2012; Riley & Segal, 2002) can be beneficial to program success.

Effective school violence prevention programs have shown results of decreased depression rates, a decrease in aggressive attitudes and behaviors, and shown improvements in students implementing nonviolent strategies and positive coping skills (Kongsuwan et al., 2012; Lim et al., 2018; Scheckner & Rollin, 2003). Utilizing a variety of means to gather and assess students as well as disseminating the information is essential (Fawson et al., 2016; Kongsuwan et al., 2012). For example, informative online educational programs designed to increase student knowledge, understanding, and awareness have been shown to be an effective method of school violence prevention (Stohlman & Cornell, 2019). Moreover, administering these programs across multiple sessions is effective (Fawson et al., 2016; Kongsuwan et al., 2012; Lim et al., 2018; Scheckner & Rollin, 2003). Additionally, having a program that incorporates both disciplinary measures as well as educational and therapeutic supports is advantageous (Nickerson & Spears, 2007). Regardless of which types of methods are employed, it is imperative that school systems establish warm, welcoming, and supportive environments for students (Eklund et al., 2017).

Summary and Conclusion

This chapter has focused on the implications of developmental theory and research for primary prevention programming. As noted, it is critical that programming takes into consideration the cognitive, social, and physical aspects of human development that might impact programming efforts and a youth's ability to focus on program activities. Second, it is important for programming to focus on the individual and contextual factors associated with increased risk for aggression, and to be sensitive to changes in these risk factors over time during childhood and adolescence. Changes in relationship contexts over time should be incorporated into programming, as different social relationships change in salience throughout development (Lee et al., 2018). Similarly, research has highlighted changing salience of different forms of aggression at various points in development and in different relationship contexts, and as a function of social opportunity (Cillessen & Mayeux, 2004). These social developmental factors should also be considered when establishing prevention programming. Finally, theory-driven research on the social-cognitive and emotional mediators of the link between risk factors for aggression and aggressive behavior suggests that programs should target these mediators. Theoretical work also underscores the importance of incorporating broader social-contextual factors into prevention programming.

Future research and practice should also consider the potential for various needs coming up to deliver programming online or in other creative, physically safe spaces such as outdoors or in a socially distanced, small group format. In 2020, it was COVID-19 that made this modification a necessity; however, in the future, it may be a different crisis. Thus, it is interesting and important for prevention programming to test the impact of traditionally implemented (face-to-face, non-socially distanced) material versus socially distanced or online programming. If programming would need to move online due to safety concerns, it is also important for programmers to ensure that participants have the electronic devices and connectivity necessary to fully participate. Regardless of the delivery mechanism, it is critical for developmental research and theory to be fully integrated into prevention programming. For maximum impact, prevention programming needs to be developmentally appropriate and relevant.

References

Ahonen, L., Loeber, R., & Pardini, D. (2015). The prediction of young homicide and violent offenders. *Justice Quarterly, 33*(7), 1265–1291. https://doi.org/10.1080/07418825.2015.1081263

Álvarez-García, D., Pérez, J. C. N., González, A. D., & Pérez, C. R. (2015). Risk factors associated with cybervictimization in adolescence. *International Journal of Clinical and Health Psychology, 15*(3), 226–235. https://doi.org/10.1016/j.ijchp.2015.03.002

Anderson, C. A., & Bushman, B. J. (2002). Human aggression. *Annual Review of Psychology, 53*, 27–51. https://doi.org/10.1146/annurev.psych.53.100901.135231

Anderson, C. A., & Huesmann, L. R. (2003). Human aggression: A social-cognitive view. In M. A. Hogg & J. Cooper (Eds.), *The handbook of social psychology, revised edition* (pp. 296–323). Sage Publications. (2007). Reprinted in M. A. Hogg & J. Cooper (Eds.) (pp. 259–287). The Sage Handbook of Social Psychology, London: Sage Publications. http://hdl.handle.net/2027.42/83427

Ang, R. P., Li, X., & Seah, S. L. (2017). The role of normative beliefs about aggression in the relationship between empathy and cyberbullying. *Journal of Cross-Cultural Psychology, 48*(8), 1138–1152. https://doi.org/10.1177/0022022116678928

Arnett, J. J. (2015). *Emerging adulthood: The winding road from the late teems through the twenties* (2nd ed.). Oxford University Press, Inc.

Arseneault, L., Bowes, L., & Shakoor, S. (2010). Bullying victimization in youths and mental health problems: 'Much ado about nothing'? *Psychological Medicine, 40*, 717–729. https://doi.org/10.1017/S0033291709991383

Arsenio, W. F., & Lemerise, E. A. (2004). Aggression and moral development: Integrating social information processing and moral domain models. *Child Development, 75*(4), 987–1002.

Baldry, A. C., Farrington, D. P., & Sorrentino, A. (2015). 'Am I at risk of cyberbullying'? A narrative review and conceptual framework for research on risk of cyberbullying and cybervictimization: The risk and needs assessment approach. *Aggression and Violent Behavior, 23*, 36–51.

Barker, E. D., Vitaro, F., Lacourse, E., Fontaine, N. M. G., Carbonneau, R., & Tremblay, R. (2010). Testing the developmental distinctiveness of male proactive and reactive aggression with a nested longitudinal experimental intervention. *Aggressive Behavior, 36*(2), 127–140. https://doi.org/10.2048/10.1002/ab.20337

Barnett, M. A., Burns, S. R., Sanborn, F. W., Bartel, J. S., & Wilds, S. J. (2004). Antisocial and prosocial teasing among children: Perceptions and individual differences. *Social Development, 13*(2), 292–310.

Bastiaensens, S., Vandebosch, H., Poels, K., Van Cleemput, K., DeSmet, A., & DeBourdeaudhuij, I. (2014). Cyberbullying on social network sites. An experimental study into bystanders' behavioural intentions to help the victim or reinforce the bully. *Computers in Human Behavior, 31*, 259–271. https://doi.org/10.1016/j.chb.2013.10.036

Bauman, S., & Del Rio, A. (2006). Preservice teachers' responses to bullying scenarios: Comparing physical, verbal, and relational bullying. *Journal of Educational Psychology, 98*(1), 219–231. https://doi.org/10.1037/0022-0663.98.1.219

Berlan, E. D., Corliss, H. L., Field, A. E., Goodman, E., & Austin, S. B. (2010). Sexual orientation and bullying among adolescents in the growing up today study. *Journal of Adolescent Health, 46*(4), 366–371.

Bierman, K., Domitrovich, C., & Gill, S. (2008). Promoting academic and social-emotional school readiness: The Head Start REDI program. *Child Development, 79*(6), 1802–1817. https://doi.org/10.1111/j.1467-8624.2008.01227.x

Björkqvist, K., Lagerspetz, K. M., & Kaukiainen, A. (1992). Do girls manipulate and boys fight? Developmental trends in regard to direct and indirect aggression. *Aggressive Behavior, 18*(2), 117–127. https://doi.org/10.1002/1098-2337(1992)18:2<117::AID-AB2480180205>3.0.CO;2-3

Bottino, S. M. B., Bottino, C., Regina, C. G., Correia, A. V. L., & Ribeiro, W. S. (2015). Cyberbullying and adolescent mental health: Systematic review. *Cadernos De Saude Publica, 31*, 463–475. https://doi.org/10.1590/0102-311X00036114

Bowlby, J. (1969). *Attachment and loss. Volume I: Attachment*. Hogarth Press.

Boxer, P., & Dubow, E. F. (2001). A social-cognitive information-processing model for school-based aggression reduction and prevention programs: Issues for research and practice. *Applied and Preventive Psychology, 10*(3), 177–192.

Boxer, P., Goldstein, S. E., Musher-Eizenman, D., Dubow, E. F., & Heretick, D. (2005). Developmental issues in the prevention of school aggression from the social-cognitive perspective. *Journal of Primary Prevention, 26*, 383–400.

Boxer, P., Musher-Eizenman, D., Dubow, E. F., Danner, S., & Heretick, D. M. (2006). Assessing teachers' perceptions for school-based aggression prevention programs: Applying a cognitive-ecological framework. *Psychology in the Schools, 43*(3), 331–344.

Boxer, P., Huesmann, L. R., Dubow, E. F., Landau, S., Gvirsman, S. D., Shikaki, K., & Ginges, J. (2013). Exposure to violence across the social ecosystem and the development of aggression: A test of ecological theory in the Israeli-Palestinian conflict. *Child Development, 84*, 163–177.

Boxer, P., Drawve, G., & Caplan, J. M. (2020). Neighborhood violent crime and academic performance: A geospatial analysis. *American Journal of Community Psychology, 65*, 343–352.

Broidy, L. M., Nagin, D. S., Tremblay, R. E., Bates, J. E., Brame, B., Dodge, K. A., Fergusson, D., Horwood, J. L., Loeber, R., Laird, R., Lynam, D. R., Moffitt, T. E., Pettit, G. S., & Vitarao, F. (2003). Developmental trajectories of childhood disruptive behaviors and adolescent delinquency: A six-site, cross-national study. *Developmental Psychology, 39*(2), 222–245. https://doi.org/10.1037/0012-1649.39.2.222

Bronfenbrenner, U. (1979). *The ecology of human development: Experiments by nature and design*. Harvard University Press.

Bronfenbrenner, U. (Ed.). (2005). *Making human beings human: Bioecological perspectives on human development*. Sage Publications Ltd..

Bronfenbrenner, U., & Evans, G. W. (2000). Developmental science in the 21st century: Emerging questions, theoretical models, research designs and empirical findings. *Social Development, 9*(1), 115–125. https://doi.org/10.1111/1467-9507.00114

Bronfenbrenner, U., & Morris, P. A. (2006). The bioecological model of human development. In R. M. Lerner & W. Damon (Eds.), *Handbook of child psychology: Theoretical models of human development* (pp. 793–828). Wiley.

Brugman, S., Lobbestael, J., Arntz, A., Cima, M., Schuhmann, T., & Dambacher, F. (2015). Identifying cognitive predictors of reactive and proactive aggression. *Aggressive Behavior, 41*(1), 51–64. https://doi.org/10.1002/ab.21573

Brunstein Klomek, A., Sourander, A., & Elonheimo, H. (2015). Bullying by peers in childhood and effects on psychopathology, suicidality, and criminality in adulthood. *The Lancet Psychiatry, 2*(10), 930–941.

Bundge, S. A., & Zelazo, P. D. (2006). A brain-based account of the development of rule use in childhood. *Current Directions in Psychological Science, 15,* 118–121.

Campbell, S. B., Spieker, S., Burchinal, M., & Poe, M. D. (2006). Trajectories of aggression from toddlerhood to age 9 predict academic and social functioning through age 12. *Journal of Child Psychology and Psychiatry, 47*(8), 791–800. https://doi.org/10.1111/j.1469-7610.2006.01636.x

Cassidy, W., Faucher, C., & Jackson, M. (2013). Cyberbullying among youth: A comprehensive review of current international research and its implications and application to policy and practice. *School Psychology International, 34*(6), 575–612. https://doi.org/10.1177/0143034313479697

Cawood, N. D. (2012). Addressing interpersonal violence in the school context: Awareness and use of evidence-supported programs. *Children & Schools, 35*(1), 41–52. https://doi.org/10.1093/cs/cds013

Chan, W. Y., Hollingsworth, M. A., Espelage, D. L., & Mitchell, K. J. (2016). Preventing violence in context: The importance of culture for implementing systemic change. *Psychology of Violence, 6*(1), 22. https://doi.org/10.1037/vio0000021

Chang, F. C., Chiu, C. H., Miao, N. F., Chen, P. H., Lee, C. M., Huang, T. F., & Pan, Y. C. (2015). Online gaming and risks predict cyberbullying perpetration and victimization in adolescents. *International Journal of Public Health, 60*(2), 257–266. https://doi.org/10.1007/s00038-014-0643-x

Chen, D. W., Fein, G. G., Killen, M., & Tam, H.-P. (2001). Peer conflicts of preschool children: Issues, resolution, incidence, and age-related patterns. *Early Education and Development, 12*(4), 523–544. https://doi.org/10.1207/s15566935eed1204_3

Chen, L., Ho, S. S., & Lwin, M. O. (2017). A meta-analysis of factors predicting cyberbullying perpetration and victimization: From the social cognitive and media effects approach. *New Media & Society, 19*(8), 1194–1213. https://doi.org/10.1177/1461444816634037

Chiodo, D., Wolfe, D. A., Crooks, C., Hughes, R., & Jaffe, P. (2009). Impact of sexual harassment victimization by peers on subsequent adolescent victimization and adjustment: A longitudinal study. *Journal of Adolescent Health, 45*(3), 246–252.

Cillessen, A. H. N., & Mayeux, L. (2004). From censure to reinforcement: Developmental changes in the association between aggression and social status. *Child Development, 75,* 147–163.

Cobbina, J. E., Galasso, M., Cunningham, M., Melde, C., & Heinze, J. (2019). A qualitative study of perception of school safety among youth in a high crime city. *Journal of School Violence, 19*(3), 277–291. https://doi.org/10.1080/15388220.2019.1677477

Côté, S., Vaillancourt, T., Barker, E. D., Nagin, D., & Tremblay, R. E. (2007). The joint development of physical and indirect aggression: Predictors of continuity and change during childhood. *Development and Psychopathology, 19*(1), 37–53. https://doi.org/10.1017/S0954579407070034

Cuellar, M. J. (2016). School safety strategies and their effects on the occurrence of school-based violence in U.S. high schools: An exploratory study. *Journal of School Violence, 17*(1), 28–45. https://doi.org/10.1080/15388220.2016.1193742

Dambacher, F., Schuhmann, T., Lobbestael, J., Arntz, A., Brugman, S., & Sack, A. T. (2015). Reducing proactive aggression through non-invasive brain stimulation. *Social Cognitive and Affective Neuroscience, 10*(10), 1303–1310. https://doi.org/10.1093/scan/nsv018

Dang, J., & Liu, L. (2020). When peer norms work? Coherent groups facilitate normative influences on cyber aggression. *Aggressive Behavior.* https://doi.org/10.1002/ab.21920

David-Ferdon, C., Vivolo-Kantor, A. M., Dahlberg, L. L., Marshall, K. J., Rainford, N., & Hall, J. E. (2016). *A comprehensive technical package for the prevention of youth violence and associated risk behaviors*. National Center for Injury Prevention and Control, Centers for Disease Control and Prevention.

Dawes, M. (2017). Early adolescents' social goals and school adjustment. *Social Psychology of Education, 20*, 299–328. https://doi.org/10.1007/s11218-017-9380-3

DeMarie-Dreblow, D., & Miller, P. H. (1988). The development of children's strategies for selective attention: Evidence for a transitional period. *Child Development, 59*, 1504–1513.

Diamond, A., Kirkham, N., & Amso, D. (2002). Conditions under which young children can hold two rules in mind and inhibit a prepotent response. *Developmental Psychology, 38*, 352–361.

Dillon, K. P., & Bushman, B. J. (2015). Unresponsive or un-noticed?: Cyberbystander intervention in an experimental cyberbullying context. *Computers in Human Behavior, 45*, 144–150. https://doi.org/10.1016/j.chb.2014.12.009

Dodge, K. A. (2006). Translational science in action: Hostile attributional style and the development of aggressive behavior problems. *Development and Psychopathology, 18*(3), 791.

Dodge, K. A., Coie, J. D., & Lynam, D. (2006). Aggression and antisocial behavior in youth. In W. Damon & N. Eisenberg (Eds.), *Handbook of child psychology* (Vol. 3, pp. 719–788). Wiley.

Dominguez, S., & Trawick-Smith, J. (2018). A qualitative study of the play of dual language learners in an English-speaking preschool. *Early Childhood Education Journal, 46*, 577–586. https://doi.org/10.1007/s10643-018-0889-7

Domitrovich, C., Cortes, R., & Greenberg, M. (2007). Improving young children's social and emotional competence: A randomized trial of the preschool 'PATHS' curriculum. *The Journal of Primary Prevention, 28*(2), 67–91. https://doi.org/10.1007/s10935-007-0081-0

Dooley, J. J., Pyżalski, J., & Cross, D. (2009). Cyberbullying versus face-to-face bullying: A theoretical and conceptual review. *Journal of Psychology, 217*, 182–188. https://doi.org/10.1027/0044-3409.217.4.182

Durlak, J. A., & Wells, A. M. (1997). Primary prevention mental health programs for children and adolescents: A meta-analytic review. *American Journal of Community Psychology, 25*, 115–152.

Eccles, J. (2009). Who am I and what am I going to do with my life? Personal and collective identities as motivators of action. *Educational Psychologist, 44*(2), 78–89.

Eccles, J. S., Lord, S. E., & Roeser, R. W. (1996). Round holes, square pegs, rocky roads, and sore feet: The impact of stage-environment fit on young adolescents' experiences in schools and families. In D. Cicchetti & S. L. Toth (Eds.), *Adolescence: Opportunities and challenges* (pp. 47–92). University of Rochester Press.

Eccles, J. S., Templeton, J., Barber, B., & Stone, M. (2003). Adolescence and emerging adulthood: The critical passageways to adulthood. In M. H. Bornstein, L. Davidson, C. L. M. Keyes, & K. A. Moore (Eds.), *Well-being: Positive development across the life course* (pp. 383–406). Lawrence Erlbaum Associates Publishers.

Eisenberg, N., & Morris, A. S. (2002). Children's emotion-related regulation. In R. V. Kail (Ed.), *Advances in child development and behavior* (Vol. 30, pp. 189–229). Academic Press.

Eisenberg, N., Cumberland, A., Spinrad, T. L., Fabes, R. A., Shepard, S. A., Reiser, M., et al. (2001). The relations of regulation and emotionality to children's externalizing and internalizing problem behavior. *Child Development, 72*(4), 1112–1134.

Eklund, K., Meyer, L., & Bosworth, K. (2017). Examining the role of school resource officers on school safety and crisis response teams. *Journal of School Violence, 17*(2), 139–151. https://doi.org/10.1080/15388220.2016.1263797

Eron, L. D. (1987). The development of aggressive behavior from the perspective of a developing behaviorism. *American Psychologist, 42*, 435–442.

Eshbaugh, E. M. (2010). Friend and family support as moderators of the effects of low romantic partner support on loneliness among college women. *Individual Differences Research, 8*, 8–16.

Euler, F., Steinlin, C., & Stadler, C. (2017). Distinct profiles of reactive and proactive aggression in adolescents: Associations with cognitive and affective empathy. *Child and Adolescent Psychiatry and Mental Health, 11*(1). https://doi.org/10.1186/s13034-0160141-4

Fawson, P. R., Broce, R., Bonner, B., & Wright, R. (2016). Adolescents' experiences: Programming implications for in-school violence prevention programs. *School Social Work Journal, 41*(1), 1–16.

Feiring, C., & Lewis, M. (1991). The transition from middle childhood to early adolescence: Sex differences in the social network and perceived self-competence. *Sex Roles, 24*, 489–509.

Fisher, C. B., Wallace, S. A., & Fenton, R. E. (2000). Discrimination distress during adolescence. *Journal of Youth and Adolescence, 29*(6), 679–695.

Frick, P. J., & Morris, A. S. (2004). Temperament and developmental pathways to conduct problems. *Journal of Clinical Child and Adolescent Psychology, 33*(1), 54–68.

Gagne, M., Lavoie, F., & Hebert, M. (2005). Victimization during childhood and revictimization in dating relationships in adolescent girls. *Child Abuse & Neglect, 29*(10), 1155–1172. https://doi.org/10.1016/j.chiabu.2004.11.009

Galen, B. R., & Underwood, M. K. (1997). A developmental investigation of social aggression among children. *Developmental Psychology, 33*(4), 589–600. https://doi.org/10.1037/0012-1649.33.4.589

Giumetti, G. W., & Kowalski, R. M. (2016). Cyberbullying matters: Examining the incremental impact of cyberbullying on outcomes over and above traditional bullying in North America. In *Cyberbullying across the globe* (pp. 117–130). Springer.

Goldstein, S. E. (2016). Adolescents' disclosure and secrecy about online behavior: Links with cyber, relational, and overt aggression. *Journal of Child and Family Studies, 25*, 1430–1440.

Goldstein, S. E., & Boxer, P. (2013). Parenting practices and the early socialization of relational aggression among preschoolers. *Early Child Development and Care, 183*(11), 1559–1575. https://doi.org/10.1080/03004430.2012.738200

Goldstein, S. E., & Tisak, M. S. (2006). Early adolescents' conceptions of parental and friend authority over relational aggression. *Journal of Early Adolescence, 26*(3), 344–364. https://doi.org/10.11777/0272431606288552

Goldstein, S. E., & Tisak, M. S. (2010). Early adolescents' social reasoning about relational aggression. *Journal of Child and Family Studies, 19*, 471–482.

Goldstein, S. E., Tisak, M. S., & Boxer, P. (2002). Preschoolers' normative and prescriptive judgments about relational and overt aggression. *Early Education and Development, 13*, 23–39.

Goldstein, S. E., Malanchuk, O., Davis-Kean, P. E., & Eccles, J. S. (2007). Risk factors for sexual harassment by peers: A longitudinal investigation of African American and European American adolescents. *Journal of Research on Adolescence, 17*, 285–300.

Goldstein, S. E., Chesir-Teran, D., & McFaul, A. (2008). Profiles and correlates of relational aggression in young adults' romantic relationships. *Journal of Youth and Adolescence, 37*(3), 251–265. https://doi.org/10.1007/s10964-007-9255-6

Goldstein, S. E., Boxer, P., & Rudolph, E. (2015). Middle school transition stress: Links with academic performance, motivation, and school experiences. *Contemporary School Psychology, 19*, 21–29.

Goldstein, S. E., Lee, C.-Y. S., Gunn, J. F., III, Bradley, S., Lummer, S., & Boxer, P. (2020). Susceptibility to peer influence during middle school: Links with social support, peer harassment, and gender. *Psychology in the Schools, 57*, 91–110.

Gorman-Smith, D., & Loeber, R. (2005). Are developmental pathways in disruptive behaviors the same for girls and boys? *Journal of Child and Family Studies, 14*(1), 15–27. https://doi.org/10.1007/s10826-005-1109-9

Grills, A. E., & Ollendick, T. H. (2010). Peer victimization, global self-worth, and anxiety in middle school children. *Journal of Clinical Child & Adolescent Psychology, 31*(1), 59–68.

Gruber, J., & Fineran, S. (2016). Sexual harassment, bullying, and school outcomes for high school girls and boys. *Violence Against Women, 22*(1), 112–133.

Guerra, N. G., & Huesmann, L. R. (2004). A cognitive-ecological model of aggression. *International Review of Social Psychology, 17*, 177–203.

Guerra, N. G., Huesmann, L. R., & Spindler, A. (2003). Community violence exposure, social cognition, and aggression among urban elementary school children. *Child Development, 74*, 1561–1576.

Guerra, N. G., Williams, K. R., & Sadek, S. (2011). Understanding bullying and victimization during childhood and adolescence: A mixed methods study. *Child Development, 82*(1), 295–310. https://doi.org/10.1111/j.1467-8624.2010.01556.x

Gunn, J. F., III, & Goldstein, S. E. (2017). Bullying and suicidal behavior during adolescence: A developmental perspective. *Adolescent Research Review, 2*(1), 77–97. https://doi.org/10.1007/s40894-016-0038-8

Hahn, R., Fuqua-Whitley, D., Wethington, H., Lowy, J., Crosby, A., Fullilove, M., Johnson, R., Moscicki, E., Price, L., Snyder, S. R., Tuma, F., Cory, S., Stone, G., Mukhopadhaya, K., Chattopadhyay, S., & Dahlberg, L. (2007). Effectiveness of universal school-based programs to prevent violent and aggressive behavior: A systematic review. *American Journal of Preventive Medicine, 33*(2 Suppl), S114–S129. https://doi.org/10.1016/j.amepre.2007.04.012

Halpern, C. T., Spriggs, A. L., Martin, S. L., & Kupper, L. L. (2009). Patterns of intimate partner violence victimization from adolescence to young adulthood in a nationally representative sample. *Journal of Adolescent Health, 45*(5), 508–516. https://doi.org/10.1016/j.jadohealth.2009.03.011

Harden, B. J., Panlilio, C., Morrison, C., Duncan, A. D., Duchene, M., & Clyman, R. B. (2017). Emotion regulation of preschool children in foster care: The influence of maternal depression and parenting. *Journal of Child and Family Studies, 26*, 1124–1134.

Haymes, E. B., Howe, E., & Peck, L. (2003). Whole-school violence prevention program: A university-public school collaboration. *Children & Schools, 25*(2), 121–127. https://doi.org/10.1093/cs/25.2.121

Hessler, D. M., & Fainsilber Katz, L. (2007). Children's emotion regulation: Self-report and physiological response to peer provocation. *Developmental Psychology, 43*(1), 27–38. https://doi.org/10.1037/0012-1649.43.1.27

Hinduja, S., & Patchin, J. W. (2010). Bullying, cyberbullying, and suicide. *Archives of Suicide Research, 14*(3), 206–221. https://doi.org/10.1080/13811118.2010.494133

Howard, D. E., Wang, M. Q., & Yan, F. (2007). Prevalence and psychosocial correlates of forced sexual intercourse among US high school adolescents. *Adolescence, 42*(168), 629–643.

Huang, Y.-Y., & Chou, C. (2010). An analysis of multiple factors of cyberbullying among junior high school students in Taiwan. *Computers in Human Behavior, 26*, 1581–1590. https://doi.org/10.1016/j.chb.2010.06.005

Hubbard, J. A., McAuliffe, M. D., Morrow, M. T., & Romano, L. J. (2010). Reactive and proactive aggression in children and adolescence: Precursors, outcomes, processes, experiences, and measurement. *Journal of Personality, 78*(1), 95–118. https://doi.org/10.1111/j.1467-6494.2009.00610.x

Hudley, C., & Graham, S. (1993). An attributional intervention to reduce peer-directed aggression among African-American boys. *Child Development, 64*, 124–138.

Huesmann, L. R. (1998). The role of social information processing and cognitive schema in the acquisition and maintenance of habitual aggressive behavior. In R. G. Geen & E. Donnerstein (Eds.), *Human aggression: Theories, research, and implications for social policy* (pp. 73–109). Academic Press. https://doi.org/10.1016/B978-012278805-5/50005-5

Huesmann, L. R., Eron, L. D., Lefkowitz, M. M., & Walder, L. O. (1984). Stability of aggression over time and generations. *Developmental Psychology, 20*(6), 1120.

Huesmann, L. R., Eron, L. D., & Dubow, E. F. (2002). Childhood predictors of adult criminality: Are all risk factors reflected in childhood aggressiveness? *Criminal Behaviour and Mental Health, 12*(3), 185–208.

Huesmann, L. R., Dubow, E. F., Eron, L. D., & Boxer, P. (2006). Middle Childhood Family-Contextual and Personal Factors as Predictors of Adult Outcomes. In A. C. Huston & M. N. Ripke (Eds.), Developmental contexts in middle childhood: Bridges to adolescence and adulthood (pp. 62–86). Cambridge University Press. https://doi.org/10.1017/CBO9780511499760.005

Huesmann, L. R., Dubow, E. F., & Boxer, P. (2009). Continuity of aggression from childhood to early adulthood as a predictor of life outcomes: Implications for the adolescent-limited and life-course-persistent models. *Aggressive Behavior, 35*(2), 136–149. https://doi.org/10.1002/ab.20300

Hunter, L., Elias, M. J., & Norris, J. (2001). School-based violence prevention: Challenges and lessons learned from an action research project. *Journal of School Psychology, 39*(2), 161–175.

Hwang, S., Machida, M., & Choi, Y. (2017). The effect of peer interaction on sport confidence and achievement goal orientation in youth sport. *Social Behavior and Personality, 45*(6), 1007–1018. https://doi.org/10.2224/sbp.6149

Jia, S., Wang, L., & Shi, Y. (2014). Relationship between parenting and proactive versus reactive aggression among Chinese preschool children. *Archives of Psychiatric Nursing, 28*(2), 152–157. https://doi.org/10.1016/j.apnu.2013.12.001

Johnson, S. L., Burke, J. G., & Gielen, A. C. (2011). Prioritizing the school environment in school violence prevention efforts. *Journal of School Health, 81*(6), 331–340. https://doi.org/10.1111/j.1746-1561.2011.00598.x

Jolliffe, D., Farrington, D. P., Loeber, R., & Pardini, D. (2016). Protective factors for violence: Results from the Pittsburgh Youth Study. *Journal of Criminal Justice, 45*, 32–40. https://doi.org/10.1016/j.jcrimjus.2016.02.007

Jones, D., Dodge, K. A., Foster, E. M., Nix, R., & Conduct Problems Prevention Research Group. (2002). Early identification of children at risk for costly mental health service use. *Prevention Science, 3*(4), 247–256.

Juvonen, J., & Gross, E. F. (2008). Extending the school grounds? Bullying experiences in cyberspace. *The Journal of School Health, 78*, 496–505. https://doi.org/10.1111/j.1746-1561.2008.00335.x

Kann, L., McManus, T., Harris, W. A., Shanklin, S. L., Flint, K. H., Queen, B., Lowry, R., Chyen, D., Whittle, L., Thornton, J., Lim, C., Bradford, D., Yamakawa, Y., Leon, M., Brener, N., & Ethier, K. A. (2018). Youth risk behavior surveillance — United States, 2017. *MMWR Surveillance Summary, 67*, 1–114. https://doi.org/10.15585/mmwr.ss6708a1

Kawabata, Y., Crick, N. R., & Hamaguchi, Y. (2013). The association of relational and physical victimization with hostile attribution bias, emotional distress, and depressive symptoms: A cross-cultural study. *Asian Journal of Social Psychology, 16*(4), 260–270. https://doi.org/10.1111/ajsp.12030

Kawabata, Y., Tseng, W. L., & Crick, N. R. (2014). Adaptive, maladaptive, mediational, and bidirectional processes of relational and physical aggression, relational and physical victimization, and peer liking. *Aggressive Behavior, 40*(3), 273–287. https://doi.org/10.1002/ab.21517

Keltner, D., Capps, L., Kring, A. M., Young, R. C., & Heerey, E. A. (2001). Just teasing: A conceptual analysis and empirical review. *Psychological Bulletin, 127*(2), 229–248. https://doi.org/10.1037//0033-2909.127.2.229

Kirova, A., & Jamison, N. M. (2018). Peer scaffolding techniques and approaches in preschool children's multiliteracy practices with iPads. *Journal of Early Childhood Research, 16*(3), 245–257.

Kloep, M., Hendry, L. B., Taylor, R., & Stuart-Hamilton, I. (2016). *Development from adolescence to early adulthood: A dynamic systematic approach to transitions and transformations.* Psychology Press.

Klomek, A. B., Marrocco, F., Kleinman, M., Schonfeld, I. S., & Gould, M. S. (2008). Peer victimization, depression, and suicidality in adolescents. *Suicide and Life-threatening Behavior, 38*(2), 166–180. https://doi.org/10.1521/suli.2008.38.2.166

Kokko, K., & Pulkkinen, L. (2005). Stability of aggressive behavior from childhood to middle age in women and men. *Aggressive Behavior: Official Journal of the International Society for Research on Aggression, 31*(5), 485–497.

Kongsuwan, V., Suttharangsee, W., Isaramalai, S., & Weiss, S. J. (2012). The development and effectiveness of a violence prevention program for Thai high school adolescents. *Pacific Rim International Journal of Nursing Research, 16*(3), 236–249.

Kowalski, R. M., & Limber, S. P. (2013). Psychological, physical, and academic correlates of cyberbullying and traditional bullying. *Journal of Adolescent Health, 53*, S13–S20. https://doi.org/10.1016/j.jadohealth.2012.09.018

Kowalski, R. M., Giumetti, G. W., Schroeder, A. N., & Lattanner, M. R. (2014). Bullying in the digital age: A critical review and meta-analysis of cyberbullying research among youth. *Psychological Bulletin, 140*, 1073–1137. https://doi.org/10.1037/a0035618

Kowalski, R. M., Limber, S. P., & McCord, A. (2019). A developmental approach to cyberbullying: Prevalence and protective factors. *Aggression and Violent Behavior, 45,* 20–32. https://doi.org/10.1016/j.avb.2018.02.009

Kozasa, S., Oiji, A., Kiyota, A., Sawa, T., & Kim, S. Y. (2017). Relationship between the experience of being a bully/victim and mental health in preadolescence and adolescence: A cross-sectional study. *Annals of General Psychiatry, 16*(1), 37–48. https://doi.org/10.1186/s12991-017-0160-4

Kwan, G. C. E., & Skoric, M. M. (2013). Facebook bullying: An extension of battles in school. *Computers in Human Behavior, 29*(1), 16–25. https://doi.org/10.1016/j.chb.2012.07.014

Ladd, G. W., Ettekal, I., & Kochenderfer-Ladd, B. (2017). Peer victimization trajectories from kindergarten through high school: Differential pathways for children's school engagement and achievement? *Journal of Educational Psychology, 109*(6), 826. https://doi.org/10.1037/edu0000177

Law, D. M., Shapka, J. D., Domene, J. F., & Gagne, M. H. (2012). Are cyberbullies really bullies? An investigation of reactive and proactive online aggression. *Computers in Human Behavior, 28*(2), 664–672. https://doi.org/10.1016/j.chb.2011.11.013

Lebrun-Harris, L. A., Sherman, L. J., Limber, S. P., Miller, B. D., & Edgerton, E. A. (2019). Bullying victimization and perpetration among US children and adolescents: 2016 National Survey of Children's Health. *Journal of Child and Family Studies, 28*(9), 2543–2557. https://doi.org/10.1007/s10826-018-1170-9

Lee, J. M., Hong, J. S., Yoon, J., Peguero, A. A., & Seok, H. J. (2018). Correlates of adolescent cyberbullying in South Korea in multiple contexts: A review of the literature and implications for research and school practice. *Deviant Behavior, 39*(3), 293–308. https://doi.org/10.1080/01639625.2016.1269568

Leff, S. S., Waasdorp, T. E., Paskewich, B., Gullan, R. L., Jawad, A. F., MacEvoy, J. P., Feinberg, B. E., & Power, T. J. (2010). The preventing relational aggression in schools everyday program: A preliminary evaluation of acceptability and impact. *School Psychology Review, 39*(4), 569–587.

Leff, S. S., Paskewich, B. S., Waasdorp, T. E., Waanders, C., Bevans, K. B., & Jawad, A. F. (2015). Friend to friend: A randomized trial for urban African American relationally aggressive girls. *Psychology of Violence, 5*(4), 433–443. https://doi.org/10.1037/a0039724

Leff, S. S., Waasdorp, T. E., & Paskewich, B. S. (2016). The broader impact of Friend to Friend (F2F): Effects on teacher–student relationships, prosocial behaviors, and relationally and physically aggressive behaviors. *Behavior Modification, 40*(4), 589–610. https://doi.org/10.1177/0145445516650879

LeVasseur, M. T., Kelvin, E. A., & Grosskopf, N. A. (2013). Intersecting identities and the association between bullying and suicide attempt among New York city youths: Results from the 2009 New York city youth risk behavior survey. *American Journal of Public Health, 103*(6), 1082–1089.

Levitt, M. J., Guacci-Franco, N., & Levitt, J. L. (1993). Convoys of social support in childhood and early adolescence: Structure and function. *Developmental Psychology, 29,* 811–818.

Lim, S. Y., Kang, N. R., & Kwack, Y. S. (2018). Effects of a class-based school violence prevention program for elementary school students. *Journal of the Korean Academy of Child & Adolescent Psychiatry, 29*(2), 54–61. https://doi.org/10.5765/jkacap.2018.29.2.54

Lindberg, S. M., Grabe, S., & Hyde, J. S. (2007). Gender, pubertal development, and peer sexual harassment predict objectified body consciousness in early adolescence. *Journal of Research on Adolescence, 17*(4), 723–742.

Linder, J. R., & Collins, W. A. (2005). Parent and peer predictors of physical aggression and conflict management in romantic relationships in early adulthood. *Journal of Family Psychology, 19*(2), 252–262. https://doi.org/10.1037/0893-3200.19.2.252

Linder, J. R., Crick, N. R., & Collins, W. A. (2002). Relational aggression and victimization in young adults' romantic relationships: Associations with perceptions of parent, peer, and romantic relationship quality. *Social Development, 11*(1), 69–86. https://doi.org/10.1111/1467-9507.00187

Litwiller, B. J., & Brausch, A. M. (2013). Cyber bullying and physical bullying in adolescent suicide: The role of violent behavior and substance use. *Journal of Youth and Adolescence, 42*, 675–684. https://doi.org/10.1007/s10964-013-9925-5

Machackova, H., & Pfetsch, J. (2016). Bystanders' responses to offline bullying and cyberbullying: The role of empathy and normative beliefs about aggression. *Scandinavian Journal of Psychology, 57*(2), 169–176. https://doi.org/10.1111/sjop.12277

Makara, K. A., & Madjar, N. (2015). The role of goal structures and peer climate in trajectories of social achievement goals during high school. *Developmental Psychology, 51*(4), 473–488. https://doi.org/10.1037/a0038801

Mallett, R. K., & Swim, J. K. (2009). Making the best of a bad situation: Proactive coping with racial discrimination. *Basic and Applied Social Psychology, 31*(4), 304–316.

Marshall, N. A., Arnold, D. H., Rolon-Arroyo, B., & Griffith, S. F. (2015). The association between relational aggression and internalizing symptoms: A review and meta-analysis. *Journal of Social and Clinical Psychology, 34*(2), 135–160. https://doi.org/10.1521/jscp.2015.34.2.135

Matlasz, T. M., Frick, P. J., Robertson, E. L., Ray, J. V., Thornton, L. C., Wall Myers, T. D., & Cauffman, E. (2020). Does self-report of aggression after first arrest predict future offending and do the forms and functions of aggression matter? *Psychological Assessment, 32*(3), 265–276. https://doi.org/10.1037/pas0000783

McAdams, C., Shillingford, M. A., & Trice-Black, S. (2011). Putting research into practice in school violence prevention & intervention: How is school counseling doing? *Journal of School Counseling, 9*(12), 1–31. http://www.jsc.montana.edu/articles/v9n12.pdf

McClelland, M. M., Acock, A. C., Piccinin, A., AnnRhea, S., & Stallings, M. C. (2013). Relations between preschool attention span-persistence and age 25 educational outcomes. *Early Childhood Research Quarterly, 28*(2), 314–324.

McClintock, M. K., & Herdt, G. (1996). Rethinking puberty: The development of sexual attraction. *Current Directions in Psychological Science, 5*(6), 178–183.

McGorry, P. D., Purcell, R., Goldstone, S., & Amminger, G. P. (2011). Age of onset and timing of treatment for mental and substance use disorders: Implications for preventive intervention strategies and models of care. *Current Opinion in Psychiatry, 24*(4), 301–306. https://doi.org/10.1097/YCO.0b013e3283477a09

McKellar, N. A., & Sherwin, H. D. (2003). Role of school psychologists in violence prevention and intervention. *Journal of School Violence, 2*(4), 43–55. https://doi.org/10.1300/j202v02n04_03

Meier, A., & Allen, G. (2009). Romantic relationships from adolescence to young adulthood: Evidence from the National Longitudinal Study of Adolescent Health. *Sociological Quarterly, 50*(2), 308–335. https://doi.org/10.1111/j.1533-8525.2009.01142.x

Merk, W., de Castro, B. O., & Koops, W. (2005). The distinction between reactive and proactive aggression: Utility for theory, diagnosis and treatment? *European Journal of Developmental Psychology, 2*(2), 197–220. https://doi.org/10.1080/17405620444000300

Merrell, K. W., Buchanan, R., & Tran, O. K. (2006). Relational aggression in children and adolescents: A review with implications for school settings. *Psychology in the Schools, 43*(3), 345–360. https://doi.org/10.1003/pits.20145

Meter, D. J., & Bauman, S. (2018). Moral disengagement about cyberbullying and parental monitoring: Effects on traditional bullying and victimization via cyberbullying involvement. *The Journal of Early Adolescence, 38*(3), 303–326.

Meyer, I. H. (2015). Resilience in the study of minority stress and health of sexual and gender minorities. *Psychology of Sexual Orientation and Gender Diversity, 2*(3), 209. https://doi.org/10.1177/0272431616670752

Mills, C. B., & Carwile, A. M. (2009). The good, the bad, and the borderline: Separating teasing from bullying. *Communication Education, 58*(2), 276–301. https://doi.org/10.1080/03634520902783666

Moffitt, T. (2007). A review of research on the taxonomy of life-course persistent versus adolescence-limited antisocial behavior. In D. Flannery, A. Vazsonyi, & I. Waldman (Eds.), *The*

Cambridge handbook of violent behavior and aggression (pp. 49–74). Cambridge University Press. https://doi.org/10.1017/CBO9780511816840.004

Mowen, T. J., & Freng, A. (2019). Is more necessarily better? School security and perceptions of safety among students and parents in the United States. *American Journal of Criminal Justice, 44*(3), 376–394. https://doi.org/10.1007/s12103-018-9461-7

Munakata, Y., Snyder, H. R., & Chatham, C. H. (2012). Developing cognitive control: Three key transitions. *Current Directions in Psychological Science, 21*, 71–77.

Murphy, B. C., & Eisenberg, N. (2002). An integrative examination of peer conflict: Children's reported goals, emotions, and behaviors. *Social Development, 11*(4), 534–557. https://doi.org/10.1111/1467-9507.00214/

National Research Council and Institute of Medicine. (2009). Preventing mental, emotional, and behavioral disorders among young people: Progress and possibilities. Committee on the prevention of mental disorders and substance abuse among children, youth, and Young adults: Research advances and promising interventions. In M. E. O'Connell, T. Boat, & K. E. Warner (Eds.), *Board on children, youth, and families, division of behavioral and social sciences and education*. The National Academies Press.

Neemann, J., Hubbard, J., & Masten, A. S. (1995). The changing importance of romantic relationship involvement to competence from late childhood to late adolescence. *Development and Psychopathology, 7*(4), 727–750.

Nickerson, A. B., & Spears, W. H. (2007). Influences on authoritarian and educational/therapeutic approaches to school violence prevention. *Journal of School Violence, 6*(4), 3–31. https://doi.org/10.1300/j202v06n04_02

Niwa, E. Y.*, Boxer, P., Dubow, E. F., Huesmann, L. R., Landau, S. F., Shikaki, K., & Gvirsman, S. (2016). Growing up amid ethno-political conflict: Aggression and emotional desensitization promote hostility to ethnic out-groups. *Child Development, 87*, 1479–1492.

Olweus, D. (1979). Stability of aggressive reaction patterns in males: A review. *Psychological Bulletin, 86*(4), 852–875. https://doi.org/10.1037/0033-2909.86.4.852

Olweus, D., & Limber, S. P. (2010). Bullying in school: Evaluation and dissemination of the Olweus Bullying Prevention Program. *American Journal of Orthopsychiatry, 80*, 124–134.

Orpinas, P., MacNicholas, C., & Nahapetyan, L. (2015). Gender differences in trajectories of relational aggression perpetration and victimization from middle to high school. *Aggressive Behavior, 41*(5), 401–412. https://doi.org/10.1002/ab.21563

Ostrov, J., Crick, N. R., & Stauffacher, K. (2006). Relational aggression in sibling and peer relationships during early childhood. *Applied Developmental Psychology, 27*(3), 241–253. https://doi.org/10.1016/j.appdev.2006.02.005

Ostrov, J. M., Kamper, K. E., Hart, E. J., Godleski, S. A., & Blakely-McClure, S. J. (2014). A gender-balanced approach to the study of peer victimization and aggression subtypes in early childhood. *Development and Psychopathology, 26*(3), 575–587.

Ostrov, J. M., Godleski, S. A., Kamper-DeMarco, K. E., Blakely-McClure, S. J., & Celenza, L. (2015). Replication and extension of the early childhood friendship project: Effects on physical and relational bullying. *School Psychology Review, 44*, 445–463.

Pardini, D. A., Raine, A., Erickson, K., & Loeber, R. (2014). Lower amygdala volume in men is associated with childhood aggression, early psychopathic traits, and future violence. *Biological Psychiatry, 75*(1), 73–80. https://doi.org/10.1016/j.biopsych.2013.04.003

Patchin, J. W., & Hinduja, S. (Eds.). (2012). *Cyberbullying prevention and response: Expert perspectives*. Routledge.

Patterson, G. R., DeBaryshe, B. D., & Ramsey, E. (1989). A developmental perspective on antisocial behavior. *American Psychologist, 44*(2), 329–335. https://doi.org/10.1037/0003-066X.44.2.329

Pellegrini, A. D., & Long, J. D. (2007). An observational study of early heterosexual interaction at middle school dances. *Journal of Research on Adolescence, 17*, 613–638. https://doi.org/10.1111/j.1532-7795.2007.00538.x

Pepler, D., Craig, W., Jiang, D., & Connolly, J. (2008). Developmental trajectories of bullying and associated factors. *Child Development, 79*, 325–338.

Perren, S., Corcoran, L., Cowie, H., Dehue, F., Mc Guckin, C., Sevcikova, A., Tsatsou, P., & Völlink, T. (2012). Tackling cyberbullying: Review of empirical evidence regarding successful responses by students, parents, and schools. *International Journal of Conflict and Violence, 6*(2), 283–292. https://doi.org/10.4119/ijcv-2919

Rademacher, A., & Koglin, U. (2019). The concept of self-regulation and preschoolers' social-emotional development: A systematic review. *Early Child Development and Care, 189*(4), 2299–2317. https://doi.org/10.1080/03004430.2018.1450251

Reid, J. B., Patterson, G. R., & Snyder, J. (2002). *Antisocial behavior in children and adolescents: A developmental analysis and model for intervention.* American Psychological Association.

Riley, P. L., & Segal, E. C. (2002). Preparing to evaluate a school violence prevention program. *Journal of School Violence, 1*(2), 73–86. https://doi.org/10.1300/j202v01n02_05

Roberts, M. C., & Peterson, L. (1984). *Prevention of problems in childhood: Psychological research and applications.* Wiley.

Russell, S. T., & Joyner, K. (2001). Adolescent sexual orientation and suicide risk: Evidence from a national study. *American Journal of Public Health, 91*(8), 1276–1281.

Russell, S. T., Sinclair, K. O., Poteat, V. P., & Koenig, B. W. (2012). Adolescent health and harassment based on discriminatory bias. *American Journal of Public Health, 102,* 493–495.

Sabbagh, M. A., Xu, F., Carlson, S. M., Moses, L. J., & Lee, K. (2006). The development of executive functioning and theory of mind: A comparison of Chinese and U.S. preschoolers. *Psychological Science, 17,* 74–81.

Sabella, R., Patchin, J., & Hinduja, S. (2013). Review: Cyberbullying myths and realities. *Computers in Human Behavior, 29,* 2703–2711. https://doi.org/10.1016/j.chb.2013.06.040

Safren, S. A., & Pantalone, D. W. (2006). Social anxiety and barriers to resilience among lesbian, gay, and bisexual adolescents. In A. M. Omoto & H. S. Kurtzman (Eds.), *Contemporary perspectives on lesbian, gay, and bisexual psychology. Sexual orientation and mental health: Examining identity and development in lesbian, gay, and bisexual people* (pp. 55–71). American Psychological Association.

Scheckner, S. B., & Rollin, S. A. (2003). An elementary school violence prevention program. *Journal of School Violence, 2*(4), 3–42. https://doi.org/10.1300/j202v02n04_02

Schnoll, J. S., Connolly, J., Josephson, W. J., Pepler, D., & Simkins-Strong, E. (2015). Same-and cross-gender sexual harassment victimization in middle school: A developmental- contextual perspective. *Journal of School Violence, 14*(2), 196–216.

Sela-Shayovitz, R. (2009). Dealing with school violence: The effect of school violence prevention training on teachers' perceived self-efficacy in dealing with violent events. *Teaching and Teacher Education, 25*(8), 1061–1066. https://doi.org/10.1016/j.tate.2009.04.010

Seldin, M., & Yanez, C. (2019). *Student reports of bullying: Results from the 2017 School Crime Supplement to the National Crime Victimization Survey. NCES 2013–329.* National Center for Education Statistics. Retrieved from https://nces.ed.gov/pubs2019/2019054.pdf

Serna, L., Nielsen, E., Lambros, K., & Forness, S. (2000). Primary Prevention with Children at Risk for emotional or behavioral disorders: Data on a universal intervention for Head Start Classrooms. *Behavioral Disorders, 26*(1), 70–84.

Shulman, E. P., Harden, K. P., Chein, J. M., & Steinberg, L. (2016). The development of impulse control and sensation-seeking in adolescence: Independent or interdependent processes? *Journal of Research on Adolescence, 26*(1), 37–44.

Smetana, J. G. (1995). Parenting styles and conceptions of parental authority during adolescence. *Child Development, 66*(2), 299–316.

Smetana, J. G. (2000). Middle-class African American adolescents' and parents' conceptions of parental authority and parenting practices: A longitudinal investigation. *Child Development, 71*(6), 1672–1686.

Smetana, J. G., & Asquith, P. (1994). Adolescents' and parents' conceptions of parental authority and personal autonomy. *Child Development, 65*(4), 1147–1162.

Smetana, J. G., & Bitz, B. (1996). Adolescents' conceptions of teachers' authority and their relations to rule violations in school. *Child Development, 67*(3), 1153–1172.

Smith, S. W., Lochman, J. E., & Daunic, A. P. (2005). Managing aggression using cognitive-behavioral interventions: State of the practice and future directions. *Behavioral Disorders, 30*(3), 227–240.

Smith, R. L., Rose, A. J., & Schwartz-Mette, R. A. (2009). Relational and overt aggression in childhood and adolescence: Clarifying mean-level differences and associations with peer acceptance. *Social Development, 19*(2), 243–269. https://doi.org/10.1111/j.1467-9507.2009.00541.x

Song, W., Qian, X., & Goodnight, B. (2018). Examining the roles of parents and community involvement and prevention programs in reducing school violence. *Journal of School Violence, 18*(3), 403–420. https://doi.org/10.1080/15388220.2018.1512415

Steinberg, L. (2008). A social neuroscience perspective on adolescent risk-taking. *Developmental Review, 28*(1), 78–106. https://doi.org/10.1016/j.dr.2007.08.002

Stohlman, S. L., & Cornell, D. G. (2019). An online educational program to increase student understanding of threat assessment. *Journal of School Health, 89*(11), 899–906. https://doi.org/10.1111/josh.12827

Sugarman, D. B., Nation, M., Yuan, N. P., Kuperminc, G. P., Ayoub, L. H., & Hamby, S. (2018). Hate and violence: Addressing discrimination based on race, ethnicity, religion, sexual orientation, and gender identity. *Psychology of Violence, 8*(6), 649–656. https://doi.org/10.1037/vio0000222

Swit, C. S., McMaugh, A. L., & Warburton, W. A. (2018). Teacher and parent perceptions of relational and physical aggression during early childhood. *Journal of Child and Family Studies, 27*(1), 118–130. https://doi.org/10.1007/s10826-017-0861-y

Tanrikulu, I. (2018). Cyberbullying prevention and intervention programs in schools: A systematic review. *School Psychology International, 39*(1), 74–91.

Tiiri, E., Luntamo, T., Mishina, K., Sillanmäki, L., Klomek Brunstein, A., & Sourander, A. (2020). Did bullying victimization decrease after nationwide school-based antibullying program? A time-trend study. *Journal of the American Academy of Child & Adolescent Psychiatry, 59*(4), 531–540. https://doi.org/10.1016/j.jaac.2019.03.023

Tisak, M. S., & Tisak, J. (1990). Children's conceptions of parental authority, friendship, and sibling relations. *Merrill-Palmer Quarterly, 1982*, 347–367.

Tisak, M. S., Tisak, J., & Goldstein, S. E. (2006). Aggression, morality, and delinquency: A social cognitive perspective. In M. Killen & J. Smetana (Eds.), *Handbook on moral development* (pp. 611–632). Lawrence Erlbaum Associates.

Tokunaga, R. S. (2010). Following you home from school: A critical review and synthesis of research on cyberbullying victimization. *Computers in Human Behavior, 26*, 277–287. https://doi.org/10.1016/j.chb.2009.11.014

Tolan, P. H., Gorman-Smith, D., & Loeber, R. (2000). Developmental timing of onsets of disruptive behaviors and later delinquency of inner-city youth. *Journal of Child and Family Studies, 9*(2), 203–220. https://doi.org/10.1023/A:1009471021975

Tremblay, R. E. (2000). The development of aggressive behavior during childhood: What have we learned in the past century? *International Journal of Behavioral Development, 24*(2), 129–141. https://doi.org/10.1080/016502500383232

Tseng, W. L., Banny, A. M., Kawabata, Y., Crick, N. R., & Gau, S. S. F. (2013). A cross-lagged structural equation model of relational aggression, physical aggression, and peer status in a Chinese culture. *Aggressive Behavior, 39*(4), 301–315. https://doi.org/10.1002/ab.21480

Ttofi, M. M., Farrington, D. P., Lösel, F., & Loeber, R. (2011). The predictive efficiency of school bullying versus later offending: A systematic/meta-analytic review of longitudinal studies. *Criminal Behaviour and Mental Health, 21*, 80–89. https://doi.org/10.1002/cbm.808

Turner, H. A., Shattuck, A., Finkelhor, D., & Hamby, S. (2017). Effects of poly-victimization on adolescent social support, self-concept, and psychological distress. *Journal of Interpersonal Violence, 32*(5), 755–780.

Underwood, M. K., Beron, K. J., & Rosen, L. H. (2009). Continuity and change in social and physical aggression from middle childhood through early adolescence. *Aggressive Behavior, 35*(5), 357–375. https://doi.org/10.1002/ab.20313

Waasdorp, T. E., & Bradshaw, C. P. (2015). The overlap between cyberbullying and traditional bullying. *Journal of Adolescent Health, 56*(5), 483–488. https://doi.org/10.1016/j.jadohealth.2014.12.002

Waasdorp, T. E., Pas, E. T., Zablotsky, B., & Bradshaw, C. P. (2017). Ten-year trends in bullying and related attitudes among 4th-to 12th-graders. *Pediatrics, 139*(6). https://doi.org/10.1542/peds.2016-2615

Wang, K., Chen, Y., Zhang, J., & Oudekerk, B. A. (2020). *Indicators of school crime and safety: 2019. NCES 2020-063/NCJ 254485.* National Center for Education Statistics, U.S. Department of Education, and Bureau of Justice Statistics, Office of Justice Programs, U.S. Department of Justice.

Webster-Stratton, C., & Reid, J. M. (2010). The Incredible Years Parents, Teachers and Child Training Series: A multifaceted treatment approach for young children with conduct problems. In J. R. Weisz & A. E. Kazdin (Eds.), *Evidence-based psychotherapies for children and adolescents* (2nd ed., pp. 194–210). Guilford Press.

Weissberg, R. P., Caplan, M., & Harwood, R. L. (1991). Promoting competent young people in competence-enhancing environments: A systems-based perspective on primary prevention. *Journal of Consulting and Clinical Psychology, 59*(6), 830–841.

Widen, S. C., & Russell, J. A. (2008). Young children's understanding of other's emotions. *Handbook of Emotions, 3*, 348–363.

Wolitzky-Taylor, M. A., Ruggiero, K. J., Danielson, C. K., Resnick, H. S., Hanson, R. F., Smith, D. W., Saundersm, B. E., & Kilpatrick, D. G. (2008). Prevalence and correlates of dating violence in a national sample of adolescents. *Journal of the American Academy of Child and Adolescent Psychiatry, 47*(7), 755–762. https://doi.org/10.1097/CHI.0b013e318172ef5f

Wolke, D., Lereya, S. T., Fisher, H. L., Lewis, G., & Zammit, S. (2014). Bullying in elementary school and psychotic experiences at 18 years: A longitudinal, population-based cohort study. *Psychological Medicine, 44*(10), 2199–2211. https://doi.org/10.1017/S0033291713002912

Wong, C. A., Eccles, J. S., & Sameroff, A. (2003). The influence of ethnic discrimination and ethnic identification on African American adolescents' school and socioemotional adjustment. *Journal of Personality, 71*(6), 1197–1232.

Woods, S., & Wolke, D. (2004). Direct and relational bullying among primary school children and academic achievement. *Journal of School Psychology, 42*(2), 135–155.

Ybarra, M. L., Strasburger, V. C., & Mitchell, K. J. (2014). Sexual media exposure, sexual behavior, and sexual violence victimization in adolescence. *Clinical Pediatric (Phila)., 53*(13), 1239–1247.

Yoon, J. S., & Kerber, K. (2003). Bullying: Elementary teachers' attitudes and intervention strategies. *Research in Education, 69*(1), 27–35. https://doi.org/10.7227/RIE.69.3

Yoon, J. S., Sulkowski, M. L., & Bauman, S. A. (2016). Teachers' responses to bullying incidents: Effects of teacher characteristics and contexts. *Journal of School Violence, 15*(1), 91–113.

Young-Jones, A., Fursa, S., Byrket, J. S., & Sly, J. S. (2015). Bullying affects more than feelings: The long-term implications of victimization on academic motivation in higher education. *Social Psychology of Education, 18*, 185–200. https://doi.org/10.1007/s11218-014-9287-1

Chapter 4
Urban School Violence: Responding with Culture and Protective Factors Among Youth of Color

Candice M. Wallace, R. Davis Dixon, Zina T. McGee, and Linda Malone-Colon

Generally, rates of violence and violent victimizations in the United States have steadily declined over the last 20 years (Federal Bureau of Investigations; Crime in the U.S., 2018; Morgan & Odekerk, 2019). Research indicates that the systemic, as well as interpersonal correlates of various types of violence (i.e., community, interpersonal, and school), are intertwined (Low & Espelage, 2014). Therefore, it is not surprising that rates of school violence have also declined. School violence is defined as aggressive and violent acts that take place on school property or on the way to or from school (Centers for Disease Control and Prevention (CDC), 2019). The National Center for Education Statistics (Wang et al., 2020) reports that the rates of students between the ages of 12 and 18 who reported being victimized at school within the last 6 months declined from 6 to 2 percent, between 2001 and 2018. This trend is consistent for male and female students of all races studied. While this trend is promising, school-related violence continues to threaten the social and educational experience for students nationwide (Kim et al., 2020; Peguero, 2011). Results from the most recent findings from the Centers for Disease Control and Prevention's Youth Risk Behavior Survey (YRBS) show that nearly 9% of high school students have reported being involved in a physical fight on school property, while 6% of students have been threatened or injured with a weapon

C. M. Wallace (✉)
Department of Psychological Science, Central Connecticut State University, New Britain, CT, USA
e-mail: candice.wallace@ccsu.edu

R. D. Dixon · L. Malone-Colon
Department of Psychology, Hampton University, Hampton, VA, USA

Z. T. McGee
Department of Social Sciences, Hampton University, Hampton, VA, USA

© The Author(s), under exclusive license to Springer Nature Switzerland AG 2023
T. W. Miller (ed.), *School Violence and Primary Prevention*,
https://doi.org/10.1007/978-3-031-13134-9_4

101

within the past 12 months of survey completion (Kann et al., 2018). Additionally, approximately 7% of students missed at least one school day within a 30-day period because they felt unsafe (Kann et al., 2018). Moreover, nearly 1 in 5 high school students have reported being bullied on school property in the last year, and about 1 in 7 have been bullied online (texting, Instagram, Facebook, or other social media) (Kann et al., 2018).

National and public attention to school violence typically focus on severe instances of behavior (e.g., mass shootings). However, less severe instances of violence such as bullying and fighting are much more common and are more likely to influence the day-to-day school experiences for youth (Eisenbraun, 2007; Greene, 2005). The factors associated with school violence are complex and varied. For instance, research suggests that experiences with bullying differ based on public versus private school attendance (Wang et al., 2020). Similarly, experiences with school violence vary based on setting and ethnic background. While students who reside in urban settings are less likely to experience the severe forms of violence that receive national attention, empirical evidence suggests that students who reside in these settings are more likely to be exposed to and victimized by community violence. In turn, community violence exposure affects experiences at school (Ozer & Weinstein, 2004). Research on school violence among youth in urban settings indicates that these youth are more likely to experience and perpetrate school violence than their suburban and rural counterparts (Wang et al., 2020).

Many of the students who reside in urban settings represent racial minorities (i.e., African Americans and Hispanics). Research on community violence among racial minorities suggests that these individuals are differentially impacted. For example, while African Americans represent 13% of the population, they represent approximately 20% of violent victimizations, generally (Morgan & Odekerk, 2019). The societal issues that are more common among ethnic minorities often result in a greater propensity for violence among these communities (Agnew, 1999; Nordberg et al., 2018). Consequently, certain students of color are more likely to be exposed to school violence. For example, African-American students are among those most likely to be bullied and victimized at school (Wang et al., 2020). African-American students are also more likely to report being in a physical fight on school property than their White or Asian peers (Wang et al., 2020). Statistics such as these indicate a thorough understanding of violence generally, and school violence specifically can only be obtained through an examination of the unique factors that impact those of different social backgrounds. This chapter examines the psychological and sociological factors that lead to school violence among urban and ethnic youth with a focus on African-American youth. We then provide support for culturally relevant variables as protective factors in community and school violence research and prevention initiatives.

Risk Factors Associated with Urban School Violence for Youth of Color

The Historical Context of School Violence

In 1975, the Senate Committee on the Judiciary ordered a report to address violence and disarray in U.S. schools. As a result, the publication of the Bayh (1975) report on school violence gained wide attention for its depiction of schools as "hotbeds of violence and vandalism." Researchers' investigations of the report later revealed that the data were skewed given the emphasis on larger schools, which were more likely to have greater levels of violence (National Institute of Education, 1978). Subsequently, the identification of school-, community-, and student-related characteristics gained larger consideration as studies later began to reveal that the problem of school violence was not as widespread as the Bayh report (Bayh, 1975) had indicated, with fewer schools demonstrating more severe levels of violence. Moreover, the publication of the *Safe Schools Study* report placed Bayh's observations under even greater scrutiny as new data began to show the manner in which certain characteristics accompanying school violence provided a greater explanation (National Center for Education Statistics, 1981). These included large school size, fewer resources, urban location, and low socioeconomic status. Additional awareness of race, gender, and punitive disciplinary policies prompted researchers to investigate with greater urgency the influence of school- and community-level factors on school violence. By detailing the impact of physical structure, social structure, and school climate, as well as economic, social, and racial dimensions, greater structural analyses of school violence emerged to determine why rates varied across school districts and what could be done to curb the levels of the most severe violence (National Institute of Education, 1978). Influences pertaining directly to unemployment, poverty, and area conditions gained less attention, as the study instead focused on aspects such as class size, student–teacher ratio, and fairness in discipline as important for decreasing school violence. Extensions of family-related and community-related stressors also became relevant in later discussions of student frustration and alienation in connections with weapon carrying and subsequent violent victimization (National Center for Education Statistics, 1981).

The years following Bayh's (1975) report on school violence have also seen increased attention placed on the linkages between exposure to violence, violent victimization, mental health, and developmental outcomes. Additionally, other studies address multi-tiered approaches to prevention and intervention, and the need to not only reduce symptoms related to violence exposure but also minimize the negative impact of school-related experiences on youth development (see Ludwig & Warren, 2009; Kilewer, 2013; McGee, 2015; McGee et al., 2017; McGee & Baker, 2002; Rawles, 2010; Taylor et al., 2010; Duru & Balkis, 2018; Cedeno et al., 2010 for examples). Moreover, the detrimental effects on both youths' physical and mental well-being have led to the continued focus on school violence as a public health concern, as questions on how best to unravel the problem cut across social, cultural, and justice-related answers. As well, other research has focused on the individual vulnerabilities significantly impacting marginalized youths' experiences with school violence (Rawles, 2010; Taylor et al., 2010; Duru & Balkis, 2018). Markedly, urban, minority youth, in particular, are disproportionately impacted by the intersection of community-level and school-level violence. As a result, discussions of the synergistic relationship between traumatic social stressors, inconsistent and inequitable school discipline, and disproportionate minority contact have recently highlighted the consequences of racial and ethnic disparities in how these youths' violent behaviors are handled in the schools. Hence, one can argue that these more recent discussions have therefore shaped the discourse on the manner in which interventions must consider multiple forms of disorder, violence, and victimization within the school environment, and the extent to which this environment in itself is reflective of daily occurrences in certain youths' communities.

Sociological and Contextual Factors Associated with Urban School Violence

Derived from the sociological foundations of youth crime and violence, researchers have succinctly pointed toward the bidirectional course of adolescent violence by analyzing incidents outside the school that originate in the school setting, and incidents occurring in the school that are initiated in the surrounding neighborhood (Mateu-Gelabert & Lune, 2003). Scholarship in this regard shows the cumulative effect of both school and neighborhood factors on adolescent violence, suggesting that school violence in itself is a highly contextual and dynamic process. Thus, adolescents do not simply assume new identities to engage in violence on school grounds. Instead, the selection of delinquent peers and weapon carrying can often mirror the structural and cultural settings overlapping between the school and neighborhood (McGee, 2003; McGee et al., 2019; Mateu-Gelabert & Lune, 2003). Similarly, studies of the sociological influences relating to school violence have continued to address such factors as prevalence and risk factors for weapon carrying and firearm violence, particularly during adolescence (see Docherty et al., 2020; Nickerson et al., 2020; McGee et al., 2019). This issue has particular relevance to school violence, since research has shown that gun-related crime disproportionately affects non-White adolescents in impoverished urban neighborhoods, and the broader correlates of gun violence are considered similar to the predictors of other serious types of violence, such as peer delinquency, gang involvement, externalizing problem behavior, and residing in disadvantaged neighborhoods (Beardslee et al., 2018). While more is known about handgun carrying among demographic subsets of populations of adolescents generally, as Docherty et al. (2020) note, the risk factors for carrying handguns to school may be similar to those for general weapon or handgun carrying. Further, as school policies and social climates might influence the presence of guns on school grounds, it is less likely that the risk factors associated with gun carrying will methodically alter over periods of time (Docherty et al., 2019).

Some research studies have addressed violence-related behaviors on school grounds within the context of juveniles reporting fear of victimization and subsequent gun-related activity, and have suggested the importance of the structural characteristics of communities and urban areas that may enhance the likelihood of violence in urban schools (McGee et al., 2017). However, others have noted that it is unclear whether other risk factors such as aggression, selling drugs, and gang activity are causes, correlates, or consequences of school gun carrying specifically. Docherty et al. (2020), for example, found a low base rate of school gun carrying among middle and high school students and suggested that addressing problem behaviors and delinquent peer networks might provide the greatest benefit in reducing gun violence. Their research points toward the need to focus on norms, attitudes, and perceptions of gun carrying and ownership. Similarly, Taylor et al. (2010), in addressing the psychometric properties of the attitudes toward street code-related violence, suggest that the level of acceptance of these attitudes varies across demographic subgroups and social contexts. Issues of violence-related attitudes have great relevance in this context since the proposed connection between schools and communities has for some time suggested that schools seldom hold distinct roles, but instead remain the products of a much larger societal problem. Additionally, it can be argued that the presence of high crime schools within high crime communities intensifies the level of fear and anxiety experienced by many students who may report weapon carrying to avenge a fight or safeguard a drug deal carried over from their immediate environments (McGee, 2015). This has particular relevance to additional studies of school violence, in particular, that have addressed fighting in school, being threatened and injured at school, and missing school days because of fear for one's safety. As scholars note that indicators of peer aggression address marked increases in bullying and victimization, children and adolescents are at a greater risk of weapon carrying (Pham et al., 2017). As a result, it has been suggested that greater familiarity should occur with the protocols and risk factors that, in turn, lead one to engage in dangerous behavior in response to fights at school, threats, and related injuries.

As a result of the interrelationship between school-level and community-level characteristics in urban areas, researchers have for some time indicated that the experiences of children and adolescents in schools reflect the availability of firearms and attitudes toward violence across families and communities (Shapiro et al., 1997; Alvarez & Bachman, 1997; Finkelhor et al., 1997). As such, another risk factor, neighborhood disadvantage, can include the proliferation of crime as fomenting deviant behaviors among youth (Patchin et al., 2006). Hence, to understand the prevalence of and risk factors associated with school violence, researchers have analyzed community context as it relates to school delinquency. Here, scholars have argued that more attention should be placed on the structural aspect of the neighborhoods as it relates to crime such as youths' exposure to community violence and school delinquency. Examinations of other contextual factors such as poverty and urban location should also be considered when examining school delinquency among youth, as those who experience economic instability are more likely to react negatively. Youth, for example, who experience educational disadvantage as a result of poverty have increased levels of criminal involvement.

Additionally, the contextual factors relating to marginalized youths' frustration and alienation in schools have prompted scholars to suggest that suspensions and expulsions drive youth further into gangs (Howell & Egley Jr, 2005; Pyrooz et al., 2014). However, research by Carson and Esbensen (2019) suggests that while the threat of gangs has resulted in school administrators instituting specific policies, less is known about the activities in which gangs are involved at school. Findings from their study on narratives of youth suggest that school administrators and teachers should use school-based disruption as intervention points to help youth exit their gang, rather than simply removing them from school. Moreover, given the number of gang "desisters" in the sample, they caution against applying the label of "gang" to youth as it may refer to a temporary status. Findings such as these present even greater caution in efforts to tease out predictors of school violence from structural hazards that may originate in the community before students enter school grounds. As such, while few studies have shown a direct connection between gang activity and school violence, scholars note that community-level and school-level gang initiation may coincide with greater concentrated gang activity in youths' immediate environments (Forster et al., 2015).

Select processes and indicators used to explain the social causes of school violence have relied heavily on some of the risk factors outlined by the Centers for Disease Control and Prevention (David-Ferdon et al., 2016). As the CDC (David-Ferdon et al., 2016) points toward structural factors such as access to weapons and environmental impact, greater research consideration has been given to both the long term and continual influences of toxic social stressors that sustain themselves within marginalized youths' environments. Thus, issues of deprived neighborhoods, food insecurities, violence in the home and community, and societal racism are thought of as correlates to the violence among urban youth, and to some extent that which spills over into the school setting (McGee, 2015).

Given this knowledge, efforts to prevent school violence that address community effects, particularly among disadvantaged youth, have also focused on street context, racial capitalism, and cultural scripts as impacting antisocial predisposition. This may be used to explain why youth, boys in particular, engage in urban violence and consistently affiliate with delinquent peers. Additionally, those demonstrating more conduct problems are at greatest risk for carrying a gun (Kodjoe et al., 2003). Hence, incidents of school violence continue to address the need to identify the societal, interpersonal, and developmental characteristics that contribute to weapon carrying (Kodjoe et al., 2003). Moreover, Docherty et al (2019) suggest that early prevention programs should target boys with severe conduct problems and those who affiliate with delinquent peers while in elementary school. Additional studies of school violence have addressed peer aggression as it occurs within the structured hierarchical school environment. Here, Gumpel and Sutherland (2010) argue that both aggression and school violence are intricately related to the school's configuration, social, and academic structure. Additionally, neither school violence nor aggression are solely dispositional. The authors highlight the need to examine situational influences that extend from communities (Gumpel & Sutherland, 2010). This has also been addressed in studies of African-American youth, for example, as scholars have noted that exposure to community violence that can spill over into schools is associated with variability in delinquent peer affiliation (Burnside et al., 2018). Hence, the intersection of exposure to violence and delinquent peer associations, as they note, provides much information for effective interventions.

Psychosocial Factors Associated with Urban School Violence

To gain a complete comprehension of school violence among urban youth of color, scholars seek to explore the dynamic relationship between environmental and individual factors associated with this phenomenon. Consistent with most human behaviors, social and contextual variables often present a ripe environment for cognitive, personality, and emotional influences on behavioral outcomes. There are numerous psychosocial correlates with aggression and violence that assist our understanding of school violence. These correlates include aggressive and impulsive traits, self-perceptions and self-control, emotional intelligence and emotional management, relational abilities, and mental health issues (Akter & Rahman, 2018; Álvarez-García et al., 2015; DeWall et al., 2007; Eysenck, 1981). Among African-American and urban youth, research indicates that some of these factors are aggravated by their sociological and contextual environment (Hurd et al., 2013; Wandersman & Nation, 1998).

Although environmental factors contribute to aggression, at a foundational level, it is easy to understand that general levels of aggression are positively associated with perpetration of school violence such that higher levels of aggression are related to more instances of school violence (Álvarez-García et al., 2015; Lochman & Wayland, 1994). We know there are biological as well as trait indicators of aggression (Barlett & Anderson, 2012; Patrick, 2008) Individuals who are inherently more aggressive are also are more likely to exhibit violent behaviors. Some children and adolescents are more aggressive and thus, more likely to engage in school violence. For example, participants who reported perpetrating school violence in high school were more likely to have higher scores on a trait aggression scale than control participants (Ragatz et al., 2011). Moreover, in middle school, boys who scored high on dispositional aggression—experiences of aggressive feelings and cognitions—were also more likely to behave aggressively in school as measured by incidents of verbal, physical, and total aggression (Ballard et al., 2004).

While the levels of aggression predict acts of school violence, other psychosocial factors are shown to predict the perpetration of violence in schools as well. At the core of research on criminal behavior lies an inability to control one's behavior (Gottfredson & Hirschi, 1990). Numerous researchers have found evidence that one of the strongest predictors of aggression and violence is a failure to engage self-restraint (DeWall et al., 2007; Vazsonyi et al., 2017; Chui & Chan, 2015). Those who struggle with self-control might also be more inclined to act impulsively. Engaging self-control often depletes regulatory resources needed to minimize impulsive behaviors (DeWall et al., 2007). Eysenck has engaged in foundational research concerning the impact of impulsivity on human behavior (Eysenck, 1981, 1994; Eysenck et al., 1984). In this work, he found that impulsivity is related to aggressive, antisocial, and violent behavior. In one study, Farrington (1989) found that impulsivity was one of the six most important predictors of aggression in children. This connection between impulsivity and aggression maintained after retesting the sample 8 years later. More recently, Jiménez-Barbero et al. (2016) found a similar link between impulsivity and externalizing behaviors. The researchers found that high impulsivity was significantly associated with externalizing behaviors and attitudes toward violence in adolescents between the ages of 12 and 15 years. Research on impulsivity also shows that African-American children show higher levels of impulsivity at 15 than their White counterparts (Assari et al., 2018; Pedersen et al., 2012). Thus, if African-American students show higher levels of impulsivity, they may than be more likely to perpetuate school violence.

Researchers have also linked locus of control to aggressive behavior. More specifically, Zainuddin and Taluja (1990) found that participants who have an internal locus of control—one that attributes their experiences to their own actions or behaviors—are less likely to be aggressive compared to those who have an external locus of control—one that attributes their experiences to outside factors such as destiny, fate, or chance. Dykeman et al. (1996) found that students from ages 10–16 were more likely to engage in violence at school when they had an external locus of control. In a study examining youth living in the urban city of Chicago, researchers found that having an internal locus of control predicted lower levels of violence perpetuation even when they controlled for individual, family, and neighborhood characteristics (Ahlin, 2014). Akter and Rahman (2018) found negative correlations between bullying behavior, locus of control and self-concept such that students displaying lower internal locus of control and self-concept were more likely to be involved in bullying.

Experiences related to social disadvantage, neighborhood disorganization, and systemic oppression have the potential to impact self-perceptions among African-American and urban youth, especially as it relates to school. Often, children who reside in impoverished settings are confronted with salient concerns related to accessing resources necessary for survival (i.e., food, money, stable shelter). As a result, academic interests and high academic achievement become secondary and are less likely to be incorporated into self-concept (Gennetian et al., 2015). When the most basic needs are unmet, African-American students may react in ways that show a lack of self-control, feelings of external locus of control, and/or increased orientation toward aggression and violence (Bernheim et al., 2015; Evans & Kim, 2013; Flouri et al., 2014; Palacios-Barrios & Hanson, 2019). More plainly, when there is a threat to the resources one needs to survive, it may become difficult to engage higher-order cognitive resources such as self-control. Moreover, experiences with discrimination as well as the internalization of stereotypes can potentially influence self-concept and self-esteem among African-American youth. In one study, researchers found that when African-American students were exposed to an experimental setting where they were racially stigmatized, they exhibited impaired self-control capacity (Inzlicht et al., 2006). Hence, these experiences with systemic issues—such as poverty and racism—correlate to the psychological factors that influence perpetuation of school violence.

Many urban children are confronted with traumatic experiences, the results of which, become integrated into their school experiences. These experiences lead to anxiety and depression (Hurd et al., 2013). The mental health issues associated with exposure to trauma are distracting and thwart students' ability to focus on academics (DePrince et al., 2009). Moreover, many students attempt to cope with mental health concerns by using externalizing behaviors. These behaviors include aggressive acts such as bullying and fighting with other students and disrespecting teachers. For example, researchers have found that when students are exposed to either direct or indirect violence, they are more likely to display externalizing behaviors (Eitle & Turner, 2002; Fleckman et al., 2016). It is clear that many students who perpetrate school violence are dealing with issues of anger, stress, and anxiety for which they are not equipped with the necessary skills to effectively manage. Thus, when conflicts with other students arise, their instinct is to fight rather than to engage in conflict resolution and problem-solving skills. Fortunately, school-based interventions that address self-concept, mental health, and honesty are shown to mitigate the perpetuation of school violence among African-American and low-income participants (Lewis et al., 2013).

Empirical evidence presents a bleak picture for urban youth of color. Given the hardships that these youth often face, it is reasonable to assume that they might be less than satisfied with life's outcomes. Children who report higher levels of hopelessness and depression are more likely to behave violently (DuRant et al., 1994). Research indicates that among students who are both perpetrators and victims of school violence, experiences with school reduce perceptions of life satisfaction (Estévez et al., 2009; Kodžopeljić et al., 2014). Thus, for urban students, experiences with school violence compound life experiences to adversely impact life satisfaction. Interestingly, researchers indicate that among students who experience school violence, satisfaction with the school experience mediates the relationship between life satisfaction and perpetration of school violence (Varela et al., 2018). Research that explores school violence and life satisfaction support these findings (Valois et al., 2006).

School Environment and Urban School Violence

As indicated by Bronfenbrenner (1994), human existence is influenced by interrelated systems that impact each other. The factors that relate to school violence mirror this theoretical proposition. Just as children bring their contextual and personal experiences to the school setting, the school setting presents circumstances that influence experiences as well. Factors surrounding the school significantly contribute to a student's perceptions of safety and security while at school. Similarly, the school environment itself significantly influences a student's perceptions of school and the probability that a student will engage in violence. The literature on the school environment suggests that two major factors contribute to school violence: the physical environment and the social environment (Johnson et al., 2012). Research that explores the impact of a school's physical environment on school violence provides mixed results. Evidence suggests that changing the physical space where maladaptive behaviors might occur or having a police presence could reduce the propensity for engaging in these behaviors among youth (Wahab & Sakip, 2019; Wilcox et al., 2006). Conversely, several studies suggest factors such as school size, class size, and the presence of physical problems do not significantly predict violent behaviors while at school (Johnson, 2009). Moreover, recent research findings suggest the presence of law enforcement at school does little to reduce rates of school violence and does not enhance feelings of safety among students (Stern & Petrosino, 2018).

Empirical evidence suggests a school's social environment might play a much larger role in perceptions of safety and the likelihood that students might engage in violent behaviors. Elements of the social environment include social norms, peer relationships, teacher/student relationships, and school management policies (including school disorder and discipline) (Johnson et al., 2012). For students of color, the social dynamics of the school including race-related dynamics (i.e., implicit discrimination) influences belongingness and engagement (Dotterer et al., 2009; Bottiani et al., 2017). Among ethnic minorities, the school setting presents one context in which prejudice and discrimination might take place. For instance, African-American students are disproportionately more likely to be punished for misbehavior and the punishment tends to be more severe (e.g., out-of-school suspension and expulsion) (Losen et al., 2015). Research also indicates that teachers often perceive the behaviors of African-American students as more disruptive and problematic than their peers (Cook et al., 2018; Gregory & Mosely, 2004). These perceptions reflect a cultural bias that criminalizes African Americans (Monroe, 2005). For African-American students, experiences with discrimination result in poor relationships with teachers and increased defiant behaviors (Cook et al., 2018; Gregory & Weinstein, 2008). Moreover, the stereotypical beliefs of African Americans might engage attribution and self-fulfilling prophecy processes such that school personnel treat African-American students in stereotype-confirming ways that elicit stereotype-confirming behaviors (i.e., school violence and disruption) (Kunesh & Noltemeyer, 2019; Rosenthal, 2002).

Attempts to modernize implementations for school violence reduction have begun to rely on the growing literature indicating that student perceptions of school fairness may be predictive of their involvement in school violence-related behavior (James et al., 2014). James et al. (2014), in a study of school violence and perceived fairness, for example, found that both perceptions of respectful treatment and social support from adults were highly associated with less self-reported violence at school. Their results suggested that guidelines designed to reduce school violence should consider the significance of effectively training teachers and other school personnel to fully engage them in the respectful, and supportive, treatment of their students. Hence, the establishment of a culture of fairness and support was deemed to be essential to reduce levels of violence at school, a consideration that further addresses the increased emphasis being placed on matters of restorative justice to curb school violence, particularly that which occurs disproportionately among minority youth.

A student's peer relationships are equally as important to perceptions of the school environment as are the relationships with teachers and other school personnel. Wang et al. (2020) report that African-American students are among those more likely to be called names, to be made fun of, and to be insulted by their peers. One study found that when individuals feel ostracized by groups they feel a lower sense of belonging which contributes to an increased level of aggression (Welton et al. 2014). Additionally, in an examination of differences between African-American and White students' perceptions of school climate and discipline, Shirley and Cornell (2012) indicate that African-American students are more likely to have peers who support aggressive behavior. African-American students are also less likely to report bullying or threats of violence to their teachers. These findings indicate African-American students with peers who adopt more normative perceptions of violence might also engage in violence themselves. Furthermore, African-American students are reluctant to report victimization and may attempt to solve the problem themselves. These attempts to rectify the problem result in increased fighting among peers.

Consequences of Urban School Violence for Youth of Color

The myriad consequences associated with school violence suggest that this phenomenon warrants increased practical and empirical examination. As such, researchers have examined the outcomes associated with school violence for the school community, including school officials, teachers, and students. Schools with higher rates of violence create an unsafe learning environment. During the 2015–2016 school year, 10% of public-school teachers reported being threatened with injury from their students and 6% of public-school teachers were attacked by a student (Musu et al. 2019). According to Dinkes (2009), teachers in urban settings report higher instances of threat from students than their suburban and rural counterparts. Being threatened or attacked while at work results in adverse mental health outcomes and performance issues for teachers (Bauer et al., 2006). A qualitative study conducted by Smith and Smith (2006) indicates that school violence contributes to the turnover of teachers in urban schools. These teachers are more likely to switch schools or professions, resulting in shortages of qualified teachers in neighborhoods that are most in need (Johnson et al., 2012).

Among high school students, approximately 6% of all students report being threatened with a weapon on school property. African-American students are among those who are most likely to be threatened with a weapon (Wang et al., 2020). These students often attend schools that place them at greater risk of being either a perpetrator or victim of violence, impacting perceptions of safety (Adams & Mrug, 2019). The perceptions of the lack of safety that derive from school violence result in increased fear among students. Akiba (2010) suggests that students who perceive they are likely to be victims of school violence are more likely to feel a sense of fear while in school settings. She also indicates that students who represent racial minorities might report higher levels of fear as they are more likely to be victims of bullying. Furthermore, schools in urban settings report higher levels of school violence which might heighten perceptions of an increased potential for victimization among students (Adams & Mrug, 2019). The impoverished setting in which many urban schools find themselves can be a source of fear for school violence among students. While these schools do not always report higher instances of school violence, a lack of resources and greater instability result in perceptions of an increased likelihood of school violence (Akiba, 2010).

Another consequence of school violence is weapon possession on school grounds. Several risk factors have been associated with the probability that a student will carry a weapon to school. For urban youth, factors such as peer affiliation and feeling unsafe contribute to incidents of carrying weapons to school (Bailey et al., 1997; Arria et al., 1997). Interestingly, recent research suggests that African American, Hispanic, and other ethnic minorities are less likely to carry a weapon to school than their White peers. However, African-American students are more likely to be threatened with a weapon on school property than are White youth (Semprevivo et al., 2020). Weapon possession in schools has the potential to intensify the severity of school violence and diminishes perceptions of school safety.

Perhaps the most disheartening consequence of school violence is the impact it has on academic outcomes for students. School violence poses a disruption to the school day that hinders the learning process (Johnson, 2009). When teachers and principals are forced to focus on issues with school violence, the time and attention needed for academics are decreased. Among students who attend schools in urban settings, these daily disruptions are exacerbated as there are higher rates of school violence (Wang et al., 2020). For the perpetrators of school violence, engaging in aggressive behaviors results in disciplinary action that hinders learning, as well. This is especially problematic for African-American students because of disproportionately harsher consequences for engaging in misbehavior. Skiba and Losen (2016) report that African-American students are more likely to be given out-of-school suspension as a form of discipline for misbehavior. When a student is sent home from school, he or she is not engaged in the academic environment and misses the critical instruction needed to perform well.

For racial minorities, school violence might compound other issues (i.e., community violence exposure and discrimination) that negatively impact academic achievement. Williams and Peguero (2013) examined whether bullying differentially impacts racial minorities. Interestingly, racial background moderates the relationship between the level of academic achievement and bullying. For high achieving, compared to low achieving, African-American students, higher rates of bullying are reported. Among all students, bullying in lower grades (ninth grade) leads to lower achievement in higher grades (12th grade). Thus, for high-achieving African-American students, bullying in earlier grades likely leads to poorer performance as they matriculate through school. Williams and Peguero (2013) suggest that racial stereotypes might explain exposure to bullying for high-achieving African-American students.

Patton et al. (2012) explored the relationship between exposure to community violence, fear, and low academic achievement among African-American male students. They reason that while schools are typically a safe haven for students who reside in urban neighborhoods, the violence that occurs in the environment surrounding schools might influence the school environment. The results of Patton and colleagues' study revealed that feeling safe in the neighborhood was inversely associated with feeling afraid at school and, these constructs are indirectly associated with hours spent studying and grades. Research on dropout rates among minority youth supports these findings. Peguero et al. (2011) examined whether school-related violence victimization is associated with drop-out rates among African-American, Hispanic, Asian-American, and White high schoolers. In this study, school-related violence victimization was not associated with dropout rates for White and Asian-American students. However, for African-American and Hispanic students, victimization while at school was associated with an increased likelihood of dropping out. Similarly, Peguero et al. (2016) demonstrate that perceptions of school disorder, including school safety, are associated with school dropout rates. These findings were more pronounced among African-American, Hispanic, and Native American young males.

Culturally Relevant Protective Factors as a Solution to Urban School Violence Among Youth of Color

The sociological circumstances and psychosocial factors that affect the school environment for minority and urban students suggest that matriculation through school is difficult. Often, minority students (particularly those of African-American descent) resort to engaging in school violence as a mechanism for coping with frustration, negative perceptions of school and self, and problematic relationships with teachers and peers. As indicated, under certain circumstances, African-American students are also more likely to be victimized. While many risk factors associated with youth violence and school violence have been identified in the literature, more recent efforts to curtail school violence suggest that an emphasis on protective factors might be equally as important (Lösel & Farrington, 2012; Miranda et al., 2019). The contextual circumstances in which many urban youths exist are difficult to change. Hence, a specific focus on protective factors that bolster coping and resiliency might reshape the course of these children's lives. The evidence presented in the remainder of this chapter highlights the relationships between protective factors and violence reduction. Furthermore, we argue that culture-based protective factors might uniquely reduce rates of school violence among minority and urban youth.

Existing literature on community violence indicates that certain culturally specific variables are related to reduced engagement in violent and maladaptive behaviors (Caldwell et al., 2004; Jagers et al., 2007b). We are suggesting a similar model be applied to school violence.

A Culture-Centered Model

Proponents of Afrocentered psychology have developed a model approach for examining the influence of culture on multiple outcomes for African Americans. These psychologists argue there are key psychosocial values that are ingrained in African-American culture. These values serve as protective buffers against the negative societal experiences that plague the African-American community. Afrocentric cultural values include spirituality, communalism, self-knowledge, and interconnectedness (Grills et al., 2015; Parham, 2009). Several studies have shown that African Americans who endorse an Afrocentric cultural value and belief system (compared to a Eurocentric one) have higher self-esteem, are more psychologically adjusted, and are less likely to engage in violent and delinquent behavior. (Tyler et al., 2005; Jagers et al., 2007a, b; Bynum et al., 2007). African Americans have uniquely relied on these factors to cope with the circumstances they have faced in the United States.

Racial Identity and Racial Socialization

Racial Socialization

Several surprising studies have indicated that while other racial minorities report lower self-esteem than Whites, African Americans report higher self-esteem and more positive self-perceptions than their White counterparts (Twenge & Crocker, 2002). Research suggests that African-American cultural values seem to protect African-Americans' sense of self from internalized discrimination (Branscombe et al., 1999; Williams & Williams-Morris, 2000). This sense of self is facilitated through socialization that teaches self-knowledge, cultural practices, and ancestral history and instills high levels of racial pride.

Scholars who explore racial socialization suggest that ethnic minorities are socialized in three distinct but overlapping ways. Cultural socialization refers to messages designed to reinforce cultural pride and historical knowledge. Ethnic socialization prepares one for coping with the prejudice and discrimination that might result from racial or cultural group belonging. Racial socialization messages focus on racism, assimilation, oppression, spirituality, and egalitarianism. These different types of racial socialization have been explored separately and under the larger umbrella of racial socialization. Most studies that explore racial socialization focus on cultural pride and/or preparation for experiences with discrimination

(Bentley et al., 2009). Taken together, theories of racial socialization suggest that what ethnic minorities learn about their racial and ethnic background, what they learn about society's perceptions of this background, and how they learn this information can prepare them to successfully negotiate the many psychosocial pressures they face.

Racial socialization has been linked with positive outcomes for African Americans. Cultural socialization helps African-American children and adolescents cope with racism and discrimination which leads to better psychological outcomes (Bynum et al., 2007). Several studies have shown that racial socialization is positively associated with self-esteem and overall feelings of wellness (Thomas et al., 2003; Spencer et al., 2003). As previously noted, feelings of self-worth and wellness are negatively associated with aggressive behaviors. Stevenson et al. (1997) explored the relationship between racial socialization, anger, and depression. This research found that racial socialization had implications for anger expression, especially among African-American boys. Children who reported a greater likelihood of being exposed to positive racial messages were also less likely to express anger. Research supports the role of anger in displays of aggression and violence in the classroom (Levinson, 2006).

Empirical evidence suggests that racial socialization has protective implications for violent and delinquent behavior (Bennett Jr, 2007). These studies have primarily explored the mitigating implications of racial socialization for community violence. Henry et al. (2015) examined socialization messages associated with cultural pride as a moderator of the relationship between community violence exposure and aggressive behavior among African-American adolescents. In this study, a relationship between community violence exposure and aggressive behavior was observed for adolescents who did not receive cultural pride messages from their mothers. This relationship was not observed among adolescents who received messages of cultural pride. The work conducted by Banerjee et al. (2015) supports this notion. These researchers indicate a relationship between community violence exposure and aggressive behaviors among those low in cultural socialization but not among those who are high in cultural socialization.

Racial Identity

Arguably, racial socialization processes help to build and maintain one's sense of racial identity. Racial identity refers to the degree to which an individual incorporates race, and perceptions of cultural components of race, into their self-concept. As it relates to racial socialization, messages about ethnic and cultural pride contribute to the likelihood that one emphasizes race in self-concept. Sellers et al. (1998) suggests a multidimensional model of racial identity where the importance of race in self-definitions (centrality), positive or negative perceptions of the race (private regard), perceptions of other's positive or negative perceptions of one's race (public regard) and beliefs of how members of one's race should behave (ideology) interact to develop racial identity. These factors can operate together or separately to influence racial identity where one component might be more or less impactful than another. Additionally, this model argues that the salience of racial identity in a given context can moderate perceptions of that context and influence behavior as a result. Among African-American students, incorporating race into self-concept and feeling proud of their race (centrality and private regard) might shape school-related efficacy. Similarly, perceptions that teachers and peers respect and appreciate your race (public regard) can positively influence your interactions with these individuals and reduce engagement in school violence.

Several studies have supported the positive effects of a strong racial identity on psychosocial outcomes for ethnic minorities. These studies have found that for African-American youth and young adults, racial identity is positively related to self-esteem and negatively related to psychological distress (Rowley et al., 1998; Sellers et al., 2003; Umaña-Taylor et al., 2002). Likewise, racial identity is related to school-related attitudes and performance (Chavous et al., 2003, 2008). Specifically, these studies suggest that racial centrality and racial pride are positively associated with favorable school attitudes and better grades. Factors such as psychological adjustment and favorable school outcomes reduce the probability of engaging in school violence (Johnson, 2009). In this regard, racial identity indirectly impacts school violence (Estévez et al., 2009).

Racial identity also has direct protective implications for violence and associated behaviors. Research conducted by Arbona et al. (1999) demonstrated that ethnic identity uniquely predicted nonfighting attitudes for African-American adolescents. These results were not observed for Hispanic adolescents implying that racial identity might function differently for African Americans than it does for other racial groups. Further, Caldwell et al. (2004) demonstrated the protective ability of racial identity by examining the relationships between racial centrality, racial discrimination, and violent behaviors among African-American adolescents. Findings suggested that for African-American males who were lower in racial centrality, racial discrimination was more likely to lead to violent behaviors than for those who were higher in racial centrality. More recently, DeGruy et al. (2012) examined racial respect as a protective moderator of the relationship between witnessing violence and engaging in violent behavior. Racial respect reflects positive attitudes related to one's cultural background and a sense of self-worth associated with one's heritage. Among the adolescents sampled in this study, racial respect was negatively associated with the intensity of violence use. Further, compared to individuals lower in racial respect, those who reported higher levels of racial respect were less impacted by witnessing violence and were less likely to engage in violent behavior as a result.

Spirituality and Religiosity

Religiosity and spirituality are integral components of the value system for African-American individuals. Chatters et al. (2009) suggest that African Americans report a higher sense of religiosity (church attendance, prayer, and other behaviors associated with a specific religion) than Whites. Among ethnic minorities, a sense of spirituality (belief in a higher power) coupled with religious practices mitigate the adverse experiences that accompany their marginalized position within the U.S. (Butler-Barnes et al., 2018). Religiosity can serve as a source of resiliency for youth development in multiple ways (Gooden & McMahon, 2016; Salas-Wright et al., 2015). Good and Willoughby (2006) demonstrate the strong positive relationship between religiosity and psychological adjustment among adolescents. Furthermore, many religions provide a core set of principles that reinforce prosocial behavior (Hardy & Carlo, 2005).

An examination of the protective benefits of religiosity and spirituality among African-American youth suggests these variables are associated with psychosocial well-being (Butler-Barnes et al., 2017; Molock et al., 2006; Petts & Jolliff, 2008). Blaine and Crocker (1995) found that African-American adolescents and emerging adults who report higher levels of religiosity and spirituality also report higher levels of self-esteem, life satisfaction, and perceived self-control; factors associated with decreased violent behavior. Several scholars suggest an Afrocentered perspective, including religiosity, is related to social and moral development as well as empathic concern for others (Jagers et al., 1997; Mattis et al., 2006). Additionally, religiosity is associated with more favorable academic outcomes among ethnic minority youth (Abar et al., 2009; Butler-Barnes et al., 2012; Sikkink & Hernandez, 2003). Kim et al. (2018) examined religiosity among urban residing, African-American youth. In this study, students who reported lower levels of religiosity also reported lower school bonding and less positive relationships with teachers.

A large body of research has demonstrated the negative association between religiosity and reductions in violent and delinquent behaviors (Salas-Wright et al., 2014, 2015, 2017). Research that specifically focuses on the association between religion and spirituality and well-being has generally found that religion negatively predicts antisocial behaviors (Mattis & Jagers, 2001). In their work with a sample of sixth-grade, urban-residing African-American youth, Jagers and Mock (1993) found that a spiritual orientation was associated with fewer reported acts of delinquency.

Communalism

Communalism is defined as "a commitment to social connectedness which includes an awareness that social bonds and responsibilities transcend individual privileges" (Boykin, 1986). According to Boykin (1983), those who espouse a communal orientation are more aware of the interdependence of people, and they pay increased attention to the social relationships they have rather than to material things. According to Hurley (1999), those who are communally oriented place an emphasis on social interactions and prioritize the group over the individual. When individuals prioritize the needs of the group, they also place the identity of the group above their individual identity. Also, Hurley asserts that this orientation makes resources, whether physical or mental, available to those affiliated with the group rather than made exclusive to one person.

When we examine the cultural practices and orientations of various cultures, there is a clear distinction between those who espouse more communal versus more individualistic beliefs. Historically, African Americans were among those cultures that endorse more communal beliefs (Grills et al., 2015). For example, on average, African Americans engage in a larger network of people who are considered family (whether they are blood-related or not). Even the notion of "it takes a village to raise a child" reflects a communal orientation that suggests an individual's development is not the sole responsibility of parents. Indeed, it is the community that assumes the duty of rearing all children.

Since research has found a preference for communal contexts among African Americans, several researchers have found that one can transfer this preference for communalism into the educational institution. The research shows that African-American students perform better when communalism informs the learning context. These findings occurred for a variety of dimensions including text recall, multiplication performance, math estimation, vocabulary, geography, and learning transfer (Boykin et al., 1997, 2004; Dill & Boykin, 2000; Hurley et al., 2005, 2009). One study has shown that African-American students academically outperformed White students when placed in a communal learning context (Hurley et al., 2009). As previously indicated, more positive academic experiences strengthen school-related attitudes and reduce the probability of engaging in violent and disruptive behaviors.

The previous research is predicated on the inference that when African-American students are placed in a context that matches their cultural orientation, they are more motivated to learn, engaged in the activity, and are therefore more likely to perform better than when they are placed in a context devoid of these characteristics. This same reasoning can be applied to school violence. Placing students of color in a context that affirms their cultural orientations and teaches them how they might best navigate their lived experiences, may create an environment such that they: (1) are more engaged, (2) see the value in positive connections with those around them and are responsible for one another, and (3) are less likely to engage in behaviors that threaten their connection to the people around them (e.g., perpetuate violence). This line of reasoning has been confirmed across several studies showing that endorsement of Afrocultural beliefs is linked to more prosocial values and less problematic behaviors (Johnson & Carter, 2020). Empirical examples of communalism bolster this claim. Humphries et al. (2000) explored the connection between communal orientations and moral reasoning. These researchers found that children and adolescents who possess higher levels of communal attitudes had a better ability to engage in moral reasoning. Moreover, Jagers et al. (2007a, b) looked specifically at the connection between communal values and violence among African-American boys. They found that those who endorsed communal values were not as likely to be violent compared to those who did not endorse those values. Comparable to other Afrocentric cultural values, evidence indicates communalism has the potential to indirectly as well as directly influence school violence.

Suggestions for Research and Practice

Suggestions for Research

Although there has been a general conversation concerning the sociological and psychosocial risk factors associated with school violence in the research literature, a more concerted effort to broach this topic for those who are most susceptible to school violence is needed. African-American students are more likely to attend schools in urban settings, and thus more likely to be exposed to community violence and unsafe school environments. They are also more likely to engage in and be victimized in the school setting. However, there is limited research that examines the factors that contribute to school violence among this and other minority populations. In response, as previously noted, increased research is focusing on the individual vulnerabilities significantly impacting marginalized youths' experiences with school violence as perpetrators and victims (Rawles, 2010; Taylor et al., 2010; Duru & Balkis, 2018). Fewer studies have explored the unique protective benefit of culture-based psychosocial factors as protectors of violence generally and school violence specifically. Future research should seek to replicate and extend the findings from existing research in this area. Future studies should also expand to explore the evolution of culture-based protective factors as the social climate changes. Furthermore, a more robust understanding of the processes that drive the impact of culture-based protective factors on community and school violence is needed. We suggest researchers focus their efforts on expanding our understanding of variables (i.e., respect, perceived social support, mattering to others, hope, and context-specific efficacy) that might mediate or moderate this relationship to mitigate school violence among urban, African American, and other ethnic minority students.

Suggestions for Intervention Efforts

Using a resilience framework for reducing rates of school violence, we suggest that prevention efforts focus on the unique cultural strengths of ethnic minority and urban youth. Existing research suggests these cultural strengths are directly and indirectly associated with community violence. These cultural factors might be associated with school violence as well. Prevention efforts designed to reduce rates of school violence should ensure that these cultural factors are incorporated into discussions, activities, and programming. While few intervention programs are distinctly tailored to specific ethnic groups, those that have adopted a culture-based framework for mitigating violent attitudes and behaviors have been met with some success (Jagers et al., 2007a, b; Wallace et al., 2018; Whaley & McQueen, 2020). Those programs that use a risk-resilience framework would likely be most beneficial as they would address some of the unique risk factors that urban and ethnic youth face while also bolstering cultural strengths that are shown to be a source of coping and resilience (Aisenberg & Herrenkohl, 2008).

Given the disproportionate rates of engagement in and exposure to school violence, we examined cultural strengths among African-American youth. While we focus on the cultural strengths of this population, we recognize that the manifestation and effectiveness of cultural protective factors might differ based on the ethnicity of the population. As a result, we suggest that prevention programs tailor themselves to the unique population they wish to serve. For instance, The Promise Program (Wallace et al., 2018), a culture and family-based community violence prevention program, was uniquely designed to address the risks that place African-American young males at disproportionate rates of violence. Developing culturally unique interventions acknowledges that prevention efforts should not take a one-fits-all approach. Alternatively, these culturally specific programs should recognize the factors associated with school violence for each population might differ. Culturally specific prevention efforts create an environment where minority youth feel included and appreciated in the school environment.

To address more recent concerns about school violence and other mental health issues, school districts across the nation are becoming increasingly focused on mental health and wellness (Hayes et al., 2019). These school systems recognize the importance of incorporating curricula that address socioemotional learning (SEL) outcomes to ensure healthy development among children. Interventions that adopt a culture-based approach often concern themselves with factors that parallel the SEL core competencies. (Collaborative for Academic, Social and Emotional Learning, 2020). For instance, SEL curricula often emphasize competence in self-awareness, social awareness, self-management, and relationship skills. Culture-based curricula that operationally define values associated with racial identity, spirituality, and communalism address these same competencies. Thus, a program that highlights communalism might also equip students with relationship skills. One that bolsters racial identity might also teach students skills in self- and social awareness. Subsequently, culture-based, school violence intervention initiatives closely align themselves with socioemotional learning goals. These programs have the potential to not only address variables associated with violent and delinquent behaviors, but they also have the potential to equip urban and ethnic students with skills needed to navigate a variety of situations that life might present.

Conclusions

As states, districts, and schools are focusing more on educating the whole child, it is important to emphasize learning contexts that honor the integrity of students' lived experiences.

More and more evidence indicates that school is not just a place for learning facts and formulas. It should be a place that develops young human beings into who they will be when they become adults. An intervention that prioritizes personal growth, strengthening identity, and building upon students' cultural orientations would surely serve to increase prosocial behaviors among these students and decrease the likelihood of engaging in school violence.

As previously outlined, many traumatic sociological experiences should be addressed among ethnic and urban students. These sociological circumstances shape psychological outcomes that can subsequently lead to maladaptive behaviors in and out of school. The school environment has the option to either add to the potential dysfunction and aggravate negative experiences or, to serve as a source of healing and resilience. Adopting evidence-based, culturally specific interventions support the latter option. New literature has emphasized healing-centered practices as opposed to trauma-informed care (Ginwright, 2018). Making this shift would abandon a deficit lens for urban and ethnic student experiences and would move toward one that focuses more on growth and wellness (Ginwright, 2018).

References

Abar, B., Carter, K. L., & Winsler, A. (2009). The effects of maternal parenting style and religious commitment on self-regulation, academic achievement, and risk behavior among African-American parochial college students. *Journal of Adolescence, 32*(2), 259–273. https://doi.org/10.1016/j.adolescence.2008.03.008

Adams, J., & Mrug, S. (2019). Individual-and school-level predictors of violence perpetration, victimization, and perceived safety in middle and high schools. *Journal of School Violence, 18*(3), 468–482. https://doi.org/10.1080/15388220.2018.1528551

Agnew, R. (1999). A general strain theory of community differences in crime rates. *Journal of Research in Crime and Delinquency, 36*(2), 123–155. https://doi.org/10.1177/0022427899036002001

Ahlin, E. M. (2014). Locus of control redux: Adolescents' choice to refrain from violence. *Journal of Interpersonal Violence, 29*(14), 2695–2717. https://doi.org/10.1177/0886260513520505

Aisenberg, E., & Herrenkohl, T. (2008). Community violence in context: Risk and resilience in children and families. *Journal of Interpersonal Violence, 23*(3), 296–315. https://doi.org/10.1177/0886260507312287

Akiba, M. (2010). What Predicts Fear of School Violence Among U.S. Adolescents? *Teachers College Record, 112*(1), 68–102. https://doi.org/10.1177/016146811011200110

Akter, S., & Rahman, S. (2018). The role of locus of control, self-concept on bullying behavior of adolescence. *International Journal of Indian Psychology, 6*(1), 30–37.

Alvarez, A., & Bachman, R. (1997). Predicting the fear of assault at school and while going to and from school in an adolescent population. *Violence and Victims, 12*(1), 69–86. https://doi.org/10.1891/0886-6708.12.1.69

Álvarez-García, D., García, T., & Núñez, J. C. (2015). Predictors of school bullying perpetration in adolescence: A systematic review. *Aggression and Violent Behavior, 23*, 126–136. https://doi.org/10.1016/j.avb.2015.05.007

Arbona, C., Jackson, R. H., McCoy, A., & Blakely, C. (1999). Ethnic identity as a predictor of attitudes of adolescents toward fighting. *The Journal of Early Adolescence, 19*(3), 323–340. https://doi.org/10.1177/0272431699019003002

Arria, A., Borges, G., & Anthony, J. C. (1997). Fears and other suspected risk factors for carrying lethal weapons among urban youths of middle-school age. *Archives of Pediatrics & Adolescent Medicine, 151*(6), 555–560. https://doi.org/10.1001/archpedi.1997.02170430021004

Assari, S., Caldwell, C. H., & Mincy, R. B. (2018). Maternal educational attainment at birth promotes future self-rated health of white but not black youth: A 15-year cohort of a national sample. *Journal of Clinical Medicine, 7*(5), 93. https://doi.org/10.3390/jcm7050093

Bailey, S. L., Flewelling, R. L., & Rosenbaum, D. P. (1997). Characteristics of students who bring weapons to school. *Journal of Adolescent Health, 20*(4), 261–270. https://doi.org/10.1016/S1054-139X(96)00283-2

Ballard, M. E., Rattley, K. T., Fleming, W. C., & Kidder-Ashley, P. (2004). School aggression and dispositional aggression among middle school boys. *RMLE Online, 27*(1), 1–11. https://doi.org/10.1080/19404476.2004.11658163

Banerjee, M., Rowley, S. J., & Johnson, D. J. (2015). Community violence and racial socialization: Their influence on the psychosocial well-being of African American college students. *Journal of Black Psychology, 41*(4), 358–383. https://doi.org/10.1177/0095798414539174

Barlett, C. P., & Anderson, C. A. (2012). Direct and indirect relations between the Big 5 personality traits and aggressive and violent behavior. *Personality and Individual Differences, 52*(8), 870–875. https://doi.org/10.1016/j.paid.2012.01.029

Bauer, J., Stamm, A., Virnich, K., Wissing, K., Müller, U., Wirsching, M., & Schaarschmidt, U. (2006). Correlation between burnout syndrome and psychological and psychosomatic symptoms among teachers. *International Archives of Occupational and Environmental Health, 79*(3), 199–204. https://doi.org/10.1007/s00420-005-0050-y

Bayh, B. (1975). Our Nation's Schools--a Report Card: "A" in School Violence and Vandalism: Preliminary Report of the Subcommittee to Investigate Juvenile Delinquency, Based on Investigations, 1971–1975, by Birch Bayh, Chairman, to the Committee on the Judiciary, United States Senate. US Government Printing Office.

Beardslee, J., Docherty, M., Mulvey, E., Schubert, C., & Pardini, D. (2018). Childhood risk factors associated with adolescent gun carrying among Black and White males: An examination of self- protection, social influence, and antisocial propensity explanations. *Law and Human Behavior, 42*(2), 110–118. https://doi.org/10.1037/lhb0000270

Bennett, M. D., Jr. (2007). Racial socialization and ethnic identity: Do they offer protection against problem behaviors for African American youth? *Journal of Human Behavior in the Social Environment, 15*(2–3), 137–161. https://doi.org/10.1300/J137v15n02_09

Bentley, K. L., Adams, V. N., & Stevenson, H. C. (2009). Racial socialization: Roots, processes & outcomes. In H. In Neville, B. M. Tynes, & S. O. Utsey (Eds.), *Handbook of African American psychology* (pp. 255–267). Sage Publications.

Bernheim, B. D., Ray, D., & Yeltekin, Ş. (2015). Poverty and self-control. *Econometrica, 83*(5), 1877–1911. https://doi.org/10.3982/ECTA11374

Bottiani, J. H., Bradshaw, C. P., & Mendelson, T. (2017). A multilevel examination of racial disparities in high school discipline: Black and white adolescents' perceived equity, school belonging, and adjustment problems. *Journal of Educational Psychology, 109*(4), 532–545. https://doi.org/10.1037/edu0000155

Boykin, A. W. (1983). The academic performance of Afro-American children. In J. Spence (Ed.), *Achievement and achievement motives* (pp. 321–371). W. Freeman.

Boykin, A. W. (1986). The triple quandary and the schooling of Afro-American children. In U. Neisser (Ed.), *The school achievement of minority children: New perspectives* (pp. 57–92). Lawrence Erlbaum.

Boykin, A. W., Jagers, R. J., Ellison, C. M., & Albury, A. (1997). Communalism: Conceptualization and measurement of an Afrocultural social orientation. *Journal of Black Studies, 27*(3), 409–418.

Boykin, A. W., Lilja, A. J., & Tyler, K. M. (2004). The influence of communal vs. individual learning context on the academic performance in social studies of grade 4–5 African- Americans. *Learning Environments Research, 7*(3), 227–244. https://doi.org/10.1007/s10984-004-3294-7

Branscombe, N. R., Schmitt, M. T., & Harvey, R. D. (1999). Perceiving pervasive discrimination among African Americans: Implications for group identification and well-being. *Journal of Personality and Social Psychology, 77*(1), 135–148. https://doi.org/10.1037/0022-3514.77.1.135

Bronfenbrenner, U. (1994). Ecological models of human development. *Readings on the Development of Children, 2*(1), 37–43.

Blaine, B., & Crocker, J. (1995). Religiousness, race, and psychological well-being: Exploring social psychological mediators. *Personality and Social Psychology Bulletin, 21*(10), 1031–1041. https://doi.org/10.1177/01461672952110004

Burnside, A., Gaylord-Harden, N., So, S., & Voisin, D. (2018). A latent profile analysis of exposure to community violence and peer delinquency in African-American adolescents. *Children and Youth Services Review, 91*, 196–203. https://doi.org/10.1016/j.childyouth.2018.06.014

Butler-Barnes, S. T., Williams, T. T., & Chavous, T. M. (2012). Racial pride and religiosity among African American boys: Implications for academic motivation and achievement. *Journal of Youth and Adolescence, 41*(4), 486–498. https://doi.org/10.1007/s10964-011-9675-1

Butler-Barnes, S. T., Martin, P. P., & Boyd, D. T. (2017). African American adolescents' psychological well-being: The impact of parents' religious socialization on adolescents' religiosity. *Race and Social Problems, 9*, 115–126. https://doi.org/10.1007/s12552-017-9199-8

Butler-Barnes, S. T., Martin, P. P., Hope, E. C., Copeland-Linder, N., & Lawrence Scott, M. (2018). Religiosity and coping: Racial stigma and psychological well-being among African American girls. *Journal of Religion and Health, 57*, 1980–1995. https://doi.org/10.1007/s10943-018-0644-9

Bynum, M. S., Burton, E. T., & Best, C. (2007). Racism experiences and psychological functioning in African American college freshmen: Is racial socialization a buffer? *Cultural Diversity and Ethnic Minority Psychology, 13*(1), 64–71. https://doi.org/10.1037/1099-9809.13.1.64

Caldwell, C. H., Kohn-Wood, L. P., Schmeelk-Cone, K. H., Chavous, T. M., & Zimmerman, M. A. (2004). Racial discrimination and racial identity as risk or protective factors for violent behaviors in African American young adults. *American Journal of Community Psychology, 33*(1–2), 91–105. https://doi.org/10.1023/B:AJCP.0000014321.02367.dd

Carson, D. C., & Esbensen, F.-A. (2019). Gangs in school: Exploring the experiences of gang-involved youth. *Youth Violence and Juvenile Justice, 17*(1), 3–23. https://doi.org/10.1177/1541204017739678

Cedeno, L. A., Elias, M. J., Kelly, S., & Chu, B. C. (2010). School violence, adjustment, and the influence of hope on low-income, African American youth. *American Journal of Orthopsychiatry, 80*(2), 213–226. https://doi.org/10.1111/j.1939-0025.2010.01025.x

Center for Disease Control and Prevention. (2019). *Preventing school violence.* https://www.cdc.gov/violenceprevention/youthviolence/schoolviolence/fastfact.html

Chatters, L. M., Taylor, R. J., Bullard, K. M., & Jackson, J. S. (2009). Race and ethnic differences in religious involvement: African Americans, Caribbean blacks and non-Hispanic whites. *Ethnic and Racial Studies, 32*(7), 1143–1163. https://doi.org/10.1080/01419870802334531

Chavous, T. M., Bernat, D. H., Schmeelk-Cone, K., Caldwell, C. H., Kohn-Wood, L., & Zimmerman, M. A. (2003). Racial identity and academic attainment among African American adolescents. *Child Development, 74*(4), 1076–1090. https://doi.org/10.1111/1467-8624.00593

Chavous, T. M., Rivas-Drake, D., Smalls, C., Griffin, T., & Cogburn, C. (2008). Gender matters, too: The influences of school racial discrimination and racial identity on academic engagement outcomes among African American adolescents. *Developmental Psychology, 44*(3), 637–654. https://doi.org/10.1037/0012-1649.44.3.637

Chui, W. H., & Chan, H. C. O. (2015). Self-control, school bullying perpetration, and victimization among Macanese adolescents. *Journal of Child and Family Studies, 24*(6), 1751–1761. https://doi.org/10.1007/s10826-014-9979-3

Collaborative for Academic, Social and Emotional Learning. (2020). *Core SEL competencies.* https://casel.org/core-competencies/

Cook, C. R., Duong, M. T., McIntosh, K., Fiat, A. E., Larson, M., Pullmann, M. D., & McGinnis, J. (2018). Addressing discipline disparities for Black male students: Linking malleable root causes to feasible and effective practices. *School Psychology Review, 47*(2), 135–152. https://doi.org/10.17105/SPR-2017-0026.V47-2

David-Ferdon, C., Vivolo-Kantor, A. M., Dahlberg, L. L., Marshall, K. J., Rainford, N., & Hall, J. E. (2016). *A comprehensive technical package for the prevention of youth violence and associated risk behaviors*. National Center for Injury Prevention and Control, Centers for Disease Control and Prevention.

DeGruy, J., Kjellstrand, J. M., Briggs, H. E., & Brennan, E. M. (2012). Racial respect and racial socialization as protective factors for African American male youth. *Journal of Black Psychology, 38*(4), 395–420. https://doi.org/10.1177/0095798411429744

DePrince, A. P., Weinzierl, K. M., & Combs, M. D. (2009). Executive function performance and trauma exposure in a community sample of children. *Child Abuse & Neglect, 33*(6), 353–361. https://doi.org/10.1016/j.chiabu.2008.08.002

DeWall, C. N., Baumeister, R. F., Stillman, T. F., & Gailliot, M. T. (2007). Violence restrained: Effects of self-regulation and its depletion on aggression. *Journal of Experimental Social Psychology, 43*(1), 62–76. https://doi.org/10.1016/j.jesp.2005.12.005

Dill, E., & Boykin, A. W. (2000). The comparative influence of individual, peer tutoring, and communal learning contexts on the text recall of African American children. *Journal of Black Psychology, 26*(1), 65–78. https://doi.org/10.1177/0095798400026001004

Dinkes, R. (2009). *Indicators of school crime and safety (2008)*. DIANE Publishing.

Docherty, M., Beardslee, J., Grimm, K. J., & Pardini, D. (2019). Distinguishing between-individual from within individual predictors of gun carrying among Black and White males across adolescence. *Law and Human Behavior, 43*(2), 144. https://doi.org/10.1037/lhb0000320

Docherty, M., Sweeten, G., Craig, T., Yang, V. J. H., Decrop, R., Beardslee, J., Piquero, A., Clark, C., & Pardini, D. (2020). Prevalence and risk factors associated with carrying a gun to school during adolescence: A statewide study of middle and high school students. *Journal of School Violence, 19*(1), 35–47. https://doi.org/10.1080/15388220.2019.1703718

Dotterer, A. M., McHale, S. M., & Crouter, A. C. (2009). Sociocultural factors and school engagement among African American youth: The roles of racial discrimination, racial socialization, and ethnic identity. *Applied Developmental Science, 13*(2), 61–73. https://doi.org/10.1080/10888690902801442

DuRant, R. H., Cadenhead, C., Pendergrast, R. A., Slavens, G., & Linder, C. W. (1994). Factors associated with the use of violence among urban black adolescents. *American Journal of Public Health, 84*(4), 612–617. https://doi.org/10.2105/AJPH.84.4.612

Duru, E., & Balkis, M. (2018). Exposure to school violence at school and mental health of victimized adolescents: The mediation role of social support. *Child Abuse & Neglect, 76*(1), 342–352. https://doi.org/10.1016/j.chiabu.2017.11.016

Dykeman, C., Daehlin, W., Doyle, S., & Flamer, H. S. (1996). Psychological predictors of school-based violence: Implications for school counselors. *The School Counselor, 44*, 35–47. Retrieved August 13, 2020, from www.jstor.org/stable/23897978

Eisenbraun, K. D. (2007). Violence in schools: Prevalence, prediction, and prevention. *Aggression and Violent Behavior, 12*(4), 459–469. https://doi.org/10.1016/j.avb.2006.09.008

Eitle, D., & Turner, R. J. (2002). Exposure to community violence and young adult crime: The effects of witnessing violence, traumatic victimization, and other stressful life events. *Journal of Research in Crime and Delinquency, 39*(2), 214–237. https://doi.org/10.1177/002242780203900204

Estévez, E., Murgui, S., & Musitu, G. (2009). Psychological adjustment in bullies and victims of school violence. *European Journal of Psychology of Education, 24*(4), 473–483. https://doi.org/10.1007/BF03178762

Evans, G. W., & Kim, P. (2013). Childhood poverty, chronic stress, self-regulation, and coping. *Child Development Perspectives, 7*(1), 43–48. https://doi.org/10.1111/cdep.12013

Eysenck, H. J. (1981). General features of the model. In *A model for personality* (pp. 1–37). Springer.

Eysenck, H. J. (1994). Personality and intelligence: Psychometric and experimental approaches. In R. J. Sternberg & P. Ruzgis (Eds.), *Personality and intelligence* (pp. 3–31). Cambridge University Press.

Eysenck, S. B., Easting, G., & Pearson, P. R. (1984). Age norms for impulsiveness, venturesomeness and empathy in children. *Personality and Individual Differences, 5*(3), 315–321. https://doi.org/10.1016/0191-8869(84)90070-9

Farrington, D. P. (1989). Early predictors of adolescent aggression and adult violence. *Violence and Victims, 4*(2), 79–100. https://doi.org/10.1891/0886-6708.4.2.79

Federal Bureau of Investigation. (2018). *Uniform crime reporting. Crime in the United States: 2018.* https://ucr.fbi.gov/crime-in-the-u.s/2018/crime-in-the-u.s.2018

Finkelhor, D., Moore, D., Hamby, S. L., & Straus, M. A. (1997). Sexually abused children in a national survey of parents: Methodological issues. *Child Abuse & Neglect, 21*(1), 1–9. https://doi.org/10.1016/S0145-2134(96)00127-5

Fleckman, J. M., Drury, S. S., Taylor, C. A., et al. (2016). Role of direct and indirect violence exposure on externalizing behavior in children. *Journal of Urban Health, 93*, 479–492. https://doi.org/10.1007/s11524-016-0052-y

Flouri, E., Midouhas, E., & Joshi, H. (2014). Family poverty and trajectories of children's emotional and behavioural problems: The moderating roles of self-regulation and verbal cognitive ability. *Journal of Abnormal Child Psychology, 42*, 1043–1056. https://doi.org/10.1007/s10802-013-9848-3

Forster, M., Grigsby, T., Unger, J., & Sussman, S. (2015). Associations between gun violence exposure, gang associations, and youth aggression: Implications for prevention and intervention programs. *Journal of Criminology*, 1–8. https://doi.org/10.1155/2015/963750

Gennetian, L. A., Wolf, S., Hill, H. D., & Morris, P. A. (2015). Intrayear household income dynamics and adolescent school behavior. *Demography, 52*(2), 455–483. https://doi.org/10.1007/s13524-015-0370-9

Ginwright, S. (2018). The future of healing: Shifting from trauma informed care to healing centered engagement. *Occasional Paper, 25.*

Good, M., & Willoughby, T. (2006). The role of spirituality versus religiosity in adolescent psychosocial adjustment. *Journal of Youth and Adolescence, 35*(1), 39–53. https://doi.org/10.1007/s10964-005-9018-1

Gooden, A. S., & McMahon, S. D. (2016). Thriving among African-American adolescents: Religiosity, religious support, and communalism. *American Journal of Community Psychology, 57*(1–2), 118–128. https://doi.org/10.1002/ajcp.12026

Gottfredson, M. R., & Hirschi, T. (1990). *A general theory of crime.* Stanford University Press.

Greene, M. B. (2005). Reducing violence and aggression in schools. *Trauma, Violence, and Abuse, 6*(3), 236–253. https://doi.org/10.1177/1524838005277406

Gregory, A., & Mosely, P. M. (2004). The discipline gap: Teachers' views on the over- representation of African American students in the discipline system. *Equity & Excellence in Education, 37*(1), 18–30. https://doi.org/10.1080/10665680490429280

Gregory, A., & Weinstein, R. S. (2008). The discipline gap and African Americans: Defiance or cooperation in the high school classroom. *Journal of School Psychology, 46*(4), 455–475. https://doi.org/10.1016/j.jsp.2007.09.001

Grills, C., Cooke, D., Douglas, J., Subica, A., Villanueva, S., & Hudson, B. (2015). Culture, racial socialization, and positive African American youth development. *Journal of Black Psychology, 42*(4), 1–31. https://doi.org/10.1177/0095798415578004

Gumpel, T. P., & Sutherland, K. S. (2010). The relation between emotional and behavioral disorders and school-based violence. *Aggression and Violent Behavior, 15*(5), 349–356. https://doi.org/10.1016/j.avb.2010.06.003

Hardy, S. A., & Carlo, G. (2005). Religiosity and prosocial behaviours in adolescence: The mediating role of prosocial values. *Journal of Moral Education, 34*(2), 231–249. https://doi.org/10.1080/03057240500127210

Hayes, D., Moore, A., Stapley, E., Humphrey, N., Mansfield, R., Santos, J., Ashworth, E., Patalay, P., Bonin, E. M., Moltrecht, B., Boehnke, J. R., & Deighton, J. (2019). Promoting mental health and wellbeing in schools: Examining Mindfulness, Relaxation and Strategies for Safety and Wellbeing in English primary and secondary schools: Study protocol for a multi-school, cluster randomised controlled trial (INSPIRE). *Trials, 20*(1), 640. https://doi.org/10.1186/s13063-019-3762-0

Henry, J. S., Lambert, S. F., & Smith Bynum, M. (2015). The protective role of maternal racial socialization for African American adolescents exposed to community violence. *Journal of Family Psychology, 29*(4), 548–557. https://doi.org/10.1037/fam0000135

Howell, J. C., & Egley, A., Jr. (2005). Moving risk factors into developmental theories of gang membership. *Youth Violence and Juvenile Justice, 3*(4), 334–354. https://doi.org/10.1177/1541204005278679

Humphries, M. L., Parker, B. L., & Jagers, R. J. (2000). Predictors of moral reasoning among African American children: A preliminary study. *Journal of Black Psychology, 26*(1), 51–64. https://doi.org/10.1177/0095798400026001003

Hurd, N. M., Stoddard, S. A., & Zimmerman, M. A. (2013). Neighborhoods, social support, and African American adolescents' mental health outcomes: A multilevel path analysis. *Child Development, 84*(3), 858–874. https://doi.org/10.1111/cdev.12018

Hurley, E. A. (1999). *Communalism among African-American students: A cultural analysis of group functioning and mathematics performance in three group learning structures* (Dissertation). Howard University, Washington, D.C.

Hurley, E., Boykin, A. W., & Allen, B. (2005). Communal versus individual learning of a math-estimation task: African American children and the culture of learning contexts. *The Journal of Psychology, 139*(6), 513–527. https://doi.org/10.3200/JRLP.139.6.513-528

Hurley, E. A., Allen, B. A., & Boykin, A. W. (2009). Culture and the interaction of student ethnicity with reward structure in group learning. *Cognition and Instruction, 27*(2), 121–146. https://doi.org/10.1080/07370000902797346

Inzlicht, M., McKay, L., & Aronson, J. (2006). Stigma as ego depletion: How being the target of prejudice affects self-control. *Psychological Science, 17*(3), 262–269. https://doi.org/10.1111/j.1467-9280.2006.01695.x

Jagers, R. J., & Mock, L. O. (1993). Culture and social outcomes among inner-city African American children: An Afrographic exploration. *Journal of Black Psychology, 19*(4), 391–405. https://doi.org/10.1177/00957984930194002

Jagers, R. J., Smith, P., Mock, L. O., & Dill, E. (1997). An Afrocultural social ethos: Component orientations and some social implications. *Journal of Black Psychology, 23*(4), 328–343. https://doi.org/10.1177/00957984970234002

Jagers, R. J., Morgan-Lopez, A. A., Howard, T. L., Browne, D. C., Flay, B. R., & Coinvestigators, A. A. (2007a). Mediators of the development and prevention of violent behavior. *Prevention Science, 8*(3), 171–179. https://doi.org/10.1007/s11121-007-0067-4

Jagers, R. J., Sydnor, K., Mouttapa, M., & Flay, B. R. (2007b). Protective factors associated with preadolescent violence: Preliminary work on a cultural model. *American Journal of Community Psychology, 40*(1–2), 138–145. https://doi.org/10.1007/s10464-007-9121-4

James, K., Bunch, J., & Clay-Warner, J. (2014). Perceived injustice and school violence: An application of general strain theory. *Youth Violence and Juvenile Justice, 13*(2), 169–189. https://doi.org/10.1177/1541204014521251

Jiménez-Barbero, J. A., Ruiz-Hernández, J. A., Llor-Zaragoza, L., Pérez-García, M., & Llor-Esteban, B. (2016). Effectiveness of anti-bullying school programs: A meta- analysis. *Children and Youth Services Review, 61*, 165–175. https://doi.org/10.1016/j.childyouth.2015.12.015

Johnson, S. L. (2009). Improving the school environment to reduce school violence: A review of the literature. *Journal of School Health, 79*(10), 451–465. https://doi.org/10.1111/j.1746-1561.2009.00435.x

Johnson, V. E., & Carter, R. T. (2020). Black cultural strengths and psychosocial well-being: An empirical analysis with Black American adults. *Journal of Black Psychology, 46*(1), 55–89. https://doi-org.ez.lib.jjay.cuny.edu/10.1177/0095798419889752

Johnson, S. M., Kraft, M. A., & Papay, J. P. (2012). How context matters in high-need schools: The effects of teachers' working conditions on their professional satisfaction and their students' achievement. *Teachers College Record, 114*(10), 1–39.

Kann, L., McMann, T., Harris, W., et al. (2018). Youth risk behavior surveillance-United States, 2017. *MMWR Surveillance Summaries, 67*(SS-8), 1–114.

Kilewer, W. (2013). The role of neighborhood collective efficacy and fear of crime in socialization of coping with violence in low-income communities. *Journal of Community Psychology, 41*(8), 920–930. https://doi.org/10.1002/jcop.21573

Kim, D. H., Harty, J., Takahashi, L., & Voisin, D. R. (2018). The protective effects of religious beliefs on behavioral health factors among low income African American adolescents in Chicago. *Journal of Child and Family Studies, 27*(2), 355–364. https://doi.org/10.1007/s10826-017-0891-5

Kim, Y. K., Sanders, J. E., Makubuya, T., & Yu, M. (2020). Risk factors of academic performance: Experiences of school violence, school safety concerns, and depression by gender. In *Child& youth care forum.* Springer.

Kodjoe, C. M., Auinger, P., & Ryan, S. A. (2003). Demographic, intrinsic, and extrinsic factors associated with weapon carrying at school. *Archives of Pediatrics & Adolescent Medicine, 157*(1), 96–103. https://doi.org/10.1001/archpedi.157.1.96

Kodžopeljić, J., Smederevac, S., Mitrović, D., Dinić, B., & Čolović, P. (2014). School bullying in adolescence and personality traits: A person-centered approach. *Journal of Interpersonal Violence, 29*(4), 736–757. https://doi.org/10.1177/0886260513505216

Kunesh, C. E., & Noltemeyer, A. (2019). Understanding disciplinary disproportionality: Stereotypes shape pre-service teachers' beliefs about black boys' behavior. *Urban Education, 54*(4), 471–498. https://doi.org/10.1177/004208591562333

Levinson, M. H. (2006). Anger management and violence prevention: A holistic solution. *ETC: A Review of General Semantics, 63*(2), 187–199. https://www.jstor.org/stable/42578632

Lewis, K. M., DuBois, D. L., Bavarian, N., Acock, A., Silverthorn, N., Day, J., et al. (2013). Effects of Positive Action on the emotional health of urban youth: A cluster-randomized trial. *Journal of Adolescent Health, 53*(6), 706–711.

Lochman, J. E., & Wayland, K. K. (1994). Aggression, social acceptance, and race as predictors of negative adolescent outcomes. *Journal of the American Academy of Child & Adolescent Psychiatry, 33*(7), 1026–1035. https://doi.org/10.1097/00004583-199409000-00014

Lösel, F., & Farrington, D. P. (2012). Direct protective and buffering protective factors in the development of youth violence. *American Journal of Preventive Medicine, 43*(2), S8–S23. https://doi.org/10.1016/j.amepre.2012.04.029

Losen, D. J, Hodson, C. L, Keith II, M. A, Morrison, K., & Belway, S. (2015). Are we closing the school discipline gap? *UCLA: The Civil Rights Project / Proyecto Derechos Civiles.* Retrieved from https://escholarship.org/uc/item/2t36g571

Low, S., & Espelage, D. (2014). Conduits from community violence exposure to peer aggression and victimization: Contributions of parental monitoring, impulsivity, and deviancy. *Journal of Counseling Psychology, 61*(2), 221–223. https://doi.org/10.1037/a0035207

Ludwig, K. A., & Warren, J. S. (2009). Community violence, school-related protective factors, and psychosocial outcomes in urban youth. *Psychology in the Schools, 46*(10), 1061–1073. https://doi.org/10.1002/pits.20444

Mateu-Gelabert, P., & Lune, H. (2003). School violence: The bidirectional conflict flow between neighborhood and school. *City & Community, 2*(4), 353–369. https://doi.org/10.1046/j.1535-6841.2003.00060.x

Mattis, J. S., & Jagers, R. J. (2001). A relational framework for the study of religiosity and spirituality in the lives of African Americans. *Journal of Community Psychology, 29*(5), 519–539. https://doi.org/10.1002/jcop.1034

Mattis, J. S., Ahluwalia, M. K., Cowie, S. E., & Kirkland-Harris, A. M. (2006). Ethnicity, culture, and spiritual development. In E. C. Roehlkepartain, P. E. King, L. Wagener, & P. L. Benson (Eds.), *The handbook of spiritual development in childhood and adolescence* (pp. 283–296).

McGee, Z. T. (2003). Community violence and adolescent development: An examination of risk and protective factors among African American youth. *Journal of Contemporary Criminal Justice, 19*(3), 293–314. https://doi.org/10.1177/1043986203254527

McGee, Z. (2015). Risk, protective factors, and symptomatology among urban adolescents: Findings of a research study on youth violence and victimization. *Journal of Offender Rehabilitation, 54*(6), 429–444. https://doi.org/10.1080/10509674.2015.1056902

McGee, Z. T., & Baker, S. R. (2002). Impact of violence on problem behavior among adolescents: Risk factors among an urban sample. *Journal of Contemporary Criminal Justice, 18*(1), 74–93. https://doi.org/10.1177/1043986202018001006

McGee, Z. T., Logan, K., Samuel, J., & Nunn, T. (2017). A multivariate analysis of gun violence among urban youth: The impact of direct victimization, indirect victimization, and victimization among peers. *Cogent Social Sciences, 3*(1), 1328772. https://doi.org/10.1080/2331188 6.2017.1328772

McGee, Z., Alexander, C., Cunningham, K., Hamilton, C., & James, C. (2019). Assessing the linkage between exposure to violence and victimization, coping, and adjustment among urban youth: Findings from a research study on adolescents. *Children, 6*, 36. https://doi.org/10.3390/children6030036

Miranda, R., Oriol, X., & Amutio, A. (2019). Risk and protective factors at school: Reducing bullies and promoting positive bystanders' behaviors in adolescence. *Scandinavian Journal of Psychology, 60*(2), 106–115. https://doi.org/10.1111/sjop.12513

Molock, S. D., Puri, R., Matlin, S., & Barksdale, C. (2006). Relationship between religious coping and suicidal behaviors among African American adolescents. *Journal of Black Psychology, 32*(3), 366–389. https://doi.org/10.1177/0095798406290466

Monroe, C. R. (2005). Why are "bad boys" always Black?: Causes of disproportionality in school discipline and recommendations for change. *The Clearing House: A Journal of Educational Strategies, Issues and Ideas, 79*(1), 45–50. https://doi.org/10.3200/TCHS.79.1.45-50

Morgan, R. E., & Odekerk, G. (2019). Criminal victimization, 2018. *Bureau of Justice Statistics. NCJ*, 253043.

Musu, L., Zhang, A., Wang, K., Zhang, J., & Oudekerk, B. (2019). *Indicators of school crime and safety: 2018*. Prepared for the National Center of Education Statistics. U.S. Department of Education. U.S. Department of Justice: Office of Justice Programs

National Center for Education Statistics. (1981). *Violence in the schools: How much and what to do?* Research Action Brief No.17, ED 208 453, 1–5. ERIC.

National Institute of Education (U.S.). (1978). *Violent schools-safe schools: The safe school study report to the Congress*. The Institute.

Nickerson, A. B., Shisler, S., Eiden, R. D., Ostrov, J. M., Schuetze, P., Godleski, S. A., & Delmerico, A. M. (2020). A longitudinal study of gun violence attitudes: Role of childhood aggression and exposure to violence, and early adolescent bullying perpetration and victimization. *Journal of School Violence, 19*(1), 62–76. https://doi.org/10.1080/15388220.2019.1703716

Nordberg, A., Twis, M. K., Stevens, M. A., & Hatcher, S. S. (2018). Precarity and structural racism in Black youth encounters with police. *Child and Adolescent Social Work Journal, 35*(5), 511–518. https://doi.org/10.1007/s10560-018-0540-x

Ozer, E. J., & Weinstein, R. S. (2004). Urban adolescents' exposure to community violence: The role of support, school safety, and social constraints in a school-based sample of boys and girls. *Journal of Clinical Child and Adolescent Psychology, 33*(3), 463–476. https://doi.org/10.1207/s15374424jccp3303_4

Palacios-Barrios, E. E., & Hanson, J. L. (2019). Poverty and self-regulation: Connecting psychosocial processes, neurobiology, and the risk for psychopathology. *Comprehensive Psychiatry, 90*, 52–64. https://doi.org/10.1016/j.comppsych.2018.12.012

Parham, T. A. (2009). Foundations for an African American psychology: Extending roots to an ancient Kemetic past. In H. Neville, B. M. Tynes, & S. O. Utsey (Eds.), *Handbook of African American psychology* (pp. 3–18). Sage Publications.

Patchin, J. W., Huebner, B. M., McCluskey, J. D., Varano, S. P., & Bynum, T. S. (2006). Exposure to Community Violence and Childhood Delinquency. *Crime & Delinquency, 52*(2), 307–332. https://doi.org.ccsu.idm.oclc.org/10.1177/0011128704267476

Patrick, C. J. (2008). Psychophysiological correlates of aggression and violence: An integrative review. *Philosophical Transactions of the Royal Society B Biological Sciences, 363*(1503), 2543–2555. https://doi.org/10.1098/rstb.2008.0028

Patton, D. U., Woolley, M. E., & Hong, J. S. (2012). Exposure to violence, student fear, and low academic achievement: African American males in the critical transition to high school. *Children and Youth Services Review, 34*(2), 388–395. https://doi.org/10.1016/j.childyouth.2011.11.009

Pedersen, S. L., Molina, B. S., Belendiuk, K. A., & Donovan, J. E. (2012). Racial differences in the development of impulsivity and sensation seeking from childhood into adolescence and their relation to alcohol use. *Alcoholism: Clinical and Experimental Research, 36*(10), 1794–1802.

Peguero, A. A. (2011). Violence, schools, and dropping out: Racial and ethnic disparities in the educational consequence of student victimization. *Journal of Interpersonal Violence, 26*(18), 3753–3772. https://doi.org/10.1177/0886260511403764

Peguero, A. A., Popp, A. M., Latimore, T. L., Shekarkhar, Z., & Koo, D. J. (2011). Social control theory and school misbehavior: Examining the role of race and ethnicity. *Youth Violence and Juvenile Justice, 9*(3), 259–275. https://doi.org/10.1177/1541204010389197

Peguero, A. A., Ovink, S. M., & Li, Y. L. (2016). Social bonding to school and educational inequality: Race/ethnicity, dropping out, and the significance of place. *Sociological Perspectives, 59*(2), 317–344. https://doi.org/10.1177/0731121415586479

Petts, R. J., & Jolliff, A. (2008). Religion and adolescent depression: The impact of race and gender. *Review of Religious Research, 49*(4), 395–414. https://www.jstor.org/stable/20447514

Pham, T., Schapiro, L., Majnu, J., & Adesman, A. (2017). Weapon carrying among victims of bullying. *Pediatrics, 140*(6), e20170353.

Pyrooz, D. C., Decker, S. H., & Webb, V. J. (2014). The ties that bind: Desistance from gangs. *Crime & Delinquency, 60*(4), 491–516. https://doi.org/10.1177/0011128710372191

Ragatz, L. L., Anderson, R. J., Fremouw, W., & Schwartz, R. (2011). Criminal thinking patterns, aggression styles, and the psychopathic traits of late high school bullies and bully-victims. *Aggressive Behavior, 37*(2), 145–160. https://doi-org.ccsu.idm.oclc.org/10.1002/ab.20377

Rawles, P. (2010). The link between poverty, the proliferation of violence and the development of traumatic stress among urban youth in the United States to school violence: A trauma informed, social justice approach to school violence. *Forum on Public Policy Online*, n. 4.

Rosenthal, R. (2002). Covert communication in classrooms, clinics, courtrooms, and cubicles. *American Psychologist, 57*(11), 839–849. https://doi.org/10.1037/0003-066X.57.11.839

Rowley, S. J., Sellers, R. M., Chavous, T. M., & Smith, M. A. (1998). The relationship between racial identity and self-esteem in African American college and high school students. *Journal of Personality and Social Psychology, 74*(3), 715–724. https://doi.org/10.1037/0022-3514.74.3.715

Salas-Wright, C. P., Vaughn, M. G., & Maynard, B. R. (2014). Buffering effects of religiosity on crime: Testing the invariance hypothesis across gender and developmental period. *Criminal Justice and Behavior, 41*(6), 673–691. https://doi.org/10.1177/0093854813514579

Salas-Wright, C. P., Vaughn, M. G., & Maynard, B. R. (2015). Profiles of religiosity and their association with risk behavior among emerging adults in the United States. *Emerging Adulthood, 3*(2), 67–84. https://doi.org/10.1177/0093854813514579

Salas-Wright, C. P., Vaughn, M. G., Maynard, B. R., Clark, T. T., & Snyder, S. (2017). Public or private religiosity: Which is protective for adolescent substance use and by what pathways? *Youth & Society, 49*(2), 228–253. https://doi.org/10.1177/0044118X14531603

Sellers, R. M., Caldwell, C. H., Schmeelk-Cone, K. H., & Zimmerman, M. A. (2003). Racial identity, racial discrimination, perceived stress, and psychological distress among African American young adults. *Journal of Health and Social Behavior, 44*(3), 302–317. https://doi.org/10.2307/1519781

Sellers, R. M., Smith, M. A., Shelton, J. N., Rowley, S. A., & Chavous, T. M. (1998). Multidimensional model of racial identity: A reconceptualization of African American racial identity. *Personality and social psychology review, 2*(1), 18–39. https://doi.org/10.1207/s15327957pspr0201_2

Semprevivo, L. K., Agnich, L. E., & Peguero, A. A. (2020). Is victimization associated with carrying a weapon? Investigating the intersection of sex and race/ethnicity. *Journal of School Violence, 19*(1), 20–34. https://doi.org/10.1080/15388220.2019.1703714

Shapiro, J. P., Dorman, R. L., Burkes, W. M., Welker, C. J., & Clough, J. B. (1997). Development and factor analysis of a measure of youth attitudes toward guns and violence. *Journal of Clinical Child Psychology, 26*(3), 311–320. https://doi.org/10.1207/s15374424jccp2603_10

Shirley, E. L., & Cornell, D. G. (2012). The contribution of student perceptions of school climate to understanding the disproportionate punishment of African American students in a middle school. *School Psychology International, 33*(2), 115–134. https://doi.org/10.1177/0143034311406815

Sikkink, D., & Hernandez, E. I. (2003). Religion matters: Predicting schooling success among Latino youth. *Interim Reports.* Institute for Latino Studies. University of Notre Dame.

Skiba, R. J., & Losen, D. J. (2016). From reaction to prevention: Turning the page on school discipline. *American Educator, 39*(4), 4–11.

Smith, D., & Smith, B. (2006). Perceptions of violence: The views of teachers who left urban schools. *The High School Journal, 89*(3), 34–42. Retrieved August 14, 2020, from www.jstor.org/stable/40364231

Spencer, M. B., Fegley, S. G., & Harpalani, V. (2003). A theoretical and empirical examination of identity as coping: Linking coping resources to the self-processes of African American youth. *Applied Developmental Science, 7*(3), 181–188. https://doi.org/10.1207/S1532480XADS0703_9

Stern, A., & Petrosino, A. (2018). *What do we know about the effects of school-based law enforcement on school safety?* WestEd.

Stevenson, H. C., Reed, J., Bodison, P., & Bishop, A. (1997). Racism stress management racial socialization beliefs and the experience of depression and anger in African American youth. *Youth & Society, 29*(2), 197–222. https://doi.org/10.1177/0044118X97029002003

Taylor, T., Esbensen, F.-A., Brick, B., & Freng, A. (2010). Exploring the measurement quality of an attitudinal scale of street code-related violence: Similarities and differences across groups and contexts. *Youth Violence and Juvenile Justice, 8*(3), 187–212. https://doi.org/10.1177/1541204010361297

Thomas, D. E., Townsend, T. G., & Belgrave, F. Z. (2003). The influence of cultural and racial identification on the psychosocial adjustment of inner-city African American children in school. *American Journal of Community Psychology, 32*(3–4), 217–228. https://doi.org/10.1023/B:AJCP.0000004743.37592.26

Twenge, J. M., & Crocker, J. (2002). Race and self-esteem: Meta-analyses comparing whites, blacks, Hispanics, Asians, and American Indians and comment on Gray-Little and Hafdahl (2000). *Psychological Bulletin, 128*(3), 371–408. https://doi.org/10.1037/0033-2909.128.3.371

Tyler, K. M., Boykin, A. W., Boelter, C. M., & Dillihunt, M. L. (2005). Examining mainstream and Afro-cultural value socialization in African American households. *Journal of Black Psychology, 31*(3), 291–310. https://doi.org/10.1177/0095798405278199

Umaña-Taylor, A. J., Diversi, M., & Fine, M. A. (2002). Ethnic identity and self-esteem of Latino adolescents: Distinctions among the Latino populations. *Journal of Adolescent Research, 17*(3), 303–327. https://doi.org/10.1177/0743558402173005

Valois, R. F., Paxton, R. J., Zullig, K. J., & Huebner, E. S. (2006). Life satisfaction and violent behaviors among middle school students. *Journal of Child and Family Studies, 15*(6), 695–707. https://doi.org/10.1007/s10826-006-9043-z

Varela, J. J., Zimmerman, M. A., Ryan, A. M., Stoddard, S. A., Heinze, J. E., & Alfaro, J. (2018). Life satisfaction, school satisfaction, and school violence: A mediation analysis for Chilean adolescent victims and perpetrators. *Child Indicators Research, 11*(2), 487–505. https://doi.org/10.1007/s12187-016-9442-7

Vazsonyi, A. T., Mikuška, J., & Kelley, E. L. (2017). It's time: A meta-analysis on the self-control-deviance link. *Journal of Criminal Justice, 48*(48–63. https://doi.org/10.1016/j.jcrimjus.2016.10.001

Wahab, A. A., & Sakip, S. R. M. (2019). An overview of environmental design relationship with school bullying and future crime. *Environment-Behaviour Proceedings Journal, 4*(10), 11–18.

Wallace, C. M., McGee, Z. T., Malone-Colon, L., & Boykin, A. W. (2018). The impact of culture-based protective factors on reducing rates of violence among African American adolescent and young adult males. *Journal of Social Issues, 74*(3), 635–651. https://doi.org/10.1111/josi.12287

Wandersman, A., & Nation, M. (1998). Urban neighborhoods and mental health: Psychological contributions to understanding toxicity, resilience, and interventions. *American Psychologist, 53*(6), 647–656. https://doi.org/10.1037/0003-066X.53.6.647

Wang, K., Chen, Y., Zhang, J., & Oudekerk, B. A. (2020). *Indicators of school crime and safety: 2019*. NCES 2020-063/NCJ 254485. Prepared for the National Center of Education Statistics. U.S. Department of Education. U.S. Department of Justice: Office of Justice Programs

Welton, E., Vakil, S., & Ford, B. (2014). Beyond bullying: Consideration of additional research for the assessment and prevention of potential rampage school violence in the United States. *Education Research International, 2014*. https://doi.org/10.1155/2014/109297

Whaley, A. L., & McQueen, J. P. (2020). Evaluating Africentric violence prevention for adolescent black males in an urban public school: An idiothetic approach. *Journal of Child and Family Studies, 29*(4), 942–954. https://doi.org/10.1007/s10826-019-016379

Wilcox, P., Augustine, M. C., & Clayton, R. R. (2006). Physical environment and crime and misconduct in Kentucky schools. *Journal of Primary Prevention, 27*(3), 293–313. https://doi.org/10.1007/s10935-006-0034-z

Williams, L. M., & Peguero, A. A. (2013). The impact of school bullying on racial/ethnic achievement. *Race and Social Problems, 5*(4), 296–308. https://doi.org/10.1007/s12552-013-9105-y

Williams, D. R., & Williams-Morris, R. (2000). Racism and mental health: The African American experience. *Ethnicity and Health, 5*(3–4), 243–268. https://doi.org/10.1080/713667453

Zainuddin, R., & Taluja, H. (1990). Aggression and locus of control among undergraduate students. *Journal of Personality and Clinical Studies, 6*(2), 211–215.

Chapter 5
Gendered Harassment in Adolescence

Christia Spears Brown, Sharla D. Biefeld, and Michelle J. Tam

A majority of youth will experience gendered harassment, specifically sexual harassment (SH) and harassment on the basis of sexual orientation, gender identity, and gender expression (SOGIE harassment) at some point in school, and these harassment experiences are related to a host of negative psychological, social, and academic outcomes (Espelage et al., 2008, 2015; Hill & Kearl, 2011; Jewell & Brown, 2014; Mays & Cochran, 2001; Leaper & Brown, 2008; Russell et al., 2010; Smith & Juvonen, 2017). Because much of that harassment happens within schools, it is especially important to understand the role of schools and teachers in preventing and mitigating (or at times, exacerbating) youth's experiences of gendered harassment.

In this chapter, we first define and document the prevalence and negative psychosocial outcomes associated with two types of gendered harassment in schools: sexual harassment and SOGIE harassment. Next, we discuss how schools may contribute to the prevalence of SH and SOGIE harassment, and how they can respond to and prevent SH and SOGIE harassment from occurring. We conclude by suggesting directions for future research.

Gendered Harassment: Prevalence in Schools and Characteristics of Victims and Perpetrators

Gendered harassment includes verbal, physical, and cyber harassment and bullying on the basis of perceived gender/sex, gender identity, and gender typicality, as well as harassment that policies heterosexual gender norms (Meyer, 2006, 2008). This

C. S. Brown (✉) · S. D. Biefeld · M. J. Tam
Department of Psychology, University of Kentucky, Lexington, KY, USA
e-mail: christia.brown@uky.edu

© The Author(s), under exclusive license to Springer Nature
Switzerland AG 2023
T. W. Miller (ed.), *School Violence and Primary Prevention*,
https://doi.org/10.1007/978-3-031-13134-9_5

includes both sexual harassment and SOGIE based harassment. While youth are in middle school and high school, gendered harassment is prevalent, affecting the vast majority of teens (Espelage & Swearer 2003; Pellegrini, 2002; Poteat et al., 2009). Although both sexual and SOGIE harassment are common in schools, they are distinct phenomena characterized by different patterns of characteristics for victims and perpetrators.

Sexual Harassment in Schools

Sexual harassment is characterized by unwanted verbal, nonverbal, and physical sexual behavior that can occur in person or online. Sexual harassment in adolescence is most frequently a peer-to-peer occurrence, typically occurring between peers who know one another and in public and visible spaces of schools, such as hallways (Charmaraman et al., 2013; Hill & Kearl, 2011; Pepler et al., 2006; Timmerman, 2003, 2005). Sexual harassment is considered a form of sexual violence; although it may seem extreme, it occurs more frequently than sexual assault, coercing someone into sexual activity, and attempted and completed rape (Ybarra & Thompson, 2018). Although peer-to-peer sexual harassment can begin in late elementary school and early middle school, research suggests that it increases as early adolescents progress through middle school and peaks around 9th to 10th grade (Pepler et al., 2006; Espelage et al., 2016).

The most common type of sexual harassment experienced by students is verbal harassment, such as hearing sexual jokes or comments and having sexual rumors spread about them (Espelage et al., 2016; Hill & Kearl, 2011). For example, Hill and Kearl (2011) found that having someone make unwelcome sexual jokes, comments, and gestures was experienced by 33% of students in their national survey. Although less frequent, physical sexual harassment, such as being touched in an unwanted sexual way, is also experienced by many youths (Espelage et al., 2016; Hill & Kearl, 2011). In a direct comparison between verbal and physical SH, Espelage et al. (2016) found that about 57% of students in their study reported experiencing some type of verbal sexual harassment, such as unwanted sexual jokes and comments or being the target of sexual rumors, and 46% reported experiencing some type of physical sexual harassment, such as being touched against their wishes, being brushed up against, blocked, grabbed, or pinched in a sexual way. A small minority, 5%, reported sexual assault, such as being kissed or touched in an unwanted way, being coerced into sexual activity, or experiencing attempted or completed rape.

Although prevalence rates of sexual harassment at school vary from study to study, in part due to methodological differences in measurement, sexual harassment appears to be a frequent occurrence for youth. One study of 18,090 high school students found that 30% of youth (37% of girls and 21% of boys) reported experiencing sexual harassment in the last year (Clear et al., 2014). Another nationally representative study found that 48% of students experienced sexual harassment in the last year, with 56% of girls and 40% of boys reporting experiencing sexual harassment (Hill & Kearl, 2011). Higher rates found by Hill and Kearl may be reflective of including some homophobic harassment, such as being called gay or lesbian in a negative way, into their definition of sexual harassment. This may especially account for the high rates reported by boys, as boys experience more homophobic harassment than any other type of harassment. When studies assess lifetime experiences with sexual harassment, results indicate that up to 90% of adolescent girls report having experienced sexual harassment at some point in school (Leaper & Brown, 2008).

For many youth, experiencing sexual harassment is a typical part of their school day. For example, a qualitative study of girls who had experienced harassment and sexual assault found that many viewed the harassment as a normal part of their life, with one 13-year-old participant saying, "it's just, like, how it goes on and everyone knows it, no one says nothing" (Hlavka, 2014, pg. 8). In one study of high school students in Australia, researchers found that sexual harassment toward girls from boys, particularly sexual jokes, name calling, and spreading of rumors, was a daily occurrence (Shute et al., 2008). Teachers and students all reported that they saw sexual harassment occur frequently (Shute et al., 2008). Hill and Kearl (2011) found that 44% of students who sexually harassed others said they did so because it was a part of school life. Taken together, research suggests that sexual harassment at school is common, public, and occurs daily.

Characteristics of Victims and Perpetrators While both boys and girls experience sexual harassment, girls are more likely to be the victim of verbal, physical, and cyber sexual harassment than boys (e.g., Hill & Kearl, 2011). In addition to gender/sex differences, sexual orientation, race, and socioeconomic status are also related to victimization rates of sexual harassment. LGBTQ students are at higher risk of being sexually harassed than heterosexual and cisgender students. For example, the 2019 National School Climate Survey found that 58.3% of LGBTQ students were sexually harassed at school in the last year, and of those students, 13.4% said that this harassment occurred often or frequently (Kosciw et al., 2020). In particular, students that identified as pansexual experienced the highest rates of sexual harassment compared to students of other sexual orientations. Additionally, girls of color and girls from low-income homes experience higher rates of sexual harassment than their White or more affluent peers, respectively (Espelage et al., 2016; Fineran & Bolen, 2006; Goldstein et al., 2007; Hill & Kearl, 2011; Mitchell et al., 2014).

Perpetration of sexual harassment is also common and frequently overlaps with victimization. Overall, 72.1% of adolescents (76.0% of boys, 68.4% of girls) reported perpetrating sexual harassment against other-gender/sex peers at least once, whereas 77.3% of adolescents (84.7% of boys, 70.3% of girls) reported perpetrating sexual harassment against same-gender/sex peers at least once (Jewell et al., 2015). In other words, while girls are more likely than boys to be the target of sexual harassment, boys are more likely to be the perpetrators (Ashbaughm & Cornell, 2008; Espelage et al., 2016; Fineran & Bennett, 1999; Gruber & Fineran, 2016; Hand & Sanchez, 2000; Hill & Kearl, 2011; Jewell et al., 2015; Pepler et al., 2006; Ybarra & Thompson, 2018).

At the individual level, certain youth are more likely to perpetrate sexual harassment than other youth. Research has shown that perpetrators of sexual harassment are often also victims of sexual and gendered harassment (Hill & Kearl, 2011; Ybarra & Thompson, 2018). For example, Ybarra and Thompson (2018) found that being the victim of sexual harassment predicted later sexual harassment perpetration. Further, when boys are victimized by sexual harassment, they are likely to perpetrate it against others, especially if they felt apathy toward others and if their beliefs about masculinity included the belief that they should be dominant in their interactions with others (Rizzo et al., 2020). In other words, when boys were the target of sexual harassment, their masculinity was usurped, by their own definition of masculinity. In response, as a way to reclaim their diminished masculinity, they sexually harassed others. Other research further suggests that, for boys, perpetrating sexual harassment appears to be a way to attain or maintain social status. Specifically, boys who are more popular, or central to their peer group, are more likely to engage in sexual harassment than their less popular peers (Jewell et al., 2015). Relatedly, teens that perpetrate sexual harassment also display less empathy than their peers who do not sexually harass (Ybarra & Thompson, 2018).

SOGIE Harassment in Schools

While sexual harassment is harassment of a sexual nature, SOGIE harassment targets individuals on the basis of: (a) their sexual orientation or perceived sexual orientation, referred to as homophobic harassment; (b) their gender identity or perceived gender identity, referred to as transphobic harassment; and (c) their gender expression or gender typicality, referred to as gender typicality harassment. SOGIE harassment can be verbal (e.g., being called homophobic epithets such as "dyke"), physical (e.g., being shoved or pushed), or relational (e.g., rumor spreading), and it can occur online or in person (Kosciw et al., 2020).

Like sexual harassment, SOGIE harassment is also a widespread issue in schools, especially in high schools. Verbal harassment is especially common, as more than half of LGBTQ high school students report hearing "gay" being used in a negative way or hearing homophobic epithets such as "fag" or "dyke" often or frequently in their schools (Human Rights Campaign, 2012; Kosciw et al., 2020; Rinehart & Espelage, 2016). Over 40% of LGBTQ students report hearing transphobic remarks such as "tranny" or "he/she" often or frequently (Kosciw et al., 2020). Lastly, more than 50% of LGBTQ students report hearing negative comments about gender expression (e.g., saying a person is not "masculine enough"; Kosciw et al., 2020). This harassment is not only perpetrated by students at schools, as more than half of LGBTQ students say they have heard teachers or staff make homophobic comments or negative comments about an individual's gender expression (Kosciw et al., 2013, 2020).

Physical SOGIE harassment is also an acute issue in schools. For example, one-third of LGBTQ students report that they have been pushed or shoved on the basis of their gender, gender identity, or sexual orientation (Earnshaw et al., 2020; Kosciw et al., 2020). Nearly, 22% of LGBTQ students say they were physically harassed on the basis of their gender expression at least once during the school year (Kosciw et al., 2020; Myers et al., 2020). Alarmingly, 11% of LGBTQ students report being physically assaulted (e.g., being punched, kicked, or attacked with a weapon) in school on the basis of their sexual orientation at least once in the last school year, and nearly 10% report being physically assaulted on the basis of their gender expression at least once in the last school year (Kosciw et al., 2020).

Lastly, relational harassment, while less commonly studied than verbal and physical harassment, is still a prevalent problem in schools. For example, over 90% of LGBTQ students say that they have felt purposefully left out or excluded by their peers, and almost three-quarters of LGBTQ youth say that they have had rumors or lies about them spread at school (Kosciw et al., 2020).

Characteristics of Victims and Perpetrators SOGIfE harassment targets sexual and gender minorities, as well as gender nonconforming or gender atypical individuals; however, heterosexual and cisgender individuals can also experience SOGIE harassment. For example, while roughly only 11% of high school students identify as lesbian, gay, or bisexual (LGB), 61% of high school students report witnessing verbal homophobic harassment, and 36% report experiencing verbal homophobic harassment (AAUW, 2001; Hill & Kearl, 2011; Lichty & Campbell, 2012). This discrepancy between the number of youth who experience homophobic harassment and those who actually identify as LGB is likely due to gender expression or gender typicality. Sexual orientation, gender identity, and gender expression are closely related, and individuals often assume a target's sexual orientation or gender identity on the basis of stereotypical gender cues (e.g., voice, dress, hair; Blashill & Powlishta, 2009; Cox et al., 2016; Kachel et al., 2018; Miller, 2018; Rieger et al., 2008). Similar to sexual harassment, the perpetrators of SOGIE harassment are also likely to be the victims of SOGIE harassment (Tam & Brown, 2020; Ybarra & Thompson, 2018).

There are also gender differences in rates of SOGIE harassment. Boys are more often the target, and the perpetrator, of SOGIE harassment than girls (Buston & Hart, 2001; D'Urso & Pace, 2019; Poteat & DiGiovanni, 2010; Poteat & Espelage, 2005; Poteat et al., 2011, 2012). This may be because boys often experience stricter gender norms and receive harsher social punishments for violating these norms than girls (Corby et al., 2007; Egan & Perry, 2001; Fagot, 1977; Lee & Troop-Gordon, 2011; Martin et al., 2017; Pauletti et al., 2017; Sandberg et al., 1993; Young & Sweeting, 2004; Zosuls et al., 2016). For girls, it may be acceptable to engage in stereotypically masculine activities or wear stereotypically masculine clothing (e.g., be a "tomboy"); conversely, boys are often punished for the smallest infractions of stereotypical gender roles (e.g., liking to dance). Indeed, sexual minority boys encounter a more hostile school climate and report feeling less safe at school than sexual minority girls (Kosciw et al., 2020). Likely rooted in a similar restriction of toxic masculinity (in which individuals labeled at birth as boys face harsh restrictions on expressions of gender), transgender girls report feeling less safe and experiencing more harassment than transgender boys (Kosciw et al., 2020).

Consequences of Gendered Harassment at School

Gendered harassment leads to negative physical, emotional, and academic outcomes for targets, perpetrators, and witnesses. It is important to note that these negative outcomes may come at a particularly sensitive point in development. During adolescence, youth explore various identities and roles (McLean & Syed, 2015; Meeus et al., 1999). Peers play a critical role in this process, and the influence of peers is especially important at this time. Similarly, rejection and harassment from peers may be especially detrimental at this age. Because the majority of this harassment is happening at school, schools have a responsibility to understand these consequences and how gendered harassment impacts their students both inside and outside of the classroom.

Targets of gendered harassment may experience a wide spectrum of responses from minor emotional upset, or appearing numb, to higher rates of PTSD and suicidality (Haskell & Randall, 2019; Bonanno & Mancini, 2012; Jewell & Brown, 2014; Mays & Cochran, 2001; Russell et al., 2010; Smith & Juvonen, 2017). On average, girls are impacted more negatively by SH than boys, whereas boys are impacted more negatively by SOGIE harassment than girls (AAUW, 1993, 2001; Fineran & Bolen, 2006; Hill & Kearl, 2011; Espelage et al., 2016). Overall, however, those that experience gendered harassment have higher rates of anxiety and suicidality than their peers who are not harassed (Jewell & Brown, 2014; Mays & Cochran, 2001; Russell et al., 2010; Smith & Juvonen, 2017). Individuals who experience SH and SOGIE harassment report lower self-esteem, more feelings of shame and worthlessness, more negative body image, and higher rates of depression, anxiety, and suicidality relative to their non-harassed peers (AAUW, 2001; Chiodo et al., 2009; Goldstein et al., 2007; Gruber & Fineran, 2016; Jewell & Brown, 2014; Mays & Cochran, 2001; Petersen & Hyde, 2009; Russell et al., 2010; Sagrestano et al., 2019; Smith & Juvonen, 2017). Targets of SH and SOGIE harassment also report a variety of somatic symptoms, including headaches and stomachaches, nausea, disordered eating, and sleep issues (Espelage et al., 2008; Hill & Kearl, 2011; Russell et al., 2010; Smith & Juvonen, 2017). These negative emotional and physical symptoms can range from moderate to severe.

Not only do targets of SH and SOGIE harassment experience physical and emotional consequences from their victimization, but they also experience negative academic outcomes (Chesire, 2004; Hill & Kearl, 2011). For example, targets of SH and SOGIE harassment report lower grades, lower school engagement, and higher school withdrawal relative to their non-harassed peers (Chesire, 2004; Hand & Sanchez, 2009; Kosciw et al., 2020; Russell et al., 2010). Additionally, school attendance and participation in extracurricular activities may decline as a result of experiencing gendered harassment. For example, in one national study, 8% of students reported quitting an activity, and 46% of adolescents that experienced sexual harassment or homophobic harassment said they did not want to go to school, because of the harassment (Hill & Kearl, 2011).

Witnessing Gendered Harassment

Although not all students are victims or perpetrators of gendered harassment, many are still exposed to gendered harassment. Prior work has found that the majority of SOGIE harassment and SH occurs in the presence of peers, primarily in public spaces such as hallways and locker rooms (Espelage & Merrin, 2016; Hill & Kearl, 2011). According to one estimate, 96% of students report having witnessed SH at school (Lichty & Campbell, 2012). Thus, students do not have to directly participate or be targeted by gendered harassment in order to be exposed to it.

Witnesses' responses to gendered harassment vary along gender/sex and are informed by their own past experiences. When witnessing SH, girls are more likely than boys to stop the harassment or to assist the victim (Hill & Kearl, 2011). Girls are also more likely to participate in social support-seeking behaviors (e.g., getting a teacher) when witnessing SOGIE harassment than boys are (Tam & Brown, 2020). Additionally, those who have experienced gendered harassment in the past are more likely to confront the harassment they witness. For example, students who are lower in same-gender typicality (who have likely been SOGIE harassed more often) and students who have experienced SH are more likely to confront perpetrators of SOGIE harassment and SH more than those higher in same-gender typicality or those who have not experienced SH (Tam & Brown, 2020).

An important impact of witnessing SH and SOGIE harassment is the school environment it creates. SH and SOGIE harassment have become so commonplace in schools that they are considered normal and expected occurrences by both students and teachers (Buston & Hart, 2001; Hill & Kearl, 2011; Kosciw et al., 2018; Meyer, 2008; Gillander Gådin & Stein, 2017). Indeed, 63% of adolescents who admit sexually harassing a peer state that they did so because "a lot of people do it" or their "friends encouraged them" (AAUW, 2001). Seeing frequent gendered harassment establishes norms that then shape peers' behaviors. Research has shown that boys perpetrate more sexual harassment when they perceive their peer groups to be accepting of sexual harassment (Dishion et al., 1996; Jewell et al., 2015; Rohlf et al., 2016). Similarly, individuals tend to perpetrate more homophobic harassment when they belong to peer groups that engage in high levels of homophobic harassment (Poteat, 2008; Poteat et al., 2015a, b). In other words, in schools, harassment behaviors do not occur in isolation, and affect not only the targets of harassment but also witnesses who then may also be potential harassers.

Youth often underestimate the negative impact of SH and SOGIE harassment on victims and minimize it, labeling it as "no big deal" (Espelage et al., 2016; Hand & Sanchez, 2000). Yet, when students routinely see their peers victimized, this creates a hostile environment at school in which students may be afraid for themselves and their friends, may feel uncomfortable, and may feel unwelcome at school (Baumeister & Leary, 1995; Gillander Gådin & Stein, 2017; Kosciw et al., 2009; Kosciw et al., 2018; Landstedt & Gådin, 2011; Tam & Brown, 2020; Witkowska & Menckel, 2005). For many youth, school becomes an unsafe and hostile environment.

The Role of Schools

Although children experience both SH and SOGIE harassment outside of school, the most common place these types of harassment occur is at school; thus, schools play a vital role in allowing gendered harassment (Espelage et al., 2016). The law is very clear that schools are required to prevent gendered harassment. The 1996 case of *Nabozny v Podlesny* found that schools can be held liable for failing to protect LGBTQ students from gendered harassment, because of guarantees of equal protection in the Fourteenth Amendment. The 1999 Supreme Court case of *Davis v Monroe County Board of Education* found that schools are also required to protect students from sexual harassment, because of Title IX of the Education Amendments which asserts that "No person in the United States shall, on the basis of sex, be excluded from participation in, be denied the benefits of, or be subjected to discrimination under any education program or activity receiving Federal financial assistance." (US Department of Education Office for Civil Rights, 2001). Thus, legally, schools are subject to losing federal funding if they do not protect students from gendered harassment.

Despite this, gendered harassment is rampant in schools. Schools play an important role in fostering acceptance of SH and SOGIE harassment in several ways. Schools and teachers tend to: (1) emphasize gender/sex as an important social category, thus increasing gender/sex stereotypes, (2) lack policies prohibiting SH and SOGIE harassment, and (3) overlook instances of SH and SOGIE harassment.

Emphasizing Gender/Sex and Increasing Stereotypes

Although the endorsement of gender stereotypes does not always result in gendered harassment, gendered harassment is rooted in gender/sex stereotypes, and the more gender/sex stereotypes youth endorse, the more they perpetrate gender harassment against their peers (Brown et al., 2020; Jewell & Brown, 2014). When teachers and schools engage in practices that increase gender/sex stereotypes, they in turn are increasing the likelihood of gendered harassment. Developmental intergroup theory suggests that stereotypes develop and are strengthened when social categories are made salient and meaningful to children (Bigler & Liben, 2006, 2007). Previous research has shown that teachers frequently emphasize gender/sex within the classroom; for example, by having certain cubbies for boys and others for girls, saying "good morning boys and girls," and calling attention to gender/sex in organizing activities. When schools and teachers increase the salience of gender/sex – by using gender/sex to sort, label, and organize students – they increase children's endorsement of gender/sex stereotypes (e.g., Bigler, 1995; Bigler & Liben, 2006, 2007; Hilliard & Liben, 2010).

Further, schools contribute to gender/sex stereotypes when they promote school activities that are heavily segregated by gender/sex. For example, organizations such as girls' and boys' scouts, girls in STEM clubs, and athletic teams separate children based on their gender/sex. In adolescence, schools and teachers continue to segregate by gender/sex with separate health classes and physical education classes. This separation, beyond increasing the salience of gender/sex categories, further discourages cross-gender/sex friendships. Positive and meaningful interactions and friendships are important components to foster positive intergroup interactions (Martin et al., 2018; Pettigrew et al., 2011; Pettigrew & Tropp, 2006). Importantly, engaging in activities *together* increases positive intergroup attitudes, more so than just group contact (Davies et al., 2011; Graham et al., 2014; Pettigrew, 1998; Pettigrew & Tropp, 2006). Thus, when schools create environments that discourage mixed-gender/sex activities, they increase youth's endorsement of gender/sex stereotypes and decrease their likelihood of cross-group friendships, indirectly contributing to high rates of acceptance and perpetration of gendered harassment (see Brown et al., 2020).

Not only are youth's gender/sex stereotypes related to their likelihood of perpetrating gendered harassment, but teachers' beliefs and responses to sexual and SOGIE harassment are also related to teachers' own biases. For example, teachers show heteronormativity biases in justifying sexual harassment. Teachers often discuss sexual harassment as a normal way for adolescent boys to show interest in romantic and sexual experiences, and this belief is informed by sexualized gender stereotypes that state boys are highly interested in sex, and girls are sexual objects (Brown et al., 2020; McMaster et al., 2002). Furthermore, the explanation of "boys being boys"'and boys simply wanting to show romantic attention to girls is a common explanation and excuse that teachers and other adults give for adolescents' sexually harassing behavior (Gillander Gådin & Stein, 2017; Sandler & Stonehill, 2005). Interestingly, when students themselves are asked why they sexually harass peers only 3% said they did so because of romantic interest (Hill & Kearl, 2011). Thus, the tolerance of SH is more closely associated with teachers' beliefs than students' motives.

Lacking Policies Prohibiting SH and SOGIE Harassment

Many schools also lack official school policies regarding SH and SOGIE harassment. For example, while Title IX has specific guidelines for addressing gender-based harassment such as requiring schools to explicitly ban SH, have policies regarding this behavior, and report SH to the Title IX officer, many schools fail to adhere to these requirements (Equal Rights Advocates, 2015). For example, one study of California schools found that many schools in the state were not in compliance with Title IX – more than 30% of schools reviewed did not have someone who received Title IX complaints, and 85% of school policies regarding SH were not easily accessible. Additionally, despite students' high reports of SH to researchers (Leaper & Brown, 2008), almost two-thirds of school districts in the U.S. reported zero instances of SH to the Office of Civil Rights (USDOE, 2016). Research on SH policies in the southeastern United States finds similar results. A majority of schools in this region have policies regarding bullying; however, we found that only 43.4% of districts mentioned sexual harassment in their code of conducts, and only 27.3% of those actually defined what sexual harassment was (Brown et al., 2022).

Similarly, schools often lack specific policies regarding SOGIE harassment, and even when these policies are present, they are rarely enforced in schools (Frost, 2017; Greytak & Kosciw, 2013; Gowen & Winges-Yanez, 2014; Kosciw et al., 2018; Russell et al., 2010). In a national survey of LGBTQ youth, few students reported that their school had policies regarding sexual orientation, and only one in 10 reported that their school had policies regarding gender identity and gender expression (Kosciw et al., 2020). Few schools have comprehensive sex education that discusses LGBTQ topics, and even fewer do so in a positive manner (Greytak & Kosciw, 2013; Kosciw et al., 2018). Just over 40% of youth in this survey report that their school administration was supportive of LGBTQ students, and only 60% of these youth attend a school that has a gay-straight alliance (Kosciw et al., 2020).

Not only is there a lack of school policies regarding gendered harassment, but many teachers feel they lack the support of school administrators to address this harassment. Many teachers feel that they do not know what to do when they witness SH and SOGIE harassment and are not supported by school administrators (Meyer, 2008; Sela-Shayovitz, 2009). For example, the majority of trainings regarding SH are focused on adult-to-student harassment and do not equip teachers on how to deal with peer-to-peer harassment (Meyer, 2008). When teachers feel unsupported by administrators and cannot rely on policies to help guide their response to seeing SH and SOGIE harassment, they are less likely to act. Similarly, research suggests that teachers have increased self-efficacy in their responses to violence at school when they are supported by the school and when they receive training on how to respond (Sela-Shayovitz, 2009). Thus, creating clear policies regarding SH and SOGIE harassment and support from the top down is vital to lessening gendered harassment.

Ignoring or Overlooking SH and SOGIE Harassment

Even when schools do have policies that prohibit SH and SOGIE harassment, teachers often fail to enforce these policies and rarely intervene to stop gendered harassment. Research suggests that teachers are *less* likely to intervene when they witness gendered harassment than when they see other types of harassment and general bullying (AAUW, 2001; Kosciw et al., 2009; Meyer, 2008). By not intervening and refusing to punish perpetrators, schools and staff communicate to students that gendered harassment is acceptable and that perpetration will go unpunished (Robinson, 2005; Gillander Gådin & Stein, 2017). Furthermore, when teachers do address SH and other gendered harassment, the punishments and consequences they assign are often lenient and ineffectual, such as giving perpetrators a "talking to" (Keddie, 2009; Meyer, 2008).

This lack of teacher support affects students' own responses to SH and SOGIE harassment. Despite the high occurrences, few students report gendered harassment to adults and teachers (Hill & Kearl, 2011; Gådin et al., 2013; Timmerman, 2003). For example, one study found that only 12% of SH victims reported it to an adult at school (Hill & Kearl, 2011). This underreporting may be, in part, related to student's lack of trust in authority figures to stop the harassment. For example, only about 12% of students feel that their schools adequately address SH and SOGIE harassment (Hill & Kearl, 2011; Kosciw et al., 2020). Students' lack of faith in schools to stop gendered harassment may also lead victims to feel hopeless that there is not any alternative to experiencing gendered harassment, and that they must "just deal with it" (Gillander Gådin & Stein, 2017; Oliver & Candappa, 2007). For example, a national survey of LGBTQ youth found that over half of these students never report harassment to family members or school staff for reasons such as not being believed (Kosciw et al., 2020).

Students may also have a desire to conceal gendered harassment from adults at school for fear of judgment and even negative consequences, such as being punished themselves (Gillander Gådin & Stein, 2017; Oliver & Candappa, 2007). For example, when students do report gendered harassment, teachers often engage in victim blaming and shift responsibility for the harassment to the victim rather than the perpetrator (Gillander Gådin & Stein, 2017; Keddie, 2009). A common example of this is punishing a girl for a dress code violation after she reports being sexually harassed. Currently, students are more aware of the school policies enforcing dress codes banning short shorts and tank tops than policies banning sexual harassment (Brown et al., 2022). Thus, for schools to actually limit gendered harassment, school and teachers need to not only have specific policies but also enforce those policies equitably.

Recommendations and Future Directions

Research has well documented that gendered harassment is common in schools and is extremely harmful to students on multiple levels including emotionally, physically, and academically. However, we continue to see high rates of perpetration of gendered harassment in middle and high schools. In order to create a safer academic environment for students, effective intervention strategies within schools should be utilized. Next, we discuss a few strategies schools can utilize to lessen gendered harassment and then suggest areas for future research.

Recommendations for Effective Intervention Strategies

Harassment intervention efforts in schools often target general bullying, but do not discuss gendered harassment (Earnshaw et al., 2018; Gruber & Fineran, 2007). When interventions ignore sexual and SOGIE harassment, it is a dangerous oversight and a missed opportunity to create safer schools. Hence, intervention efforts to decrease general bullying should also target gendered harassment and should directly address SH and SOGIE harassment. As suggested by the bully sexual violence pathway (Espelage et al., 2012, 2015) and the bioecological theory of sexual harassment (Brown et al., 2020), interventions to lessen gender harassment must directly and explicitly address SOGIE harassment and should begin when children are young. When bullying interventions do not discuss gendered harassment, it suggests that this type of harassment is acceptable behavior and further increases its normalization (Gillander Gådin, 2012; Larkin, 1994). However, if gendered harassment is treated as equally harmful as general bullying, it may become less accepted and normalized.

Furthermore, preventing gendered harassment, particularly sexual harassment, may hinge on preventing homophobic and gender typicality-based harassment when children are young, as these precede sexual harassment and are correlated with perpetrating high rates of sexual harassment (Espelage et al., 2012, 2015). For example, research suggests that middle schoolers' homophobic bullying and general bullying were predictors of sexual harassment behaviors 3 years later, such that those that engaged in high level of homophobic bullying also later engaged in higher levels of sexual harassment (Espelage et al., 2012). Additionally, in one study, boys who bullied their peers were almost five times more likely to sexually harass their peers 2 years later, and those who also engaged in homophobic harassment were more likely to sexually harass their peers than those that reported low levels of homophobic harassment (Espelage et al., 2015). Thus, general bullying, homophobic harassment, and sexual harassment prevention should not be considered separate, but instead predictive of one other.

Schools may also lessen gendered harassment by making sure gender/sex equity is valued and fostered. Rinehart and Espelage (2016) found that having high levels of gender equity (reported by teachers and staff) was associated with less gendered harassment, both SH and homophobic harassment, reported by students. One way to foster greater gender/sex equity is by promoting positive cross-gender/sex interactions, as those are related to better intergroup attitudes and may increase empathy for peers of another gender/sex (Martin et al., 2017).

Finally, students themselves have many important insights for how to lessen SH and SOGIE harassment in their schools. For example, students suggest that they should be able to anonymously report sexual harassment, in particular, thus circumventing some negative social impacts (Hill & Kearl, 2011). Students also suggest that schools punish perpetrators in a consistent fashion, have a designated person that students can talk to regarding sexual harassment, and have in-class discussions regarding gendered harassment (Plan International & PerryUndem, 2018).

Recommendations for Future Research

Given how common sexual and SOGIE harassment is in schools, there is clearly much work to do to understand how schools can help change the school climate. We suggest several areas of future research. First, researchers should examine early predictors for perpetrating gendered harassment (i.e., characteristics emerging in elementary school). This would facilitate designing early and effective interventions. For example, it is important to examine how cross-gender/sex friendships in elementary school might increase empathy for other gender/sex children and might lead to lower rates of harassment perpetration in adolescence.

We also suggest research address how to best empower teachers and administrators to address SH and SOGIE harassment. Research has shown that teachers who feel supported by their administration are more likely to intervene when they witness gender harassment. Thus, future research should investigate how to best assist teachers and administrators in consistently enforcing policies against gendered harassment.

Although effective prevention of gendered harassment should be a major goal of researchers, policy-makers, and educators, there are many children who have already experienced gendered harassment. As previously discussed in this chapter, children suffer many negative consequences from perpetrating, witnessing, and being victims of gendered harassment; thus, future research should also focus on how to lessen these negative consequences and support children when they do experience SH and SOGIE harassment. Furthermore, many perpetrators of gendered harassment were themselves victims and future research should investigate the mechanisms that may underlie this connection and ways to disrupt the cyclical violence of being victimized and then victimizing others (Pauletti et al., 2014; Tam et al., 2019; Ybarra & Thompson, 2018).

Lastly, future research should also focus on online harassment, especially in light of the 2020 COVID-19 pandemic and physical isolation many students experienced. In the early spring of 2020, the COVID-19 pandemic circled the globe and in the U.S. schools began shutting down and learning became completely remote. Even prior to the COVID-19 pandemic, the majority of adolescents in the US had access to a smartphone and 45% reported being online almost constantly (Anderson & Jiang, 2018). Many of these online interactions include gendered harassment. Prior to COVID-19, one national survey estimated that about 41% of women and 22% of men have experienced online SH (Kearl, 2018). Furthermore, in the 2019 GLSEN school climate survey, 45% of LGBTQ students reported experiencing online harassment or cyberbullying in the last year (Kosciw et al., 2020). Thus, future research should focus on how increased online interactions and decreased in-person interactions impacted the prevalence of gendered harassment online, and the subsequent impact on students.

Conclusion

Homophobic slurs, unwanted touching, unwelcome sexual jokes, and other forms of gender-based harassment and violence are pervasive in school hallways and classrooms. This harassment has lasting negative impacts; however, it is widely ignored by adults. Schools play an important role in fostering the acceptance of SH and SOGIE harassment through: (1) emphasizing gender/sex and reinforcing stereotypes, (2) absence of policies prohibiting SH and SOGIE harassment, and (3) teachers' tendency to overlook these types of harassment. Moving forward, attention needs to be given to interventions that lessen gendered harassment in schools and help youth feel safe and secure while learning.

References

American Association of University Women. (2001). *Hostile hallways: Bullying, teasing, and sexual harassment in school*. American Association of University Women.

American Association of University Women. Educational Foundation, & Harris/Scholastic Research. (1993). *Hostile hallways: The AAUW survey on sexual harassment in America's schools*. American Association of University Women.

Anderson, M., & Jiang, J. (2018). Teens, social media & technology 2018. *Pew Research Center, 31*(2018), 1673–1689. Retrieved from: http://publicservicesalliance.org/wp-content/uploads/2018/06/Teens-Social-Media-Technology-2018-PEW.pdf

Ashbaughm, L. P., & Cornell, D. G. (2008). Sexual harassment and bullying behaviors in sixth graders. *Journal of School Violence, 7*(2), 21–38. https://doi.org/10.1300/J202v07n02_03

Baumeister, R. F., & Leary, M. R. (1995). The need to belong: Desire for interpersonal attachments as a fundamental human motivation. *Psychological Bulletin, 117*(3), 497.

Bigler, R. S. (1995). The role of classification skill in moderating environmental influences on children's gender stereotyping: A study of the functional use of gender in the classroom. *Child Development, 66*(4), 1072–1087. https://doi.org/10.1111/j.1467-8624.1995.tb00923.x

Bigler, R. S., & Liben, L. S. (2006). A developmental intergroup theory of social stereotypes and prejudice. In *Advances in child development and behavior* (Vol. 34, pp. 39–89). JAI. https://doi.org/10.1016/S0065-2407(06)80004-2

Bigler, R. S., & Liben, L. S. (2007). Developmental intergroup theory: Explaining and reducing children's social stereotyping and prejudice. *Current Directions in Psychological Science, 16*(3), 162–166. https://doi.org/10.1111/j.1467-8721.2007.00496.x

Blashill, A. J., & Powlishta, K. K. (2009). Gay stereotypes: The use of sexual orientation as a cue for gender-related attributes. *Sex Roles, 61*, 783–793. https://doi.org/10.1007/s11199-009-9684-7

Bonanno, G. A., & Mancini, A. D. (2012). Beyond resilience and PTSD: Mapping the heterogeneity of responses to potential trauma. *Psychological Trauma: Theory, Research, Practice, and Policy, 4*(1), 74–83. https://doi.org/10.1037/a0017829

Brown, C. S., Biefeld, S. D., & Elpers, N. (2020). A bioecological theory of sexual harassment of girls: Research synthesis and proposed model. *Review of General Psychology, 24*(4), 299–320. https://doi.org/10.1177/1089268020954363

Brown, C. S., Biefeld, S. D., & Bulin, J. (2022). High school policies about sexual harassment: What's on the books and what students think. *Journal of Social Issues*, 1–20. https://doi.org/10.1111/josi.12505

Buston, K., & Hart, G. (2001). Heterosexism and homophobia in Scottish school sex education: Exploring the nature of the problem. *Journal of Adolescence, 24*(1), 95–109. https://doi.org/10.1006/jado.2000.0366

Charmaraman, L., Jones, A. E., Stein, N., & Espelage, D. L. (2013). Is it bullying or sexual harassment? Knowledge, attitudes, and professional development experiences of middle school staff. *Journal of School Health, 83*(6), 438–444. https://doi.org/10.1111/josh.12048

Chesire, D. J. (2004). *Test of an integrated model for high school sexual harassment.* Illinois State University. https://doi.org/10.2307/1128339

Chiodo, D., Wolfe, D. A., Crooks, C., Hughes, R., & Jaffe, P. (2009). Impact of sexual harassment victimization by peers on subsequent adolescent victimization and adjustment: A longitudinal study. *Journal of Adolescent Health, 45*(3), 246–252. https://doi.org/10.1016/j.jadohealth.2009.01.006

Clear, E. R., Coker, A. L., Cook-Craig, P. G., Bush, H. M., Garcia, L. S., Williams, C. M., et al. (2014). Sexual harassment victimization and perpetration among high school students. *Violence Against Women, 20*(10), 1203–1219.

Corby, B. C., Hodges, E. V., & Perry, D. G. (2007). Gender identity and adjustment in black, Hispanic, and white preadolescents. *Developmental Psychology, 43*(1), 261. https://doi.org/10.1037/0012-1649.43.1.261

Cox, W. T., Devine, P. G., Bischmann, A. A., & Hyde, J. S. (2016). Inferences about sexual orientation: The roles of stereotypes, faces, and the gaydar myth. *The Journal of Sex Research, 53*(2), 157–171. https://doi.org/10.1080/00224499.2015.1015714

D'Urso, G., & Pace, U. (2019). Homophobic bullying among adolescents: The role of insecure-dismissing attachment and peer support. *Journal of LGBT Youth, 16*(2), 173–191. https://doi.org/10.1080/19361653.2018.1552225

Davies, K., Tropp, L. R., Aron, A., Pettigrew, T. F., & Wright, S. C. (2011). Cross-group friendships and intergroup attitudes: A meta-analytic review. *Personality and Social Psychology Review, 15*(4), 332–351. https://doi.org/10.1177/1088868311411103

Dishion, T. J., Spracklen, K. M., Andrews, D. W., & Patterson, G. R. (1996). Deviancy training in male adolescent friendships. *Behavior Therapy, 27*(3), 373–390. https://doi.org/10.1016/S0005-7894(96)80023-2

Earnshaw, V. A., Reisner, S. L., Menino, D. D., Poteat, V. P., Bogart, L. M., Barnes, T. N., & Schuster, M. A. (2018). Stigma-based bullying interventions: A systematic review. *Developmental Review, 48*, 178–200. https://doi.org/10.1016/j.dr.2018.02.001

Earnshaw, V. A., Menino, D. D., Sava, L. M., Perrotti, J., Barnes, T. N., Humphrey, D. L., & Reisner, S. L. (2020). LGBTQ bullying: A qualitative investigation of student and school health professional perspectives. *Journal of LGBT Youth, 17*(3), 280–297.

Egan, S. K., & Perry, D. G. (2001). Gender identity: A multidimensional analysis with implications for psychosocial adjustment. *Developmental Psychology, 37*(4), 451. https://doi.org/10.1037/0012-1649.37.4.451

Equal Rights Advocates. (2015). *Ending harassment now: Keeping our kids safe at school.* https://cdn.atixa.org/website-media/atixa.org/wp-content/uploads/2015/12/12193459/Ending-Harrasment-Now-Keeping-Our-Kids-Safe-At-School.pdf

Espelage, D. L., & Swearer, S. M. (2003). Research on school bullying and victimization: What have we learned and where do we go from here? *School Psychology Review, 32*(3), 365–383. https://doi.org/10.1080/02796015.2003.12086206

Espelage, D. L., Aragon, S. R., Birkett, M., & Koenig, B. W. (2008). Homophobic teasing, psychological outcomes, and sexual orientation among high school students: What influence do parents and schools have? *School Psychology Review, 37*(2), 202–216. https://doi.org/10.1080/02796015.2008.12087894

Espelage, D. L., Basile, K. C., & Hamburger, M. E. (2012). Bullying perpetration and subsequent sexual violence perpetration among middle school students. *Journal of Adolescent Health, 50*(1), 60–65. https://doi.org/10.1016/j.jadohealth.2011.07.015

Espelage, D. L., Basile, K. C., De La Rue, L., & Hamburger, M. E. (2015). Longitudinal associations among bullying, homophobic teasing, and sexual violence perpetration among middle school students. *Journal of Interpersonal Violence, 30*(14), 2541–2561. https://doi.org/10.1177/0886260514553113

Espelage, D. L., Hong, J. S., Rinehart, S., & Doshi, N. (2016). Understanding types, locations, & perpetrators of peer-to-peer sexual harassment in U.S. middle schools: A focus on sex, racial, and grade differences. *Children and Youth Services Review, 71*, 174–183. https://doi.org/10.1016/j.childyouth.2016.11.010

Fagot, B. I. (1977). Consequences of moderate cross-gender behavior in preschool children. *Child Development*, 902–907. https://doi.org/10.2307/1128339

Fineran, S., & Bennett, L. (1999). Gender and power issues of peer sexual harassment among teenagers. *Journal of Interpersonal Violence, 14*(6), 626–641. https://doi.org/10.1177/088626099014006004

Fineran, S., & Bolen, R. M. (2006). Risk factors for peer sexual harassment in schools. *Journal of Interpersonal Violence, 21*(9), 1169–1190. https://doi.org/10.1177/0886260506290422

Frost, D. M. (2017). The benefits and challenges of health disparities and social stress frameworks for research on sexual and gender minority health. *Journal of Social Issues, 73*(3), 462–476.

Gådin, K. G. (2012). Sexual harassment of girls in elementary school: A concealed phenomenon within a heterosexual romantic discourse. *Journal of Interpersonal Violence, 27*(9), 1762–1779. https://doi.org/10.1177/0886260511430387

Gådin, K. G., Weiner, G., & Ahlgren, C. (2013). School health promotion to increase empowerment, gender equality and pupil participation: A focus group study of a Swedish elementary school initiative. *Scandinavian Journal of Educational Research, 57*(1), 54–70. https://doi.org/10.1080/00313831.2011.621972

Gillander Gådin, K., & Stein, N. (2017). Do schools normalise sexual harassment? An analysis of a legal case regarding sexual harassment in a Swedish high school. *Gender and Education, 31*(7), 920–937. https://doi.org/10.1080/09540253.2017.1396292

Goldstein, S. E., Malanchuk, O., Davis-Kean, P. E., & Eccles, J. S. (2007). Risk factors of sexual harassment by peers: A longitudinal investigation of African American and European American adolescents. *Journal of Research on Adolescence, 17*(2), 285–300.

Gowen, L. K., & Winges-Yanez, N. (2014). Lesbian, gay, bisexual, transgender, queer, and questioning youths' perspectives of inclusive school-based sexuality education. *The Journal of Sex Research, 51*(7), 788–800. https://doi.org/10.1080/00224499.2013.806648

Graham, S., Munniksma, A., & Juvonen, J. (2014). Psychosocial benefits of cross-ethnic friendships in urban middle schools. *Child Development, 85*(2), 469–483. https://doi.org/10.1111/cdev.12159

Greytak, E. A., & Kosciw, J. G. (2013). Responsive classroom curriculum for lesbian, gay, bisexual, transgender, and questioning students. In E. S. Fisher & K. Komosa-Hawkins (Eds.), *Creating safe and supportive learning environments: A guide for working with lesbian, gay, bisexual, transgender, and questioning youth and families* (pp. 156–174). Routledge/Taylor & Francis Group.

Gruber, J. E., & Fineran, S. (2007). The impact of bullying and sexual harassment on middle and high school girls. *Violence Against Women, 13*(6), 627–643. https://doi.org/10.1177/1077801207301557

Gruber, J., & Fineran, S. (2016). Sexual harassment, bullying, and school outcomes for high school girls and boys. *Violence Against Women, 22*(1), 112–133. https://doi.org/10.1177/1077801215599079

Hand, J. Z., & Sanchez, L. (2000). Badgering or bantering? Gender differences in experience of, and reactions to, sexual harassment among US high school students. *Gender & Society, 14*(6), 718–746. https://doi.org/10.1177/089124300014006002

Haskell, L., & Randall, M. (2019). *The impact of trauma on adult sexual assault victims*. Justice Canada.

Hill, C., & Kearl, H. (2011). *Crossing the line: Sexual harassment at school.* American Association of University Women.

Hilliard, L. J., & Liben, L. S. (2010). Differing levels of gender salience in preschool classrooms: Effects on children's gender attitudes and intergroup bias. *Child Development, 81*(6), 1787–1798. https://doi.org/10.1111/j.1467-8624.2010.01510.x

Hlavka, H. R. (2014). Normalizing sexual violence: Young women account for harassment and abuse. *Gender & Society, 28*(3), 337–358. https://doi.org/10.1177/0891243214526468

Human Rights Campaign. (2012). *Growing up LGBT in America. HRC youth survey report key findings.* Retrieved from: https://assets2.hrc.org/files/assets/resources/Growing-Up-LGBT-in-America_Report.pdf?_ga=2.97314263.918503027.1615932336-852452177.1615932336

Jewell, J. A., & Brown, C. S. (2014). Relations among gender typicality, peer relations, and mental health during early adolescence. *Social Development, 23*(1), 137–156. https://doi.org/10.1111/sode.12042

Jewell, J., Brown, C. S., & Perry, B. (2015). All my friends are doing it: Potentially offensive sexual behavior perpetration within adolescent social networks. *Journal of Research on Adolescence, 25*(3), 592–604. https://doi-org.ezproxy.uky.edu/10.1111/jora.12150

Kachel, S., Simpson, A. P., & Steffens, M. C. (2018). "Do I sound straight?": Acoustic correlates of actual and perceived sexual orientation and masculinity/femininity in men's speech. *Journal of Speech, Language, and Hearing Research, 61*(7), 1560–1578. https://doi.org/10.1044/2018_JSLHR-S-17-0125

Kearl, H. (2018). *The facts behind the# metoo movement: A national study on sexual harassment and assault (executive summary).* Retrieved from: http://www.stopstreetharassment.org/wp-content/uploads/2018/01/Executive-Summary-2018-National-Study-on-Sexual-Harassment-and-Assault.pdf http://hdl.handle.net/20.500.11990/790

Keddie, A. (2009). 'Some of those girls can be real drama queens': Issues of gender, sexual harassment and schooling. *Sex Education, 9*(1), 1–16. https://doi.org/10.1080/14681810802639863

Kosciw, J. G., Greytak, E. A., & Diaz, E. M. (2009). Who, what, where, when, and why: Demographic and ecological factors contributing to hostile school climate for lesbian, gay, bisexual, and transgender youth. *Journal of Youth and Adolescence, 38*(7), 976–988. https://doi.org/10.1007/s10964-009-9412-1

Kosciw, J. G., Palmer, N. A., Kull, R. M., & Greytak, E. A. (2013). The effect of negative school climate on academic outcomes for LGBT youth and the role of in-school supports. *Journal of School Violence, 12*(1), 45–63. https://doi.org/10.1080/15388220.2012.732546

Kosciw, J. G., Greytak, E. A., Zongrone, A. D., Clark, C. M., & Truong, N. L. (2018). *The 2017 National School Climate Survey: The experiences of lesbian, gay, bisexual, transgender, and queer youth in our nation's schools.* Gay, Lesbian and Straight Education Network (GLSEN). 121 West 27th Street Suite 804, New York, NY 10001.

Kosciw, J. G., Clark, C. M., Truong, N. L., & Zongrone, A. D. (2020). *The 2019 National School ClimateSurvey: The experiences of lesbian, gay, bisexual, transgender, and queer youth in our nation's schools.* NewYork: GLSEN.

Landstedt, E., & Gådin, K. G. (2011). Experiences of violence among adolescents: Gender patterns in types, perpetrators and associated psychological distress. *International Journal of Public Health, 56*(4), 419–427. https://doi.org/10.1007/s00038-011-0258-4

Larkin, J. (1994). Walking through walls: The sexual harassment of high school girls. *Gender and Education, 6*(3), 263–280. https://doi.org/10.1080/0954025940060303

Leaper, C., & Brown, C. S. (2008). Perceived experiences with sexism among adolescent girls. *Child Development, 79*(3), 685–704. https://doi.org/10.1111/j.1467-8624.2008.01151.x

Lee, E. A. E., & Troop-Gordon, W. (2011). Peer processes and gender role development: Changes in gender atypicality related to negative peer treatment and children's friendships. *Sex Roles, 64*(1–2), 90–102. https://doi.org/10.1007/s11199-010-9883-2

Lichty, L. F., & Campbell, R. (2012). Targets and witnesses: Middle school students' sexual harassment experiences. *Journal of Early Adolescence, 32*(3), 414–430. https://doi.org/10.1177/0272431610396090

Martin, C. L., Andrews, N. C., England, D. E., Zosuls, K., & Ruble, D. N. (2017). A dual identity approach for conceptualizing and measuring children's gender identity. *Child Development, 88*(1), 167–182. https://doi.org/10.1111/cdev.12568

Martin, C. L., Fabes, R. A., & Hanish, L. D. (2018). Differences and similarities: The dynamics of same- and other-sex peer relationships. In W. M. Bukowski, B. Laursen, & K. H. Rubin (Eds.), *Handbook of peer interactions, relationships, and groups* (pp. 391–409). The Guilford Press.

Mays, V. M., & Cochran, S. D. (2001). Mental health correlates of perceived discrimination among lesbian, gay, and bisexual adults in the United States. *American Journal of Public Health, 91*(11), 1869–1876.

McLean, K. C., & Syed, M. U. (Eds.). (2015). *The Oxford handbook of identity development.* Oxford Library of Psychology.

McMaster, L. E., Connolly, J., Pepler, D., & Craig, W. M. (2002). Peer to peer sexual harassment in early adolescence: A developmental perspective. *Development and Psychopathology, 14*(1), 91–105. https://doi.org/10.1017/S0954579402001050

Meeus, W., Iedema, J., Helsen, M., & Vollebergh, W. (1999). Patterns of adolescent identity development: Review of literature and longitudinal analysis. *Developmental Review, 19*(4), 419–461. https://doi.org/10.1006/drev.1999.0483

Merrin, G. J. (2016). *Violence victimization among sexual minority high school students: Impact of school disorganization on mental health outcomes.* Available at: https://espelagelab.web.unc.edu/conferences/2016

Meyer, E. J. (2006). Gendered harassment in North America: School-based interventions for reducing homophobia and heterosexism. In C. Mitchell & F. Leach (Eds.), *Combating gender violence in and around schools* (pp. 43–50). Trentham Books.

Meyer, E. J. (2008). Gendered harassment in secondary schools: Understanding teachers' (non) interventions. *Gender and Education, 20*(6), 555–570. https://doi.org/10.1080/09540250802213115

Miller, A. E. (2018). Searching for gaydar: Blind spots in the study of sexual orientation perception. *Psychology & Sexuality, 9*(3), 188–203. https://doi.org/10.1080/19419899.2018.1468353

Mitchell, K. J., Ybarra, M. L., & Korchmaros, J. D. (2014). Sexual harassment among adolescents of different sexual orientations and gender identities. *Child Abuse & Neglect, 38*(2), 280–295. https://doi.org/10.1016/j.chiabu.2013.09.008

Myers, W., Turanovic, J. J., Lloyd, K. M., & Pratt, T. C. (2020). The victimization of LGBTQ students at school: A meta-analysis. *Journal of School Violence, 19*(4), 421–432. https://doi.org/10.1080/15388220.2020.1725530

Oliver, C., & Candappa, M. (2007). Bullying and the politics of 'telling'. *Oxford Review of Education, 33*(1), 71–86. https://doi.org/10.1080/03054980601094594

Pauletti, R. E., Cooper, P. J., & Perry, D. G. (2014). Influences of gender identity on children's maltreatment of gender-nonconforming peers: A person× target analysis of aggression. *Journal of Personality and Social Psychology, 106*(5), 843. https://doi.org/10.1037/a0036037

Pauletti, R. E., Menon, M., Cooper, P. J., et al. (2017). Psychological androgyny and children's mental health: A new look with new measures. *Sex Roles, 76*, 705–718. https://doi.org/10.1007/s11199-016-0627-9

Pellegrini, A. D. (2002). Bullying, victimization, and sexual harassment during the transition to middle school. *Educational Psychologist, 37*(3), 151–163. https://doi.org/10.1207/S15326985EP3703_2

Pepler, D. J., Craig, W. M., Connolly, J. A., Yuile, A., McMaster, L., & Jiang, D. (2006). A developmental perspective on bullying. *Aggressive Behavior: Official Journal of the International Society for Research on Aggression, 32*(4), 376–384. https://doi.org/10.1002/ab.20136

Petersen, J. L., & Hyde, J. S. (2009). A longitudinal investigation of peer sexual harassment victimization in adolescence. *Journal of Adolescence, 32*(5), 1173–1188. https://doi.org/10.1016/j.adolescence.2009.01.011

Pettigrew, T. F. (1998). Intergroup contact theory. *Annual Review of Psychology, 49*(1), 65–85. https://doi.org/10.1146/annurev.psych.49.1.65

Pettigrew, T. F., & Tropp, L. R. (2006). A meta-analytic test of intergroup contact theory. *Journal of Personality and Social Psychology, 90*(5), 751. https://doi.org/10.1037/0022-3514.90.5.751

Pettigrew, T. F., Tropp, L. R., Wagner, U., & Christ, O. (2011). Recent advances in intergroup contact theory. *International Journal of Intercultural Relations, 35*(3), 271–280. https://doi.org/10.1016/j.ijintrel.2011.03.001

Plan International & PerryUndem. (2018). *The state of gender equality for U.S. adolescents: Full research finding from a national survey of adolescents.* https://www.planusa.org/docs/state-of-gender-equality-2018.pdf

Poteat, V. P. (2008). Contextual and moderating effects of the peer group climate on use of homophobic epithets. *School Psychology Review, 37*(2), 188–201. https://doi.org/10.1080/02796015.2008.12087893

Poteat, V. P., & DiGiovanni, C. D. (2010). When biased language use is associated with bullying and dominance behavior: The moderating effect of prejudice. *Journal of Youth and Adolescence, 39*(10), 1123–1133. https://doi.org/10.1007/s10964-010-9565-y

Poteat, V. P., & Espelage, D. L. (2005). Exploring the relation between bullying and homophobic verbal content: The Homophobic Content Agent Target (HCAT) Scale. *Violence and Victims, 20*(5), 513–528. https://doi.org/10.1891/vivi.2005.20.5.513

Poteat, V. P., Espelage, D. L., & Koenig, B. W. (2009). Willingness to remain friends and attend school with lesbian and gay peers: Relational expressions of prejudice among heterosexual youth. *Journal of Youth and Adolescence, 38*(7), 952–962. https://doi.org/10.1007/s10964-009-9416-x

Poteat, V. P., Kimmel, M. S., & Wilchins, R. (2011). The moderating effects of support for violence beliefs on masculine norms, aggression, and homophobic behavior during adolescence. *Journal of Research on Adolescence, 21*(2), 434–447. https://doi.org/10.1111/j.1532-7795.2010.00682.x

Poteat, V. P., O'Dwyer, L. M., & Mereish, E. H. (2012). Changes in how students use and are called homophobic epithets over time: Patterns predicted by gender, bullying, and victimization status. *Journal of Educational Psychology, 104*(2), 393. https://doi.org/10.1037/a0026437

Poteat, V. P., Rivers, I., & Vecho, O. (2015a). The role of peers in predicting students' homophobic behavior: Effects of peer aggression, prejudice, and sexual orientation identity importance. *School Psychology Review, 44*(4), 391–406. https://doi.org/10.17105/spr-15-0037.1

Poteat, V. P., Yoshikawa, H., Calzo, J. P., Gray, M. L., DiGiovanni, C. D., Lipkin, A., ... & Shaw, M. P. (2015b). Contextualizing Gay-Straight Alliances: Student, advisor, and structural factors related to positive youth development among members. *Child Development, 86*(1), 176–193. https://doi.org/10.1111/cdev.12289

Rieger, G., Linsenmeier, J. A., Gygax, L., & Bailey, J. M. (2008). Sexual orientation and childhood gender nonconformity: Evidence from home videos. *Developmental Psychology, 44*(1), 46. https://doi.org/10.1037/0012-1649.44.1.46

Rinehart, S. J., & Espelage, D. L. (2016). A multilevel analysis of school climate, homophobic name-calling, and sexual harassment victimization/perpetration among middle school youth. *Psychology of Violence, 6*(2), 213. https://doi.org/10.1037/a0039095

Rizzo, A. J., Banyard, V. L., & Edwards, K. M. (2020). Unpacking adolescent masculinity: Relations between boys' sexual harassment victimization, perpetration, and gender role beliefs. *Journal of Family Violence,* 1–11. https://doi.org/10.1007/s10896-020-00187-9

Robinson, K. H. (2005). Gender and Education Reinforcing hegemonic masculinities through sexual harassment: Issues of identity, power and popularity in secondary schools. *Gender and Education, 17*(1), 19–37. https://doi.org/10.1080/0954025042000301285

Rohlf, H., Krahé, B., & Busching, R. (2016). The socializing effect of classroom aggression on the development of aggression and social rejection: A two-wave multilevel analysis. *Journal of School Psychology, 58*, 57–72. https://doi.org/10.1016/j.jsp.2016.05.002

Russell, S. T., Horn, S., Kosciw, J., & Saewyc, E. (2010). Safe schools policy for LGBTQ students and commentaries. *Social Policy Report, 24*(4), 1–25. https://doi.org/10.1002/j.2379-3988.2010.tb00065.x

Sagrestano, L. M., Ormerod, A. J., & DeBlaere, C. (2019). Peer sexual harassment predicts African American girls' psychological distress and sexual experimentation. *International Journal of Behavioral Development, 43*(6), 492–499. https://doi.org/10.1177/0165025419870292

Sandberg, D. E., Meyer-Bahlburg, H. F., Ehrhardt, A. A., & Yager, T. J. (1993). The prevalence of gender-atypical behavior in elementary school children. *Journal of the American Academy of Child & Adolescent Psychiatry, 32*(2), 306–314. https://doi.org/10.1097/00004583-199303000-00010

Sandler, B. R., & Stonehill, H. M. (2005). *Student-to-student sexual harassment K-12: Strategies and solutions for educators to use in the classroom, school, and community.* Rowman & Littlefield Education.

Sela-Shayovitz, R. (2009). Dealing with school violence: The effect of school violence prevention training on teachers' perceived self-efficacy in dealing with violent events. *Teaching and Teacher Education, 25*(8), 1061–1066. https://doi.org/10.1016/j.tate.2009.04.010

Shute, R., Owens, L., & Slee, P. (2008). Everyday victimization of adolescent girls by boys: Sexual harassment, bullying or aggression? *Sex Roles, 58*(7–8), 477–489. https://doi.org/10.1007/s11199-007-9363-5

Smith, D. S., & Juvonen, J. (2017). Do I fit in? Psychosocial ramifications of low gender typicality in early adolescence. *Journal of Adolescence, 60*, 161–170. https://doi.org/10.1016/j.adolescence.2017.07.014

Tam, M. J., & Brown, C. S. (2020). Early adolescents' responses to witnessing gender-based harassment differ by their perceived school belonging and gender typicality. *Sex Roles, 1–14.* https://doi.org/10.1007/s11199-020-01126-0

Tam, M. J., Jewell, J. A., & Brown, C. S. (2019). Gender-based harassment in early adolescence: Group and individual predictors of perpetration. *Journal of Applied Developmental Psychology, 62*, 231–238. https://doi.org/10.1016/j.appdev.2019.02.011

Timmerman, G. (2003). Sexual harassment of adolescents perpetrated by teachers and by peers: An exploration of the dynamics of power, culture, and gender in secondary schools. *Sex Roles, 48*(5), 231–244. https://doi.org/10.1023/A:1022821320739

Timmerman, G. (2005). A comparison between girls' and boys' experiences of unwanted sexual behavior in secondary schools. *Educational Research, 47*(3), 291–306. https://doi.org/10.1080/00131880500287641

U.S. Department of Education, Office of Civil Rights. (2001). *Revised sexual harassment guidance: Harassment of students by school employees, other students, or third parties.* Title IX. Retrieved from https://www2.ed.gov/about/offices/list/ocr/docs/shguide.html#_edn1

U.S. Department of Education, Office of Civil Rights. (2016). *2013–2014 Civil Rights Data Collection. Number of allegations of harassment or bullying reported to responsible school employees, by type of allegation: School Year 2013–14.* Retrieved from: https://ocrdata.ed.gov/StateNationalEstimations/Estimations_2013_14

Witkowska, E., & Menckel, E. (2005). Perceptions of sexual harassment in Swedish high schools: Experiences and school-environment problems. *The European Journal of Public Health, 15*(1), 78–85.

Ybarra, M. L., & Thompson, R. E. (2018). Predicting the emergence of sexual violence in adolescence. *Prevention Science, 19*(4), 403–415. https://doi.org/10.1007/s11121-017-0810-4

Young, R., & Sweeting, H. (2004). Adolescent bullying, relationships, psychological well-being, and gender-atypical behavior: A gender diagnosticity approach. *Sex Roles, 50*, 525–537. https://doi.org/10.1023/B:SERS.0000023072.53886.86

Zosuls, K. M., Andrews, N. C. Z., Martin, C. L., et al. (2016). Developmental changes in the link between gender typicality and peer victimization and exclusion. *Sex Roles, 75*, 243–256. https://doi.org/10.1007/s11199-016-0608-z

Chapter 6
Intergenerational Experiences of Bullying, Violence, Support and Survival Skills in Schools

Dai Williams

The human potential for coercion, control and violence affects the personal safety of everyone, of all ages, in most societies. Through history control cultures have created powerful corporations and empires often at a high cost for individuals and communities – part of the dark side of mankind. Human survival depends on the ability of individuals and groups to develop survival skills and resilience needed to live in controlling and violent cultures. But how?

This chapter explores the following areas:

1. What concerns you about bullying and violence?
2. Practical coping strategies for individuals
3. Bullying and different kinds of challenges – from abuse to cultures of violence
4. Practical coping strategies for families and friends
5. What is going on? Confidence, control and respect in relationships
6. Practical issues for professionals, leaders and authorities and for major incidents
7. Long-term responses to bullying and violence – post-trauma transitions
8. The importance of maintaining boundaries for students and communities
9. Emerging threats to children in the twenty-first century
10. New visions, techniques, opportunities and resources
11. Conclusions: contributions of intergenerational experiences to child development.

If you are seeking immediate ideas you can use for yourself, or to help a friend or your child, then start with sections "What Concerns You About Bullying and Violence?" and "Practical Coping Strategies for Individuals – Immediate Issues and Personal Development to Enhance Resilience". If you are a parent or teacher with direct responsibilities for your children's welfare, we also explore further issues and resources. Teachers, counsellors, leaders and other professionals, researchers or

D. Williams (✉)
Eos Career Services, Surrey, UK

T. W. Miller (ed.), *School Violence and Primary Prevention*,
https://doi.org/10.1007/978-3-031-13134-9_6

policy-makers will already understand the features and causes of bullying. I hope that some of my clients' reflections on adult experiences of bullying at school and work, and our mentoring discussions to resolve them, may offer fresh ideas and sources that may be adapted for training or practical support to students.

Civilisation relies on the responsibilities of all citizens to be alert to the safety, potential vulnerability and well-being of others and to confront and contain abuse and violence. Laws set boundaries to extreme behaviour but surviving and overcoming bullying affects everyone – me, you, our families, friends, schools and work organisations, communities and society.

We learn and share personal and organisational skills to survive aggression and thrive in healthy relationships. Societies have done this for millennia relying on wisdom passed down through generations (Gluckman, 1956). Modern education and research can add understanding and better practice – especially for families and communities fragmented by conflicting ideologies, technology, war, disasters and migration. But intergenerational experiences passed on informally by parents, grandparents and communities are still crucial to social evolution.

Experiences of bullying and violence in schools have many links to challenging, violent and abusive adult behaviour in families, work and community organisations – sometimes coming from collective cultures of abuse and violence as well as deviant and dangerous individuals.

Figure 6.1 illustrates key relationships and support potentially available to individuals in one generation from birth to parenthood, and their effects as role models and for social support in families, schools and communities. Ironically, these may

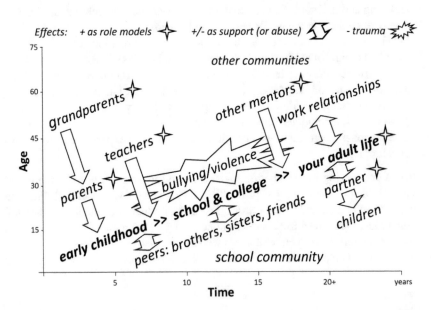

Fig. 6.1 Intergenerational experiences and effects on bullying at school and work. (Adapted with permission of ABC-CLIO, LLC, from Williams (2012), Chap. 12, Fig. 12.2, p. 279; permission conveyed through Copyright Clearance Center, Inc)

also be pathways for physical and mental abuse. How can children learn which relationships to trust and which to avoid?

Figure 6.1 illustrates intergenerational experiences and their potential positive and negative effects on bullying in school and work. This format was originally developed by the author to illustrate intergenerational effects of military service (Williams, 2012).

These notes explore examples of bullying, violence, coercion and fear in childhood and adult life and related survival skills. These cases include reflections on school and adult life events, taken from my life and work in human resources with international staff, students and managers, and as an occupational psychologist working with career counselling clients.

The examples have been anonymised to respect privacy. They are chosen to explore how and why bullying, violence and coercive control develop, to increase awareness of hazardous situations and relationships, and to share and develop survival skills and resilience for young people and adults. You can compare these reflections with your own experiences.

These notes offer practical tips for readers from young people and parents to grandparents. Tricky! Better ways to understand and respond to bullying, over-control and violence are important for adults everywhere – from workers to refugees, from prison staff and prisoners to politicians, from celebrities to priests – and whether they help or abuse children.

These thoughts and suggestions must also be credible and usable by the professional teachers, leaders and counsellors who run school communities in different countries. These techniques and reflections may appear rather basic or traditional for specialist practitioners, researchers and policy advisers who are developing new therapies, training and best practice guidelines for safeguarding in schools and society. They offer some of the more useable and understandable theories and practices we have collected and shared with several hundred clients and other practitioners from varied cultures and professions over 40 years.

What Concerns You About Bullying and Violence?

Your Situation

While you read these notes about other people's experiences, they may take you on a journey through your own situation now, in the past and in the future. You may find it useful to make some notes about your current situation, for example, for these questions:

- What attracted you to read this paper?
- In a few words how do you feel today? Put an X on the scale below:

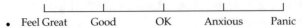

- Feel Great   Good   OK   Anxious   Panic
- Are there any immediate issues that concern you now?
- Are you concerned about your own situation, or for someone else, or both?
- If you are concerned for someone else are they family, friends or others?
- Do you have anyone to talk to for help?
- Who has helped you the most this year?
- Is there something you are looking forward to, or a person to meet, this week?
- Are you responsible for someone else's safety, e.g. as a parent, teacher or manager?

Your Resources

Do you have special skills or experience to help other people?

Do you have specialist support or supervision you can call on quickly or regularly?

Some schools, organisations and communities have expert resources to help students, staff and families. They may also have strict procedures and rapid response procedures for dealing with incidents such as bullying, violence or other abuse and safeguarding issues (see section "Practical Issues for Professionals, Leaders and Authorities and for Major Incidents" and Brymer et al., 2012).

Many websites offer advice and support within countries or states. However, some websites and many social media links may be unsafe or predatory. Schools and other trusted local organisations can play a vital role in providing lists of respected resources, e.g. for children and parents.

However, some readers may have urgent needs but very few or no trusted local resources, e.g. communities recently affected by wars, epidemics like COVID-19, or natural disasters such as earthquakes, storms or floods. Some of you, or the people you help, may be outside the law as refugees, in criminal communities or trafficked as slaves, so too frightened to ask for help.

Even in developed countries like the UK, professional resources are very limited for individual care and support, counselling, therapy or protection against bullying, violence, coercive control or domestic violence. Public services for child mental health have waiting lists of months or years in the UK, except at high cost for private clients or from charities. Law moves too slowly.

Me, You, Us, Now

If you or someone you care about (me, you and us) are in a situation which seems to be getting out of control, you need to regain some control now. The next section suggests immediate questions and actions you can use right now to stabilise your own confidence and reduce threats until more support is available.

Practical Coping Strategies for Individuals – Immediate Issues and Personal Development to Enhance Resilience

If you feel you are being bullied now or are afraid of bullying or violence, there are some things you can do right now, for yourself. The other sections will show how other people may be able to help and encourage you. You can start with the Checklist in Box 6.1.

Box 6.1: The Eos Life–Career Checklist

If you are coping with problems, it is useful to know what is OK in your life as well.

Circle each answer that applies to you. 'Yes' and 'No' are not necessarily good or bad – this depends on the question being asked.

How do you feel today?

In control of your life?	*yes/sometimes/no*
Do you or your family have enough money to eat and pay bills?	*yes/sometimes/no*
Emotionally supported by a friend or relative?	*yes/sometimes/no*
Keen to do new things?	*yes/sometimes/no*
Fit and healthy?	*yes/sometimes/no*
Confident about most decisions?	*yes/sometimes/no*
Tired with difficulty sleeping?[a]	*yes/sometimes/no*
Worried, anxious or panicky?[a]	*yes/sometimes/no*

Circumstances (for you or your family)

Do you, your parents or partner have a steady paid job?	*yes/sometimes/no*
Do you/they have other income, e.g. rent, pension or benefits?	*yes/sometimes/no*
Do you have a home, flat or other safe place to sleep?	*yes/sometimes/no*
Do you/they have any debts that concern you?	*yes/sometimes/no*
Is your/their study, work or home at risk this month/year?	*yes/sometimes/no*
Do you have any special hobbies, sports or leisure interests?	*yes/sometimes/no*

Current interests:...

Recent Life Events (for you or your family)

Have you or your family had any of the following situations in the last 2 years?

What happened and when did it start (month/year)?

New school, job, opportunity or achievement….............................	*yes/no*
Accident, injury or illness (include COVID-19)................................	*yes/no*
New friendship, relationship, marriage or birth of a child..............	*yes/no*
Leaving school, home or college...	*yes/no*
Redundancy/early retirement...	*yes/no*
Unemployment or exclusion from school.......................................	*yes/no*
Reduced household income...	*yes/no*
New course, teacher/new job, manager or organisation change.......	*yes/no*
Moving home, school or work location..	*yes/no*

Box 6.1 (continued)

Bereavement...	*yes/no*
End of friendship, separation or other sense of loss...........................	*yes/no*
Any relative(s) who rely on you...	*yes/no*
Sources of Help	
Who has helped or encouraged you in the last year?..	
Review	

Look at the answers you have circled. If you feel an answer is OK or good put a ✓ beside it. If you are not sure, put a *?*. If you are not happy about the answer, put an X.
You may want to do something about items marked with a *?* or an X. See the *Life-Career First Aid* tips in the next section. For [a] items, see Eos notes on *coping with stress*, and for recent life events, see notes *on coping with change* and *transitions* online at www.eoslifework.co.uk/themes.htm. The Life–Career Checklist (Williams 2009) and Career First Aid notes are client briefing notes (Williams 2000b)
(Copyright © Eos Career Services)

Life–Career First Aid[1]

Your Checklist answers are for you to explore and keep. You can do the first section again after a few days, compare your answers and see what changes. Your answers are confidential for you to keep. You can discuss them with a parent, teacher, counsellor or other persons you trust if you wish. Or keep them in a journal.

If professional support is not available for students, parents and other adults coping with school, career or personal crisis situations, then some of the following *Life Career First Aid* suggestions may be useful. They are also available online at www.eoslifework.co.uk/c1staid.htm (Williams 2000b). They were developed as self-help skills for career counselling clients. They may be useful for a wide range of life, study and career situations. They are practical life skills for confidence, fitness, decision making, stress and transition management (coping with trauma, loss or change).

Ideally, we have satisfying studies and careers which give us a sense of achievement. But when events begin to get out of control in your life – at school, home or the street – it can feel like a jungle. Your first priority is *survival*. These are some *basic survival rules*:

1. **What is the problem – concern or crisis?**
   If we have an obvious problem, we become concerned. Concerns motivate us to find answers. Unresolved issues cause more problems. These can become a vicious circle and potentially a crisis. Our first task is to stabilise the situation, with help or advice from others if needed.

---

[1] Copyright © Eos Career Services.

2. **Take care of yourself and manage stress**

How can we stabilise a study or career crisis? The first step is to manage the symptoms of stress to help you get back in control and to think clearly. Three key tasks are *fitness, training for stressful situations* and *relaxation* (stress dumping). Regular, quality *exercise* (walking, cycling, swimming, etc.) for half an hour each day can make a big difference, especially if sleep is affected. This can save you an hour a day with clearer thinking and fewer mistakes.

Take care of yourself, family and friends who may also be stressed. Take care when biking, driving or working. Try to *stay calm* when others get angry. Practice *relaxing* and calm breathing several times a day and before stressful tasks, e.g. on the road, classes, meetings or interviews. Take regular breaks and find 'still moments' in your day.

3. **Seek help and information for immediate problems**

Check facts and seek help. Some situations need *prompt action* or *referral* for expert advice, e.g. legal or financial advice, medical advice for illness or severe distress, counselling for relationships and advice from someone you trust and respect in difficult school, college or work situations. Early action may prevent a problem from getting worse. If you help other people learn to recognise your limits and refer them to others.

4. **Buy time for major decisions**

Stress can affect our judgement and our ability to think ahead. *Buy time*, take a break and reschedule tasks. If possible, *put off major decisions* for a few weeks until you can think clearly again. This applies to stressed groups and families as well as individuals. You may feel you want to escape. But *try not to quit* your course, job or relationships – at least until you have checked all your options. If you must make a major decision under stress check your options with someone you trust.

5. **Check your options**

By checking options, even hypothetical ones, we can make *better quality decisions* and *feel more in control*. Many problems have more than one solution. For example, you have options to struggle on at school or work if you feel ill or take a day off, to act now or later, to have a main plan and a fallback position (always have a Plan B). When we are under stress, it is even more important to check options to reduce the chance of making mistakes or to try other options. Checking several options and discussing them with others helps to sharpen your ideas about what really matters to you.

6. **Do not give up – your future starts today**

Hard times show us life from a new perspective. It is a chance to rediscover *what we really value* and *who our real friends are*. Have courage. Even when things seem at their worst, new opportunities may be near. The darkest hour is just before dawn. Remember how you survived previous changes or disappointments. Sometimes, we need a crisis to let go of old ways and come to terms with a new reality.

7. **Eat your elephant a spoonful at a time**

   Sometimes a major problem seems to be blocking us completely. Find the smallest, easiest thing that you can do successfully and try it. Small victories give us confidence to move forward again.

8. **Support your friends**

   Harassment and scapegoating are common in stressed organisations and communities. Confront them firmly and stand by your friends or you may be next.

9. **Have something you can look forward to**

   Plan things you enjoy, time for yourself and to be with people you like. Your future starts today.

These questions and ideas may help you to feel calmer and stronger in yourself – *to feel more in control of your life*. Your inner strength may help you to develop a kind of invisible force field around yourself. It lets you see and speak to the world, and to listen to other people, but keeps unkind words and abuse outside.

There is an age-old saying, 'Sticks and stones may break my bones, but words will never hurt me'. In modern words, 'Don't let them get to you'. You already have some natural skills for meeting new people, making new friends and being careful with people that you do not know.

Topics to Explore

This chapter has several topics that may help you recognise the hazards of bullying and abuse, ways of responding to difficult people, and ways of helping others. These include:

- *Learning from experience – your own* and examples of *other people's experiences*
- Valuing the *support of family and friends* and giving them support too
- Our inner sense of control, levels of confidence and staying in control
- How we relate to and influence in our world – other people, things and events
- *Transactions* and conversations with other people (*Transactional Analysis*)
- *Boundaries* and how to respect them
- Important *life events* and the changes or *transitions* that may follow them

It also has sections for other people who may give you support, e.g. parents and teachers, and for school leaders (Head Teachers) and other people with special skills or you may be one of these supporters. A lot of people work together to try to make schools safe for learning and fun for growing up in. And they can work together for rapid response and support when something unexpected happens. A lot of these ideas come from older people who were bullied when they were children, or later were bullied at work. We can learn from them exchanging important survival tips between generations. Skip to the most interesting sections for you.

Examples of Individual Cases of Bullying and Violence in Schools

Note: the cases discussed throughout the chapter were real observed or reported events. They have been completely de-identified to protect privacy and confidentiality.

Case A: Village School – Peer Bullying and Isolated Violence

A small village primary school with 30 children. The playtime had stopped. Something bad had happened. Two boys aged about 8 had grabbed a girl with curly blond hair. They had pulled out a handful of her hair. Although they were young children, this was a serious physical attack causing severe pain. The respected head-mistress suspended classes for the whole school while she had a long disciplinary meeting with the boys. Finally, she addressed the silent children in the playground. She described the incident and her rare decision to smack the two boys and send them home. She set a boundary, a sanction and an example: bullying and violence would not be tolerated in her school. This was many years ago. Corporal (physical) punishment is now banned in the United Kingdom.

Case B: Secondary School – Peer Bullying of a New Student and Peer Support

A large state secondary school, entrance age 11. During the morning break, a second-year student (aged 12) attacks a younger first-year student (aged 11) soon after he joined the school. Another second-year student sees the attack and takes a flying tackle at the bully – peer intervention and support. Both are given one-hour detention for fighting. There was usually good discipline and bullying was rare – a safe modern school with no corporal punishment.

Bullying and Different Kinds of Challenges – From Abuse to Cultures of Violence

The Diverse Range of Bullying, Abuse and Violence in Schools and Society

The first two examples, Cases A and B, were isolated incidents. Teachers responded with prompt discipline. The incidents were both related to attacks on weaker students, one gender-related and one age-related. These illustrate common boundary and discipline issues for young people, and challenges for teachers responding to violence in schools.

Bullying and violence may take many different forms with different actors and in different settings. Our priority concern in these notes is bullying and violence in school settings, often as remembered by adults. *Many of the relationships in Fig. 6.1 – with*

family, friends and communities – are channels for good role models and support.
They can include parents, teachers and grandparents plus siblings and friends. But
sometimes they can be channels for abuse as well as support. And then abuse in one
relationship or social setting may cascade into others or spread into whole cultures,
e.g. in religious or politically divided communities.

There are various definitions of bullying, but three key elements as given in the
US Centers for Disease Control and Prevention's (CDC) uniform definition of bullying among youths (from Gladden et al., 2014) are important and are as follows:

> Bullying is a form of youth violence and an adverse childhood experience (ACE). CDC
> defines bullying as any unwanted aggressive behavior(s) by another youth or group of
> youths, who are not siblings or current dating partners, that involves an observed or per-
> ceived power imbalance, and is repeated multiple times or is highly likely to be repeated.
> Bullying may inflict harm or distress on the targeted youth including physical, psychologi-
> cal, social, or educational harm (CDC, 2021).

Bullying can include cyberbullying (Campbell, 2017). It can also affect witnesses or
bystanders. Bystanders can discourage or encourage bullying or scapegoating and
can be traumatised too. Bullies can also be victims of prior or ongoing abuse, e.g.
at home.

In practical terms, the occurrence of bullying and violence covers a diverse
range, from isolated one-to-one incidents to large-scale, ongoing cultures of violence, illustrated as follows:

- Isolated incidents of *verbal abuse*
- Isolated incidents of *physical violence*
- Unwanted and inappropriate *sexual encounters* – touching, sexting, to assault
- Incidents involve *one-on-one* bully/victim encounters
- Incidents involve small, medium or larger *groups scapegoating vulnerable individuals*
- Bullying involves chronic *psychological abuse* – *verbal attacks* denigrating gen-
  der, race, faith, colour and/or stressful *social exclusion* from friends and
  peer groups
- Bullying involves *repeated physical abuse* causing injury and pain, combined
  with *threats and actual physical violence* to create ongoing fear or terror
  for victims
- *Endemic bullying and violence*, by groups or gangs, and intergroup conflict and
  violence often between ethnic, political or religious factions, often sanctioned
  and encouraged by adult organisations
- *Official* and *unofficial abuse and violence by adults*, e.g. *corporal punishment* by
  teachers and prefects (senior students) sanctioned as part of official disciplinary
  procedures
- *Covert sexual abuse* by individual adults, widespread physical and sexual abuse
  in privileged institutions over generations, e.g. by faith communities in the UK,
  Ireland, Canada and Australia and probably many other countries, and genital
  mutilation in some cultures.

Have you experienced, or observed any of these situations? *How can individuals, parents and communities help individual children to survive and thrive in human societies where bullying, violence and abuse are endemic?* Clear summaries with useful links are available online, e.g. #StopBullying (CDC, 2019). In practice, human individuals and communities are astonishingly innovative and adept at navigating societal conflicts and cultures of violence. In larger communities, social anthropologists like Gluckman (1956) have explored these issues for decades to find the natural coping strategies that communities have evolved over millennia.

Cultures of Violence

The following example illustrates how an individual child responded creatively to a school culture of violence:

Case C: Secondary Boarding School – School Culture of Violence

A young adult professional had good qualifications and potential. But during his life review discussion he described challenging experiences at his secondary school. After a normal early education with a stable family his parents sent him to a boarding (residential) school from ages 11 to 16 years.

This school had many students from military families whose parents were overseas. The school had a very robust (challenging) culture of violence with extensive bullying from older to younger students in each year. He did not want to participate in the bullying but to survive he needed to establish credibility with the gangs.

His survival strategy was to organise shoplifting expeditions from the school to local areas. The gangs left him alone and he was not caught or prosecuted. He survived for 2–3 years before he moved to a healthier college environment.

This is a serious account of an endemic culture of violence. Brutalising younger students groomed them to join in and maintain the culture of violence throughout the school. It was reported by a young adult so had happened 10–15 years earlier. These *cultures of violence* were typical of many schools in the UK in the twentieth century and still exist in many countries.

His parents seemed unaware of the hazards they were exposing their child to in an expensive school. Perhaps they accepted it from their own childhood experiences – good experience for toughening up young men to be prepared for military service during and after two World Wars. The film 'if…' (Paramount Pictures 1968) was an accurate parody of this UK private school culture in the 1950s and 1960s and its potential for extreme violence. This may apply in other cultures.

Education standards and national law reforms in the UK outlawed *corporal punishment* (CP) from UK state schools in 1987. For private schools, it was banned in 1999 in England and Wales (30 years after 'if…'!), 2000 in Scotland and 2003 in Northern Ireland. Many schools had anticipated the legislation and abandoned CP voluntarily several years earlier (Farrell, 2021).

Intergenerational Transmission of Cultures of Bullying and Violence

State legislation is necessary to start to address *national cultures of violence* including corporal punishment. But these may have brutalised generations of parents, resulting in *domestic violence* against women and children which is likely to continue until the last generation of brutalised children has reached old age.

Traditions of domestic violence against women and children have also continued among incoming communities from other countries that still sanction corporal punishment and beating in schools, domestic violence in homes and as state punishment.

These *cultures of domestic violence* against women and children continue to brutalise many young people particularly in economically stressed communities, contributing to ongoing street violence, and to random incidents of violence in schools.

In many countries, long-standing *ethnic and religious conflicts* are perpetuated by intergenerational traditions. These conflicts are often violent and are sustained by paramilitary organisations. In these environments, adults provide role models for training and developing children who will progress to join active fighting groups, often with initiation rituals as rites of passage for admission to full adult membership. These will usually involve weapons.

Gun and Knife Cultures

In many cultures, schools may play a direct role in *conflict readiness and weapon training* prior to military service with the state. In the Middle East and Africa, training may be associated with religious communities such as Sunni and Shia, or other tribal allegiances, e.g. in Iraq, Syria, Afghanistan, the Balkans, Israel and Palestine. But many private schools in the UK still have military Cadet Forces, too, with weapons training. In the USA, carrying guns is a constitutional right.

One possible advantage of cultures of violence in schools where firearms are allowed is that weapons training is likely to include strict safety procedures and some degree of discipline for their safe use, e.g. removing ammunition until it is needed on the range.

However, if students and young adults can store weapons at home, there is effectively no control over their access to the weapon itself and to the ammunition it needs. So teenage students can have access to operational assault rifles and the ammunition they need. This creates the potential for lethal attacks in schools, or other target locations like worship spaces, e.g. churches or mosques.

Strict police enforcement of gun control laws in the UK may have contributed to a shift to *knife culture* a few years ago. Some communities are pushing back against this trend e.g. Art Against Knives in London.

Radicalisation and De-escalation

For an individual school community – of parents and students, and of teachers, school leaders and governors – these external environmental factors may create opportunities for random acts of violence. But if the lone wolf threat is quite disciplined or focussed they may also be more predictable. In the United Kingdom, this has led UK police to be more vigilant and to develop violence reduction and prevention projects like 'PREVENT'.

In the UK, these community violence reduction and prevention strategies may have pre-empted quite a few potential attacks. Some programs include liaisons with schools and teachers to identify potential offenders. But some radicalised young people have still committed terror attacks or murders after de-radicalisation training.

Gang Cultures

Gang cultures may not only perpetuate criminal violence but also provide some practical protection to young people in fragmented communities and violent neighbourhoods. The anthropological function of gangs suggests that long-term strategies to reduce bullying and violence for children in schools need to understand evolving gang and street culture in cities. Violence reduction in communities and schools needs wider parallel initiatives in communities to harness, or at least to recognise the future potential of social support and discipline of gangs to channel and contain bullying and violence in schools and communities.

Community Psychology initiatives in the UK have begun to develop *dialogues with gangs and youth communities* in London and other parts of the United Kingdom to offer mental health awareness and reduce violence, especially knife crime. MAC (Music and Change)-UK, launched in 2008 by Clinical Psychologist Dr. Charlotte Howard, developed with young people from the streets. Dr. Sally Zlotowitz (CEO of Art Against Knives) coordinated the emerging Community Psychology network in the UK and with MAC-UK (Zlotowitz et al., 2016).

With an approach called INTEGRATE, they run a series of innovative but professionally grounded youth mental health projects 'to generate youth lead solutions, co-produce projects and employ those with lived experience. They draw on evidence-based psychological practice and attempt to tackle the root causes of mental ill-health by changing wider social, economic and health policy that creates exclusion and inequality' (MAC-UK, 2020). See also New initiatives to support vulnerable, violent and excluded young people and their families in section "New Visions, Techniques, Opportunities and Resources".

Practical Coping Strategies for Families and Friends

Seeing a brother or sister, or close friend being bullied, abused or violently attacked – at home, school or in the street – can be deeply distressing and sometimes traumatising. In some cases, you as a family member or friend may be at risk from the same person or group which is likely to increase your own stress or distress. In worst cases, the threat may be from another family member, e.g. an older sibling, parent or other near relatives.

In other cases, you may not know what kind of abuse is occurring, or who it is coming from. However, you may be alerted by serious changes in your relative or friend's behaviour, e.g. they may become withdrawn, quiet, stop smiling, show signs of crying, substance abuse (drink or drugs) or self-harm. How can you help?

First, *take care of yourself*. Consider all the questions and suggestions for individuals in section "Practical Coping Strategies for Individuals – Immediate Issues and Personal Development to Enhance Resilience", including the *Life–Career Checklist* and *Career First Aid* suggestions, including your own fitness that will help you to manage your own stress to be calmer and more supportive. And you can explore potential sources of expert help and advice who can advise you on how best to help your relative or friend.

Getting Professional Support

Explore other friends, relatives, teachers or doctors that you think you can trust, or who know and care about the person who you think is in trouble or needs help. Ask if they will listen to your concerns in confidence. Most professionals have strict rules of confidentiality. For example, medical professionals and therapists cannot discuss someone else's condition – at least without their (or their parents') permission.

However, you can ask a professional to *listen* to your concerns because you may have the vital information they may not be aware of, e.g. about bullying, substance abuse (drugs or alcohol) or self-harm. They are unlikely to tell you how they use your information. But you may see that they give your friend more urgent and appropriate support as in this example.

Case D: Alerting Professionals
A highly valued technical expert had been off sick from work for 2 months. A close friend was concerned that the person's doctor was not aware of his heavy drinking habit in addition to his medication. The friend was advised to seek a listening consultation with the doctor on his friend's behalf. The doctor agreed to listen but correctly declined to discuss his patient. He subsequently changed the treatment programme. The sick friend stabilised and returned to work a few weeks later.

Children or adults in complex situations, e.g. suffering bullying, violence or coercive control may need specialist support from several professionals. Ideally, at least one key support worker knows all the others who are involved. Any one resource who fails to cooperate and support can undo the work of several others at severe risk to the vulnerable person being supported.

Supporting Your Friends and Family

Try to maintain regular contact with the person or friend you are concerned for. *Social and emotional support* from a trusted friend or relative is one of the most important enabling factors for people coping with mental distress, trauma, loss and change, see notes on Transition in section "Long-Term Responses to Bullying and Violence – Post-trauma Transitions" (Williams, 1999a, c).

If the abuse, bullying or violence is occurring in your school (or for adults in a workplace) then a group of friends may have more power and influence to confront or deter the individual or group perpetrator(s) – that are causing the violence or abuse. This is very important; see Life–Career First Aid advice item 8 in section "Practical Coping Strategies for Individuals – Immediate Issues and Personal Development to Enhance Resilience". If they continue unchallenged, you may become a victim too. This advice was added in response to the following adult bullying episode, Case E.

Case E: Victimised Specialist – Vulnerability to Bullying During a Loss Transition and Without Peer Support

An older manager was redeployed to run a department of specialist staff for which he had little experience. He decided to impose authority by intimidating and bullying the specialist staff one by one. Most were able to stand up to him. One had suffered a personal loss a few months earlier. The manager used repeated criticism and humiliation for several weeks until whenever he came into the room the victim felt paralysed and shook with fear. Other staff did not intervene. After 6 weeks, the specialist made a suicide attempt and then decided to quit.

Parent Responsibility for Choice and Conduct of School

Parents expect to trust schools to safeguard their children from all kinds of abuse. Many parents will send children to expensive private schools expecting better education opportunities. But cost or brand (e.g. religious schools) is not a guarantee of a safe culture or teacher quality. This case is a chilling reminder of the need for parent vigilance and ongoing support to children at school:

Case F: Long-Term Career Effects of Primary Teacher Violence

During a career mentoring programme a young adult client achieved a top score on numerical ability but showed no interest in career options that might use this, e.g. science or finance. In the life review conversation, he reported violent abuse by his maths teacher in a private school when he was age 9. The teacher would hold him by the hair or ear and ask him to answer arithmetic questions. Each time he got a wrong answer the teacher slapped his face. This trauma appeared to have deeply affected his future study choices. The assessments gave him positive feedback to understand his block and explore wider options. Jung's concept of Shadow was suggested for further reading (Johnson, 1991).

It was curious that his parents were unaware of the sadistic, potentially paedophile behaviour of the teacher. It is a serious warning to parents to maintain an active interest in their children's experiences at school and to listen to unusual incidents or complaints.

In the twenty-first century, child safeguarding is taken far more seriously in UK education. Teachers and health professionals must now report bruised or injured children as possible victims of domestic abuse – a new fear for parents. But in less regulated cultures, the ongoing risks of abuse and violence by teachers or other adult staff must be monitored, for example, in aid programmes for regions traumatised by conflict or natural disasters.

This case also illustrated how a long-term effect of childhood trauma can cause many adults to avoid education and career opportunities for which they might have repressed talents. This can be important for individual adults, for universities and higher education colleges selecting students, and for employers and human resources teams.

Hidden talents may be obvious once recognised. Psychometric testing can be a quick and valuable way of revealing hidden talents but does need skilled interpretation. Some high-ability adult clients had turbulent early school experiences because they got bored quickly in class. This could be complicated by other factors like dyslexia, ADHD or autism outside the range of normal expected classroom behaviour in schools with limited educational support resources.

Parents and students may find independent career and educational psychology assessments helpful if exploring apparent anomalies between interests, skills and formal exam results. Frustrations and stress may make these students more vulnerable to being targeted for bullying or scapegoating, or occasionally to react with disruptive or violent behaviour. Do not give up on them!

What Is Going on? Confidence, Control and Respect in Relationships

Confidence and Our Inner Sense of Control

How we feel about ourselves – our *confidence* or *inner sense of control* – is an essential anchor to our personal behaviour, and to our relationships with other people. This basic aspect of human potential is identified in many similar concepts such as self-respect, self-control, self-discipline, independence, agency, autonomy, dignity, courage or well-being (Skinner, 1996; Bandura, 2006). Our Confidence or inner sense of control can take years to develop on a spectrum from low to high see

Table 6.1 Inner sense of control or confidence: how do you feel today?

High confidence/internal		Adaptable		Low confidence/external	
Rebel, over-confident?	Independent self-motivated	Confident team player	Cautious tolerant	Anxious vulnerable	Dependent helpless, fear

Table 6.1 but can change from day to day, even in minutes. This inner sense of control may be crushed by external forces, people and experiences such as bullying, that may cause feelings of submission, dependence, failure, fear, helplessness or despair. So, it is a vital area for personal development for children and adults (Table 6.1).

Children with different levels of confidence within a group may be obvious to parents, teachers and other students. Significant changes for individuals or groups of children, e.g. loss of confidence or distress, may indicate a cause for concern, vigilance and support.

This *inner strength* is important to our sense of identity and behaviour – our confidence to act. It may be partly related to our underlying personality but will vary significantly depending on recent and current experiences. Julian Rotter (1966) referred to this as *Locus of Control*, ranging from *internal*, e.g. confident entrepreneurs, to *external*, e.g. refugees, slaves or prisoners. Palmer and Dryden described Locus of Control as a coping construct, a continuum (in Woolfe and Dryden, 1996, 533–4).

We develop our inner control through childhood, learning from role models in our families – our parents, grandparents, siblings and others, in our education – teachers, friends and older students, in our community – from ethnic, faith and political cultures, and from sport, leisure, public and social media.

Some of these influences can be positive, helping us to develop our inner strength and confidence, a sense of purpose, and resilience to respond to challenging people or situations. But many cultures restrict this human potential for inner strength and dignity. They may diminish the value of individuals and groups because of for example gender, colour, ethnicity, religion and social class. Such *control cultures* cultivate obedience and submission, e.g. for political control, and coercion or slavery for commercial or sexual exploitation.

Parents may be forced to impose these abusing control cultures and behaviours on their children, e.g. female genital mutilation (FGM), or may help children to survive and overcome them by cultivating tolerance and outer compliance while maintaining inner strength and dignity. Oppressed communities may develop astonishing resilience in societies where bullying is endemic from dominant groups.

As part of our sense of well-being, our inner sense of control can fluctuate dramatically during periods of transition after trauma loss or change including bullying, with the potential to recover later, see section "Long-Term Responses to Bullying and Violence – Post-trauma Transitions".

Outer Influence and Assertiveness – How Do We Treat Others?

While our inner sense of control concerns how we feel within ourselves, our *outer sense of control* is our *ability to influence* the world around us – how we relate to other people and seek to control people, things and events. This potential for *assertiveness* and *aggression* covers a huge range of behaviour – from mystic or rescue workers, through organisers, leaders and entrepreneurs, to coercive control and war criminals.

We learn to assert our own needs from birth, to discover our power to influence other people and how to use this appropriately in different situations. Beels et al. (1992) distinguished between unassertive, assertive (appropriate) and aggressive (inappropriate) behaviours. But these can be seen as different levels of outer influence or control that we move between in different situations, e.g. between home, school, work and play, see Table 6.2.

These descriptions illustrate a spectrum of adult human control behaviour. Young children are likely to be less assertive. But children learn quickly from experience how parents, other adults and older children control them – from gentle, caring support and respect to bullying and extreme violence. This is a crucial aspect of the *intergenerational experiences* shown in Fig. 6.1. Children must learn the important differences between low and appropriate influence or assertiveness and the hazardous progression through over-control into aggression, bullying and violence (Beels et al., 1992).

Children must also learn how to recognise and respect their own and other people's *boundaries* in different roles and situations, see Table 6.2 above, and explained in more detail in Table 6.3 in section "The Importance of Boundaries for Students and Communities" and in Table 6.3, e.g. in games and sports. Bullying behaviour, at school, in the street, at home, at work or online violates other people's boundaries. It may involve individuals or groups. So where do children learn to bully?

Table 6.2 Outer influence – levels of assertiveness and control. How do we treat others?

Less assertive		Appropriate influence		Over control, aggression	
Un-controlling cautious, kind compassion	Respecting consulting, supporting	Respecting firm but fair inspiring	Operational control directing	Over-control bullying domination harassing	Autocratic coercive-control violence
Boundaries: Safe		Negotiable		Hazardous	Dangerous

Cultural Contexts for Control Behaviours

Cultures, faiths and media create widely different expectations on parents, teachers and children. Simple psychological scales as shown in Tables 6.1 and 6.2 are only a starting point to understanding control behaviour. Many cultures place high expectations on academic success, others on physical performance and others on commercial success. Some societies place high status on competition, aggression and violence, but then sanction or imprison children and young people who act out the same principles in school, on the street or on social media.

Each child inherits remarkable potential to influence their world. But how this potential is nurtured and channelled will depend on their family, social and economic status, culture, faith, media and effects of past and current trauma – even before they start school. An abused child may exhibit distressed, controlling or bullying behaviour to others within their first year at school, possibly within days or weeks. Others may show vulnerability or fear (low inner sense of control) and be quickly recognised as potential targets for abuse and bullying. Some may live in fear at home or on the street, then act out their distress as aggression in a safer environment like school, or after school on the street.

Developing a child's awareness of the spectrum of helpful and unhelpful outward relating behaviours with others will help develop their own effective relating behaviours, and help them to recognise and understand dangerous others. Learning to support each other and weaker group members against abuse are essential social skills in families and schools. Many excellent programs of assertiveness training and alternatives to violence are available.

Parenting and Control in Relationships

How can we help children to develop awareness of healthy and appropriate control behaviour and skills? Parents and grandparents play a vital role in developing and maintaining healthy relationships with their children. Ideally parents and family can demonstrate respecting, supportive relationships and advise children on how to cope with challenging or abusive relationships, see Fig. 6.1.

Parents can help children to develop their inner confidence (sense of control) and confidence in talking with other people (outer relating). They can help them to develop respecting relationships, from gentle, supportive, caring concern to highly dynamic but respecting team cooperation, motivation and leadership – respecting, firm but fair, and operational control, see Table 6.2.

Parents and teachers can help young children develop skills to recognise, deflect and stabilise unhelpful or hazardous relationships. These are relationships that may violate their personal boundaries (see section "The Importance of Boundaries for Students and Communities") with abuse, bullying, coercion, sexual grooming or violence.

Unfortunately, the traumatic effects of a bullying parent can last for decades. It can also spill over into work relationships see the example in Case H.

Ironically, informal social networks including gangs may provide essential survival skills for children in hostile urban environments which parents and schools may not even recognise, or where families are hazardous. Recognising sexual predators, drug dealers, and hostile gang territories are life or death learning needs for many children. Teams and gangs may provide understanding and peer support for children in hazardous families or communities. But they may involve other potential hazards of violence or exploitation.

Self-Awareness: Do I Over-Control or Bully?

A career development exercise gave this adult client an alert to possible over-controlling behaviour at work. He was likely to use a similar approach at home as a parent:

Case G: Entrepreneur – Self-awareness of High-control Behaviour

A senior real estate manager had difficulties with staff. He was highly driven and described a strong need to control his organisation. Feedback from assessment exercises indicated that as an independent person (internal sense of control) he would not like to work for himself as a strongly dominating or controlling person. 'That could be a problem', he reflected.

We discussed alternative approaches to management such as firm but fair control, delegation and situational leadership to increase trust and respect. Experienced supervisors constantly adjust the amount of control they exert depending on the situation and the different skills and experience of team members. They give firm direction to inexperienced people in hazardous situations, and delegate fully to more experienced staff (*firm but fair* or balanced control). If an emergency occurs direct *operational control* is needed over all staff until the situation is under control.

In 1963, Field Marshal Montgomery talking to our school said that leaders can rule by status, fear or respect. For a leader to gain authority, they must use power appropriately to win respect. This was quite different from traditional military leadership cultures of bullying and fear. This approach may also apply to adults and children. Parents and teachers need to win their children's respect, not demand it.

Using Transactional Analysis (TA) in Parenting and Other Relationships

The scales in Tables 6.1 and 6.2 indicate tendencies for an internal sense of control, and for outward influence and control or assertiveness when relating to other people. But relationships operate in real time, with a flow or exchange of messages in words and actions (eye contact, facial expressions, gestures or physical contacts) called *transactions*. How do we see, or feel, and recognise warning signs of controlling and potentially abusive behaviour? And what options do we have to avoid or respond to violence and abuse?

In the 1950s, Dr Eric Berne proposed an approach for helping people with challenging relationships called *Transactional Analysis (TA)* (Berne, 1961; Harris, 1973; Stewart & Joines, 2012). It is directly relevant to understanding relationships in families, schools and communities and some of the dynamics of abuse, bullying and violence.

Transactional Analysis suggests that individuals have several 'ego states' (internal moods or levels) – *Parent, Adult* and *Child* – and a repertoire of actions and responses that we learn as children first from our parents (and grandparents) and later from other contacts, e.g. at school.

So when two people meet and talk, each one may start from one of the three levels. This can be represented by two sets of three circles (like traffic lights) and the levels abbreviated to P (Parent), A (Adult) and C (Child) – see Fig. 6.2.

We learn many different Parent scripts in childhood, from actual parents and other authority figures. *Nurturing Parent* is appropriate for emotional support but may encourage unhealthy dependency. *Controlling Parent* is appropriate for urgent

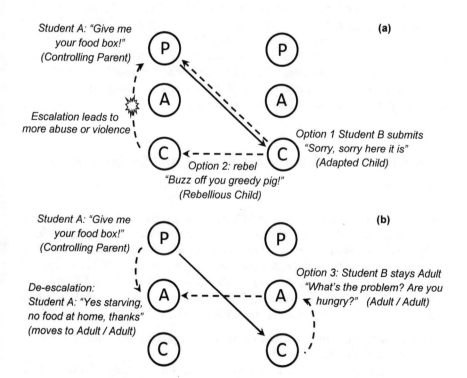

Fig. 6.2 Transactional analysis examples of parent adult child options responding to threat

warnings and commands but potentially autocratic or toxic, violating other people's boundaries with abuse, violence or coercive control (entrapment). These Parent scripts interact with different Child Scripts, e.g. *Adapted Child* (obedient or submissive, sometimes rebellious) with negative *Parent/Child* consequences (Fig. 6.2(a)). *Free Child* and fun-loving *Child/Child* banter adds joy to friendships but can slide into scapegoating or excluding behaviour. *Adult/Adult* transactions are respectful and supportive, with information sharing and mutual problem solving, see Fig. 6.2(b). This illustrates an option to deflect abuse by *staying adult* and can turn a hostile encounter into cooperation. This can be valuable in de-escalating, rebalancing and resolving abusive relationships (see following examples).

For real Parents, Teachers, School Counsellors and students, there is a wide literature explaining TA and how to apply it in many settings, e.g. for families, schools, work and community organisations. These are available in books, e.g. Stewart and Joines (2012) and internet videos and may be part of many professional interventions to reduce conflict, abuse and violence in schools, e.g. for individuals and groups in staff or parent awareness and development programmes.

From individual mentoring discussions with my clients, their inner and outer sense of control (compared with the scales in Tables 6.1 and 6.2) suggest behaviours like aspects of the TA Parent/Adult/Child ego-states. An individual's internal sense of control, and outer control behaviours will fluctuate over months depending on recent events. However, our TA states can change much faster in different situations.

Conversations about appropriate and inappropriate types and levels of control may be part of professional development programmes for teachers, counsellors and managers. Control is a key area of school culture – for management, communications and security, and for codes of discipline for students and staff. Ironically, over-control (or coercive control including violent or corporal punishment) may increase rebellion. Authority needs both power and respect.

Adult Experiences of Workplace Bullying and Coping Strategies with Bullies

The following examples of adult experiences of bullying at work gave me opportunities to learn more about the dynamics of bullying relationships using transactional analysis with other techniques. These included life-review conversations about experiences from early childhood, different kinds of parents, schools and traumas. In some cases, *Carl Jung's concept of Shadow* also offered a metaphor for recurring echoes of childhood trauma including bullying when they re-emerged in adult life and work, as described in Robert Johnson's book *Owning Your Own Shadow* (1991).

Case H: Conflict at Work – How to Stay Adult Against Controlling Parent Behaviour and Childhood Shadow

An experienced professional was referred for stress counselling. She was having severe difficulties with a new manager who frequently criticised her. When the manager entered the room she would sigh and make disapproving noises. This triggered panic for the professional who would burst into tears.

In her life review the client recalled endless criticism as a child from her mother. The boss's domineering entrance evoked similar responses. Discussion included awareness of the TA Parent/Adult/Child model for 'staying adult', Jung's concept of Shadow, and to remind herself that 'she is not my mother' for future encounters. The client returned to work more confidently and moved to a senior role the next year.

Case I: Engineer and Manager – Staying Adult to Win Respect with a Controlling Boss

A specialist design engineer faced a serious professional dilemma. He had discovered a potentially lethal design flaw in the company's product for high-performance vehicles. However, whenever he tried to discuss it with his manager he was silenced. He was conflicted between keeping his job and a potentially fatal accident if the product failed.

We discussed the Parent/Adult/Child TA model. They were both exceptional engineers. So he planned an Adult/Adult approach with more confidence (not showing fear) and by asking technical questions. They had a dialogue (a rare event), shared the issue and resolved the design problem. Their relationship became stronger.

These cases illustrated practical ways to use awareness of confidence and assertiveness together with transactional analysis (TA) to restore clients' ability to cope with bullying situations. It gave them new options for engaging with coercive or bullying individuals. These may be helpful for parents and teachers for awareness of their own behaviours and as role models for children and students. They give great opportunities for role-playing exercises to increase awareness and skills. School support specialists may already use similar ideas in individual support sessions with survivors of bullying or violence, and for engaging with aggressive or over-controlling students.

Practical Issues for Professionals, Leaders and Authorities and for Major Incidents

Containing and reducing bullying and violence in schools is an essential part of most education and training programmes in the education sector, for teachers, leaders, counsellors, psychologists and other specialists. At a basic level, teachers need practical skills to maintain good order in classes and social spaces, with duties of care for student health, safety and welfare. Teachers and students usually work within a larger system. The school is a complex and potentially supportive organisation with people, physical resources, rules and culture. Remote learning during the COVID-19 pandemic has altered some of these assumptions.

Pastoral Skills

Ideally, schools have stable psychological environments conducive to learning, personal and social development. But schools are also complex and dynamic environments where each student has differing needs and abilities, directly affected by their home, family and community environments. Individuals and groups face predictable challenges, e.g. examinations, unexpected challenges from family life events (illness, separation or bereavement) and school incidents (see Transitions).

So, individual teachers need pastoral skills to prepare and support students through a wide range of stresses and crises, as well as subject knowledge and teaching skills. And they need to be aware of the family and community context that the children live in and come from, e.g. poverty, stable or fragmented extended families, diversity and conflict.

Rules and Boundaries (see also section "The Importance of Boundaries for Students and Communities")

School rules usually set clear boundaries between expected, acceptable and unacceptable behaviour, and sanctions for breaking them that should be known and understood by all students. It follows that *a prime role of school leaders and governing bodies is to review these boundaries and sanctions* as new challenges emerge from within and outside the school, e.g. the advent of mobile phones and social media.

Bullying and violence are *threats to the welfare of individuals*, sometimes obvious, sometimes covert. They may also represent *boundary violations that threaten the stable operation of the school as an organisation* including the possibility of continuing, repeated or proliferating attacks by other disaffected students.

School Leaders have special responsibilities for *trauma risk management* needed for bullying and violent incidents, both from internal and sometimes external attackers.

These are likely to include:

Prevention:
• Anticipation of potential threats of bullying and violence
Risk assessment of each type of threat, with expert advice and support
Training for staff
Education and awareness of threats and rules for staff, students and families

Detection:
• Reporting channels, e.g. for victims, witnesses, family, support groups
Security systems and alarms.
Monitoring key indicators, e.g. sickness, absence, study performance, self-harm, etc.

Response: (and see Psychological First Aid)

- Levels of response for victim and perpetrator – from discrete enquiry to full emergency

Roles and authorities – who to involve, when, and how.

Investigation, options, decisions

Follow-up and support
- For victim and perpetrator, teacher, witnesses and families. Consider *Non-violent Resistance (NVR)* conflict resolution awareness and skills. Include monthly reviews for at least 6, ideally 12 months (for potential post-trauma transition effects).

Case J: Teacher's Skilful De-escalation and Reconciliation Response in a City School

A grandparent reported a recent incident for her granddaughter aged 10, usually confident, fit and popular. Another girl, also aged 10, perhaps less popular, began a campaign of verbal abuse. Threats escalated until the girl had to hide in the toilets for fear of violence. She has a good relationship with her mother, so she reported the incident to her at home. The mother contacted the school.

The school was aware that the other girl was having problems in her home life and requested tolerance (not exclusion). The teacher had conversations with both girls to restore normal dialogue. Then she set them a joint project to prepare a presentation on bullying to their class. This response acknowledged the stresses and distress of both girls and gave them social support and relating skills. They comfortably co-exist with no further issues.

Responding to Extreme Violence and Trauma in the Twenty-First century

Unfortunately, school violence is also developing *new levels of trauma such as terrorist attacks in many countries.*

Trauma is an inevitable risk in military organisations with potential to trigger complex mental health problems including PTSD and other conditions. In the UK, *Trauma Risk Management (TRiM)* programs (Greenberg et al., 2008) have been adopted in many parts of the military and civilian emergency services since 2006. This is a versatile approach that aims to increase mental health awareness in all personnel, de-stigmatise mental health symptoms of trauma and encourage social support.

The Eos Career First Aid tips in section "What Concerns You About Bullying and Violence?" were designed for personal use by individuals coping with trauma stress and change. But professional teachers, counsellors, consultants, leaders (head teachers) and other authorities need more sophisticated methods for response to major trauma incidents affecting children, schools and communities.

In the USA, the tragedies of 9/11 and random acts of extreme violence in schools have triggered the development of detailed guidelines for *Psychological First Aid.*

Psychological First Aid (PFA)

Gerald Juhnke, Darcy Granello and Paul Granello give a detailed guide to the concept of *Psychological First Aid* (PFA) in their recent book *School Bullying and Violence* (2020, p 176–236). The earlier 2006 PFA guide, a publication of the National Child Traumatic Stress Network and the National Center for PTSD, was updated with a new edition (Brymer et al., 2012). The PFA Field Operations Guide and Juhnke et al.'s (2020) supplementary suggestions for implementation offer a detailed and advanced methodology for professional specialists supporting severe traumas in schools.

The introduction to the 2nd edition describes *Psychological First Aid for Schools (PFA-S)* as 'an evidence-informed intervention model to assist students, families, school personnel, and school partners in the immediate aftermath of an emergency. PFA-S is designed to reduce the initial distress caused by emergencies, and to foster short- and long-term adaptive functioning and coping' (Brymer et al., 2012).

Juhnke et al. (2020) summarise the PFA approach in two chapters. Chapter 7 of their book describes *the first four core actions* which are as follows:

Core Action 1: Contact and engagement
Core Action 2: Safety and comfort
Core Action 3: Stabilisation
Core Action 4: Information gathering

Then, Chap. 8 describes *the Advanced Core Actions*:

Core Action 5: Practical assistance
Core Action 6: Connection with social supports
Core Action 7: Information on coping
Core Action 8: Linkage with collaborative service

This is a practical framework for sequencing specialist support from brief conflict encounters up to major traumatic incidents involving lethal violence and multiple casualties. It is valuable to school leaders and potentially other organisations running services or events for children that might be targets for major incidents as part of their disaster planning responsibilities.

Juhnke et al.'s (2020) guide to advanced best practice illustrates higher-level responses involving a cluster of professionals – counsellors, social workers, family therapists, psychologists, etc. – with more specialist advice than this paper can offer and based on experiences of more severe incidents. Students and parents living in states with advanced disaster response resources may be reassured to know that this level of planning has been developed.

They illustrate immediate practical situations and sample dialogues (vignettes) between support specialists, victims, witnesses and parents. Although these are structured, they are also light touch encounters, responding to individual's needs, not over-prescribed. They stress the underlying humanistic psychology approach:

'PFA is health based and does not focus on psychopathology. In other words, those who developed PFA believed most survivors are resilient ... many survivors will adequately cope with whatever event they experienced without developing debilitating, long-term, trauma related symptoms ... a broad continuum from mild to severe symptoms. This stands in stark contrast to those who view school bullying and violence survivors as 'broken' and in need of 'fixing'. (Juhnke et al., 2020, pp. 176–177).

The Advanced Core Actions also address the important roles of mobilising the potential social and emotional support systems illustrated in Fig. 6.1 to be available for survivors and their families. This also includes distributing coping information about potential post-violence reactions.

Schools that practise emergency response drills may explain the main features of the PFA approach to parents and students. Parents living in states or countries with limited or no disaster response services may find the best practice advice in Juhnke et al. (2020) well worth reading in case parts of it can be adapted to emergency response plans in their local community.

Shadows from the Past: Reflections on Violence from Teachers

The practical challenges of disaster management in schools are a clear and urgent priority for School Leaders. However, another long-term source of bullying and violence in schools needs ongoing vigilance. This involves *teacher violence*. In the UK, this has been greatly reduced by changes in the law banning corporal punishment in schools (and for parents disciplining children at home). But the potential for teacher violence and abuse is likely to continue in the many states and countries that still permit corporal punishment.

In section "Practical Coping Strategies for Families and Friends", Case F encouraged parents to pay attention to potential signs of abuse when children return from school, including possible adult or teacher abuse. These are some more incidents of teacher violence from my case history.

Case K: Primary School Teacher Pupil Conflict Flashes into Teacher Violence
A class of 10-year-old children sit in their desks shocked by the scene. The rebellious student aged 10 was usually a likeable boy but from a poor and dysfunctional family. His face was often puffy and tearful. The head teacher was usually fair, but they had got into an argument. The teacher got his cane to punish the boy who was now shouting, crying and crawling along the floor, holding an arm up to protect himself. The teacher was chasing him and thrashing him with the stick. A few months later the student's older brother (aged 16) committed sexual assaults on other children. The teacher seemed unaware of the boy's abusing home environment. He did not use the cane again. This incident occurred many years before corporal punishment was banned in the UK, but it illustrates the hazards of conflict between teachers and distressed students. Referring to Fig. 6.1, this case illustrates how the normal support channels – from the teacher and elder siblings – could be

undermined by unreported bullying and ongoing physical and sexual abuse in a family also stressed by poverty.

It also illustrates how a disagreement or misunderstanding between normally reasonable people can flash into individual or group anger and potentially violence. Non-violent conflict resolution, non-violent resistance and violence management training skills are crucially important for teachers and many other professionals working with the public and distressed communities.

Case L: Long-Term Career Effects of School Corporal Punishment
A student brought a new home-made guitar to school. During a quiet French dictation class run by a strict teacher, the guitar broke with a loud crash. The class collapsed with laughter, but the teacher thought it was a deliberate provocation. The student was given three strokes of the cane. He developed a strong antipathy to abuse of power by authorities channelled in protests and later in advocacy roles.

These historical examples of the systematic use of violence as a means of social control in schools may shock twenty-first-century teaching professionals. But they have long-lasting effects on the attitudes of many parents and grandparents who grew up under older regimes. And like sexual abuse, these will be ongoing hazards in relationships of trust with children, exacerbated by *new technologies*, e.g. social media and internet pornography. These subvert the major progress in human rights and dignity in the education systems of many but not all advanced economies.

Long-Term Responses to Bullying and Violence – Post-trauma Transitions

Not all traumas cause PTSD (post-traumatic stress disorder). However, many may cause short-term responses over several weeks, and potentially an extended post-traumatic period of *transition*. Transition psychology has explored human responses to trauma loss and change after major life events, good as well as bad, for several decades. It evolved in the 1960s and 1970s from research into bereavement (Kubler–Ross model), culture shock, e.g. for international students, and for Peace Corps volunteers, and then for redundancy and other career changes.

Several different models of transition have been proposed ranging from career events, through culture shock and organisational change, e.g. Hopson and Adams (1976); Hopson et al. (1991); Sugarman (1986, 2001); and Furnham and Bochner (1986). Schlossberg et al. (1995) suggested another model useful for therapeutic interventions.

We have worked with the notion of culture shock since 1971 and the Transition Cycle included in Leonie Sugarman's lectures in 1978 and books on Life-Span Development (1986, 2001). We have used *the Transition Cycle* in Fig. 6.3, adapted in 1999 (Williams, 1999a) from Hopson and Adams (1976), in international student and recruit briefings since 1983 and with career counselling clients since 1986. It is summarised in my paper *Life events and career change: transition psychology in practice* (Williams, 1999a) and in a symposium with organisational psychologists Peter Herriot, Richard Plenty and Ashley Weinberg, in *Human Responses to Change* (Williams, 1999c). Prof. Tom Miller (2010) collated a wide selection of more recent papers on transition in his *Handbook of Stressful Transitions Across the Lifespan* including the pychological after effects of mass trauma (Williams, 2010).

The *Life/Career Checklist* includes a list of recent life events that may start a period of transition for individuals traumatised by bullying or violence, which may also affect family members, friends and teachers in severe cases such as school shootings or other terrorist incidents.

The *Transition Cycle* in Fig. 6.3 may have several phases lasting up to a year, sometimes longer, with variations in the early stages depending on whether the trigger event was a positive or negative event leading through periods of honeymoon or denial. These may protect the individual from the full impact of the event or change for 3–4 months – important over millennia for personal survival after major traumas. Minimising or Denial of the severity of the incident is likely to be important to survivors affected by bullying or severe violence. It buys time to come to terms (to adjust) with the full implications of the event.

Unfortunately, the denial phase may give the appearance that the survivor has come to terms with the event after 3–4 months. Then many support systems including schools and work organisations may lose interest in their progress. But the new reality may gradually undermine the individual's confidence and sense of identity with contradictions between his/her previous 'safe' view of the world and their recent or ongoing experiences. The cognitive dissonance this causes can lead to growing anxiety and depression, recognised as 'common mental health disorders' or 'adjustment disorder'.

This may lead to a period of severe distress or crisis typically 6 months after a major life event, least expected by the individual or those around them. They may seek to quit their studies or relationships as an escape, but this may not solve their distress. This transition crisis period needs maximum tolerance and support by families, friends and their schools, and to avoid making unwise decisions while distressed. This is why the Career First Aid tips include checking options and buying time for major decisions.

The transition cycle appears to be a developmental process which has evolved to help humans to survive and thrive – particularly after major traumas or losses. We may need to go through a phase of distress before we can identify attitudes or beliefs disrupted by events, and that must be let go before we can come to terms with the new reality.

Life review conversations with several hundred clients reporting many transitions have suggested the following enabling and inhibiting factors in Box 6.2 can assist us to work through the transition crisis and recovery phases.

Box 6.2: Factors that Enable or Inhibit Successful Recovery During Periods of Transition

Enabling factors	Inhibiting factors
Economic security	Economic insecurity
Emotional security/support	Emotional insecurity/isolation
Good health	Poor health
Prior transition skills	Lack of transition skills or awareness
Valuing the past	Hostile study or work environment
Supportive study or work environment	Lack of transition awareness or support in family or school
Transition awareness and support in family and school.	

Adapted from Williams (1999a)

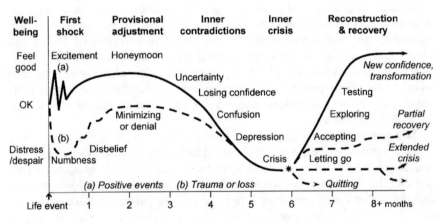

Fig. 6.3 The transition cycle: phases of vulnerability and development after trauma loss and change (Williams, 1999a, adapted with permission of John Wiley & Sons, from Hopson & Adams (1976), Chap. 1, Fig. 1.2, p. 13; permission conveyed through Copyright Clearance Center, Inc)

However, with good social and emotional support and basic security (food, shelter, mobility), individuals often resolve the transition crisis phase within a few weeks, without medication or therapy unless they are severely distressed. This turning point can lead to a remarkable recovery phase – not just back to normal but often with new energy, insights and sociability.

This can appear to be a miracle of self-healing. But the transition process appears to be an innate psychological resource that enables humans to grow and develop through times of change. While most medical models tend to focus on the pathological problems such as more severe PTSD after experiences of trauma, the transition model identifies a key feature of natural human resilience, sometimes referred to as post-traumatic growth.

Transition awareness would be useful as part of the school curriculum and parent education programmes, for students ideally from age 10 or before they face the major transition from junior to secondary school. Children may have experienced several significant life events by that age – starting school, birth of siblings and possible vicarious transitions from parents' life events, e.g. relocation, job changes, births, deaths and sometimes separation.

Parents act as role models for transition coping behaviour without knowing it which could be an asset or a hindrance to young children. Children may be particularly vulnerable to bullying or self-harm during transition crisis periods, e.g. 4–6 months after changing schools or after family traumas. Teachers could be alert for this.

Bullying, violence and other antisocial behaviour, truancy and mental health crises may also be symptoms of transition crisis behaviour for individuals and groups sharing the same loss or change at the same time. The *life event items* in the Life–Career Checklist (section "Practical Coping Strategies for Individuals – Immediate Issues and Personal Development to Enhance Resilience") may be important. So, bullies, victims and survivors may already have been unconsciously working through a period of transition when an incident occurs – by them or to them.

In Case E, described earlier the target of the predatory manager had suffered a serious loss several months earlier. While other staff in the department were able to withstand his taunts and critical comments, this individual was already in a period of confusion and distress, and unable to withstand additional harassment. This case led to the '*Support Your Friends*' advice in the Career First Aid section.

For parents, teachers and specialist counsellors, the potential crisis phase of transitions 5–6+ months after major life events – trauma loss or change, or after good events like moving to a new school or birth of a younger sibling, are higher risk periods for being targets of bullying, scapegoating or violence, and at higher risk of severe mental distress than their peers or classmates. Some cases may behave more aggressively or over-react to minor jokes or banter with violence. In these cases, the apparent bully may also be a 'victim'.

This is why the *Life–Career Checklist* includes a set of questions about recent life events for themselves or immediate family, and why the *Career First Aid* tips encourage individuals to take extra care if they or friends are showing signs of distress.

Major incidents of severe violence or hostage situations are likely to cause post-trauma transitions for many people affected, whereas long-lasting PTSD may only affect about 15% of trauma survivors. It is possible that some of the delayed onset mental health crises diagnosed as severe PTSD may partly involve transition crisis behaviour, then diagnosed as adjustment disorder.

Unfortunately, medical interventions with medication may possibly impair and delay the letting go, healing and recovery phases that appear to be natural processes in transition. Likewise, 'spontaneous remission' and post-traumatic growth may be part of a natural developmental process that most people experience 10 or 20 or more times in a lifetime, like updating our psychological software after significant life events. This is a fascinating and optimistic area for enquiry in educational and developmental psychology research and practice.

The Importance of Boundaries for Students and Communities

Our team supported 300 international students aged 18–30 years studying in over 30 colleges and universities. We provided 2-day cultural briefings when they first arrived in the UK before they went on to their study locations. This included briefings about UK laws, customs and health, including sexual health. Many students came from countries with strict religious rules with clear right or wrong codes, e.g. for dress and relationships. It was important to alert them to more ambiguous sexual behaviour in the UK. Young people may wear revealing clothes, but this did not mean they were available for sex. Sex with children under 16 years of age is strictly illegal although they may look older. Also for driving most UK drivers exceed the speed limits which may suggest to foreign drivers that this is normal. But this is hazardous.

The challenge of preparing these cross-cultural briefings required *a new way to describe interpersonal boundaries* to explain the many ambiguous rules and confusing social behaviour in UK culture. Instead of rules and practices being simply right or wrong, we explained that there may also be an ambiguous danger zone between right and wrong.

Learning About Boundaries – how to recognise them, negotiate them and to respect other peoples has become increasingly important in the last thirty years as human rights have gained more importance, e.g. since the end of Apartheid in South Africa and the end of the Soviet regime in Russia from 1989 onwards, greater concern for safeguarding of children, and gradual recognition of equal opportunities for women, for people of colour and for LGBTQ communities. In 2008 Professor Tom Miller's book School Violence and Primary Prevention (Miller 2008) was a major survey of school violence issues. In Chapter 10 he and Lane Veltkamp highlighted boundary issues for students and teachers in the Chapter Boundary Violations: Harrassment, Exploitation, and Abuse with particular the importance of awareness and concern for sexual boundary violations among staff and managers (Miller and Veldkamp, 2008). These notes started from sexual health awareness briefings for young international students coming to study in the UK.

Schools are places where children from diverse ethnic, cultural and faith communities meet in large numbers and where multiple boundary issues will arise. These are challenging for teachers and school authorities to regulate. And they are very challenging for children to learn and manage, depending on their own identity and the guidance, role modelling and support they get from their parents, siblings, extended families and communities.

Bullying and violence in schools, and in the streets and communities they are part of will frequently emerge around boundary issues. A pair of trainers on phone wires may indicate invisible gang territories and boundaries.

We have tried to find better ways of helping clients to recognise boundary issues and how to manage them. For adult career counselling clients, a key issue in the 1990s was the question of the *life-work boundary*, or boundaries, particularly for working time. For schools, this might be modified as the *life-learning boundary*.

We explored this subject in an article called *Managing the life-work boundary* (Williams, 2000a). Instead of simply Right/Wrong (safe or illegal), this suggested two intermediate stages to give four stages – *Safe, Negotiable, Hazardous and Dangerous* (usually unlawful) (see Table 6.3).

These stages may be applied to any boundary issue but for adult working life six domains are important: Time, Money, Physical Health, Metal Health, Relationships and Identity (e.g. gender and race).

For young people in schools and colleges, this view of boundaries can be adapted to the activities and issues in Table 6.3. The list of items can be altered or extended ideally by students themselves to explore options between safe and dangerous or illegal behaviour, including rights to explore negotiable areas, and call out hazardous or dangerous behaviours, thus reclaiming individual and group agency. This dialogue also includes the school that traditionally sets behaviour boundaries. Also for more formal negotiations with communities, media and the state for defining legal boundaries and sanctions for violating them.

Table 6.3 Life and learning boundary issues and personal well-being in schools

Life zone	Safe	Negotiable	Hazardous	Dangerous	School culture
Time	Own and family	School hours	Homework, paid work	Unlimited demands	*Study and travel time*
Money and food	Sufficient for needs	Scholarships, assistance	Poverty, hunger, insecurity	Exploitation, starvation	*Fees and benefits*
Physical health	Healthy and fit	Energy and effort	Fatigue and strain	Accident or injury	*Health and sport/fitness*
Mental health	Calm, fulfilled	Stimulated, motivated	Anxiety, stress	Panic, anger or violence	*Expectations, conflicts*
Relationships	Support and cooperation	Respect, direction	Over-control	Harassment, abuse	*Power, control*
Identity (*gender, faith race*)	Valued, shared	Dignity, respected	Devalued, prejudiced	Scapegoating or excluded	*Values, art customs*

Adapted from Williams (2000a)

Bullying, harassment and reactions to them are manifestations of violations of personal boundaries in hazardous or dangerous boundary areas (see Table 6.2) and, e.g. in relationships or on controversial identity issues such as gender, faith and race. They will have serious impacts on mental and potentially physical health whether external wounding, eating disorders or self-harm. In some cases, violence may be triggered as a panic or escape response for individuals who are under extreme duress.

Time conflicts may be a major issue for many students with competing demands between study time expected in school and at home and during COVID home study.

Boundaries, Laws and Criminal Behaviour

The line at which boundaries are drawn must be clear and recognisable for children and young people. At some point, boundaries are defined in law as criminal behaviour. The *Age of Criminal Responsibility* (ACR) varies between nations, recommended at 12 years of age by international legal standards. In 2007, the UN Committee on the Rights of the Child (UN CRC) declared an ACR of less than 12 years *'not to be internationally acceptable'* (UN CRC 2007 as cited in Browne & Bunn, 2018). The ACR in England, Wales and Northern Ireland is currently 10 years, but it was raised to 12 in Scotland in 2019.

In the USA, the lower age for delinquency varies between states, where it is not specified in 33 states and is between 6 and 10 years in the other states, with a Federal view at 7 years. 'Delinquent acts are law violations of children and older youth that would be considered a crime if committed by an adult' (Zang, 2017).

Dangerous behaviours may also be illegal, potentially violating criminal or civil laws and jurisdiction may pass from the school to the police. Carrying a gun may be hazardous but not illegal in some countries, a loaded gun is dangerous, and firing it to injure or kill someone a criminal act.

Parents and teachers must educate children to recognise boundaries and the consequences of crossing them.

Bullying and low-level violence – without injury – are pastoral and disciplinary issues, partially explained by basic psychological methods. But malicious criminal behaviour needs additional professional interpretations, e.g. by forensic psychologists, psychiatrists and legal experts.

Helping children to learn, recognise and respect boundaries is a special responsibility for parents and teachers. In strong faith-based cultures, parents and teachers may also need to work with religious authorities who will have additional rules and boundaries of their own.

Emerging Threats to Children in Schools in the Twenty-First Century

These reflections have been collected to offer ideas that may be of immediate practical use to parents, teachers, school leaders and specialists coping with bullying, violence and other challenging behaviour in schools now in the twenty-first century. It is frankly frightening to see the daily hazards faced by children, their parents and teachers around the world.

Extreme Violence

From lethal attacks with assault rifles in US schools to terrorist bombs in girls' schools in Afghanistan, to mass kidnappings of students in sub-Saharan Africa require teachers and police with courage, military skills of organisation and protection to prevent or mitigate attacks, and compassionate skills and professional support to restore traumatised students, staff, schools and communities after major incidents.

Substance Abuse and Other Self-Harm

Substance abuse with illegal drugs and alcohol are endemic problems in many countries. But they have developed to epidemic proportions assisted by new technologies for production and distribution. And in many communities, increasing numbers of young people who find themselves entrapped and powerless resort to self-harm as a way of indicating some token gestures of control or despair.

Pornography

While extreme attacks get international media coverage, increasing a climate of fear, *more insidious threats* have infiltrated societies around the World from modern information technology. The flood of online *pornography* available to and targeted at children, was an early effect of the growth of the internet – the Pandora's box effect.

Malicious Use of Social Media

The depraving and corrupting influence of internet pornography continues but seems almost forgotten as public concern increases to confront the *malicious use of social media*. It has become a key channel for subverting younger populations in many ways and countries. This can be small-scale local, harassment or intimidation by friends who may become bullies or abusers, up to larger-scale attacks to groom or radicalise young people. Subversion may be for religious, political or ethnic campaigns to harass, abuse, and radicalise children and young people from their earliest access to *mobile phones*.

The COVID-19 Pandemic

In 2020 and 2021, the global pandemic has added major challenges for schools and families. In many countries, education has had to rely on internet communications and some children have spent months isolated from teachers and friends. Stress levels from poverty, hunger and fear have added tension for many families, with increasing risks of domestic abuse, violence and self-harm. Threats to pass the virus to younger, weaker or medically vulnerable children, e.g. by spitting are another channel for bullying in the pandemic. Unfortunately lockdowns during the pandemic have increased pressure on families with increased risks of domestic violence bullying and other abuse. Schools and communities may choose to arrange systematic reviews of the experiences and potential traumas of the pandemic for all children and families, and arrange transition recovery support groups or schemes.

Climate Change

Perhaps the largest threat to children throughout the World is the emerging issue of climate change. In practical terms, this may be an underlying factor in many more immediate issues – from extreme temperatures in classrooms during heat waves to natural disasters like fires, storms and floods that may destroy schools. This threat is so profound and diverse that it has been ignored or denied by many political leaders. But it is now being recognised as abnormal weather events increase every year. This will affect children in all schools into the future in many ways, some acute, some gradual.

By increasing ambient levels of stress and anxiety, climate change is likely to increase anxiety for individuals and tensions in groups, with potential increases in anger and violence [see Fear and violence in stressed populations (Williams, 1999b)].

However, with careful encouragement, children can and do adapt to changing physical and social environments often faster than adults. Several of the suggestions here may be used to enable the natural resilience of individual students and school communities, e.g. the Life–Career First Aid principles. And aspects of the Transition process may be fundamental to enabling individuals, families and communities to recover and adapt after specific climate-related emergencies, and after the migrations, these will eventually require.

New Visions, Techniques, Opportunities and Resources

From Nightmares to Inspirations – School Communities and Open Systems

The advent of social media has proliferated almost instant and mostly unmoderated feedback in every aspect of social life. This may provide almost instant gratification but also undefended vulnerability. This has been ruthlessly exploited by global data corporations, criminal organisations and predatory political and religious organisations.

In systems theory terms (von Bertalanffy, 1968), complex systems including human society, rely on feedback for self-regulation and stability.

> 'Closely connected with system theory is… communication. The general notion in communication theory is that of information. A second central concept of the theory of communication and control is that of feedback'. (von Bertalanffy, 1968)

If feedback is not moderated it can escalate, destabilise and potentially disrupt the systems it should be enabling, as seen in the IT-driven US stock market crash of 1987.

Ludwig von Bertalanffy's General Systems Theory was intended as much for new insights into social, psychological and biological systems, as for information science and every other technical system.

Courageous researchers, policy-makers and practitioners are finding new insights for stabilising the chaotic effects of unmoderated feedback in social media in new systems perspectives, e.g. *Dynamic Systems Theories* among other Theories of Adolescent Development summarised by Barbara and Philip Newman (Newman and Newman 2020). New technologies have driven economic and social change far faster that human societies or legal systems can understand their impacts, or ways to harness their effects. Systems theories, principles and best practices need to be as widely understood as the devices that exploit them.

Healthy Systems and Online Resources

New technologies are not all good or bad – it depends on how they are used. Despite the hazards of the internet and social media, it can offer healthy systems that provide information, support and online learning sources.

Two examples with international access are *The Recovery College* and *Future Learn.*

The Recovery College Approach to Community Mental Health Needs

The Recovery College is a growing network of local and online courses in the UK for *child and adult mental health support*, mostly run by regional NHS (National Health Service) authorities. It can be valuable to help parents caring for children with mental health challenges, e.g. anxiety, ADHD and more complex conditions, some of which may increase students' vulnerability to bullying and violence.

> 'When we think about the word recovery, most of us think about 'getting better'. However, in mental health, recovery is a journey towards a meaningful and fulfilling life, achieving a sense of wellbeing. It's personal and unique to each person, everyone will progress at different speeds, in different directions and to different destinations' (Recovery College Online, 2022).

Ideally, the Recovery College experience involves real face-to-face meetings in small groups, with peers who may share similar issues but are further along the recovery journey, coordinated by fully qualified mental health professionals.

Recovery College Online resources include guest courses for children and young people (https://lms.recoverycollegeonline.co.uk/). But like other online resources, parents or teachers need to check the sponsoring organisations (e.g. regional NHS) to avoid potentially predatory cloned websites or platforms.

Recovery College sites suggest the *CHIME framework* for mental health recovery developed by Leamy et al. (2011) from a wide survey of best practice. These five areas are: *connectedness, hope and optimism, identity, meaning and purpose, and empowerment.*

Online Learning Resources, e.g. the Future Learn Open College Platform

Future Learn is an online learning centre based in the UK but drawing together students and specialists in many subject areas from around the World. It also has a low-cost model to make its courses accessible to the widest audience, from free short courses to realistic cost fees for graduate and professional level programmes, offered by specialist centres.

Some of these programmes are suitable for parents, others for teachers and medical professionals for topical issues of current concern, e.g. for *cyberbullying*,

Future Learn provides portals to centres like EUI in Europe for example the Religion, radicalisation, resilience course facilitated by Triandafyllidou and

Magazzini (2021). And to QUT – Queensland University of Technology in Australia, from short courses like *Bullying in Schools: How Should Teachers Respond?* to professional development modules for teachers *Trauma-Aware Education: Teaching Students Who Have Suffered Complex Trauma*. Courses are developed by specialists like Prof. Marilyn Campbell (e.g. The Australian perspective: Efforts to counter cyberbullying 2017) and network with specialists in other countries from Ireland, Europe and Canada.

Leaders, researchers and policy-makers will find these sources potentially useful for quality summaries of issues and resources and for networking with research centres and programmes in other countries. For example, the *Religion, Radicalisation, Resilience* programme is part of the GREASE project run by the Robert Schuman Centre for Advanced Studies in the European University Institute (*EUI*).

New Initiatives to Support Vulnerable, Violent and Excluded Young People and Their Families

In many countries, individuals and groups of psychologists have recognised that traditional methods of delivering professional support to large populations of disaffected young people are incapable of meeting escalating mental health education and support needs – in schools and on the streets. There are too few resources, long delays for therapy and a total loss of trust in official agencies among gangs, or in communities traumatised by wars and religious or political conflicts.

Two recent initiatives illustrate radically different approaches for outreach to largely traumatised, often violent children and young people – the MAC-UK project in London, and the NVR (Non-Violent Resistance) projects in Israel, Gaza and Europe.

Community Psychology Initiatives – MAC-UK (Music and Change), London

As mentioned earlier, Community Psychology initiatives led by Dr. Charlotte Howard and Dr. Sally Zlotowitz have begun to develop dialogues with gangs and youth communities in London to offer mental health awareness and reduce violence, especially knife crime. This approach is radically different from traditional Clinical Psychology reaching out to vulnerable and marginalised individuals and groups in their community contexts e.g. working with young mothers addressing their psycho-social needs, and housing activists in low-income areas (Walker, Zlotowitz, Zoli, 2022).

MAC-UK's vision is 'to create social equality by radically transforming excluded young people's access to mental health services. Excluded young people are not the problem – in fact, they hold the solutions to the problems they face' (MAC-UK, 2020). Their mission is to help (community mental health) services to 'take what we know works in the clinic, out to meet young people where they are at'.

The MAC-UK (2020) approach includes valuing *the lived experience* of young people as experts in their own lives which needs to be valued by the services supporting them. They work closely with related projects and agencies (*co-production*) to provide support with, rather than to or for, young people and their communities.

They see 'putting relationships back into the science of health care and social care as central to the solution. Trust is the foundation for transformed public services. [And they] work to address the systems that perpetuate the health, social and economic inequalities experienced by excluded groups' (MAC-UK, 2020).

Dr. Howard, the pioneer of MAC-UK, described her community psychology approach to engaging with youth violence in London: 'Everything I have learnt about youth violence has come from young people and from trying to encourage others to listen to them. And I'm convinced that Politics is a big part of the problem. If we are to solve this issue, it has to be enabled by Politicians, not owned by them' (MAC-UK, 2018).

These initiatives complement violence reduction work inside schools to stabilise communities.

Non-violent Resistance (NVR)

The principles of Non-Violent Resistance evolved in the twentieth century from people like Gandhi for resistance to colonial domination in India, and later in the USA by Martin Luther King and others against racial oppression in the USA and by peace movements against nuclear weapons proliferation. Instead of traditional violent rebellions against controlling regimes (mass Parent/Child disputes in TA terms), they sought change through non-violent protests (using Adult/Adult responses).

Gandhi's ideas represented 'a peace psychology that seeks to elucidate psychological processes involved in the prevention and mitigation of destructive conflict, violence, dominance, oppression and exploitation' – an antidote to fear (Christie et al., 2001).

Psychology Professor Haim Omer (from a traumatised holocaust refugee family) started to adapt the NVR approach to work with families and challenging children. His aim was to empower parents (many traumatised) to restore constructive relations with disruptive or violent children.

Parts of the NVR approach honour aspects of traditional Nurturing Parent behaviour in TA terms – Nurturing, Acceptance and Empathy.

These are balanced by aspects of the Controlling Parent state in TA – Firmness Structure and setting Boundaries. Omer's interpretation addresses and values aspects of differing personalities – potentially adaptable and inclusive.

Parents and carers report increased confidence in their parenting, a greater sense of agency (control) or presence, improved relationships within the family and improved behaviour. He extends the same principles to empower teachers. In the toughest test, a clinical psychologist working with traumatised families in Gaza, Dr. Ahmed abu-Tawahani, adopted many of the same approaches.

The NVR approach addresses many of the same issues of bullying and violence in schools explored here, and with some similar methods but with well-developed training and mentoring programmes, better explained in Omer's books (2021) and websites, e.g. NVR Practitioners Consortium: https://nvrpc.org.uk/what-is-nvr%3F.

Conclusions: Contributions of Intergenerational Experiences to Child Development

So what can the experiences of adult life stories and reflections on childhood in the twentieth century offer that is relevant to children, schools, families and communities in the global chaos of the twenty-first century? How can memories of bullying and violence from three to four generations, up to 60–80 years ago, be relevant today?

Well, these living memories still include World War II, which traumatised most of the largest countries in the World, and many smaller ones with physical devastation and mass migrations of refugee populations. Yet most of these populations survived and eventually thrived. Their collective experiences offer cautions, wisdom and hope.

Curiously cultures of violence moved from the defeated countries in WWII to thrive in the victorious nations, partly to motivate new generations to become fighting populations with military training for the new Cold War. They were strongly reinforced by the western media – films and TV – 'lest we forget'.

The atrocities of WWII such as the holocaust were attributed to the losing countries. But they echoed on through the next generation as young war heroes and casualties became parents and teachers (Williams, 2012). Despite their own war traumas, many tried to encourage strength and resilience balanced with compassion for their children and students.

Older generations tend to create hierarchies. In succeeding generations, this led their children to question old pre-war values and seek fairer societies.

This post-war recovery started major social changes in many countries leading to greater respect and concern for the welfare of children, women, education and human rights. These changes have evolved slowly. Banning corporal punishment in UK schools, and in homes, took over 40 years – two generations. Domestic and school violence continues but traditional boundaries that sanctioned men's rights to abuse women and children have begun to move.

Deeply embedded cultures of violence and other destructive traditions and beliefs take generations to change. But each new generation of parents and teachers plays vital roles in choosing what values and behaviour must change for your children and communities.

So learning how to understand, confront and change anti-social behaviour with firm but fair, non-violent behaviours, unconditional positive regard and more inclusive attitudes will give each new generation of children more resilience to trauma and abuse. These are the positive learnings passed down through recent generations out of bitter experiences in the past – the positive legacy of intergenerational experiences – such as this question:

Children and young people need love and stability. Are we doing all we can to uphold and sustain parents and others who carry the responsibility for providing this care?

No one said life would be easy but with inner strength and mutual support, new generations will survive bullying and violence, and thrive, learning from our traumas and changing how to grow through theirs.

Acknowledgements The Life–Career Checklist and Career First Aid notes are Copyright © Eos Career Services with fair use permissions.

References

Bandura, A. (2006). Toward a psychology of human agency. *Perspectives on Psychological Science, 1*, 164–180. and at https://albertbandura.com

Beels, C., Hopson, B., & Scally, M. (1992). *Assertiveness – A positive process*. Mercury & Lifeskills Communications Ltd.

Berne, E. (1961). *Games people play*. Grove Press.

Browne, P., & Bunn, S. (2018). *Age of criminal responsibility*. Houses of Parliament POSTNOTE No 577 June 2018. London, https://researchbriefings.files.parliament.uk/documents/POST-PN-0577/POST-PN-0577.pdf

Brymer, M., Taylor, M., Escudero, P., Jacobs, A., Kronenberg, M., Macy, R., Mock, L., Payne, L., Pynoos, R., & Vogel, J. (2012). *Psychological first aid for schools: Field operations guide* (2nd ed.). National Child Traumatic Stress Network. Available at: https://www.nctsn.org/resources/psychological-first-aid-schools-pfa-s-field-operations-guide

Campbell, M. (2017). The Australian perspective: Efforts to counter cyberbullying. In *Bullying and cyberbullying: Prevalence, psychological impacts and intervention strategies* (pp. 201–208). Nova Publishers. ISBN 9781536100648.

CDC. (2019). *#StopBullying*. Accessed 2021 at: https://www.cdc.gov/injury/features/stop-bullying/index.html

CDC – Centers for Disease Control and Prevention. (2021). *Fast fact: Preventing bullying*. Accessed at: https://www.cdc.gov/violenceprevention/youthviolence/bullyingresearch/fast-fact.html

Christie, D. J., Wagner, R. V., & Winter, D. D. (2001). *Peace, conflict, and violence – Peace psychology for the 21st century*. Prentice Hall.

Farrell, C. (2021). World corporal punishment research. *Corporal punishment in UK schools*. Accessed October 2021: https://www.corpun.com/counuks.htm

Furnham, A., & Bochner, S. (1986). *Culture shock*. Methuen.

Gladden, R. M., Vivolo-Kantor, A. M., Hamburger, M. E., & Lumpkin, C. D. (2014). *Bullying surveillance among youths: Uniform definitions for public health and recommended data elements, version 1.0*. National Center for Injury Prevention and Control, Centers for Disease Control and Prevention and U.S. Department of Education. Available at: https://www.cdc.gov/violenceprevention/pdf/Bullying-Definitions-FINAL-a.pdf

Gluckman, M. (1956). *Custom and conflict in Africa*. Basil Blackwell.

Greenberg, N., Langston, V., & Jones, N. (2008). Trauma Risk Management (TRiM) in the UK armed forces. *Journal of the Royal Army Medical Corps, 154*(2), 123–126. Found at: http://www.kcl.ac.uk/kcmhr/publications/assetfiles/interventions/Greenberg2008.pdf

Harris, T. A. (1973). *I'm OK – You're OK*. Random House.

Hopson, B., & Adams, J. D. (1976). Towards an understanding of transition. In J. D. Adams, J. Hayes, & B. Hopson (Eds.), *Transition: Understanding and managing personal change*. Martin Robertson.

Hopson, B., Scally, M., & Stafford, K. (1991). *Transitions – The challenge of change*. Mercury & Lifeskills.

Johnson, R. A. (1991). *Owning your own shadow: Understanding the dark side of the psyche*. Harper Collins.

Juhnke, G. A., Granello, D. H., & Granello, P. F. (2020). *School bullying and violence. Interventions for mental health specialists*. OUP.

Leamy, M., Bird, V., Le Boutillier, C., Williams, J., & Slade, M. (2011). Conceptual framework for personal recovery in mental health: Systematic review and narrative synthesis. *The British Journal of Psychiatry, 199*, 445–452. https://doi.org/10.1192/bjp.bp.110.083733

MAC-UK. (2018). *We took to the streets of London to talk to young people – Here's what they said* [Internet]. Available at: https://mac-uk.org/news/we-took-to-the-streets-of-london-to-talk-to-young-people-heres-what-they-said/

MAC-UK. (2020). *Our work. MAC-UK community psychology website*. Available at: https://mac-uk.org/our-work/ and https://mac-uk.org/vision-mission-and-values/

Miller, T. W. (2008). *School violence and primary prevention*. Springer. https://doi.org/10.1007/978-0-387-77119-9

Miller, T. W. (2010). *Handbook of stressful transitions across the lifespan*. Springer. https://doi.org/10.1007/978-1-4419-0748-6

Miller, T. W., & Veltkamp, L. J. (2008). Boundary violations: Harassment, exploitation and abuse. In T. W. Miller (Ed.), *School violence and primary prevention* (pp. 201–213). Springer. https://doi.org/10.1007/978-0-387-77119-9_10

Newman, B.M., & Newman, P.R. (2020). Theories of Adolescent Development. Academic Press.

Omer, H. (2021). *Non-violent resistance: A new approach to violent and self-destructive children*. Cambridge University Press. And notes at www.haimomer-nvr.com

Recovery College Online (UK NHS). (2022). *What is recovery? Information and advice for service users, carers and staff about recovery in mental health*. Accessed at: https://www.recoverycollegeonline.co.uk/recovery-wellbeing/recovery/about/

Rotter, J. B. (1966). General expectations for internal versus external control of reinforcement. *Psychological Monograph, 609*, 1–28.

Schlossberg, N. K., Waters, E. B., & Goodman, J. (1995). *Counseling adults in transition*. Springer.

Skinner, E. A. (1996). A guide to constructs of control. *Journal of Personality and Social Psychology, 71*(3), 549–570.

Stewart, I., & Joines, V. (2012). *TA today: A new introduction to transactional analysis*. Lifespace.

Sugarman, L. (1986). *Life-span development: Concepts, theories and interventions*. Methuen.

Sugarman, L. (2001). *Life-span development: Frameworks, accounts and strategies*. Psychology Press.

Triandafyllidou, A., & Magazzini, T. (2021). *EUI course facilitators for: Religion, radicalisation, resilience*. Accessed via Future Learn at: https://www.futurelearn.com/courses/religion-radicalisation-resilience

UN Committee on the Rights of the Child (CRC). (2007). *General Comment No. 10 (2007): Children's rights in juvenile justice (para 32)*. Accessed at https://www.refworld.org/docid/4670fca12.html

von Bertalanffy, L. (1968). *General system theory: Foundations, development, applications*. George Braziller.

Walker, C., Slotowitz, S., Zoli, A., et al (eds.), (2022). *The palgrave handbook of innovative community and clinical psychologies*. Palgrave Macmillan. Springer Nature https://doi.org/10.1007/978-3-030-71190-0_1

Williams, D. (1999a). Life events and career change: Transition psychology in practice. In *BPS occupational psychology conference blackpool proceedings* (pp. 288–293). Accessed Sept 2010 at www.eoslifework.co.uk/transprac.htm.

Williams, D. (1999b). *Fear and violence in stressed populations.* Accessed at: http://www.eoslifework.co.uk/gturmap.htm

Williams, D. (1999c). Human responses to change. *Futures, 31*(1999), 609–616.

Williams, D. (2000a). *Managing the life-work boundary.* Accessed at http://www.eoslifework.co.uk/boundaries.htm

Williams, D. (2000b). *Career first aid. Eos client briefing notes.* Accessed at: http://www.eoslifework.co.uk/c1staid.htm

Williams, D. (2009). The life-career checklist – Issues and priorities for clients managing life or career crisis and change. In *BPS occupational psychology conference, blackpool, 2009. Abstracts* (pp. 140–142). Accessed at: www.eoslifework.co.uk/pdfs/LCC.pdf

Williams, D. (2010). Surviving and thriving: How transition psychology may apply to mass traumas and changes. In T. W. Miller (Ed.), *Handbook of stressful transitions across the lifespan.* Springer. https://doi.org/10.1007/978-1-4419-0748-6_27

Williams, D. (2012). Forgotten heroes? Health and well-being issues and resources for UK veterans and their families in the twenty-first century. In T. W. Miller (Ed.), *The praeger handbook of veterans' health* (Vol. 1). ABC-CLIO.

Woolfe, R., & Dryden, W. (1996). *Handbook of counselling psychology* (pp. 533–534). Sage. (Ch. 24 Palmer, S. Developing Stress Management Programmes, for individuals, families & organisations. Locus of Control, social support, work relationships).

Zang, A. (2017). U.S. age boundaries of delinquency 2016. *Juvenile Justice GPS (Geography, Policy, Practice & Statistics).* Accessed at: http://www.ncjj.org/Publication/U.S.-Age-Boundaries-of-Delinquency-2016.aspx

Zlotowitz, S., Barker, C., Moloney, O., & Howard, C. (2016). Service users as the key to service change? The development of an innovative intervention for excluded young people. *Child and Adolescent Mental Health, 21*(2), 102–108. https://doi.org/10.1111/camh.12137

Part II
Factors and Forms of School Violence

Chapter 7
Updated Perspectives on Linking School Bullying and Related Youth Violence Research to Effective Prevention Strategies

Dorothy L. Espelage and Susan M. Swearer

Bullying, a subset of aggression, has been an international focus of scholarship for several decades and has been declared as public health concern globally (Espelage, 2015; Hymel & Espelage, 2018; Kann et al., 2018). An abstract literature search with the terms "adol*" and "bully*" yielded 382 peer-reviewed journal articles from 2001 through 2010, and an astounding 1585 articles from 2011 through 2020.

Defining Bullying: Past and Present

Over the years, there have been significant advances in our understanding of adolescent bullying, although, within the past decade, serious attention has been given to addressing definitional issues in the adolescent bullying literature. The term "bullying" originated in Germany in 1538 as, "a browbeating individual who is especially cruel to others who are weaker" (Volk et al., 2014). However, among bullying researchers, the most familiar and widely cited definition was conceptualized and derived by Dan Olweus. Olweus (1993) first proposed and defined bullying in the 1970s as a subcategory of aggression characterized by three critical components, including: (1) intentionality, (2) repetition, and (3) a power imbalance where perpetrators have some advantage over their victims (e.g., physical size or strength, status, competence, and numbers) and victims have difficulty defending themselves (Olweus, 1993). This definition has been widely adopted by many adolescent

D. L. Espelage (✉)
School of Education, University of North Carolina at Chapel Hill, Chapel Hill, NC, USA
e-mail: espelage@unc.edu

S. M. Swearer
College of Education and Human Sciences, University of Nebraska – Lincoln, Lincoln, NE, USA

© The Author(s), under exclusive license to Springer Nature Switzerland AG 2023
T. W. Miller (ed.), *School Violence and Primary Prevention*,
https://doi.org/10.1007/978-3-031-13134-9_7

aggression scholars around the world (e.g., Felix et al., 2011; Juvonen et al., 2003; Ybarra et al., 2012); however, the ways in which these components are assessed vary widely. However, bullying researchers agree that when the three components of repetition, severity, and a perceived or observed power imbalance are present in an aggressive incident (i.e., bullying), there is an amplification of harm perceived by the target (Van der Ploeg et al., 2015; Van Noorden et al., 2016; Ybarra et al., 2014).

Within the last decade, there has been a concerted effort among scholars to reach a consensus on how bullying should be defined, operationalized, and assessed, how it differs from other forms of aggression (e.g., dating violence), and how it relates to other forms of violence across early and late adolescence (Rodkin et al., 2015; Volk et al., 2017). In 2011, the US Centers for Disease Control and Prevention (CDC) convened a group of international scholars and unanimously agreed that "Bullying is any unwanted aggressive behavior(s) by another youth or group of youths who are not siblings or current dating partners that involves an observed or perceived power imbalance and is repeated multiple times or is highly likely to be repeated. Bullying may inflict harm or distress on the targeted youth including physical, psychological, social, or educational harm" (Gladden et al., 2014, p. 7).

Bullying can include verbal, social (exclusion), physical, and electronic forms of aggression, ranging from name-calling, rumors/exclusion, threats of physical harm, physical attacks, and extortion. Bullying can occur face to face (offline) or online through cell phones or computers and in video/computer games. Finally, some bullying behaviors may overlap with aggression that meets the legal definition of harassment, but not all incidents of harassment constitute bullying. Given that bullying co-occurs with other forms of aggression and school violence (Espelage et al., 2012, 2018a, b; Rodkin et al., 2015), educators and scholars should not limit themselves to the traditional definition, but examine aggression and bullying in a comprehensive manner. Finally, assessment of victimization should not be limited to peer-on-peer experiences but should be assessed for all members of the school environment, including teachers, school staff, and paraprofessionals (Espelage et al., 2013a; Reddy et al., 2018).

Central to studying bullying behavior is how it is used to discriminate and victimize someone based on the intersection of one's identities which include but are not limited to race, gender, socioeconomic status (SES), disability, immigrant status, sexual orientation, transgendered status, and religion. This form of violence is often called bias-based aggression (or bias-based bullying) and is when a term or action relating to a marginalized identity is used pejoratively (Bradshaw & Johnson, 2011). Although any individual can be targeted and feel harm caused by bullying, this form of violence is reliably directed at individuals and identity groups who are perceived to be "different" in undesirable ways from the dominant culture of space or what is expected from a person of their identities. As such, youth who are physically larger, gender expansive, disabled, homeless or have low SES, religious minorities, or a person who is Black, Indigenous or of Color tend to be targeted for bullying (Earnshaw et al., 2018; Garnett et al., 2014). Intentional or unconscious, these actions are used to uphold societally determined social hierarchies and police individuals for not complying (Payne & Smith, 2016; Volk et al., 2014). For example, when an individual is or is perceived to be part of a sexual minority group, they are often subjected to discrimination and homophobic bullying (Camodeca et al., 2019; Espelage et al., 2018c; Hatchel et al., 2019; Poteat et al., 2012; Rivers, 2011; Russell et al., 2012). Also, racial minorities or immigrant youth frequently encounter racial or xenophobic bullying due to the dominant biases held regarding their physical traits, skin color, cultural differences, or language use (Koo et al., 2012; Peguero, 2012).

Social-Ecology of Bullying and Associated Youth Violence

Bronfenbrenner's (1977) seminal ecological systems' framework has been proposed as the preferred framework for examining the determinants of bullying and peer victimization, and other forms of youth violence. This framework postulates that bullying is an outcome within the multiple-level systems (microsystem, meso-system, exosystem, and macrosystem) in which they occur (Bronfenbrenner, 1977) and supports the need for multifaceted approaches to research on bullying (Espelage, 2015; Hong & Espelage, 2012; Rose et al., 2015). As Bronfenbrenner (1977) had envisioned, an individual youth is positioned at the center of a series of nested systems structures, including classrooms and schools. Structures or locations where children have direct contact are referred to as the *microsystem*, including family, peers, community, and schools. The interaction between components of the microsystem is referred to as the *mesosystem*. An example of a mesosystem is the interrelations between the family and school, such as parental involvement in their child's school. The *exosystem* is the social context with which the child does not have direct contact, but which affects him or her indirectly through the microsystem. Examples would be teacher or staff perceptions of the school environment and opportunities for professional development around bullying, school violence, or school climate. The *macrosystem* level is commonly regarded as a cultural "blueprint," which may determine the social structures and activities at the various levels (Bronfenbrenner, 1977). This level includes organizational, social, cultural, and political contexts, which influence the interactions within other system levels (Bronfenbrenner, 1977). The final level of the ecological framework, the *chronosystem* level, includes consistency or change (e.g., historical or life events) of the individual and the environment over the life course (e.g., changes in family structure).

A social-ecological explanation of bullying suggests that youth become involved in bullying as perpetrators, victims, perpetrator–victims, or bystanders as a result of complex interactions between their own individual characteristics and those of their families, schools, peers, and society. Therefore, targeting multiple levels of the social ecology can both help improve the general social environments where youth spend their time and reduce bullying by bolstering protective aspects of the system.

Prevention, Intervention, and Policy Efforts

As noted, bully prevention and intervention efforts have grown exponentially over the years. Within the previous decade, there was a significant increase in legislative efforts to prevent bullying in schools; today, anti-bullying laws are prevalent in all 50 states (Cascardi et al., 2018; Cornell & Limber, 2015). However, given that research on bullying and violence prevention laws in schools has focused on content analyses of these laws (Cornell & Limber, 2015; Stuart-Cassel et al., 2011), it is unclear to what degree these laws and policies are effective and what the factors are that might contribute to their successful implementation (Flannery et al., 2016).

Violence prevention programs, especially those in the school settings, most often target one type of youth aggression (e.g., bullying perpetration) exclusively even though empirical findings suggest that youth aggression co-occurs with other types of youth aggression (Debnam et al., 2016; Espelage et al., 2015a, 2021; Foshee et al., 2015, 2016). Several longitudinal study findings also suggest that adolescents who frequently show signs of aggressive behaviors, such as bullying, are at increased odds of being involved in other types of aggressive behaviors, for example, dating violence and sexual harassment (Espelage et al., 2012, 2015a, 2018a, b). Therefore, targeting multiple forms of youth aggressive behaviors affecting adolescents, particularly middle and high schoolers is highly suggested (Connolly et al., 2015).

There has been a considerable growth in prevention programs for bullying and concomitant types of youth violence (e.g., sexual violence, teen dating violence) in the United States. The existing violence prevention programs in schools within the past decade include a wide array of programs. Such programs include the universally based, whole-school approach, which focuses on the entire school community (Storer et al., 2017); socio-emotional learning, which focuses on social skills training, coping skills, or de-escalation approach (Espelage et al., 2013b); and bystander intervention (Nickerson et al., 2014; Polanin et al., 2012). However, the efficacy and effectiveness of the existing programs remain unclear, as there are only a small number of randomized controlled trials that test the efficacy or effectiveness of programs that are specifically designed to reduce bullying or target the consequences of bullying.

Meta-Analytic Studies: Traditional Bullying

Within the area of bullying among children and adolescents, several meta-analytic studies were conducted in the last decade that have had significant impacts on the ways in which bullying is addressed globally. For example, Ttofi and Farrington (2011) found program elements that were associated with decreases in rates of bully perpetration included parent training/meetings, improved playground supervision, disciplinary methods, classroom management, teacher training, classroom rules, whole-school anti-bullying policy, school conferences, information for parents, and cooperative group work. Decreases in rates of victimization were associated with the following program elements: disciplinary methods, parent training/meetings, use of videos, and cooperative group work. Further, the duration and intensity of the program for children and teachers were significantly associated with a decrease in perpetration and victimization.

In two separate 2019 meta-analyses, Gaffney et al. (2019a, b) included a review of 100 bully prevention program evaluations and randomized clinical trials, with 72% being conducted outside the United States. Additionally, 65 different anti-bullying programs were evaluated, with four programs representing 38% of the total sample. The Olweus Bully Prevention Program was the most commonly evaluated (18%), generally through age cohort designs (Gaffney et al., 2019b), resulting in larger effect sizes in Norway, when compared to evaluations in the United States (Gaffney et al., 2019a). Of the 12 countries that had multiple evaluations, the United States had the fourth largest reduction in bully perpetration (1.38 OR; Range 0.86 OR (Netherlands) to 1.59 OR (Spain)) and seventh-largest reduction in victimization (1.17 OR; Range 0.88 OR (Cypress) to 1.62 OR (Italy; Gaffney et al., 2019b). Overall, Gaffney and colleagues (2019b) found reductions of perpetration by approximately 19–20% and victimization by approximately 15–16%.

Although promising, these meta-analyses also pointed to several gaps in the area of bullying prevention efforts. First, these meta-analyses revealed smaller effect sizes for randomized clinical trials (RCT) designs in comparison to non-RCT designs (Gaffney et al., 2019b; Ttofi & Farrington, 2011). This suggests that studies conducted in less authentic educational environments (e.g., those with a higher degree of researcher involvement), elicited stronger effects than those conducted in more applied settings (Bradshaw, 2015; Ttofi & Farrington, 2011). Moreover, another systematic review of bullying prevention programs concluded that research conducted outside of the United States and studies with racially and ethnically homogeneous samples were significantly more likely to report significant findings (Evans et al., 2014).

Meta-Analytic Study: Traditional and Cyberbullying

In a recent meta-analysis of the effects of school-based programs on both traditional and cyberbullying, Polanin et al. (2021a, b) included a total of 50 studies and 320 extracted effect sizes spanning 45,371 participants. Results indicated that programs reduced cyberbullying perpetration ($g = -0.18$, SE = 0.05, 95% CI [-0.28, -0.09]) and victimization ($g = -0.13$, SE = 0.04, 95% CI [-0.21, -0.05]). Results indicated that when programs have an explicit focus on targeting cyberbullying, reductions were also noted for traditional bullying. We strongly encourage developers of bully prevention programs or those that are revising their programs to include specific and elaborate content on cyberbullying, given its rising prevalence and associations with other forms of aggression.

Meta-Analytic Study: Teen Dating Violence

Concerning bullying that is linked to teen dating violence and sexual violence, even fewer studies evaluating the effectiveness of sexual violence prevention using a randomized design can be found in the research literature (Foshee et al., 2012). Also, a recent meta-analytic study on dating violence and sexual violence programs for middle and high school students reported that although existing programs influence knowledge and improve attitudes, these programs are not affecting these behaviors to a significant extent (De La Rue et al., 2017). These patterns of findings seem to suggest that developing and implementing effective violence prevention and intervention programs are likely to be more challenging in the United States than in other countries (Evans et al., 2014).

Tiered Prevention and Intervention Approaches

In the prevention literature, the terms "primary," "secondary," and "tertiary" refer to specific prevention and intervention strategies designed to reduce problem behavior in youth. Perhaps the most widely recognized model that embraces this three-tiered model is the Multitiered System of Supports (MTSS; Cowan et al., 2013), under which Positive Behavioral Intervention and Supports is a framework for behavioral prevention and intervention efforts in schools (PBIS; Sprague & Golly, 2004; Sprague & Walker, 2005). PBIS is a system-based, behaviorally focused prevention and intervention set of strategies designed to improve educational outcomes and social development for all students. PBIS frameworks indicate that approximately 80% of students will need primary prevention strategies, 15% will need secondary prevention strategies, and 5% will need tertiary prevention strategies.

Applied to the social-ecological problem of bullying where bullying is conceptualized as emerging from different domains of a child's lives (e.g., individual, school, peer, family), the goal of primary prevention is to reduce the number of new cases of bullying. The idea is that through whole-school and classroom-wide strategies, new incidents of bullying can be curtailed. Fifteen percent of students will need secondary prevention strategies designed to reduce engagement in bullying. These might be the students who are involved in bullying as a bystander or students who are involved in bullying less frequently or less severely. Finally, tertiary prevention strategies are designed for the 5% of students who are involved in frequent and intense bullying behaviors. These are the students who might have concomitant psychological problems (i.e., depression and anxiety) as a result of their involvement in bullying behaviors (Davis et al., 2019; Polanin et al., 2021a, b; Walters & Espelage, 2018). The goal of tertiary prevention is to reduce complications, severity, and frequency of bullying behaviors. While not an exhaustive list, Fig. 7.1 outlines three bullying prevention and intervention initiatives that illustrate the MTSS framework. A description of these three initiatives will be provided in the next section of this chapter.

Fig. 7.1 Bullying
prevention and intervention
in a Multitiered System of
Supports

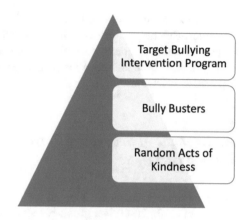

An Example of Primary Prevention for Bullying Behaviors: Random Acts of Kindness

The Random Acts of Kindness Foundation was established in 1995 (www.ran-domactsofkindness.org). The mission of the Random Acts of Kindness Foundation is to "make kindness the norm" by promoting resiliency, kindness, and well-being in schools, homes, workplaces, and communities (Schonert-Reichl & Arruda, 2016). All of their programs follow a simple framework: Share, Inspire, Empower, Act, and Reflect. The goal of their school curriculum, Kindness in the Classroom, is to enhance children's social and emotional competence through skill-building activities that promote positive social behaviors and school adjustment. With its focus on creating a culture of kindness, Kindness in the Classroom is an excellent example of primary prevention for bullying behaviors.

The Kindness in the Classroom is a year-long (36 weeks) curriculum that focuses on six kindness concepts: Respect, Caring, Inclusiveness, Integrity, Responsibility, and Courage. Six weeks is dedicated to each concept, with 4 weeks of lessons and 2 weeks of projects presented. Lessons are designed to be presented once a week, ranging from 30–45 min in length. Each lesson follows the structure of their Kindness framework. First, students share with their peers on what they have learned and experienced with others since the previous lesson. By listening to others' experiences, students' learning is reinforced and are more likely to continue spreading kindness. Second, lessons are designed to inspire both students and teachers through various activities and role-play scenarios.

To empower their students, teachers facilitate class-wide and small group discussions to give students the tools needed to find ways to express kindness in their daily lives. Existing opportunities to act with kindness are found throughout the lessons, but students demonstrate their ideas and skills by completing unit projects. Students work to bring real, tangible kindness into the world through projects involving one of the six kindness concepts. Finally, at the end of each lesson and project, teachers guide students to reflect on what they have learned and identify how being kind impacts their own lives, as well as the lives of those around them.

In a randomized controlled trial conducted by the University of British Columbia (Schonert-Reichl & Arruda, 2016), Kindness in the Classroom significantly improved students' emotional and social competence, including empathy/sympathy and intrinsic prosocial motivation, while also significantly decreasing antisocial and aggressive behaviors.

An Example of Secondary Prevention for Bullying Behaviors: Bully Busters

Bully Busters: A Teacher's Manual for Helping Bullies, Victims, and Bystanders (Newman et al., 2000) is a group-based, psychoeducational program developed to target teachers' skills and self-efficacy in reducing bullying behaviors. The focus of Bully Busters is to alter the school environment by changing teachers' and school administrators' responses and creating a school culture that encourages peer action to reduce or eliminate the problem of bullying.

As such, this program falls under both primary and secondary levels of prevention. This program was created based on three core assumptions: changing the environment is more powerful than changing individuals, prevention is better than intervention, and changing the environment requires support and understanding among teachers (Horne et al., 2011). There are four versions of the program: Bully Busters: A Teacher's Manual for Helping Bullies, Victims, and Bystanders – Grades 6–8 (Newman et al., 2000), Bully Busters: A Teacher's Manual for Helping Bullies, Victims, and Bystanders – Grades K–5 (Horne et al., 2003), Helping Bullies, Victims, and Bystanders: A Parent's Guide to Bully Busters (Horne et al., 2008), and Empowering Teen Peers to Prevent Bullying: The Bully Busters Program for High School (Horne et al., 2012). The high school program has a different structure than the other school-age programs, with the emphasis on adult facilitators and older students as peer leaders, rather than the teacher-led modality.

The Bully Busters Program is implemented through a staff development training workshop, which is then followed by teacher support groups. The workshop provides information on the social-ecological model on which the program is based, and the specific classroom materials and activities included. The workshop is comprised of seven modules, each composed of an overview, rationale, objectives to be accomplished, discussions, and student activities that are related to the topic. Module One is designed to help teachers and students recognize the extent of the problem of bullying, provide a common definition, dispel myths about bullying, and develop classroom exercises to help students understand bullying. The second module focuses on the development of bullying, the variety of forms it can take, gender differences in bullying behaviors, and common myths and misconceptions. Module Three examines how to recognize the types of victims and victimization of bullying and effects of victimization and prepares teachers to conduct skills training to help students learn effective methods to report and manage the bullying problem.

Recommendations and interventions for bullying behaviors are the focus of the fourth module, which provides teachers with specific strategies to create a bully-free classroom, including empathy skills education, social skills training, anger control skills, and classroom management techniques. The fifth module expands students' skills development through the instruction of strategies to implement with victims of bullying, such as victim support, interventions for specific types of victims, and group assimilation. Module Six focuses on aiding teachers in the role of prevention of bullying via characteristics of schools and teachers that lead to bullying reduction and different recommendations to prevent bullying and victimization. This module also includes student activities that focus on building problem-solving and decision-making skills to prevent conflict. Module Seven addresses teacher-coping skills, relaxation training, and emotion management, with the goal of teachers applying the skills, then teaching those skills to their students. After all of the modules are completed, a follow-up assessment of teachers' knowledge and self-efficacy is administered, as well as a student and teacher survey of bullying in their school.

After the workshop, the Bully Buster Teacher Support Teams are composed and organized. In addition to reviewing the modules, the Support Teams fulfill several roles: they serve as a reminder to continue addressing bullying behaviors, provide opportunities to discuss problematic situations in the classroom or with specific students, and offer the chance to evaluate what is working and what is not effective in the prevention of bullying behaviors. A study conducted by Newman-Carlson and Horne (2004) found that the treatment program effectively increased teachers' knowledge of intervention skills, teachers' self-efficacy, and reduced classroom bullying through measurement of disciplinary referrals.

An Example of Tertiary Prevention for Bullying Behaviors: Target Bullying Intervention Program

The Bullying Intervention Program (T-BIP; Swearer & Givens, 2006) is an individual cognitive-behavioral intervention for use with students who bully others. The guiding premise behind T-BIP is twofold. First, we are guided by the reality that the social-cognitive perceptions of students involved in bullying interactions are as critical as are the aggressive behaviors, because the perceptions and cognitions of the participants serve to underlie, perpetuate, and escalate bullying interactions (Doll & Swearer, 2005; Swearer & Cary, 2003). Second, there is compelling research that suggests that homogeneous group interventions are not helpful for aggressive youth and in fact, may be damaging (Dishion et al., 1999). Based on these two underlying premises, the T-BIP was developed as a mechanism for school counselors and school psychologists to work directly with students who bully others.

The T-BIP is in part based upon two decades of research on school bullying under the research project, "Target Bullying: Ecologically-Based Prevention and

Intervention for Schools." Target Bullying is a participatory research project whereby university researchers and school personnel and families work together to understand the bullying phenomenon. The T-BIP was developed by the request of a middle school principal who experienced the fact that in-school suspension, suspension, and expulsion were ineffective strategies for reducing bullying behaviors. Research has also found that zero-tolerance policies are not effective in curbing aggressive behaviors (Casella, 2003) and that expulsion is equally ineffective in reducing aggressive behavior (Gordon, 2001). Thus, the interventions typically employed in school settings (group treatment, zero tolerance, and expulsion) are ineffective in dealing with bullying behaviors.

The T-BIP is an alternative to in-school suspension for bullying behaviors that is being implemented in a Midwestern public school district. When a student is referred for bullying behaviors, the typical protocol is that the student is sent to in-school suspension. In the T-BIP, parents are given a choice: in-school suspension or the T-BIP. In all cases ($n = 272$) since the program's inception in 2005, parents have chosen T-BIP. In order to participate in the T-BIP, active parental consent and student assent are obtained. Then, the T-BIP is scheduled according to the same policies and procedures that the school uses to schedule in-school suspension.

The T-BIP is a three-hour one-on-one cognitive–behavioral intervention session with a masters-level student therapist under the supervision of a licensed psychologist. There are three components to the T-BIP: (1) assessment, (2) psychoeducation, and (3) feedback. The assessment component consists of widely used measures to assess experiences with bullying, depression, anxiety, cognitive distortions, school climate, and self-concept. The assessment component lasts approximately 1 h. The psychoeducation component lasts about 2 h and consists of the student therapist presenting an engaging and youth-friendly PowerPoint presentation about bullying behaviors. The presentation is followed by a short quiz to assess understanding. This is followed by several worksheet activities about bullying behavior that are used from Bully Busters (Newman et al., 2000) or virtual reality learning experiences for students ages 13 and older. Finally, the student therapist and the referred student watch videos about bullying. The session ends with a debriefing component where the referred student talks about his or her experiences with bullying and impressions of T-BIP. Based on the assessment data and the interactions with the referred student, a bullying intervention treatment report is written. Recommendations are based on the data collected. The treatment report is reviewed with the parents, student, and school personnel during a face-to-face solution-oriented meeting.

Since mid-fall 2005, there have been 272 participants in grades one through eleven. The mean age was 11.45 years (range: 7–17 years old). For race/ethnicity, 50.4% of participants identified as White, 16.9% Biracial, 8.8% Black/African American, 9.6% Latino/Hispanic, 4% Native American, 1.1% Middle Eastern, 0.4% Asian American, 0.4% Eastern European, and 4% identifying as other. Twelve participants (4.4%) did not complete the race or ethnicity items. In terms of self-reporting engagement in bullying, 41.2% of participants reported that they bullied others, were bullied, and observed bullying (bully-victim-bystanders), 9.6% of participants reported they both bullied others and were bullied (bully-victims); 5.9%

reported they bullied others (bully); 5.6% reported they observed bullying (bystander); 3.6% reported they were victimized only (victim); and 3.6% reported that they were not involved at all in bullying. In terms of psychosocial functioning, eight participants endorsed clinical levels of depression and five participants endorsed clinical levels of anxiety. Participants endorsed a range of cognitive distortions and behavioral problems. The variety of presenting problems acknowledged by the participants suggests that homogeneous group interventions for students who bully others are likely to be ineffective. At the tertiary level, it appears that individually focused interventions for bullying are likely to be more efficacious than group forms of treatment (Dishion et al., 1999).

How to Implement Prevention Strategies?

The most effective prevention and intervention programming will exist when a coordinated effort exists between primary, secondary, and tertiary strategies. As previously mentioned, MTSS (Cowan et al., 2013) is an example of coordinating these strategies. Clearly, coordinating school, family, and community prevention and intervention efforts is essential in reducing aggressive and bullying behaviors in students (Sprague & Walker, 2005). However, despite the fact that there are more than 300 violence prevention programs (Howard et al., 1999), there is little guidance for school personnel and parents on how to implement these programs.

Successful implementation of any prevention or intervention strategy depends in large part on the people involved. Any program will fail if the adults in the system are not supportive. If the adults in the school are enthusiastic, positive, and emotionally healthy and have a unified focus on doing what is in the best interests of students, then the school climate will be a healthy and positive environment. This environment in itself will help create a prevention-oriented atmosphere and will help prevent problems before they start. At the primary prevention level, strategies that help promote a positive school climate, positive relationships in the school, and positive home–school relationships are vital.

Teachers in the school must be supported in their classroom management strategies and classroom-based interventions. Secondary prevention strategies are more likely to be successful when teachers are supported in their work and they are able to identify the students who are struggling. When schools adhere to a unified referral system for at-risk students, they decrease the likelihood that a student might fall through the cracks or does not get additional help (i.e., social skills training). Positive relationships between teachers, administrators, and school support staff (i.e., school social workers, school psychologists) are critical.

Schools must support their counseling departments, as these personnel are trained in working with difficult students. At the tertiary level, there are many interventions that can be utilized in working with students who are involved in bullying behaviors. These interventions typically occur at the individual level, such as individual therapy. However, small group work, such as support groups, and family therapy may also be effective. It is incumbent upon counseling departments to have a solid referral system for teachers and parents and to develop strong links to providers in the community. Primary, secondary, and tertiary prevention and intervention efforts that are coordinated, positive, supportive, and data-based are vital for the reduction of bullying behaviors in our schools.

Leveraging Technology to Inform Bullying and Youth Violence Prevention

Increasingly, the prevention of bullying and other forms of youth violence are leveraging technology and multimedia. Given the limited efficacy of physical bullying prevention programs, a need exists for a novel, theoretically informed, prevention programming. Several studies have employed video technology to deliver prevention curricula, and their use can be an effective way to deliver content and demonstrate skills on a large scale while keeping costs of implementation low. One example of a study using video to deliver social-emotional learning prevention curriculum is the Second Step program (Espelage et al., 2013b). The Second Step lessons were accompanied and supported by a media-rich DVD which included interviews with students and demonstrations of skills. The videos were used to reinforce skills acquisition during the program delivery which supported other prevention strategies (Espelage et al., 2013b).

However, given the need to reinforce social-emotional learning competencies outside of the classroom/school, Ybarra et al. (2016) developed a 7-week middle school text-messaging program called *BullyDown* that included SEL content and encouraged bystander intervention. Results of a small pilot study indicated that there were reductions in bullying in the intervention condition (Ybarra et al., 2016). Bully prevention through text messaging is particularly innovative and has the potential to advance bully prevention, where they may be failing. First, BullyDown will be delivered outside of school. By engaging with the content in a non-academic setting, youth may be more likely to apply their new behaviors across contexts, including bullying scenarios that take place on the way to and from school and other places where youth congregate. This also has the advantage of giving youth the opportunity to learn SEL components and interact with someone else in the program (i.e., a Text Buddy) without a potential perpetrator sitting at a desk nearby. It also bypasses situations when school-based programming is not viewed as "cool" by some students, resulting in their under-engagement in program activities, which can implicitly reinforce negative social norms. Second, in school-based intervention programs, school personnel are often called upon to implement the content. To do so, they need to be extensively trained to maximize efficacy. Increasingly, financial resources for training are simply not available in US public schools. BullyDown is administered through text messaging, bypassing training, and competition with professional development time. Third, compared to in-person interventions that may be vulnerable to variable implementation fidelity, all youth in the program receive the same content in the same order, thereby ensuring fidelity. Compared to "apps" that require a smartphone and data, all cell phones are text messaging-capable and therefore, all students who have a cell phone would be able to participate. Fourth, the meta-analytic results described above reflect the best-case scenario. Although all states require schools to implement bullying prevention programming, there is significant variation in what is mandated, resulting in a wide spectrum of programming offered in schools across the US. In the FGs, we conducted in the BullyDown development process, very few youths talked about a comprehensive bullying prevention curriculum in their school. BullyDown can be delivered as a "booster" outside of school time that enhances whatever programming is being offered by schools. In doing so, one of the benefits of BullyDown is that it helps to ensure all youth are exposed to the basic tenets of a bullying prevention curriculum. Finally, given the focus on victimization that most of the current prevention programs have, BullyDown's focus on perpetration is innovative.

Virtual reality (VR) has also been utilized as a tool for bully prevention. To explore VR as a violence prevention tool, Ingram et al. (2019) used a pseudo-randomized controlled design to pilot test the effects of a VR-enhanced bullying prevention program compared to the currently used bullying prevention programming in two Midwestern US middle schools. The enhanced program included professionally designed VR scenarios that place students into situations as if they were witnessing them in real life (e.g., at the party or in the hallway watching an altercation). This in-vivo experience decreases all four dimensions of psychological distance (spatial, social, temporal, hypothetical) that the traditional bullying curriculum does not. These activities include reflecting on character identification, perspective-taking discussion questions, and creating short films aimed to evoke empathy. Results indicated that students in the VR condition reported increases in self-reported empathy and greater willingness to intervene to help a victim of bullying. VR and other programs that use multimedia should be considered as a complement to other school-based prevention efforts.

Conclusions

Bullying involvement among school-aged children continues to be a public health concern and co-occurs with other forms of youth violence, including bias-based aggression, sexual violence, and teen dating violence. Involvement with these forms of youth violence is associated with mental health issues, psychiatric symptoms, academic challenges, and peer relation issues. Research on school-based bullying has burgeoned over the last few decades, and much has been learned about the etiological theories regarding why youth become involved and how bullying is a precursor and antecedent to other forms of aggression. It is clear that bullying involvement is a multifaceted phenomenon that originates as a result of a complex interaction between individual youth and their environments. Multitiered prevention and intervention approaches have shown promise in reducing bullying. We discussed examples of primary, secondary, and tertiary approaches to bully prevention and encourage preventionists to consider how to leverage technology to improve transfer of skills to contexts outside of the classroom or school.

As prevention scientists who have collectively been engaged in bully prevention efforts for over 50 years, we have learned many lessons including:

- Bullying co-occurs with other forms of violence and cannot be examined in isolation.
- Minoritized youth (e.g., gender/sexual minority youth, students with disabilities) are particularly at-risk for bullying involvement, but often do not focus on prevention efforts.
- Bully prevention needs to involve all stakeholders – parents, teachers, administrators, coaches, and faith-based leaders, not just students.
- Bully prevention in the United States is not as successful as in other countries, and even within the United States, success varies depending on school districts.
- Efficacy of bully prevention efforts is directly tied to implementation fidelity. Programs need to be implemented as intended if they are to sustain positive outcomes.
- Bully prevention should be integrated into all aspects of school culture and community.

Acknowledgments The authors would like to thank Sam Kesselring, a doctoral student at the University of Nebraska, and Lincoln, for her research and editorial work on this chapter.

References

Bradshaw, C. P. (2015). Translating research to practice in bullying prevention. *American Psychologist, 70*(4), 322. https://doi.org/10.1037/a0039114

Bradshaw, C. P., & Johnson, R. M. (2011). The social context of bullying and peer victimization: An introduction to the special issue. *Journal of School Violence, 10*(2), 107–114.

Bronfenbrenner, U. (1977). Toward an experimental ecology of human development. *American Psychologist, 32*(7), 513–531.

Camodeca, M., Baiocco, R., & Posa, O. (2019). Homophobic bullying and victimization among adolescents: The role of prejudice, moral disengagement and sexual orientation. *European Journal of Developmental Psychology, 16*(5), 503–521. https://doi.org/10.1080/1740562 9.2018.1466699

Cascardi, M., King, C. M., Rector, D., & DelPozzo, J. (2018). School-based bullying and teen dating violence prevention laws: Overlapping or distinct? *Journal of Interpersonal Violence, 33*(21), 3267–3297. https://doi.org/10.1177/0886260518798357

Casella, R. (2003). Zero tolerance policy in schools: Rationale, consequences, and alternatives. *Teachers College Record, 105*, 872–892. https://doi.org/10.1111/1467-9620.00271

Connolly, J., Josephson, W., Schnoll, J., Simkins-Strong, E., Pepler, D., MacPherson, A., Weiser, J., Moran, M., & Jiang, D. (2015). Evaluation of a youth-led program for preventing bullying, sexual harassment, and dating aggression in middle schools. *Journal of Early Adolescence, 35*(3), 403–434. https://doi.org/10.1177/0272431614535090

Cornell, D., & Limber, S. P. (2015). Law and policy on the concept of bullying at school. *American Psychologist, 70*, 333–343.

Cowan, K. C., Vaillancourt, K., Rossen, E., & Pollitt, K. (2013). *A framework for safe and successful schools* [Brief]. National Association of School Psychologists. http://www.nasponline.org/resources/handouts/Framework_for_Safe_and_SuccessfulSchool_Environments.pdf

Davis, J. P., Merrin, G. J., Ingram, K. M., Espelage, D. L., Valido, A., & El Sheikh, A. (2019). Bully victimization, depression, & school belonging among middle school youth: Disaggregating between- and within-person longitudinal effects. *Journal of Child and Family Studies, 28*(9), 2365–2378.

De La Rue, L., Polanin, J. R., Espelage, D. L., & Pigott, T. D. (2017). A meta-analysis of school-based interventions aimed to prevent or reduce violence in teen dating relationships. *Review of Educational Research, 87*(1), 7–34.

Debnam, K. J., Waasdorp, T. E., & Bradshaw, C. P. (2016). Examining the contemporaneous occurrence of bullying and teen dating violence victimization. *School Psychology Quarterly, 31*(1), 76–90.

Dishion, T. J., McCord, J., & Poulin, F. (1999). When interventions harm: Peer groups and problem behavior. *American Psychologist, 54*(9), 755–764. https://doi.org/10.1037/0003-066X.54.9.755

Doll, B., & Swearer, S. M. (2005). Cognitive behavior interventions for participants in bullying and coercion. In R. B. Mennuti, A. Freeman, & R. Christner (Eds.), *Cognitive behavioral interventions in educational settings*. Brunner-Routledge.

Earnshaw, V. A., Reisner, S. L., Menino, D. D., Poteat, V. P., Bogart, L. M., Barnes, T. N., & Schuster, M. A. (2018). Stigma-based bullying interventions: A systematic review. *Developmental Review, 48*, 178–200.

Espelage, D. L. (2015). Emerging issues in school bullying research and prevention science. In E. T. Emmer & E. Sabornie (Eds.), *Handbook of classroom management: Research, practice, and contemporary issues* (pp. 76–93). Taylor & Francis.

Espelage, D. L., Basile, K. C., & Hamburger, M. E. (2012). Bullying perpetration and subsequent sexual violence perpetration among middle school students. *Journal of Adolescent Health, 50*(1), 60–65. https://doi.org/10.1016/j.jadohealth.2011.07.015

Espelage, D. L., Anderman, E., Brown, V., Jones, A., Lane, K., McMahon, S. D., et al. (2013a). Understanding and preventing violence directed against teachers: Recommendations for a national research, practice, and policy agenda. *American Psychologist, 68*, 75–87. https://doi.org/10.1037/a0031307

Espelage, D. L., Low, S., Polanin, J. R., & Brown, E. C. (2013b). The impact of a middle school program to reduce aggression, victimization, and sexual violence. *Journal of Adolescent Health, 53*(2), 180–186. https://doi.org/10.1016/j.jadohealth.2013.02.021

Espelage, D. L., Basile, K. C., De La Rue, L., & Hamburger, M. E. (2015a). Longitudinal associations among bullying, homophobic teasing, and sexual violence perpetration among middle school students. *Journal of Interpersonal Violence, 30*(14), 2541–2561. https://doi.org/10.1177/0886260514553113

Espelage, D. L., Hong, J. S., Rao, M. A., & Thornberg, R. (2015b). Understanding the ecological factors associated with bullying across the elementary to middle school transition in the United States. *Violence & Victims, 30*(3), 470–487. https://doi.org/10.1891/0886-6708. VV-D-14-00046

Espelage, D. L., Basile, K. C., Leemis, R. W., Hipp, T. N., & Davis, J. P. (2018a). Longitudinal examination of the bullying-sexual violence pathway across early to late adolescence: Implicating homophobic name-calling. *Journal of Youth and Adolescence, 47*(9), 1880–1893. https://doi.org/10.1007/s10964-018-0827-4

Espelage, D. L., Davis, J., Basile, K. C., Rostad, W. L., & Leemis, R. W. (2018b). Alcohol, prescription drug misuse, sexual violence, and dating violence among high school youth. *Journal of Adolescent Health, 63*(5), 601–607.

Espelage, D. L., Merrin, G. J., & Hatchel, T. (2018c). Peer victimization & dating violence among LGBTQ youth: The impact of school violence & crime on mental health outcomes. *Youth Violence and Juvenile Justice, 16*(2), 156–1783. https://doi.org/10.1177/1541204016680408

Espelage, D. L., Ingram, K. M., Hong, J. S., & Merrin, G. J. (2021). Bullying as a developmental precursor to sexual and dating violence across adolescence: Decade in review. *Trauma, Violence, & Abuse,* 15248380211043811.

Evans, C. B. R., Fraser, M. W., & Cotter, K. L. (2014). The effectiveness of school-based bullying prevention programs: A systematic review. *Aggression and Violent Behavior, 19*(5), 532–544. https://doi.org/10.1016/j.avb.2014.07.004

Felix, E. D., Sharkey, J. D., Green, J. G., Furlong, M. J., & Tanigawa, D. (2011). Getting precise and pragmatic about the assessment of bullying: The development of the California bullying victimization scale. *Aggressive Behavior, 37*(3), 234–247.

Flannery, D. J., Todres, J., Bradshaw, C. P., Amar, A. F., Graham, S., Hatzenbuehler, M., Masiello, M., Moreno, M., Sullivan, R., Vaillancourt, T., Le Menestrel, S. M., & Rivara, F. (2016). Bullying prevention: A summary of the report of the National Academies of Sciences, Engineering, and Medicine. *Prevention Science, 17,* 1044–1053. https://doi.org/10.1007/s11121-016-0722-8

Foshee, V. A., McNaughton Reyes, H. L., Ennett, S. T., Cance, J. D., Bauman, K. E., & Bowling, J. M. (2012). Assessing the effects of families for safe dates, a family-based teen dating abuse prevention program. *Journal of Adolescent Health, 51*(4), 349–356. https://doi.org/10.1016/j.jadohealth.2011.12.029

Foshee, V. A., McNaughton, R. L., Tharp, A. T., Chang, L. Y., Ennett, S. T., Simon, T. R., et al. (2015). Shared longitudinal predictors of physical peer and dating violence. *Journal of Adolescent Health, 56,* 106–112.

Foshee, V. A., McNaughton Reyes, H. L. M., Chen, M. S., Ennett, S. T., Basile, K. C., DeGue, S., Vivolo-Kantor, A. M., Moracco, K. E., & Bowling, J. M. (2016). Shared risk factors for the perpetration of physical dating violence, bullying, and sexual harassment among adolescents exposed to domestic violence. *Journal of Youth and Adolescence, 45,* 672–686. https://doi.org/10.1007/s10964-015-0404-z

Gaffney, H., Farrington, D. P., & Ttofi, M. M. (2019a). Examining the effectiveness of school-bullying intervention programs globally: A meta-analysis. *International Journal of Bullying Prevention, 1*(1), 14-31. https://doi.org/10.1007/s42380-019-0007-4

Gaffney, H., Ttofi, M. M., & Farrington, D. P. (2019b). Evaluating the effectiveness of school-bullying prevention programs: An updated meta-analytical review. *Aggression and Violent Behavior, 45,* 111–133. https://doi.org/10.1016/j.avb.2018.07.001

Garnett, B. R., Masyn, K. E., Austin, S. B., Miller, M., Williams, D. R., & Viswanath, K. (2014). The intersectionality of discrimination attributes and bullying among youth: An applied latent class analysis. *Journal of Youth and Adolescence, 43*(8), 1225–1239.

Gladden, R. M., Vivolo-Kantor, A. M., Hamburger, M. E., & Lumpkin, C. D. (2014). *Bullying surveillance among youths: Uniform definitions for public health and recommended data elements, version 1.0.* National Center for Injury Prevention and Control, Centers for Disease Control and Prevention.

Gordon, A. (2001). School exclusions in England: Children's voices and adult solutions? *Educational Studies, 27*(1), 69–85. https://doi.org/10.1080/03055690020002143

Hatchel, T., Polanin, J., & Espelage, D. L. (2019). Suicidal thoughts and behaviors among LGBTQ youth: Meta-analyses and a systematic review. *Archives of Suicide Research, 25,* 1–37.

Hong, J. S., & Espelage, D. L. (2012). A review of research on bullying and peer victimization in school: An ecological systems analysis. *Aggression and Violent Behavior, 17,* 311–312. https://doi.org/10.1016/j.avb.2012.03.003

Horne, A. M., Bartolomucci, C. L., & Newman-Carlson, D. (2003). *Bully busters: A teacher's manual for helping bullies, victims, and bystanders – Grades K-5.* Research Press.

Horne, A. M., Stoddard, J., & Bell, C. (2008). *A parent's guide to understanding and responding to bullying: The bully busters approach.* Research Press.

Horne, A. M., Bell, C. D., Raczynski, K. A., & Whitford, J. L. (2011). Bully busters: A resource for schools and parents to prevent and respond to bullying. In D. L. Espelage & S. M. Swearer (Eds.), *Bullying in North American schools: A social-ecological perspective on prevention and intervention* (2nd ed., pp. 227–240). Routledge.

Horne, A. M., Nitza, A., Dobias, B. F., Joliff, D. L., Raczynski, K. A., & Voors, W. (2012). *Empowering teen peers to prevent bullying: The bully busters program for high school*. Research Press.

Howard, K. A., Flora, J., & Griffin, M. (1999). Violence-prevention programs in schools: State of the science and implications for future research. *Applied & Preventative Psychology, 8*(3), 197–215. https://doi.org/10.1016/S0962-1849(05)80077-0

Hymel, S., & Espelage, D. L. (2018). Preventing aggression and youth violence in schools. In T. Malti & K. Rubin (Eds.), *Handbook of child and adolescent aggression: Emergence, development and intervention*. Guilford Press.

Ingram, K. M., Espelage, D. L., Valido, A., Heinhorst, J., & Joyce, M. (2019). Pilot trial of a virtual reality enhanced bullying prevention curriculum. *Journal of Adolescence, 71*, 72–83.

Juvonen, J., Graham, S., & Schuster, M. A. (2003). Bullying among young adolescents: The strong, the weak, and the troubled. *Pediatrics, 112*(6), 1231–1237.

Kann, L., McManus, T., Harris, W. A., Shanklin, S. L., Flint, K. H., Queen, B., et al. (2018). Youth risk behavior surveillance—United States, 2017. *MMWR Surveillance Summaries, 67*(8), 1–114.

Koo, D. J., Peguero, A. A., & Shekarkhar, Z. (2012). The "model minority" victim: Immigration, gender, and Asian American vulnerabilities to violence at school. *Journal of Ethnicity in Criminal Justice, 10*(2), 129–147. https://doi.org/10.1080/15377938.2011.609405

Newman, D. A., Horne, A. M., & Bartolomucci, C. L. (2000). *Bully busters: A teacher's manual for helping bullies, victims, and bystanders*. Research Press.

Newman-Carlson, D., & Horne, H. M. (2004). Bully busters: A psychoeducational intervention for reducing bullying behaviors in middle school students. *Journal of Counseling & Development, 82*(3), 259–267. https://doi.org/10.1002/j.1556-6678.2004.tb00309.x

Nickerson, A. B., Aloe, A. M., Livingston, J. A., & Feeley, T. H. (2014). Measurement of the bystander intervention model for bullying and sexual harassment. *Journal of Adolescence, 37*(4), 391–400. https://doi.org/10.1016/j.adolescence.2014.03.003

Olweus, D. (1993). *Bullying at School*. Blackwell Publishing.

Payne, E., & Smith, M. J. (2016). Gender policing. In *Critical concepts in queer studies and education* (pp. 127–136). Palgrave Macmillan.

Peguero, A. A. (2012). Schools, bullying, and inequality: Intersecting factors and complexities with the stratification of youth victimization at school. *Sociological Compass, 6*, 402–412.

Polanin, J. R., Espelage, D. L., & Pigott, T. D. (2012). A meta-analysis of school-based bullying prevention programs' effects on bystander intervention behavior. *School Psychology Review, 41*(1), 47–65.

Polanin, J. R., Espelage, D. L., Grotpeter, J. K., Spinney, E., Ingram, K. M., Valido, A., ... & Robinson, L. (2021a). A meta-analysis of longitudinal partial correlations between school violence and mental health, school performance, and criminal or delinquent acts. *Psychological Bulletin, 147*(2), 115. https://doi.org/10.1037/bul0000314

Polanin, J. R., Espelage, D. L., Grotpeter, J. K., Ingram, K., Michaelson, L., Spinney, E., et al. (2021b). A systematic review and meta-analysis of interventions to decrease cyberbullying perpetration and victimization. *Prevention Science*, 1–16.

Poteat, V. P., O'Dwyer, L. M., & Mereish, E. H. (2012). Changes in how students use and are called homophobic epithets over time: Patterns predicted by gender, bullying, and victimization status. *Journal of Educational Psychology, 104*(2), 393–406. https://doi.org/10.1037/a0026437

Reddy, L., Espelage, D. L., Anderman, E., Kanrich, J., & McMahon, S. (2018). Addressing violence against educators through measurement and research. *Aggression and Violent Behavior, 42*, 9–28.

Rivers, I. (2011). *Homophobic bullying: Research and theoretical perspectives*. Oxford University Press.

Rodkin, P. C., Espelage, D. L., & Hanish, L. D. (2015). A relational framework for understanding bullying: Developmental antecedents and outcomes. *American Psychologist, 70*(4), 311.

Rose, C. A., Nickerson, A. B., Stormont, M., & Burns, M. (2015). Advancing bullying research from a social-ecological lens: An introduction to the special issue. *School Psychology Review, 44*(4), 339–352. https://doi.org/10.17105/15-0134.1

Russell, S. T., Sinclair, K. O., Poteat, V. P., & Koenig, B. W. (2012). Adolescent health and harassment based on discriminatory bias. *American Journal of Public Health, 102*(3), 493–495.

Schonert-Reichl, K. A., & Arruda, J. W. (2016). *Random acts of kindness – UBC summary report of research: Preliminary findings*. Random Acts of Kindness Foundation. https://assets.randomactsofkindness.org/downloads/RAK_UBC_Executive_Summary_Report.pdf

Sprague, J. R., & Golly, A. (2004). *Best behavior: Building positive behavior supports in schools*. Sopris West Educational Services.

Sprague, J. R., & Walker, H. M. (2005). *Safe and healthy schools: Practical prevention strategies*. Guilford Press. https://doi.org/10.1016/j.childyouth.2017.01.018

Storer, H. L., Casey, E. A., & Herrenkohl, T. I. (2017). Developing "whole school" bystander interventions: The role of school-settings in influencing adolescents response to dating violence and bullying. *Children and Youth Services Review, 74*, 87–95.

Stuart-Cassel, V., Bell, A., & Springer, J. F. (2011). *Analysis of state bullying laws and policies*. Office of Planning, Evaluation and Policy Development, U.S. Department of Education.

Swearer, S. M., & Cary, P. T. (2003). Perceptions and attitudes toward bullying in middle school youth: A developmental examination across the bully/victim continuum. *Journal of Applied School Psychology, 19*(2), 63–79. https://doi.org/10.1300/J008v19n02_05

Swearer, S. M., & Givens, J. E. (2006). *Designing an alternative to suspension for middle School bullies* [Paper presentation]. National Association of School Psychologists 37th Annual Convention, Anaheim.

Ttofi, M. M., & Farrington, D. P. (2011). Effectiveness of school-based programs to reduce bullying: A systematic and meta-analytic review. *Journal of Experimental Criminology, 7*(1), 27–56.

Van der Ploeg, R., Steglich, C., Salmivalli, C., & Veenstra, R. (2015). The intensity of victimization: Associations with children's psychosocial well-being and social standing in the classroom. *PLoS One, 10*, e0141490.

Van Noorden, T. H., Bukowski, W. M., Haselager, G. J., Lansu, T. A., & Cillessen, A. H. (2016). Disentangling the frequency and severity of bullying and victimization in the association with empathy. *Social Development, 25*, 176–192.

Volk, A. A., Dane, A. V., & Marini, Z. A. (2014). What is bullying? A theoretical redefinition. *Developmental Review, 34*, 327–343.

Volk, T., Veenstra, R., & Espelage, D. L. (2017). So you want to study bullying?: A theoretical and methodological primer to enhance the validity, transparency, and compatibility of bullying research. *Aggression and Violent Behavior, 36*, 34–43.

Walters, G. D., & Espelage, D. L. (2018). From victim to victimizer: Hostility, anger, and depression as mediators of the bullying victimization–bullying perpetration relationship. *Journal of School Psychology, 68*, 73–83.

Ybarra, M. L., Boyd, D., Korchmaros, J. D., & Oppenheim, J. K. (2012). Defining and measuring cyberbullying within the larger context of bullying victimization. *Journal of Adolescent Health, 51*(1), 53–58.

Ybarra, M. L., Espelage, D. L., & Mitchell, K. J. (2014). Differentiating youth who are bullied from other victims of peer-aggression: The importance of differential power and repetition. *Journal of Adolescent Health, 55*, 293–300.

Ybarra, M. L., Prescott, T. L., & Espelage, D. L. (2016). Stepwise development of a text messaging-based bullying prevention program for middle school students (BullyDown). *JMIR mHealth and uHealth, 4*(2), e60. https://doi.org/10.2196/mhealth.4936

Chapter 8
School-Related Violence During the COVID-19 Pandemic

Thomas W. Miller

Introduction

A global pandemic involving COVID-19, including several mutations and the Omicron variants of the virus, has, during the period from 2019 through 2022, generated unprecedented challenges for parents, children, teachers, school administrators, healthcare providers, and our world community. Based on the data collected internationally, the World Health Organization declared the presence of the Coronavirus, labeled COVID-19, a disease of pandemic proportion in March 2020 (WHO, 2020b, March 11). A pandemic declaration can result in increased levels of stress, anxiety, panic, and functional depression for some individuals (Farrington & Baldry, 2010). Guidelines were developed in accordance with World Health Organization protocols and subsequently distributed worldwide to address the nature of this pandemic (WHO, 2020a, March 30).

Recognized is the realization that these unusual circumstances create significant uncertainty and strain in the lives of many families. The twenty-first century has been witness to a variety of youth-oriented violence which has resulted in a serious problem globally. Such violence spreads lasting and harmful effects on its victims and their families, friends, and communities (CDC, 2019; Human Rights Watch, 2020). What we do know is that it will take time and sound research to learn and understand the impact of being out of school, being in the home, and the potential for child abuse amid a global pandemic in the twenty-first century.

T. W. Miller (✉)
Department of Psychiatry, College of Medicine, Department of Gerontology, College of Public Health, University of Kentucky, Lexington, KY, USA

Institute for Collaboration on Health, Intervention, and Policy, University of Connecticut, Storrs, CT, USA
e-mail: tom.miller@uconn.edu

T. W. Miller (ed.), *School Violence and Primary Prevention*,
https://doi.org/10.1007/978-3-031-13134-9_8

217

Violence in the Home with School-Aged Children

Episodes of violence in the homes of perpetrators are likely to occur during periods where families are in close and quarantined quarters for extended period of time. School personnel are often the eyes and ears of such episodes of violence in the homes but when there is no school during a pandemic that opportunity is lost. Teachers, school administrators, safety officers, and school-based healthcare providers have been out of the reach of such potential children who are abused during this period of time. The global pandemic referred to as the COVID-19 pandemic is this century's defining health crisis and includes the continued presence of some aspects of school-related violence.

While initially, children seemed less likely to experience severe symptoms of or mortality from COVID-19 infection, those in high-risk home situations faced increased adversity as governments worldwide implemented restrictive prevention and control measures (Raman et al., 2020).

Recommendations for children's health including those in high-risk homes for abuse and neglect during COVID-19 have been developed from several sources (Cuevas-Parra & Stephano, 2020; UNICEF, 2020, Klein et al., 2020) as well as the United Nations and the International Pediatric Association. The results of having to quarantine in small living quarters with parents who may be unemployed present several challenges for children especially those at risk for any form of neglect, maltreatment, or abuse. This type of situation may result eventually in more serious psychosocial and mental health issues that would require more professional treatment interventions. Estimates suggested that more than 1.5 billion children were out of school during this period of the pandemic, and widespread job losses along with economic insecurity for many families could result in higher rates of potential maltreatment, exploitation, and abuse of children (Human Rights Watch, 2020).

Importance of a Safety Signal

Safety signals are present for several individuals, although they may not always be aware of their safety signals. These safety signals are learned cues that predict the nonoccurrence of an aversive event (Miller, 2020). As such, safety signals are the potent inhibitors for anticipated stressful situations that may be present in the lives of children who are victims of abuse, neglect, or exploitation. Clinical researchers who have been examining this phenomenon within the conceptualization of safety signal learning have found that traumatized persons who are able to use safety cues are able to inhibit fear or better prepare themselves for anticipated victimization (Miller, 2020). For many children, the need for a safety signal alerts them to maintain an awareness of various forms of domestic violence and trends which may result from quarantines, lockdowns, and other measures used to mitigate the spread of COVID-19 (Human Rights Watch, 2020). Peterman et al. (2020) identified direct and indirect pathways through which pandemics could increase the risk for violence against women and children including: "(1) economic insecurity and poverty-related stress, (2) quarantines and social isolation, (3) disaster and conflict-related unrest and instability, (4) exposure to exploitative relationships due to changing demographics, (5) reduced health service availability and access to first responders, and (6) inability to temporarily escape" or to cope with the victimization.

The Public Health Perspective During a Pandemic

The necessary direction for prevention interventions during a pandemic period emerges from the strength of public health policies and perspectives. Researchers have examined the potential and the incidents of child abuse and maltreatment during a period of being quarantined in the home and where in-person schooling was restricted or unavailable. Emerging during this period of time were prevention intervention programs that examined how children think and feel about abuse and maltreatment in their lives. Programs such as these focused on enhancing interpersonal and emotional skills that improve communication, conflict management, and problem-solving for at-risk students (CDC, 2017). The approaches by design are considered "universal," because they are delivered to all students in a particular grade and at a specific school-age level according to the Community Preventive Services Task Force (2005) and educational researchers Farrington and Baldry (2010). These programs focused on either general concepts related to violence in the public sector or specific forms of violence that include bullying, maltreatment, or dating violence (Hahn et al., 2007; Robert Wood Johnson Foundation, University of Wisconsin Population Health Institute, 2014; Centers for Disease Control and Prevention, 2017).

With the development and implementation of universal school-based violence prevention programs introduced and made available during the second decade of the twenty-first century, the state of Oregon (Oregon Revised Statutes, 2015) has "enacted a law requiring school districts to incorporate bullying prevention into existing student training programs … to reduce both violence and victimization among students" (Robert Wood Johnson Foundation, University of Wisconsin Population Health Institute, 2014, as cited in CDC, 2017). With application to the pandemic period that affected school activities, Kann et al. (2016) provided the results of their research in support of the value of targeted prevention interventions that may aid school districts with planning for effective interventions. Their research was based on school-related youth violence which was culled from data collected on a nationwide survey of high school students. Results revealed that about 6 percent of the students completing the survey reported not going to school on one or more days in a thirty-day period preceding the survey because they "felt unsafe at school or on their way to and from school" (Kann et al., 2016, as cited in CDC, 2017).

The National Center for Injury Prevention and Control (2013, as cited in CDC, 2017) reported that "more than 200,000 school-aged youth between the ages of 5 and 18 sustained non-fatal injuries from physical assaults, and nearly 2000 were killed in homicides." According to the CDC (2021), youth violence is a serious public health issue "that can have lasting harmful effects on victims and their families, friends, and communities." Among the various forms of school-related violence is the intentional use of media-related challenges to students. Such violence has resulted in the behavior likely to cause physical and/or psychological harm to others.

School-related violence refers to harmful behaviors that may have their beginning in preschool experiences and continue into high school and even into college. School-related violence includes both verbal and physical behaviors that involve disruptive and problem behaviors, among others. It includes a victimizer who employs bullying, slapping, or hitting that results in emotional and in some cases physical harm to the victim. There have been a number of published educational research studies (Cicchetti et al., 2000; Danese et al., 2020).

In an effort to examine the benefits of school-based programs targeting school-based violence, the Community Preventive Services Task Force (2005, as cited by CDC, 2017) found that "universal school-based violence prevention programs were associated with reductions in violent behavior at all grade levels. Median relative reductions were about 30 percent for high school students, 7 percent for middle school students, 18 percent for elementary school students, and 32 percent for pre-kindergarten and kindergarten students. The review also found that the programs appeared to be effective in reducing violent behavior among students in all school environments, regardless of socioeconomic status, race and ethnicity, or crime rate. The evidence also shows that specific programs have been associated with reductions in delinquency and alcohol and substance abuse, and improvements in academic performance" (Washington State Institute for Public Policy, 2015, as cited by CDC, 2017).

Public Health Policy

The Children's Bureau of the U.S. Department of Health and Human Services (2020) notes that teachers, educators, safety officers, nurses, and social workers are mandated by law to report a child who shows the symptoms or signs associated with child abuse, exploitation, or maltreatment. During a pandemic with stay-at-home mandates, children at risk do not have exposure to the screeners for such experiences. As a result, they rarely have the opportunity to tell a teacher; counselor; school nurse, psychologist or social worker; pediatrician; neighbor; or another trusted adult about what they are experiencing. As a consequence, a majority of child abuse cases in United States fail to be reported and remain unrecognized. Hager (2020) has argued that child abuse and maltreatment need further scrutiny because close to "90 percent of children who are killed as a result of abuse or neglect did not have previous cases with a child protective services agency." This may be explained by the fact that such maltreatment and abuse are most likely to occur in the privacy of the child's home or school location. Staffing shortages in social agencies charged with monitoring child maltreatment are sometimes a cause of failure to report such incidents as effort to keep families with at-risk children intact is a primary goal.

The Global Perspective on School-Related Violence Associated with the Pandemic Period

The current generation has much to learn from the multiplicity of challenges during a global pandemic. Events like this global pandemic can be very stressful (Miller, 2010) has been a tremendous strain on our spectrum of agencies from government, school, and healthcare systems. The End Violence Against Children organization has focused on the aggravating circumstances that have been brought on by the pandemic and curbing the risks that occur during this time period that includes loneliness, stress in the home, domestic violence, and isolation of families and their children (Bradbury-Jones & Isham, 2020).

Efforts within the United Kingdom have addressed children at risk in families where spousal and child abuse have been identified through the UK's Domestic Violence Helpline. There is emerging evidence of an increased number of domestic homicides in the United Kingdom since the lockdown restrictions were enacted (Ingala Smith, 2020, as cited in Bradbury-Jones & Isham, 2020). During the extended period of this pandemic, there has been increased usage of services like helplines as well as the need for social service visits both in the United States and abroad.

As a result of quarantine restrictions worldwide, several countries have reported lockdowns and stay-at-home orders. Internationally based researchers have been examining this issue and have reported that family violence including intimate partner violence, child abuse, elder abuse, and sexual violence can escalate during and after large-scale disasters or crises (New Zealand Family Violence Clearinghouse, 2020). Several governmental agencies and other organizations and networks such as End Violence Against Children, New Zealand Family Violence Clearinghouse, the US Centers for Disease Control and Prevention, the Alliance for Child Protection in Humanitarian Action (2020), UNICEF, and the World Health Organization are imposing necessary prevention intervention measures to try to flatten the curve of COVID-19 and the accompanying risks of abuse, exploitation, and neglect of children and adolescents.

For those children and adults who are living and surviving in abusive relationships, this period of months and years has been a very trying time. These homes have not provided a safe place in which to live. Researchers have begun to address this issue (Domenico et al., 2020; López & Rodó, 2020; Augeraud-Veron, 2020). From their investigations, perhaps we should begin with the home and family situation and the necessity of at-risk children staying home from the safety of school.

The combination of mandates, lockdown, and quarantine restrictions have provided perpetrators increased opportunities to act out during the period of this pandemic which has resulted in increased incidents of maltreatment and abusive situations that have been identified in poor and at-risk communities.

Considerations for Preventing Child Maltreatment During a Global Pandemic

There is still much to learn, but at this writing, there are some actions that might be taken to counter abusive and controlling episodes of exploitation, abuse, and violence that may benefit victims during this pandemic. It is important that potential victims are given the opportunity to be asked directly in the absence of school personnel, and on repeated occasions, about whether they feel safe. This may fall on family members, neighbors, and friends who are aware of the potential for abuse and exploitation, in their home and when they are with potential perpetrators. All these efforts reflect on the international efforts of the public health domain. From a public health perspective, the safety and protection of victims of abuse and exploitation require education, training, and experience for first responders and agency staff. What emerges is the need for both the private and public sectors to cooperate through education and training that focus on understanding the emotional, physical, and psychological signals that victims indicate when they are unsafe and in a victim–victimizer relationship. Both health and legal services also need to be readily available for victims and for agencies to utilize. For prevention purposes, these efforts need to extend to both public and private community-based organizations that are both professional and voluntary in nature. Child maltreatment and psychological harm has been the object of several research studies that have introduced prevention intervention strategies (Allan et al., 2014; Dodge 1993; Gardner et al., 2019; Seddighi et al., 2019; Sheridan & McLaughlin 2014; Alliance for Child Protection in Humanitarian Action 2020). Bradbury-Jones and Isham (2020) have noted that national, regional, and local governments must realize the responsibility they have especially during a pandemic period for protecting and supporting the necessary and essential services to those children and their families who may be at risk for child maltreatment abuse and neglect.

Hager (2020) addresses the importance of parental and professional care for children in at-risk and vulnerable families. In several states and communities, public service announcements in multiple media "have been encouraging untrained members of the public to look for signs of abuse among struggling families" (Hager, 2020). Noted is the realization that as Americans experience unemployment and jobless conditions because of the quarantine and isolation associated with the pandemic, increased stress and tension occur in many homes, but most notably in those homes that are identified as at-risk. As a result of those increased tensions in low-income homes, there is a heightened likelihood of abuse, maltreatment, and neglect in these homes. Because of lockdowns, shelter-in-place, and quarantining, educational institutions at all levels were closed for extended periods of time. These institutions serve as safety zones for children who experience maltreatment in their homes. As a consequence of the closures, parents were tasked with full-time childcare, which raised the potential for stress, tension, and abuse in the home. Educational researchers, healthcare professionals, and clinicians have recognized that there is insufficient evidence-based decision-making research identifying triggers and causative factors when it comes to preparing for an unexpected global pandemic. With the noted virtual efforts within the school setting, school closures, stay-at-home requirements, and necessary quarantines have resulted in fewer eyes on our children, especially those at high risk. While the school setting provides a safe place for children, first-line school-based personnel such as teachers, counselors, psychologists, administrators, and social workers who are mandated by law to report any signs of child maltreatment were not available to identify potential child victims of maltreatment or abuse.

Another concern when addressing the needs of children at risk for maltreatment during a global pandemic is parental burnout. According to Griffith (2020), "research on parental burnout has suggested that parents who experience burnout are more likely to engage in child abuse and neglect," usually in the family home setting. Burnout is conceptualized as a syndrome that results from chronic stress that has not been successfully managed. Burnout is often marked by reduced energy and exhaustion for the necessary parent-caring required for successful caring and management of children in the family setting. For parents in general and for parents living in low-income and at-risk homes, burnout during periods like this can result in significant levels of parental-related stress in that family setting. The challenges these parents face often involve the usual childcare issues along with the availability of resources needed for the demands of parenting and the resources available for at-risk parents to meet those demands. More specifically, regional and local organizations work to provide support to at-risk youth and families through several programs. These programs often include dropout prevention programs, alternative educational programs, family education and counseling, and assistance to parents in managing children who are involved with the juvenile justice system.

Advances in SMART technology, internet access, and the media have also played a significant role in the potential for violence during the pandemic. Sibling and peer victimization has shown itself through various media platforms and is a growing problem associated with social media use during out-of-school periods. During the pandemic, social media activities increased substantially, and it has become a significant public health concern. Cyber-vengeance can take several forms and has been associated with face-to-face confrontations, concern about going to school, and physical or psychological altercations (Garett et al., 2016). Garett et al. (2016) initially examined the relationship and association between social media and cyberbullying, concluding that victims experienced various levels of harassment from peers and/or siblings resulting in emotional and psychological anxiety and depression. They argue that because of the variability in defining and measuring the various levels of harassment experienced by victims, standardized instruments and further crafted and well-designed research models suitable for replication are required.

Health Care and Educational Needs During the Pandemic

Access to both the health care and to the educational needs of children is a critical issue for parents, teachers, and healthcare providers during a pandemic. Virtual and telehealth and telecare options are expanded to address some of these needs, yet more is needed in this area. This will require research that generates what portals are needed and how they may best be adapted to the needs of children, adolescents, and adults at all socioeconomic levels and in a variety of our communities. It will require safe and secure means of transmittal and delivery of these services. In both education and in health care, various models must be explored and prepared for future situations that require their usage. Some of the barriers currently experienced can be remedied by regulatory changes which expand services and reimbursement for telehealth-delivered care and treatment. Given user and provider willingness to utilize virtual models when appropriate, goals of achieving greater access for many can be accomplished.

This pandemic has had a devastating impact on the education needs of children at all levels of formal education. It has not been surprising that trends in both math and reading achievement scores have dropped, while mental health challenges have increased. There is the need for cognitive tools that can adapt to virtual learning that address social, emotional, memory, and language skills along with self-regulation skills that can benefit social development during such events and periods of isolation for school-aged children.

The impact and the complexity that social media has provided have affected family functioning especially in at-risk families during the pandemic. As Cuartas (2020) along with Hager (2020) have documented, it is clear that a pandemic can trigger significant social and economic distress for the global population. When this occurs, the likelihood of increased incidents of child abuse, maltreatment, and neglect will surface. Most vulnerable are low-income families who are struggling to make ends meet, facing homelessness, and experiencing deficits in the ability to provide for these children who require basic caring, as well as food, clothing, shelter, and healthy living conditions.

Certain Lessons Learned During the Global Pandemic

The global pandemic of the twenty-first century has created an awareness among the current generation to better recognize and understand the importance of the complexity of our ecological world. Within this framework, the family, the healthcare system, and the educational system all have learned significant roles and responsibilities that must be met in a time of stress and crisis. The emergence of COVID-19 created many disruptions to our daily lives. It affected physical and mental activities; our use of time, space, sleep, and lifestyle behaviors; and our ability to function under a restrictive life pattern. Giuntella et al. (2021) report that the Centers for Disease Control and Prevention has estimated that approximately one-third of Americans were experiencing clinical degrees of anxiety and depression as a result of adapting to the nature and course of the pandemic.

The general population has reacted to the pandemic in multiple ways ranging from denial to isolation and withdrawal from external contacts. For many, the result of isolation has produced outcomes that have included anxiety and depression, along with external stressors that emerged from governmental reports and sources as noted through the Centers for Disease Control and Prevention, authored by Hacker et al. (2021), on the impact of COVID-19 on mental and physical health. The planning and preparation noted through governmental agencies and the generated guidelines demonstrated that their learning process was limited by the shifts required to adapt to and accommodate the variants of the original coronavirus. COVID-19 and its effects on lifestyle resulted in a mixture of public reactions including distrust, uncertainty, ambivalence, and doubt about the future. This has brought about economic and social vulnerability experienced by some during the onset and extensive time period of the pandemic. The pandemic impacted the normal functioning of children, families, teachers, peers, and significant others with signs of fear, restlessness, loss of interest in usual activities, limited ability to concentrate, and acting out (Brooks et al., 2020; Cuartas, 2020; Danese et al., 2020). Consequences such as these become an additive burden and tend to overload adult caregivers, which compromises their ability to respond appropriately to their children's needs and distress. When this occurs, it often results in provoking more negative, impulsive, and even aggressive responses in children at home or in the school setting (Cuartas, 2020; Center on the Developing Child at Harvard University, 2016; Anderson et al., 2020; Giuntella et al., 2021).

As we transition to some level of normalcy over time, there are residuals of the pandemic that will continue to affect our lives. The cumulative effects of this twenty-first century pandemic will likely have a long-term effect on this generation. The combination of long-term inequities in education along with what has been described as unfinished learning during the pandemic for school-aged children, especially for the earlier grades, will impact these children perhaps throughout their lives. At the same time, educators must be recognized for the efforts they expended from the onset of the pandemic to the present. They have laid the groundwork and provided a foundation for the lessons to be learned from this very unexpected experience. The lessons learned beg our attention to the following considerations:

- The required shifts and special needs of all children and their physical, social, and psychological development must be addressed for future planning and application during periods like a global pandemic.
- Parents and caregivers must be provided the necessary training and education to develop the ability to recognize the child's concerns physically and emotionally

and respond accordingly. This requires advanced preparation, education, and training. The lesson learned is that social agencies need to provide such advanced preparation, education, and training for parents who are caregivers in at-risk families.

- School administrators, teachers, and school staff all need education focusing on the initial quarantine and screening process. Educational scientists and researchers need to generate evidence-based models on how to manage a child's feelings, along with social and emotional development during a period of isolation,
- Public health agencies and service providers should utilize the benefits of multiple international perspectives in addressing an understanding of the needs of children, vulnerable families, and the general public in providing the necessary education and training to adapt to future pandemics and similar occurrences.
- The utilization of various forms of the virtual medium through telehealth and tele-education must be examined further. While there is controversy over the use of some virtual services in education during the pandemic, research is needed to address a roadmap for virtual models of education and health care that can be available for use during periods that include but are not limited to the pandemic.
- Further clinical and evidence-based research studies should be developed in addressing the maltreatment, exploitation, and abuse of children and adults during a pandemic event. Special attention to appropriate prevention interventions is needed.
- First responders and social services staff require evidence-based and well-designed models for providing the necessary information for family caregivers and vulnerable families. Curriculum development that is easily understood and disseminated must be a priority.
- With respect to the safety and protection of victims of harassment, abuse, and exploitation, there is a need to develop a standardized curriculum for the required education, training, and experience needed by first responders and agency staff in providing positive prevention interventions where needed.
- Community organizations and individuals in the private and public sectors need to cooperate through education and training that focuses on understanding the emotional, physical, and psychological signals that victims indicate when they are unsafe and in a victim–victimizer relationship.
- Health and legal services need to be crafted and readily available for victims during a period such as the pandemic.
- Recognizing that the current childcare services, especially for vulnerable families, is not adequate at this time, state, county, and city governments need to develop policies and procedures that address childcare services required during a period like a pandemic. Once policies and procedures are established, implementation of such procedures is necessary.
- Public, private, and nonprofit organizations should prepare to offer various services to at-risk families and caregivers that provide advocacy resources, safe housing options, peer support, and mentoring services.
- International, national, regional, and local governments must realize their responsibility for educating, protecting, and supporting services that provide crisis and

therapeutic intervention services to children, parents, teachers, and healthcare providers who are charged with the responsibility to care for vulnerable children and their families during an event such as a global pandemic.

References

Allan, N. P., Capron, D. W., Lejuez, C. W., Reynolds, E. K., MacPherson, L., & Schmidt, N. B. (2014). Developmental trajectories of anxiety symptoms in early adolescence: The influence of anxiety sensitivity. *Journal of Abnormal Child Psychology, 42*, 589–600. https://doi.org/10.1007/s10802-013-9806-0

Alliance for Child Protection in Humanitarian Action. (2020). *Technical note: Protection of children during the coronavirus pandemic.* Retrieved from https://alliancecpha.org/en/COVD19

Anderson, R. M., Heesterbeek, H., Klinkenberg, D., & Hollingsworth, T. D. (2020). How will country-based mitigation measures influence the course of the COVID-19 epidemic? *The Lancet, 395*, 931–934. https://doi.org/10.1016/S0140-6736(20)30567-5

Augeraud-Veron. (2020). Lifting the Covid lockdown: Different scenarios for France. *Mathematical Modelling of Natural Phenomenon, 15*, 40–45.

Bradbury-Jones, C., & Isham, L. (2020). The pandemic paradox: The consequences of COVID-19 on domestic violence. *Journal of Clinical Nursing, 29*(13–14), 2047–2049. https://doi.org/10.1111/jocn.15296

Brooks, S. K., Webster, R. K., Smith, L. E., Woodland, L., Wessely, S., Greenberg, N., & Rubin, G. J. (2020). The psychological impact of quarantine and how to reduce it: Rapid review of the evidence. *The Lancet, 395*, 912–920.

CDC, National Center for Injury Prevention and Control. (2013). Web-based Injury Statistics Query and Reporting System (WISQARS). Available at https://www.cdc.gov/injury/wisqars/index.html

Center on the Developing Child at Harvard University. (2016). *Building core capabilities for life: The science behind the skills adults need to succeed in parenting and in the workplace.* Available at www.developingchild.harvard.edu

Centers for Disease Control and Prevention. (2017). *School-based violence prevention: Interventions changing the context.* Available at https://www.cdc.gov/policy/hst/hi5/violenceprevention/index.html

Centers for Disease Control and Prevention. (2019). *Preventing school violence.* Available at https://www.cdc.gov/violenceprevention/pdf/yv-factsheet508.pdf

Centers for Disease Control and Prevention. (2021). *Violence prevention: Prevention strategies.* https://www.cdc.gov/violenceprevention/youthviolence/prevention.html

Cicchetti, D., Toth, S. L., & Maughan, A. (2000). An ecological–transactional model of child maltreatment. In A. Sameroff, M. Lewis, & S. Miller (Eds.), *Handbook of developmental psychopathology* (2nd ed., pp. 689–722). Kluwer Academic Publishers. https://doi.org/10.1007/978-1-4615-4163-9_37

Community Preventive Services Task Force. (2005). *School-based programs to reduce violence.* Available at https://www.thecommunityguide.org/findings/violence-school-based-programs

Cuartas, J. (2020). Heightened risk of child maltreatment amid the COVID-19 pandemic can exacerbate mental health problems for the next generation. *Psychological Trauma: Theory, Research, Practice, and Policy, 12*(S1), S195–S196. https://doi.org/10.1037/tra0000597

Cuevas-Parra & Stephano (2020). Co-Researching With Children in the Time of COVID-19: Shifting the Narrative on Methodologies to Generate Knowledge Patricio Cuevas-Parra First Published December 21, 2020 Research Article https://doi.org/10.1177/1609406920982135.

Danese, A., Smith, P., Chitsabesan, P., & Dubicka, B. (2020). Child and adolescent mental health amidst emergencies and disasters. *The British Journal of Psychiatry, 216*, 159–162.

Dodge, K. A. (1993). Social-cognitive mechanisms in the development of conduct disorder and depression. *Annual Review of Psychology, 44*, 559–584. Available at https://doi.org/10.1146/annurev.ps.44.020193.003015

Domenico, L. D., Pullano, G., Colizza, V., et al. (2020). Impact of lockdown on Covid-19 epidemic in Ile-France and possible exit strategies. *BMC Medicine, 18*, 240–247.

Farrington, D., & Baldry, A. (2010). Individual risk factors for school bullying. *Journal of Aggression, Conflict and Peace Research, 2*(1), 4–16.

Gardner, M. J., Thomas, H. J., & Erskine, H. E. (2019). The association between five forms of child maltreatment and depressive and anxiety disorders: A systematic review and meta-analysis. *Child Abuse & Neglect, 96*, 104082. https://doi.org/10.1016/j.chiabu.2019.104082

Garett, R., Lord, L. R., & Young, S. D. (2016). Associations between social media and cyberbullying: A review of the literature. *mHealth, 2*, 46. https://doi.org/10.21037/mhealth.2016.12.01

Giuntella, O., Hyde, K., Saccardo, S., & Sadoff, S. (2021). Lifestyle and mental health disruptions during COVID-19. *Proceedings of the National Academy of Sciences of the United States of America, 118*, e2016632118. Available at https://doi.org/10.1073/pnas.2016632118

Griffith, A. K. (2020). Parental burnout and child maltreatment during the COVID-19 pandemic. *Journal of Family Violence.* https://doi.org/10.1007/s10896-020-00172-2

Hacker, K. A., Briss, P. A., Richardson, L., Wright, J., & Petersen, R. (2021). COVID-19 and chronic disease: The impact now and in the future. *Preventing Chronic Disease, 18*, 210086. https://doi.org/10.5888/pcd18.210086

Hager, E. (2020). Is child abuse really rising during the pandemic? *The Marshall Project.* Available at https://www.themarshallproject.org/2020/06/15/is-child-abuse-really-rising-during-the-pandemic

Hahn, R., Fuqua-Whitley, D., Wethington, H., et al. (2007). Effectiveness of universal school-based programs to prevent violent and aggressive behavior: A systematic review. *American Journal of Preventive Medicine, 33*(2), S114–S129.

Human Rights Watch. (2020, April 9). *COVID-19 and children's rights.* Available at https://www.hrw.org/news/2020/04/09/covid-19-and-childrens-rights

Ingala Smith, K. (2020). *Counting dead women. Coronavirus doesn't cause men's violence against women.* Available at https://kareningalasmith.com/2020/04/15/coronavirus-doesnt-cause-mens-violence-against-women/

Kann, L., McManus, T., Harris, W. A., et al. (2016). Youth risk behavior surveillance — United States, 2015. *MMWR Surveillaince Summaries, 65*(SS-6):1–174. https://doi.org/10.15585/mmwr.ss6506a1

Klein, J. D., Koletzko, B., El-Shabrawi, M. H., et al. (2020). Promoting and supporting children's health and healthcare during COVID-19 – International Paediatric Association Position Statement. *Archives of Disease in Childhood, 105*, 620–624.

López, L., & Rodó, X. (2020). The end of social confinement and Covid 19 re-emergence risk. *Natural Human Behaviour, 4*, 746–755.

Miller, T. W. (Ed.). (2010). *Handbook of stressful transitions across the lifespan.* Springer. https://doi.org/10.1007/978-1-4419-0748-6

Miller, T. W. (2020). A safety signal's significance with the COVID-19 coronavirus. *SF Journal of Medicine and Research, 1*(2), 1010.

New Zealand Family Violence Clearinghouse. (2020). National Centre for family and whanau violence research and information. Available at https://nzfvc.org.nz/

Oregon Revised Statutes, 2015 Edition, with 2016 Amendments. (2016) § 339.359: Harassment, intimidation and bullying: training programs. Available at https://oregon.public.law/statutes/ors_339.359

Peterman, A., Potts, A., O'Donnell, M., Thompson, K., Shah, N., Oertelt-Prigione, S., & Gelder, N. V. (2020). *Pandemics and violence against women and children.*

Center for Global Development. Available at https://www.cgdev.org/publication/pandemics-and-violence-against-women-and-children

Raman, S., Harries, M., Nathawad, R., on behalf of International Society for Social Pediatrics & Child Health (ISSOP) COVID-19 Working Group, et al. (2020). Where do we go from here? A child rights-based response to COVID-19. *BMJ Paediatrics Open, 4*, e000714. https://doi.org/10.1136/bmjpo-2020-000714

Robert Wood Johnson Foundation, University of Wisconsin Population Health Institute. (2014). *County health rankings & roadmaps: School-based programs to reduce violence and bullying.* Available at https://www.countyhealthrankings.org/take-action-to-improve-health/what-works-for-health/strategies/school-based-violence-bullying-prevention-programs

Seddighi, H., Salmani, I., Javadi, M. H., & Seddighi, S. (2019). Child abuse in natural disasters and conflicts: A systematic review. *Trauma, Violence & Abuse*, 1524838019835973. https://doi.org/10.1177/1524838019835973

Sheridan, M. A., & McLaughlin, K. A. (2014). Dimensions of early experience and neural development: Deprivation and threat. *Trends in Cognitive Sciences, 18*, 580–585. Available at https://doi.org/10.1016/j.tics.201409.001

U.S. Department of Health & Human Services, Administration for Children and Families, Administration on Children, Youth and Families, Children's Bureau. (2020). *Child maltreatment 2018.* Available at https://www.acf.hhs.gov/cb/report/child-maltreatment-2018

UNICEF. (2020). *COVID-19: Children at heightened risk of abuse, neglect, exploitation and violence amidst intensifying containment measures.* Available at https://www.unicef.org/press-releases/covid-19-children

Washington State Institute for Public Policy. (2015). *Good behavior game. Benefit-cost results.* Available at http://www.wsipp.wa.gov/BenefitCost/Program/82.

World Health Organization. (2020a, March 30). *WHO releases guidelines to help countries maintain essential health services during the COVID-19 pandemic.* Available at https://www.who.int/news/item/30-03-2020-who-releases-guidelines-to-help-countries-maintain-essential-health-services-during-the-covid-19-pandemic

World Health Organization. (2020b, March 11). *WHO Director-General's opening remarks at the media briefing on COVID-19 – 11 March 2020.* Available at https://www.who.int/director-general/speeches/detail/who-director-general-s-opening-remarks-at-the-media-briefing-on-covid-19%2D%2D-11-march-2020

Chapter 9
Sexual Exploitation, Abuse, and Trafficking of School-Aged Children

Annie Farmer

Introduction

In July of 2019, I stood in front of a federal courthouse in Manhattan after speaking at the bail hearing for Jeffrey Epstein. I was somewhat shocked to see the throng of people with microphones and cameras, asking questions and snapping photos. It had been almost a quarter-century since my unfortunate encounter with Epstein and Ghislaine Maxwell. For much of that time, it had been my impression that many people, including members of media and law enforcement, had known about his sexual abuse of girls and young women and had little concern. However, by the summer of 2019, something had shifted. Epstein had been arrested, and news outlets that once mentioned his "young prostitutes" now discussed the "young victims." As I stood outside the courthouse, I realized that people were paying attention and seeing this case in a new way.

Several researchers have noted what Conte describes as the "ebb and flow in this country's willingness to acknowledge and respond to the problem of child sexual abuse" (Olafson et al., 1993, p. 26). After the phenomenon gained the public's attention in the 1980s leading to an explosion in research and advocacy efforts, the 1990s brought a cultural backlash with many voicing doubt about the validity of these concerns. In the past two decades, recognition of the prevalence of child sexual abuse has gradually increased as the media has focused more attention on abuse within large institutions and on presenting the stories of survivors of powerful perpetrators. Social movements such as #MeToo have led many individuals to speak out about their abuse experiences, including abuse suffered as children. The cultural denial of these crimes appears to be lessening once again. Yet, even as

A. Farmer (✉)
Private Practice, Austin, TX, USA
e-mail: drfarmer@anniefarmer.com

© The Author(s), under exclusive license to Springer Nature
Switzerland AG 2023
T. W. Miller (ed.), *School Violence and Primary Prevention*,
https://doi.org/10.1007/978-3-031-13134-9_9

231

documentaries providing more nuanced portrayals of survivors' experiences have been viewed by tens of millions, misconceptions about the nature of this type of abuse persist.

The media attention given to Jeffrey Epstein's arrest created the opportunity to have a broader conversation about the issue of child sexual exploitation. However, coverage of the story has often been sensationalized and politicized in ways that distract from some of the central issues. There has also been a recent spike in the online spread of misinformation about child sex trafficking. False narratives about these often avoided or misunderstood topics have gained traction, highlighting the confusion that persists about what these crimes look like, how best to describe them, and how often they occur.

The purpose of this chapter is to clarify some of these issues. I will define key terms that come up frequently in the context of child sexual abuse and exploitation, discuss what current research indicates about the prevalence of these crimes, and present information that refutes common misconceptions about the nature of these offenses. I will also review what is known about how to recognize the signs that a child is a victim of abuse and respond appropriately before concluding with a brief review of a few specific approaches aimed at preventing these crimes.

Child Sexual Abuse and Exploitation Terminology

The use of inconsistent language to describe sexual crimes against children has long been problematic for those working on researching, preventing, and prosecuting these offenses (Goldman & Padayachi, 2000). The same terms are often used to mean slightly different things (Murray et al., 2014), new terminology is frequently being introduced to describe crimes that involve the use of rapidly developing technologies, and older terminology is falling out of favor as more attention is given to the ways language can stigmatize and harm the children it describes (Greijer & Doek, 2016). In 2014 an inter-agency working group composed of representatives from 18 NGO and UN agencies focused on child welfare was established to address these issues. After more than a year of discussion and consultation with a broad coalition of experts, the group congregated in Luxembourg to approve the *Terminology Guidelines for the Protection of Children from Sexual Exploitation and Sexual Abuse*. Often referred to as the Luxembourg Guidelines, the resulting document highlights the "significant challenges for policy development and programming, development of legislation, and data collection" that result from a lack of consensus on terminology and includes recommendations about which terms are most clear, which should be avoided, and which should be used with caution (Greijer & Doek, 2016, p. 1).

Child

While it may appear self-evident, the first term that is sometimes a source of confusion in conversations centered on child sexual abuse and exploitation is the word *child*. In common English, this term is often used to refer to those under the age of puberty, but it can also describe any person under the age of legal majority (Merriam-Webster, n.d.). The Convention on the Rights of the Child (CRC) defines a child as a human being under 18 years of age (UN General Assembly, 1989). The authors of the Luxembourg guidelines recommend the use of the word child to refer to individuals under age 18 (Greijer & Doek, 2016). They note that other commonly used terms such as youth, adolescent, or teenager may include 18- and 19-year-olds and emphasize the importance of using specific language that highlights the particular rights and protections afforded to individuals that are not legal adults.

Child Sexual Abuse

Child sexual abuse (CSA) is a label utilized in many legal and policy contexts both domestically and internationally. It functions as an umbrella term that can include many different types of harm, but discrepancies exist in exactly how it is applied. Legal interpretations are inconsistent, but organizations focused on promoting health and providing services to victims of these crimes have generally opted for more inclusive definitions. The World Health Organization describes CSA as "the involvement of a child in sexual activity that he or she does not fully comprehend, is unable to give informed consent to, or for which the child is not developmentally prepared and cannot give consent, or that violates the laws or social taboos of society." They specify that this activity can be initiated by an adult or by "another child who by age or development is in a relationship of responsibility, trust, or power".

The Centers for Disease Control and Prevention define child sexual abuse as "any completed or attempted (non-completed) sexual act, sexual contact with, or exploitation (i.e., non-contact sexual interaction) of a child by a caregiver" (Leeb et al., 2008). Each of these categories of abuse is then further explained: sexual acts include contact involving penetration of the mouth or sexual organs of either the abuser or child; sexual contact includes "intentional touching, directly or through clothing of the genitalia, anus, groin, breast, inner thigh, or buttocks" done in the context of abuse but not in the context of routine care for a child's wellbeing. Importantly, exploitation is considered a form of abuse whether or not sexual contact is involved. This may include things like exposing a child to sexual materials, filming a child in a sexual manner, or coercing the child to enter into sex acts or sexual touching with others.

The authors of the Luxembourg Guidelines echo this broad definition of the term child sexual abuse to include both contact and non-contact forms of abuse and specify that this can include perpetration by other children as well as adults. Such abuse does not require an element of exchange between the victim and the perpetrator. They also note that explicit force is unnecessary, nor is the child's awareness of the experience as an act of abuse. The implication is that if a child has not reached the age of sexual consent, such activity is inherently harmful and, therefore, abusive, without evidence of coercion or force being required (Greijer & Doek, 2016).

Child Sexual Exploitation

While child sexual exploitation (CSE) is a form of child sexual abuse, it is a label used to specifically refer to crimes in which there is an element of exchange between victim and perpetrator or in which a person (either the perpetrator or a third-party) benefits in some way, beyond personal sexual gratification, from the child's sexual activity. It is a broad term that can include all of the forms of exploitation discussed below. While in theory, all types of child sexual exploitation are subsumed under the umbrella of child sexual abuse, in practice, many governments and organizations use the phrase child sexual exploitation and abuse.

Commercial sexual exploitation of children (CSEC) is sometimes used interchangeably with CSE. However, the Luxembourg Guidelines suggest that this term is best used to describe those crimes where the benefit to the person exploiting the child is monetary (Greijer & Doek, 2016). CSEC may be used as a synonym for child sex trafficking but can include other forms of child sexual exploitation that result in economic gains, such as the sale of explicit images of children, child sex tourism, and child marriage (Albanese, 2007; Miller-Perrin & Wurtele, 2017).

Child sex trafficking (CST) is defined by the National Center for Missing and Exploited Children as "the recruitment, harboring, transportation, provision, obtaining, or advertising of a minor child for the purpose of a commercial sex act, which involves the exchange of anything of value – such as money, drugs, or a place to stay – for sexual activity" (2020). Although many are confused by the term, trafficking does not necessitate travel of any kind – not across state lines or international boundaries (Miller-Perrin & Wurtele, 2017). The phrase *Domestic Minor Sex Trafficking* (DMST) is utilized to specifically highlight the commercial sexual exploitation of children in the United States, particularly when they are exploited in the context of prostitution (Thorn, 2020). In the past, the terms child prostitution/ child prostitute/child sex worker were commonly employed to describe this situation; however, the concern that these could imply the child's consent or the responsibility has led most organizations and governments to move away from this wording and toward language that better captures the exploitation that is inherent to these situations (Greijer & Doek, 2016). The terms *survival sex* and *transactional sex* are sometimes used to describe a particular form of CST in which a young person is not coerced into sex by someone like a pimp but engages in sex with others to provide for their needs – whether this be shelter, food, or other material items. There is a debate about whether this language helps draw attention to the ways this may be a different experience in comparison with engaging in these activities for the benefit of a third party (Lutnick, 2016) or whether it may obscure the fact that those people choosing to engage in sex with these minors are still committing child sexual abuse (Greijer & Doek, 2016). In her book, Domestic Minor Sex Trafficking: Beyond Victims and Villians, Lutnick uses the term *sex trades* in place of trafficking or prostitution, arguing that it describes the activity of trading sex for some form of payment without including any underlying assumptions about the people who are involved (2016).

Online Child Sexual Exploitation and Abuse

The exponential growth of information and communication technologies has created new opportunities for those who commit sexual crimes against children in the last two decades. The terms *online child sexual exploitation* and *online sexual abuse* have both been used to describe offenses that involve the Internet at some point. This includes when images of abuse created offline are shared or sold online or when a child is groomed or solicited online and then abused in person (ECPAT, 2020). The Luxembourg guidelines emphasize that the Internet offers a means to exploit children, but online abuse is not a distinct type of abuse (Greijer & Doek, 2016). Given the increasing integration of technology into our lives, a significant proportion of CSE and CSA fits this description. However, there are instances when highlighting the online aspect of abuse is particularly important as technology is central to how it is perpetrated. The live streaming of CSA, for example, is a growing problem in which "abuse video is transmitted instantaneously to the viewer, who can watch, engage, and even direct abuse while it is occurring" (ECPAT, 2020). Any device with a web-enabled camera can be used for this purpose (cellphones, laptops, gaming consoles). Perpetrators can share the video via any platform with video chat services (NSCEP, 2016). This type of "on-demand" exploitation can be particularly challenging to detect and prosecute as a record of the abuse is not necessarily created or exchanged.

Child Sexual Abuse/Exploitation Images/Material

While the term "child pornography" is still employed in the US legal system and therefore referenced in many government documents, individuals and organizations working to stop this type of crime have widely adopted the term child sexual abuse material (CSAM) to describe content that depicts sexually explicit activities involving a child (Thorn, 2020). They argue that this term better captures the fact that each image is a record of a crime. Describing such imagery as pornography, which is increasingly widely consumed and typically depicts consenting adults, may normalize this material. The Luxembourg Guidelines recommend that the term child sexual abuse material be reserved for material depicting acts of sexual abuse and/or focusing on the genitalia of the child. The term child sexual exploitation material is recommended to describe all other sexualized material depicting children (Greijer & Doek, 2016). While some organizations refer to images rather than material, material is a more inclusive term as it can include audio files in addition to still photographs or video footage.

Within the broader category of child sex abuse and exploitation materials, distinctions are made based on how they are created. Materials created by youth represent a growing proportion of CSAM and are often referred to as self-generated abuse material (Netclean report, 2018). A small portion of this material consists of what has been deemed "innocent images," for example, photos that a family member takes of a child at the beach or that a child takes without any sexual intent (Netclean, 2018). A larger portion of these materials come about due to "sexting," or the interpersonal exchange of self-produced sexualized images via cell phone or the Internet (Döring, 2014). Sexting can be a normative sexual behavior in adolescence (Symons et al., 2018), but can also be exploited by both peers and adults. A crime occurs when images that are produced voluntarily are then non-consensually shared with people beyond the intended recipient. There is also the potential for unwanted exposure to sexual imagery when a child receives unsolicited explicit photos from peers or adults. Research suggests that many young people creating and sending sexual imagery to romantic partners feel coerced to do so. This may often overlap with other abusive behavior in unhealthy teen relationships (Wolak et al., 2018).

Sextortion

Once someone has shared sexually explicit photos of themselves, they become vulnerable to a crime that has come to be referred to as "sextortion." In these scenarios, perpetrators threaten to expose sexual images a victim has provided if additional images, sexual favors, or other requests are not met (Wolak et al., 2018). The phrase *sexual extortion of a child* is recommended in the Luxembourg guidelines as a clearer alternative to sextortion, but many law enforcement and victim-serving organizations continue to use the more colloquial term. In 2016, a National Strategy for Child Exploitation Prevention and Interdiction was delivered to Congress. It included the results of a threat assessment survey of over 1000 law-enforcement and victim-services organizations throughout the United States. Respondents indicated that sexual extortion was the most significantly growing threat to children, with over 60% reporting witnessing an increase in this type of abuse (NSCEP). The threat assessment also describes these cases as generally having more minor victims per offender than all other child sexual exploitation offenses, with many forensic investigations revealing that an offender has been communicating with and cataloged materials from hundreds of potential victims all over the world.

In a 2018 study that surveyed 1385 victims of this form of sexual exploitation, 572 of whom were under age 18 at the time, over half of minor victims reported that they knew their perpetrators in person (Wolak et al., 2018). Many identified them as romantic partners. Victims under the age of 18 were more likely than adult victims to be pressured into sending initial images, to be threatened for over 6 months, and to be encouraged by perpetrators to harm themselves. Half did not disclose these incidents to anyone, and very few reported these crimes to officials (Wolak et al., 2018). Given the complexity of balancing the need to protect young people with the need to respect their rights and agency, some law-enforcement organizations are emphasizing the importance of making responses to these cases proportional, taking context into account, and working to reduce stigma for the youth who are involved (College of Policing, 2016).

Grooming

Another term that frequently appears in discussions of child sexual abuse and exploitation is grooming, a deliberate process by which offenders gradually prepare victims for abuse through manipulation. Based on examinations of common offender behavior, researchers have developed a variety of models of grooming. Some of these have focused on a set of common stages that are moved through during this preparation period, such as van Dam's five-stage model in which he proposes that a perpetrator first identifies a vulnerable child, then engages that child in a peer-like environment, desensitizes the child to touch, isolates the child, and finally makes the child feel responsible (2001). Others have proposed that grooming behavior can best be understood by categorization into common subtypes, for example, personal, familial, and institutional grooming (McAlinden, 2006) or physically grooming the victim, psychologically grooming the victim and family, and grooming the social environment and community (Leberg, 1997). In their review of several descriptions of this process, Bennett and O'Donohue argue that heterogeneity in definitions of grooming creates problems in understanding, preventing, and prosecuting these crimes (2014). To promote consistent identification of this behavior, they encourage the adoption of a simplified definition of grooming as "antecedent inappropriate behavior that functions to increase the likelihood of future sexual abuse" (p. 969).

Research with perpetrators and victims of abuse provides examples of various behaviors frequently employed for this purpose. In a review of the literature on sexual misconduct by female teachers, Knoll found that these perpetrators repeatedly used special attention or rewards to bribe the students they targeted. This tactic had a powerful effect on children's cognitions and motivations (2010). Shannon's 2008 study of police reports of sexual crimes against children in Sweden that included an element of online interaction found that sexual desensitization through talking inappropriately about sex with a child was a common element in both situations that were limited to online encounters and those which also included an in-person meeting (2008). Intentional boundary violations such as walking in when a child is undressing or using "accidental touch" have also been reported by child sex offenders to be techniques used to prepare a child for abuse (Elliott et al., 1995).

Grooming behavior is not limited to interactions with the victim but may also involve the child's environment. Perpetrators of CSAE have often worked to occupy positions of trust in the community and are described as helpful and charming (Craven et al., 2006). They are often people with insider status (van Dam, 2001). This may come with work in settings that provide the opportunity to be with children, such as schools, churches, or youth sports leagues. It may also come from intentionally forming relationships with the family of a child that is viewed as vulnerable and, therefore, a potential victim. In fact, around 60% of children who are sexually abused are abused by people the family trusts (Finkelhor, 2012; Whealin, 2007). This type of grooming not only creates the opportunity for abuse to occur, but strong relationships with the family and community can also mean that if a child does report abuse that they will be less likely to be believed as the perpetrator is seen as more believable (Craven et al., 2006).

While grooming is not always present in child sex abuse or exploitation, it is a common feature across categories of abuse, in crimes that occur in person and virtually, in cases where children are abused for an individual's sexual gratification and where there is commercial trafficking. Law enforcement investigators report that grooming is present in a significant portion of cases involving self-generated CSAM. In cases where children are groomed to provide CSAM, requests often escalate into threats and cross into behavior that would be classified as sextortion (Netclean, 2018; Koops et al., 2018).

In a novel 2018 study prompted by the discovery of a YouTube video containing what the authors referred to as "child-produced sexual imagery," Granno, Mosca, & Walravens-Evans document a disturbing trend involving social media and grooming. The original video that prompted their research showed a girl under age 10 performing a yoga pose that required her to be on her hands and knees. Based on the video's comments, there appeared to be sexual interest in the content from adult male viewers. By systematically using search terms related to the original video, they located many similar videos that appeared to be created by girls ages 6–14 but have predominately adult male viewers. Within these videos' comment sections, males provided rewards for the child producers by offering praise and "likes." They also requested additional content, often encouraging more explicit poses or clothing. Given the way commenters worked in unison to encourage the production of additional sexually implicit imagery, Granno and her colleagues termed this phenomenon *collective grooming*. They note that beginning in 2014, there has been a steep increase in the use of search terms that they linked to this content and observed that such material is challenging to detect, given that it is not overtly sexual and the search terms used to locate these images are not sexual either.

Prevalence Rates

While many studies have attempted to estimate how many children will experience child sexual abuse and exploitation, several factors have made it difficult to accurately gauge this figure. Crime data reflect the differences in laws between jurisdictions, and survey data have been collected using criteria that range from very open to very restrictive. As researchers have conducted studies using different definitions of abuse, unsurprisingly, results have varied significantly and led to stark differences in estimated prevalence rates (Douglas & Finkelhor, 2005). Methodological differences and differing time periods of studies can also contribute to wide-ranging results making it difficult to compare findings.

The low disclosure rates of child sexual abuse and exploitation are also a significant hurdle in accurately determining how many children are victims of these crimes. A recent study based on phone interviews with 13,052 children and parents found that among 10- to 17-year-olds, over 65% of sexual abuse episodes were not reported to parents or any adult (Gewirtz-Meydan & Finkelhor, 2020). Less than 20% of all cases were reported to the police. This finding is consistent with many previous studies which have found that children are more likely to keep their abuse a secret than to tell others about it (Bottoms et al., 2007; London et al., 2005, 2008).

In their 2018 white paper on child sexual abuse prevalence studies, Townsend and Rheingold identified and reviewed 16 such studies of American youth and found six that used consistent definitions and methodologies. They noted that these studies, conducted between 2000 and 2011, were also remarkably consistent in their findings. Their meta-analysis of these six papers, which focused on contact-abuse only, resulted in the estimated prevalence rate of 7.5–11.7%. This suggests that approximately one in 10 American children will be sexually abused by the age of 18. Broken down by gender, that is one in seven girls and one in 25 boys. Only two of the studies asked participants questions about experiences with non-contact forms of abuse and exploitation. Inclusion of these forms of abuse leads to an estimated overall prevalence rate of 27.4–27.8%, with 20.2% of boys and 34.9% of girls experiencing child sexual abuse by the age of 18.

In their 2012 meta-analysis of original investigations of child-reported experiences of sexual abuse conducted internationally, Barth and colleagues found similar but slightly elevated patterns of results. Based on the 32 studies that met inclusion criteria, the pooled prevalence estimate was 15% of girls experiencing sexual abuse and 8% of boys. The nine studies they identified that specifically asked about non-contact abuse found pooled prevalence estimates of 31% for girls and 17% for boys.

Accurate estimates of the commercial sexual exploitation of children are especially complicated to determine. The covert nature of these crimes, the lack of a uniform reporting system, the fear of retribution from traffickers, and the fact that children may not self-identify as trafficked contribute to the challenge (Miller-Perrin & Wurtele, 2017). In her book, Domestic Minor Sex Trafficking: Beyond Victims and Villains, Lutnick critiques the often-cited estimate that 100,000–300,000 young people are at risk of trafficking (Estes & Weiner, 2005) as being methodologically flawed (2016). She argues that this estimate has repeatedly been misused by the media, government, and advocacy groups to describe the number of young people not at risk of but currently involved in commercial sexual exploitation in the United States (2016). She argues that it is not possible to assess prevalence rates accurately based on the existing studies, and valid data is difficult to gather given that when asked about the sex trade, young people "have good reason not to acknowledge their involvement, such as concerns about being judged, stigmatized, or arrested" (p. 23). Despite these issues, some organizations attempt to make more conservative estimates based on numbers of youth arrested for prostitution offenses or those reported missing. The National Center for Missing and Exploited Children reports that of the 26,300 endangered runaways reported to them last year, approximately one out of six were likely sex trafficking victims (2020).

While reports to law enforcement in the United States about some types of child sex crimes have been dropping since they peaked in the 1990s, the last two decades have seen an exponential increase in reports of child sexual abuse materials circulating online (Thorn, 2020). In the year 1998, there were approximately 3000 reports of online CSAM to the National Center for Missing and Exploited Children, the organization that serves as the national clearinghouse for reports from the public and technology companies that detect images on their platforms (Keller & Dance, 2019). In 2018, reports topped 18 million reports, with technology companies reporting a record 45 million unique images, in the form of photos and videos, of child sexual abuse. These reports include recirculated images that have been previously identified and new images of exploitation and abuse. While such material was created, sold, and traded before the digital era, the explosion of social media, the advent of the "dark web," and advances in encryption and cloud storage systems have made it easier for criminals "to produce, access, and share child sexual abuse materials; to find like-minded offenders; and reduce their risk of detection" (ECPAT, 2020). In a 2019 *New York Times* investigative series on the growing problem of CSAM online, journalists reported that those who work in the field see disturbing trends in the imagery that is detected (Keller & Dance, 2019). Across law enforcement agencies, investigators have reported more images of younger victims and graphic abuse. Due to the overwhelming number of cases reported through the NCMEC cyber tipline, the FBI has had to triage cases and primarily focus on investigations of infants' and toddlers' images. A 2016 report from the UK's Internet Watch Foundation corroborates this alarming trend – 53% of the images they detected involved the abuse of children under the age of ten, and 28% of the imagery involved rape and sexual torture (Bursztein et al., 2019).

Misconceptions about Child Sexual Abuse and Exploitation

With the COVID-19 global pandemic underway, Americans spent more time at home and more time online in the summer of 2020. In this context, a conservative political activist posted his suspicions that some expensive cabinets sold by an online retailer, with names like Yaritza and Alivya, were actually being used as shipping containers to sell children (Spring, 2020). He posted his comment in June, and by mid-July, the idea that missing children were being trafficked via these cabinets was spreading across all social media platforms and across the globe. An analysis using Google Trends shows that searches for the term child sex trafficking began to climb in early June and then shot to an all-time high in early August with four of the top five related queries involving Wayfair, the furniture company's name. People were suddenly up in arms about the horror of child sex trafficking, sharing and posting millions of times, and in doing so, spreading false rumors about missing children whom people were speculating might be associated with these crimes (Dickson, 2020).

According to those who work in victim-services organizations, the problem is that the spread of such misinformation reinforces common myths about CSEA that obscure important facts about how these crimes actually occur and can inadvertently divert resources away from those that need them. In an interview on National Public Radio (White, 2020), Megan Cutter, director of the US National Human Trafficking Hotline, emphasized the importance of learning what these crimes actually look like from trusted sources. She reported that the hotline was overwhelmed by reports following the Wayfair conspiracy, with many callers repeating the same information they had seen online from viral posts about missing children. Unfortunately, this meant that people seeking assistance or with first-hand information about a crime would have had more difficulty getting through. Similar thoughts were echoed in my recent conversation with Katelyn Brewer, president, and CEO of Darkness to Light, a nonprofit organization focused on preventing child sexual abuse (November 16, 2020, personal communication). She expressed her belief that the attention being paid to these types of conspiracy theories about child sexual exploitation is part of a larger pattern of people wanting to see CSAE as something that happens far away to other people. She argues that while this may be a more comfortable narrative for many people, it conflicts with what has been learned about these crimes over the last few decades and consequently keeps people from understanding how to help keep those children in their homes and communities safe.

In contrast to such narratives that suggest children are most at risk of abuse or exploitation from strangers, research suggests that in 91% of reported cases, perpetrators of CSAE crimes are someone the child or family knows (Finkelhor & Shattuck, 2012). Abusers are often trusted members of the community in positions with access to children, for example, coaches, doctors, neighbors, teachers, or members of their religious community. The younger the victim, the more likely it is that the perpetrator is actually a family member. In 50% of known CSAE cases where the victim is under 6 years old, the abuser is a relative. This is also true in 23% of cases with 12- to 17-year-old victims (Snyder, 2000). The majority of children known to be exploited in the production of child sexual abuse materials live at home when this happens, and a parent is often the producer of this material (National Institute of Justice, 2007).

The promotion of the image of children being violently forced into abuse and exploitation is also problematic. While there certainly are cases in which physical violence is used to gain access to a victim, it is well established in the literature that grooming and/or coercion are more commonly used to attain this goal (Albanese, 2007). In the case of CSEC, traffickers often target vulnerable children by spending time in locations they frequent, connecting with them through social media, or using peers or classmates to help groom targets (Department of Education, 2015). Findings from qualitative studies on domestic child sex trafficking suggest that a common pattern is that of an older male pimp, initially acting like a boyfriend, working to lure, coerce, and manipulate a younger female adolescent into involvement in the commercial sex industry (Williamson & Prior, 2009). Enticements may also take the form of offers to help the child with his or her career or education, or false promises to be a benefactor. In her research on domestic minor sex trafficking, Lutnick conducted in-depth interviews with caseworkers at large youth-serving organizations (2016). She found that in addition to the youth who were coerced by romantic partners, caseworkers saw other common patterns in how youth became engaged in having sex for payment, including neglect at home and need to help care for siblings with the money earned, homelessness keeping youth from working and having independent housing, homophobia, and transphobia leading to LGBTQ youth being homeless and becoming involved in the sex trade due to a lack of options or desire to affirm their sexual or gender identity. In a 2016 survey of 260 survivors of DMST, one in six respondents reported being trafficked before 12. Family members were almost exclusively responsible for the initial trafficking of those younger than 10, most commonly fathers or step-fathers.

While no child or community is immune to these crimes, some argue that not enough attention has been made to educate the public about the factors that place some children at higher risk of being targeted by a sexual predator. Family structure is a significant predictor of vulnerability. Children in foster care are ten times more likely to be sexually abused than children being raised by both biological parents (Sedlak et al., 2010). For children residing with a single parent and that parent's live-in partner, the risk is 20 times as great. A family's socioeconomic status also contributes to the likelihood of the child becoming a victim of CSEA, with children three times as likely to be abused from homes classified as low SES and/or in which the parents are not in the workforce (Sedlak et al., 2010). Race and ethnicity also factor into risk as Black children are nearly twice as likely to experience CSAE as White children, and Hispanic children are at slightly greater risk than Non-Hispanic White Children. Reported incidences of CSA are almost double for children with disabilities when compared to children with no disability (Berliner, 2011).

A recent study of individuals aged 16 and older who were involved in commercial sex work highlights some particular risk factors for CSEC (Fedina et al., 2019). Of the 273 participants currently trading sex, 115 were identified as current or former child sex trafficking victims. The authors found that previous experiences of abuse (emotional and/or sexual), ever running away from home, having family members involved in sex work, and having friends that purchase sex, were all factors that were significantly associated with being trafficked as a child. Among youth who have run away, the risks are uneven. Research suggests that lesbian, gay, and bisexual runaway adolescents are more likely to experience physical and sexual child abuse and to engage in survival sex than those who identified as heterosexual (Tyler et al., 2004). Although research on CSEC has primarily looked at the experiences of cisgender youth, studies that have focused on young transgender women have found that approximately 60% report having traded sex for some form of payment (Lutnick, 2016). Race and ethnicity also play a role in the risk of involvement in commercial sexual exploitation. Based on the 2014 FBI Uniform Crime Report data, 52% of all juveniles arrested for commercial sex acts were African-American children.

Another common misconception related to CSEC is that children who have been trafficked are hoping to be saved. Many young people who are exploited in the context of prostitution do not identify as victims (Miller-Perrin & Wurtele, 2017). Trafficked youth often come from a background of adversity, and traffickers may be perceived as fulfilling their unmet needs, both physical and emotional (Hopper, 2017). In cases where traffickers are family members, who may themselves have also been trafficked at some point, children may perceive their behavior as normal or fear betraying them. If traffickers are viewed as romantic partners, there is a significant likelihood of trauma bonding. This response is characterized by positive feelings such as loyalty and gratitude, dependence on, and a desire to protect the trafficker. In addition, a significant number of children are involved in commercial sexual exploitation in some form but are not being trafficked by a third party. In these cases, young people may feel they have found a successful strategy for meeting their needs and be resistant to the idea of needing to get out of the situation (Lutnick, 2016).

Just as there are misconceptions about how abuse and exploitation typically occur and who is targeted, there are many false narratives about who perpetrates these crimes. For example, not all adults who engage in this behavior are pedophiles. Pedophilia, by definition, is a psychological condition based on sexual attraction to pre-pubescent children (hebephilia is the term used to describe people who prefer pubescent minors) (Schaefer et al., 2010). Research suggests that approximately 50% of the adults who sexually abuse children are pedophiles; the other half of perpetrators do so for various reasons but without a specific attraction to children (Tenbergen et al., 2015). They may struggle with impulse control disorders, have antisocial personality traits, or not have the social and emotional skills to attract a romantic partner of appropriate age. Although at lower rates, women are also perpetrators of sexual abuse and exploitation, and research has indicated that they acknowledge pedophilic attraction at approximately the same rate as men (Fromuth & Conn, 1997).

As many as 40% of children who are sexually abused are not abused by adults at all, but by older or more powerful children (Finkelhor, 2012). When children under the age of 6 are assaulted, 43% of the time, the perpetrator is also a child, and 14% of these children are under age 12 themselves (Snyder, 2000). Many of these minors do not go on to reoffend. In a 2016 meta-analysis, Caldwell reviewed 106 data sets examining sexual recidivism rates among more than 33,000 youth and found a mean 5-year recidivism rate of 2.75%. These appear more often to be crimes of opportunity that occur in the context of nurturing activities such as babysitting.

Those who purchase and view CSAM were once believed to exhibit a distinct pattern of criminality. The prevailing theory was that most of these offenders exclusively engaged in viewing CSAM but did not commit offenses themselves; however, emerging research has called that into question (Carey, 2019). Bourke & Hernandez found that among inmates completing a voluntary treatment program, those incarcerated for possession of CSAM without a history of hands-on abuse were more likely than not to admit to undetected abuse histories (Bourke & Hernandez, 2009). In another study, investigators interviewed 127 offenders after their arrests for possession of CSAM and found less than 5% admitted to having ever perpetrated abuse. However, when agents followed up with polygraph-assisted interview methods, an additional 53% of the sample admitted to hands-on CSA (Bourke et al., 2014).

Consequences for Survivors

The evidence of negative consequences for some children who experience sexual abuse and exploitation is extensive and well-documented. The medical and scientific community has recognized the numerous ways that child sexual abuse can negatively affect one's health by ranking child sexual abuse 12th among 67 preventable risk factors contributing to the U.S. burden of disease (U.S. Burden of Disease Collaborators, 2013). Given the variety of experiences included under the umbrella of child sexual abuse, however, the effects are not uniform (Olafson, 2011). Among the factors that interact to influence how significantly a child's health will be affected by this trauma are the age of onset of the abuse, the severity of abuse, the use of force, and the relationship between the victim and the perpetrator (De Bellis et al., 2011). Individual factors such as a previous history of trauma may also influence how someone responds to CSA and make it difficult to isolate the effects of one experience of victimization from another. A recent study conducted across multiple sites found that among the 229 sexually abused 8- to 14-year-olds in the sample, children reported a mean of 2.6 additional traumas. Twenty-six percent of the children reported having been physically abused, 37% reported being in a serious accident, 58% reported witnessing domestic violence, and 70% had experienced a traumatic loss such as a family member's death.

Emotional and behavioral issues are common sequelae of child sexual abuse. Research has shown that posttraumatic stress reactions, anxiety, depression, and suicide attempts are all much more common in children who have been sexually abused (Leeb et al., 2011; Kilpatrick et al., 2003; Pérez-González & Pereda, 2015). Children's efforts to cope with the trauma of abuse may lead to behaviors that can become problematic. Adolescents with a history of child sexual abuse have been found in multiple studies to be much more likely to struggle with substance misuse (Kilpatrick et al., 2003; Shin et al., 2010).

This group also exhibits higher rates of delinquency, engagement in health-risking sexual behavior, teen pregnancy, and running away from home (Smith et al., 2006; Siegel & Williams, 2003; Kellogg et al., 1999). CSA often predicts a decline in children's academic performance and an increase in the risk of dropping out of school (Daignault & Hebert, 2009).

Higher risks of mental and physical health problems among survivors of CSA persist into adulthood. One study of young women in their early twenties found that those who were sexually abused as children were four times more likely than their non-abused peers to be diagnosed with an eating disorder (Fuemmeler et al., 2009). In a study focused on middle-aged women, researchers found that those who were sexually abused as children were twice as likely to be obese and twice as likely to suffer from depression as those who were not abused (Rohde et al., 2008). Research also suggests that both men and women with this history report significantly higher rates of substance problems and suicide attempts (Simpson & Miller, 2002; Kendler et al., 2000). While paths to illness are not well understood, there is also strong evidence that adults with a history of child sexual abuse are more likely to develop several health problems; one study comparing those with a CSA experience to be 30% more likely than their non-abused peers to have a serious medical condition such as diabetes, cancer, heart problems, stroke, or hypertension (Sachs-Ericsson et al., 2005). Even when CSA survivors do not experience long-term physical or mental health consequences, there remains an increased risk for subsequent sexual victimization and altered beliefs about self, others, and the world (Fargo, 2009; Ogloff et al., 2012; Olafson, 2011).

More attention is now being paid to the particular challenges that victims face when abuse is recorded and shared online. In a recent survey of CSAM survivors, respondents indicated that the distribution of their images impacts them differently than the hands-on abuse they suffered because the distribution never ends, and as others view a child's trauma, the victimization continues (Canadian Center for Child Protection, 2018). Many reported living with the constant fear of being recognized by those who have viewed the material, with one survivor stating, "I am very skeptical in dealing with people and look for any sign that could indicate that this person has seen it" (p. 167). 30% of respondents reported that they had been recognized at some point and that this experience was further traumatizing. In the United States, laws require agencies involved in prosecuting individuals who have possession of CSAM images to alert the family (or the victim after he or she reaches age 18) when his or her images are involved in a crime (National Center for Missing & Exploited Children, 2019). This policy is designed to help those who have survived these crimes to seek civil restitution in these cases; however, these notifications can be painful reminders of the continued spread of their abuse.

Recognizing Child Sexual Abuse and Exploitation

Learning to recognize the red flags of child sexual abuse and exploitation is an important part of caring for children in our communities. Early identification of abuse can prevent further harm and provide children and families the opportunity for treatment when needed. Because children are unlikely to disclose that they have

Table 9.1 Signs of child sexual abuse

"Too perfect" behavior	Unexplained anger
Withdrawal	Rebellion
Fear	Having nightmares
Depression	Bedwetting in children who had previously outgrown it
Being cruel to animals	Self-injury
Bullying or being bullied	Running away
Fire-setting	Falling grades at school
Showing sexual behavior/using sexual language at an early age	Using alcohol or drugs at an early age

Source: Adapted from Darkness to Light (n.d.)

Table 9.2 Signs of Involvement in CSEC (Children's Bureau, 2019)

Frequent, unexplained absences from school
Repeatedly running away from home
Unexplained bruises or scars
Signs of drug addiction
Sudden changes in clothes, friends, or access to money
Having a "boyfriend" or "girlfriend" who is noticeably older and/or controlling

Source: 2019/2020 Prevention Resource Guide

been sexually abused, it is imperative to know the most common signs. Children are more likely to display emotional and behavioral signals than to show physical signs of the abuse, but any physical evidence of abuse is important to document (Johnson, 2004). Physical signs can include bruises, bleeding, redness, rashes, swelling in the genital area, urinary tract infections, and other problems such as chronic stomach pain and headache (Children's Bureau, 2019). Some of the common emotional and behavioral indicators are listed in Table 9.1.

As commercial sexual exploitation is one form of child sexual abuse, any of the indicators listed above could be present in these cases. In a conversation about how people who are concerned about the problem of CSEC can best help, Megan Cutter, of the US National Human Trafficking Hotline, encourages the public to focus on "proximity and context" (White, 2020). In other words, people should be paying attention to the youth around them and looking out for changes in their situations or behavior. Some additional signs that could signal involvement in commercial sexual exploitation are listed in Table 9.2.

Once abuse or exploitation is suspected, responding appropriately is crucial. All 50 states include mandated reporting statutes that designating that certain groups of professionals are required to report instances of suspected or known child abuse to either child welfare organizations or law enforcement (Child Welfare Information Gateway, 2019a, b). In 18 states and Puerto Rico, the law requires all persons to report suspected abuse or neglect. Teachers are among those most likely to make reports of abuse that go on to be substantiated (Sedlak et al., 2010). However, a survey of teachers indicated that 24% had never received any guidelines on their state's mandated reporting requirements. In a survey of 577 mandated reporters regularly in contact with youth, almost 60% had no training to recognize the signs of domestic minor sex trafficking (Hartinger-Saunders et al., 2017). Many appeared to lack awareness of the dynamics involved. Nearly 25% reported that child sex trafficking does not occur in their communities, and 21% reported that most victims were children brought to the US from other countries. About 1 in 10 of those surveyed believe that laws regarding child sexual exploitation do not include adolescents. A lack of knowledge of reporting policies and inaccurate beliefs about abuse and exploitation continue to be obstacles to removing children from dangerous situations and connecting them with appropriate resources.

When individuals come across child sexual abuse materials or evidence of child sexual exploitation online, this should also be reported to law enforcement whether or not any victims are known or identifiable. One way of doing this is through the National Center for Missing and Exploited Children's cyber tipline: http://www.missingkids.com/CyberTipline. This online form asks questions about the type and location of material and forwards this information to the appropriate law enforcement agencies. Many social media companies also have internal ways of flagging inappropriate content that users can employ to make sure that content is taken down from these platforms more rapidly.

Responding to Disclosures of Abuse

The type of response a child receives when disclosing abuse can make a significant difference for the child. A supportive response, especially from a primary caregiver who communicates that the child is believed, has been linked to better outcomes for sexually abused or exploited children, including less self-blame (Melville et al., 2014; Cohen & Mannarino, 2000). Research has also demonstrated that whether a mother receives support following the discovery of CSA is predictive of her child's outcomes following treatment (Cohen & Mannarino, 1998). Advocacy organizations working with this issue have identified the following best practices when responding to a child that has disclosed abuse:

- Listen calmly without overreacting
- Express that you believe the child and that what happened was not the child's fault
- Praise the child for his or her courage and express gratitude for the disclosure
- Ask open-ended questions and allow silence to encourage a child to share the experience, but do not ask leading questions or push for details

- Tell the child you will be there to help figure out the next steps and find support (Darkness to Light, n.d.)

In a 2019 study, Quayle and Cariola used a vignette-based questionnaire to gather information on adolescents' views of how to best respond to situations in which youth-produced sexual images are non-consensually shared. They recruited participants aged 14–18 who self-identified as taking and distributing nude or nearly nude images of themselves. The authors found that what young people found helpful "from parents or carers was being reassuring and respecting privacy, along with offering to work with the young person to resolve the problem together. Parents or carers talking to others about what had happened was seen to be important but only when the young person's permission had been secured." Others have argued that the topic of sexting and online safety should be included in youth health education and prevention programs.

There is a need for additional research to establish how to best support sexually exploited and abused children in their recovery and reintegration. Children's needs will differ greatly based on how they are affected by their traumatic experiences, and a broad range of interventions may be beneficial. Several studies have examined which psychotherapy interventions are most effective in addressing the mental health struggles that some children will face after experiencing trauma. The treatment modality that has the most evidence of reducing symptoms of depression, anxiety, and posttraumatic stress in this population, is cognitive behavioral therapy (Macdonald et al., 2016; Wetherington et al., 2008). However, clinicians working with abuse survivors point out that this approach may be a better fit for adolescents than young children who may require therapies that incorporate more creative and nonverbal elements (Radford et al., 2015). The cultural context is also a crucial consideration. A qualitative study that involved interviews with 213 representatives from organizations working with survivors of child sexual exploitation in Asia reported that many respondents expressed concern about applying Western methods to address the psychological needs of the youth they served as they may not be appropriate given differences in cultural beliefs and values (Rafferty, 2018).

Qualitative studies with adult survivors of child sexual abuse and exploitation provide some insight into important areas to consider in offering various forms of treatment. A meta-synthesis of eight research articles exploring people's healing experiences identified several common themes, including disconnecting oneself from the experience of abuse, disclosing as a beginning to healing, the need to establish identity through a process of self-reflection, experiencing comfort through connection with other survivors of CSA, and accepting this experience as part of life. In his interviews with 25 young people (13–23 years old) in the UK about what had been or would be helpful to them in moving on from experiences of sexual exploitation, Gilligan (2016) noted that many expressed significant fear of additional harm from those involved in their trafficking and the need for safe spaces to stay. Subjects also emphasized the need for those who work with them at agencies to be "friendly, flexible, persevering, reliable and non-judgmental" (p. 115). They expressed significant doubt that law enforcement and state social workers would protect, respect, or listen to them.

Given the significant level of care often needed by children who have been repeatedly exploited in the context of trafficking, residential treatment centers offering rehabilitative services tailored to this population are beginning to open in some areas. The Refuge is a 45-bed facility in Central Texas, serving 11- to 19-year-old girls who have been involved in DMST (The Refuge, 2020). They opened in 2018 and began offering services using a holistic treatment model. The refuge's *Circle of Care* model includes eight domains in which goals are set and reviewed quarterly: medical, physical, psychological, educational, spiritual, social/relational, independent living and job skills, and community connections. Through the treatment center's partnerships with the community, residents can attend a university-sponsored onsite charter school and have psychiatric care supervised by providers at a local medical school. Youth move through housing options that provide increased levels of independence as they gain comfort in their surroundings and develop more autonomy. Residents also have the option to explore their own interests in ways that have likely not been possible previously with onsite arts programming, yoga and sports facilities, and an equine therapy center. While this model has not yet been evaluated through research, the partnership with a local university allows for data to be collected that will help evaluate the efficacy of this approach.

Prevention of Child Sexual Abuse and Exploitation

In the United States, the last few decades have seen increased efforts to prevent child sexual abuse and exploitation through a variety of wide-ranging strategies. Legislative reforms, new law enforcement policies, and school-based educational initiatives have all been employed to tackle this complex issue. There has been a decline in the number of reports to law enforcement of child sexual abuse since documented cases peaked in the 1990s (Wolak et al., 2008). This reduction has been widely celebrated, but some question whether it is due to the success of prevention efforts or just a product of overall drops in crime rates and improvements in child welfare (Finkelhor, 2009). Others note that it is difficult to gauge the true magnitude of change due to challenges around low disclosure rates and problematic prevalence estimates (Olafson, 2011).

The Child Abuse Prevention and Treatment Act (CAPTA), originally passed by the federal government in 1974 and reauthorized in 2010, was an important legislative step in protecting children's rights. More recently, the Preventing Sex Trafficking and Strengthening Families Act of 2014 and the Justice for Victims of Trafficking Act of 2015 have earmarked additional resources toward developing policies and procedures to "identify, document, and provide appropriate services" to children who are at risk of or involved in commercial sexual exploitation (Child Welfare Information Gateway, 2019a, b). While these are promising steps toward reducing child sex crimes, the 2019 New York Times investigation into the epidemic proliferation of online child sex abuse materials illustrates how creating laws alone is not enough (Keller & Dance, 2019). Their reporting exposed that the United States Congress had recognized the problem of CSAM and outlined a national strategy for child exploitation prevention and interdiction in the PROTECT Our Children Act of 2008 (Providing Resources, Officers, and Technology to Eradicate Cyber Threats to Our Children). Yet 11 years later, the justice department had completed just two of the six monitoring reports mandated by the law and had not appointed an official to lead the charge against these online crimes. In addition, the federal government had repeatedly provided only about half of the $60 million the law earmarked to fund the state and local law enforcement efforts each year. One of the bill's sponsors, Florida representative Debbie Wasserman Schultz, was not even aware of the scale of the government's failures before being contacted for the story. Legislative action is one important piece of reducing the number of children who are harmed through sexual abuse and exploitation, but legislation without government follow-through does little to aid prevention efforts.

While most people working with this complex issue agree that criminal justice initiatives are vital to reducing abuse rates, there are conflicting opinions on which strategies and services are most beneficial. In his 2009 review of child abuse prevention methods, David Finkelhor, director of the Crimes Against Children Research Center, notes that the management of child sexual offenders (through registration and community notifications) has taken up tremendous community resources. Such strategies are limited in their potential effectiveness because only a small minority of CSA cases, approximately 10%, involve previously known offenders. He connects this finding to research suggesting that offenders tend to engage in abuse repeatedly before getting caught but have relatively low recidivism rates when compared with those who commit other types of crime (Smallbone et al., 2008). Given the even lower recidivism rates for juvenile offenders, management strategies that are stigmatizing and thus become an obstacle to reintegration and stability can be particularly problematic and may ultimately work against the goals of these laws. Finkelhor suggests that resources may be better invested in detecting and apprehending unidentified offenders and developing assessments to identify individuals at high risk of reoffending for more intensive management (2009).

The other primary form that prevention efforts have taken is education. Curriculums have focused primarily on teaching children and have been delivered in schools where lessons are typically presented within a framework of other personal safety skills (Brown & Saied-Tessier, 2015). Goals include teaching children to recognize situations that may be harmful, strategies for leaving such situations, and for sharing information about any abuse or uncomfortable behavior with a trusted adult. While these lessons have been widely implemented in the past, some have raised concerns that these curriculums could confuse children, make them distrustful of adults, or place too much pressure on children to stay up and say no to offenders (Finkelhor, 2009). Evidence of the prevention of abuse is challenging to establish. However, one long-term study found that female college students who had participated in this type of education within their schools were significantly less likely to have experienced CSA than girls who had not (Gibson & Leitenberg,

2000). One meta-analysis based on 24 studies conducted internationally with 5802 participants demonstrated that such training increased children's knowledge about this topic with no demonstrated increase in anxiety or fear (Walsh et al., 2015). While critics' fears about children's exposure to these curriculums have not been backed up by research, additional benefits have been found (Finkelhor, 2009). One meta-analysis reports evidence that the delivery of these curriculums results in increased disclosure. Another found a reduction in self-blame among children who received the curriculum and were later sexually abused. Given that attributions about the cause of abuse are related to recovery from this trauma, education that reduces shame and self-blame can have long-term benefits for children (Andrews, 1995).

Along with training that aims to prevent young people from becoming victims of CSA, there has been a call for more efforts to develop tools that prevent juveniles from becoming sexual abuse offenders (Letourneau et al., 2017). Researchers have argued that given this population is already less prone to reoffend, first offenses could likely be prevented. One tool developed for this purpose is *Help Wanted, a* training created by researchers at the Moore Center for the Prevention of Child Sexual Abuse, Johns Hopkins Bloomberg School of Public Health. The lessons target adolescents and young adults who self-identify as being attracted to children. The training includes five short video modules that cover the definition of CSA, consequences for child victims and perpetrators, how to make decisions about whether to disclose the attraction to others, how to cope with the attraction, and how to build a positive self-image and healthy sexuality. It is available for free online, and no data is collected about users to ensure their privacy (https://www.helpwantedprevention.org/).

More attention is now also being paid to the importance of training adults to prevent CSA. The *Stewards of Children* training developed by the nonprofit organization Darkness to Light includes 2 hours of instruction that emphasizes the responsibility adults have to protect children in their communities and integrates research findings with video clips from interviews with adult CSA survivors (Letourneau et al., 2016). The program is based on a five-step model. Instruction covers the following five areas: facts about child sexual abuse and exploitation, how to minimize the opportunity for it to occur, how to talk about bodies, sex, and appropriate boundaries with children and adults, how to recognize possible physical and emotional signs that a child is being abused, and how to respond if a child discloses abuse or when abuse is discovered or suspected. While prevention is challenging to prove, there is a growing body of evidence that the training influences behavior change among attendees. In October 2015, a one-year follow-up survey of 79,544 Texas educators who had taken the training, alone or in tandem with Texas Mandated Reporter training, demonstrated that educators increased their reports of child sexual abuse to authorities by 283% as compared with their career averaged reports in the year before training (Townsend & Haviland, 2016).

The Children's Bureau produces an annual guide full of tip sheets distributed by youth and family-serving organizations. In their 2019/2020 Prevention Resource

Guide, they include an educational handout for families that outlines several strategies parents can use to prevent child sexual abuse, including:

- Ensure that organizations, groups, and teams that your children are involved with minimize one-on-one time between children and adults. Ask how staff and volunteers are screened and supervised.
- Make sure your children know that they can talk to you about anything that bothers or confuses them.
- Teach children accurate names of private body parts and the difference between touches that are 'okay' and 'not okay.'
- Empower children to make decisions about their bodies by allowing them age-appropriate privacy and encouraging them to say 'no' when they do not want to touch or be touched by others—even in nonsexual ways.
- Teach children to take care of their own bodies (e.g., bathing or using the bathroom) so they do not have to rely on adults or older children for help (Children's Bureau, 2019).

With an increased awareness of the risks that children face in the online environment, new programs are being developed to prevent harm in this context. The National Center for Missing and Exploited Children has an online safety education program called NetSmartz that includes a library of developmentally appropriate resources such as videos and activities on topics like sexting and sextortion. They are designed to educate young people about potential online risks and to empower parents with tools to discuss these topics in a nonjudgmental way with their children. UNITAS is an organization that creates digital comics based on survivors' experiences of sex trafficking and other forms of exploitation. These are then shared on social media, where so many children are first targeted for grooming and exploitation. Other nonprofits with expertise in this area are working to develop tools that harness technology's power to address issues such as CSAM and online sexual exploitation that have grown exponentially in the digital environment. Thorn has developed tools such as Safer, a service that uses machine learning and image identification techniques to help companies find, remove, and report child sexual abuse material on their networks. They also run an online deterrence program in which messages are sent directly to people searching for CSAM, educating them about the risks of their behavior, interfering with their sense of anonymity, and encouraging them to seek help (2020).

In her article on the prevention of child trafficking specifically, Rafferty argues for the need to adopt a human-rights-based approach in this work (2013). She outlines several strategies that align with the four pillars that the UN has espoused in their efforts to fight all types of human trafficking: "(a) the primacy of human rights (b) prevention of trafficking by addressing root causes (c) the extension of protection and assistance to all victims (instead of criminalization), and (d) the punishment of perpetrators and redress of victims." (p. 565) These methods of prevention vary from strengthening legal frameworks to encouraging the participation of children in developing solutions. Research with survivors of CSEC has demonstrated that young people have important insights about their experiences that have implications for prevention efforts. In one qualitative study involving young people who had been sexually exploited, participants discussed how being without care and attention from the adults in their lives left them vulnerable to exploitation (Hallett, 2016). They also described how narrow "protections" initiated by the government in response to exploitation often do not address underlying vulnerabilities and therefore leave them feeling ignored or unacknowledged. The author argues that the study's results provide support for the investment in early intervention strategies that provide additional resources to families in order for them to provide better care to these children before abuse and exploitation can occur.

Conclusion

The public's understanding of child sexual abuse and exploitation has been complicated by the lack of consensus on issues like appropriate terminology, accurate prevalence rates, and the most effective prevention strategies. However, significant efforts have been made globally to move toward using shared language and definitions that allow for more confidence in assessing the size of the problem and the best methods for combatting it. As the research base grows and survivors describe their experiences and struggles, clear patterns have emerged in how these crimes occur, how they are connected, and who is most at risk. These findings conflict with many myths about CSA and CSE that continue to be promoted and distract people from knowing how to keep themselves, their families, and communities safe. The truth about child sex crimes can be disturbing, and the temptation for us to deny or minimize them is strong. Steven J. Grocki, chief of the child exploitation and obscenity section at the US Department of Justice, described society's reticence to tackle the problem of child sexual abuse imagery by saying, "They turn away from it because it's too ugly of a mirror" (Keller & Dance, 2019). With more victims than ever coming forward, sharing their stories, and requesting acknowledgment, it is vital that we not turn away from this problem anymore.

References

Albanese, J. (2007). *Commercial sexual exploitation of children: What do we know and what do we do about it?*. National Institute of Justice. https://www.ncjrs.gov/pdffiles1/nij/215733.pdf

Andrews, B. (1995). Bodily shame as a mediator between abusive experiences and depression. *Journal of Abnormal Psychology, 104*(2), 277–285.

Bennett, N., & O'Donohue, W. (2014). The construct of grooming in child sexual abuse: Conceptual and measurement issues. *Journal of Child Sexual Abuse, 23*, 957–976.

Berliner, L. (2011). Child sexual abuse: Definitions, prevalence, and consequences. In J. E. B. Myers (Ed.), *The APSAC handbook on child maltreatment* (3rd ed., pp. 215–232). Sage.

Bottoms, B., Rudnick, A., & Epstein, A. (2007). A retrospective study of factors affecting the disclosure of childhood sexual and physical abuse. In M. E. Pipe, M. E. Lamb, Y. Orbach, & C. Cederborg (Eds.), *Child sexual abuse: Disclosure, delay, and denial* (pp. 175–194). Lawrence Erlbaum Associates.

Bourke, M. L., & Hernandez, A. E. (2009). Butner study redux: A report of the incidence of hands-on child victimization by child pornography offenders. *Journal of Family Violence., 24*(3), 183–191.

Bourke, M., Fragomeli, L., Detar, P., Sullivan, M., Meyle, E., & O'Riordan, M. (2014). The use of tactical polygraph with sex offenders. *Journal of Sexual Aggression, 21*(3), 1–14. https://doi.org/10.1080/13552600.2014.886729

Brown, J., & Saied-Tessier, A. (2015). *Preventing child sexual abuse.* NSPCC.

Bursztein, E., Bright, T., DeLaune, M. Eliff, D. M., Hsu, N., Olson, L. Shehan, J., Thakur, M., & Thomas, K. (2019). *Rethinking the detection of child sexual abuse imagery on the Internet.* Google, National Center for Missing and Exploited Children (NCMEC), & Thorn. https://dl.acm.org/doi/10.1145/3308558.3313482

Carey, B. (2019, September 29). Preying on children: The emerging psychology of pedophiles. *The New York Times.* https://www.nytimes.com/2019/09/29/us/pedophiles-online-sex-abuse.html

Children's Bureau. (2019). *A healthy family for every child.* Available at: https://www.acf.hhs.gov/cb

Child Welfare Information Gateway. (2019a). *Responding to child victims of human trafficking.* U.S. Department of Health and Human Services, Administration for Children and Families, Children's Bureau.

Child Welfare Information Gateway. (2019b). *Mandatory reporters of child abuse and neglect.* https://www.childwelfare.gov/pubPDFs/manda.pdf

Cohen, J. A., & Mannarino, A. P. (1998). Factors that mediate treatment outcome of sexually abused preschool children: Six- and 12-month follow up. *Journal of the American Academy of Child and Adolescent Psychiatry, 37*, 44–51.

Cohen, J. A., & Mannarino, A. P. (2000). Predictors of treatment outcome in sexually abused children. *Child Abuse & Neglect, 24*(7), 983–994. https://doi.org/10.1016/S0145-2134(00)00153-8

College of Policing. (2016). *Police action in response to youth produced sexual imagery ('Sexting').* http://www.college.police.uk/News/College-news/Documents/Police_action_in_response_to_sexting_-_briefing_(003).pdf

Craven, S., Brown, S., & Gilchrist, E. (2006). Sexual grooming of children: Review of literature and theoretical considerations. *Journal of Sexual Aggression, 12*(3), 287–299. https://doi.org/10.1080/13552600601069414

Daignault, I. V., & Hebert, M. (2009). Profiles of school adaptation: Social, behavioral, and academic functioning in sexually abused girls. *Child Abuse & Neglect, 33*, 102–115.

Darkness to Light. (n.d.). *Stewards of children [online training].* https://www.d2l.org/education/stewards-of-children/

De Bellis, M. D., Spratt, E. G., & Hooper, S. R. (2011). Neurodevelopmental biology associated with childhood sexual abuse. *Journal of Child Sexual Abuse, 20*(5), 548–587.

Department of Education. (2015). *Human trafficking in America's schools.* https://safesupportive-learning.ed.gov/human-trafficking-americas-schools

Dickson, E. J. (2020, July 14). A Wayfair child-trafficking conspiracy theory is flourishing on TikTok, despite it being completely false. *Rolling Stone.* https://www.rollingstone.com/culture/culture-news/wayfair-child-trafficking-conspiracy-theory-tiktok-1028622/

Döring, N. (2014). Consensual sexting among adolescents: Risk prevention through abstinence education or safer sexting? *Cyberpsychology: Journal of Psychosocial Research on Cyberspace, 8*(1). https://doi.org/10.5817/cp2014-1-9

Douglas, E., & Finkelhor, D. (2005). *Child sexual abuse fact sheet.* Crimes Against Children Research Center. http://unh.edu/ccrc/factsheet/pdf/childhoodSexualAbuseFactSheet.pdf

ECPAT International. (2020). *Summary paper on online child sexual exploitation.* ECPAT International. https://www.ecpat.org/wp-content/uploads/2020/12/ECPAT-Summary-paper-on-Online-Child-Sexual-Exploitation-2020.pdf

Elliott, M., Browne, K., & Kilcoyne, J. (1995). Child sexual abuse prevention: What offenders tell us. *Child Abuse and Neglect, 19*, 579–594.

Estes, R. J., & Weiner, N. A. (2005). The commercial sexual exploitation of children in the United States. In S. W. Cooper, R. J. Estes, A. P. Giardino, N. D. Kellogg, & V. Vieth (Eds.), *Medical, legal, and social science aspects of child sexual exploitation: A comprehensive review of pornography, prostitution, and Internet crimes.* G.W. Medical Publishing, Inc.

Fargo, J. D. (2009). Pathways to adult sexual revictimization: Direct and indirect behavioral risk factors across the lifespan. *Journal of Interpersonal Violence, 24,* 1771–1791.

Fedina, L., Williamson, C., & Perdue, T. (2019). Risk factors for domestic child sex trafficking in the United States. *Journal of Interpersonal Violence, 34*(13), 2653–2673. https://doi.org/10.1177/0886260516662306

Finkelhor, D. (2009). The prevention of childhood sexual abuse. *The Future of Children, 19*(2), 169–194. https://doi.org/10.1353/foc.0.0035

Finkelhor, D. (2012). *Characteristics of crimes against juveniles.* Crimes against Children Research Center.

Finkelhor, D., & Shattuck, A. (2012). *Characteristics of crimes against juveniles.* Crimes Against Children Research Center. Retrieved from http://unh.edu/ccrc/pdf/CV26_Revised%20 Characteristics%20of%20Crimes%20against%20Juveniles_5-2-12.pdf

Fromuth, M. E., & Conn, V. E. (1997). Hidden perpetrators: Sexual molestation in a nonclinical sample of college women. *Journal of Interpersonal Violence, 12*(3), 456–465. https://doi.org/10.1177/088626097012003009

Fuemmeler, B. F., Dedert, E., McClernon, F. J., & Beckham, J. C. (2009). Adverse childhood events are associated with obesity and disordered eating: Results from a U.S. population-based survey of young adults. *Journal of Traumatic Stress, 22,* 329–333.

Gewirtz-Meydan, A., & Finkelhor, D. (2020). Sexual abuse and assault in a large national sample of children and adolescents. *Child Maltreatment, 25*(2), 203–214. https://doi.org/10.1177/1077559519873975

Gibson, L. E., & Leitenberg, H. (2000). Child sexual abuse prevention programs: Do they decrease the occurrence of child sexual abuse? *Child Abuse & Neglect, 24*(9), 1115–1125. https://doi.org/10.1016/S0145-2134(00)00179-4

Gilligan, P. (2016). Turning it around: What do young women say helps them to move on from child sexual exploitation? *Child Abuse Review, 25,* 115–127. https://doi.org/10.1002/car.2373

Goldman, J. D., & Padayachi, U. K. (2000). Some methodological problems in estimating incidence and prevalence in child sexual abuse research. *The Journal of Sex Research, 37*(4), 305–314. https://doi.org/10.1080/00224490009552052

Greijer, S., & Doek, J. (2016). *Terminology guidelines for the protection of children from sexual exploitation and sexual abuse.* Terminology and Semantics Interagency Working Group on Sexual Exploitation of Children. http://luxembourgguidelines.org

Hallett, S. (2016). 'An uncomfortable comfortableness': 'Care', child protection and child sexual exploitation. *The British Journal of Social Work, 46*(7), 2137–2152. https://doi.org/10.1093/bjsw/bcv136

Hartinger-Saunders, R. M., Trouteaud, A. R., & Matos Johnson, J. (2017). Mandated reporters' perceptions of and encounters with domestic minor sex trafficking of adolescent females in the United States. *The American Journal of Orthopsychiatry, 87*(3), 195–205. https://doi.org/10.1037/ort0000151

Hopper, E. K. (2017). Polyvictimization and developmental trauma adaptations in sex trafficked youth. *Journal of Child & Adolescent Trauma., 10,* 161–173. https://doi.org/10.1007/s40653-016-0114-z

Johnson, C. F. (2004). Child sexual abuse. *Lancet, 364,* 462–470.

Keller, M. H., & Dance, G. J. (2019, September 29). The Internet is overrun with images of child sexual abuse. What went wrong? *New York Times.* https://www.nytimes.com/interactive/2019/09/28/us/child-sex-abuse.html

Kellogg, N. D., Hoffman, T. J., & Taylor, E. R. (1999). Early sexual experience among pregnant and parenting adolescents. *Adolescence, 43,* 293–303.

Kendler, K. S., Bulik, C. M., Silberg, J., Hettema, J. M., Myers, J., & Prescott, C. A. (2000). Childhood sexual abuse and adult psychiatric and substance use disorders in women: An epidemiological and Cotwin control analysis. *Archives of General Psychiatry, 57*(10), 953–959. https://doi.org/10.1001/archpsyc.57.10.953

Kilpatrick, D. G., Ruggiero, K. J., Acierno, R., Saunders, B. E., Resnick, H. S., & Best, C. L. (2003). Violence and risk of PTSD, major depression, substance abuse/dependence, and comorbidity: Results from the National Survey of Adolescents. *Journal of Consulting and Clinical Psychology, 71*, 692–700.

Knoll, J. (2010). Teacher sexual misconduct: Grooming patterns and female offenders. *Journal of Child Sexual Abuse, 19*, 371–386.

Koops, T., Dekker, A., & Briken, P. (2018). Online sexual activity involving webcams—An overview of existing literature and implications for sexual boundary violations of children and adolescents. *Behavioral Sciences & the Law, 36*, 182–197.

Leberg, E. (1997). *Understanding child molesters: Taking charge*. Sage Publications.

Leeb, R. T., Paulozzi, L., Melanson, C., et al. (2008). *Child maltreatment surveillance: Uniform definitions for public health and recommended data elements, version 1.0*. Centers for Disease Control and Prevention, National Center for Injury Prevention and Control. Retrieved from: http://www.cdc.gov/violenceprevention/pdf/cm_surveillance-a.pdf

Leeb, R., Lewis, T., & Zolotor, A. J. (2011). A review of physical and mental health consequences of child abuse and neglect and implications for practice. *American Journal of Lifestyle Medicine, 5*(5), 454–468.

Letourneau, E. J., Nietert, P. J., & Rheingold, A. A. (2016). Brief report: Initial assessment of a prevention program effect on child sexual abuse reporting rates in selected South Carolina counties. *Child Maltreatment, 21*(1), 74–79.

Letourneau, E. J., Schaeffer, C. M., Bradshaw, C. P., & Feder, K. A. (2017). Preventing the onset of child sexual abuse by targeting young adolescents with universal prevention programming. *Child Maltreatment, 22*(2), 100–111. https://doi.org/10.1177/1077559517692439

London, K., Bruck, M., Ceci, S. J., & Shuman, D. W. (2005). Disclosure of child sexual abuse: What does the research tell us about the ways that children tell? *Psychology, Public Policy, and Law, 11*(1), 194–226.

London, K., Bruck, M., Wright, D. B., & Ceci, S. J. (2008). Review of the contemporary literature on how children report sexual abuse to others: Findings, methodological issues, and implicationsfor forensic interviewers. *Memory, 16*(1), 29–47. http://www2.fiu.edu/~dwright/pdf/disclosure.pdf

Lutnick, A. (2016). *Domestic minor sex trafficking – beyond victims and villains*. Columbia University Press.

Macdonald, A., Pukay-Martin, N. D., Wagner, A. C., Fredman, S. J., & Monson, C. M. (2016). Cognitive-behavioral conjoint therapy for PTSD improves various PTSD symptoms and trauma-related cognitions: Results from a randomized controlled trial. *Journal of Family Psychology, 30*(1), 157–162. https://doi.org/10.1037/fam0000177

McAlinden, A. (2006). "Setting 'em up": Personal, familial and institutional grooming in the sexual abuse of children. *Social & Legal Studies, 15*(3), 339–362.

Melville, J. D., Kellogg, N. D., Perez, N., & Lukefahr, J. L. (2014). Assessment for self-blame and trauma symptoms during the medical evaluation of suspected sexual abuse. *Child Abuse & Neglect, 38*(5), 851–857. https://doi.org/10.1016/j.chiabu.2014.01.020

Merriam-Webster. (n.d.). Child. In *Merriam-Webster.com dictionary*. Retrieved November 29, 2020, from https://www.merriam-webster.com/dictionary/child

Miller-Perrin, C., & Wurtele, S. K. (2017). Sex trafficking and the commercial sexual exploitation of children. *Women & Therapy, 40*(1–2), 123–151. https://doi.org/10.1080/02703149.2016.1210963

Murray, L. K., Nguyen, A., & Cohen, J. A. (2014). Child sexual abuse. *Child and Adolescent Psychiatric Clinics of North America, 23*(2), 321–337. https://doi.org/10.1016/j.chc.2014.01.003

National Center for Missing and Exploited Children. (2019). *Captured on film: survivors of child sex abuse material are stuck in a unique cycle of trauma.* https://www.missingkids.org/content/dam/missingkids/pdfs/Captured%20on%20Film.pdf

National Center for Missing and Exploited Children. (2020). *Child sex trafficking identification resource.* https://www.missingkids.org/content/dam/missingkids/pdfs/CST%20Identification%20Resource.pdf

National Institute of Justice. (2007). *Commercial sexual exploitation of children: What do we know and what do we do about it? (Publication NCJ 215733).* US Department of Justice. Office of Justice Programs.

Netclean. (2018). *The Netclean report: A report about child sexual abuse crime.* https://www.netclean.com/netclean-report-2018/

Ogloff, J. R. P., Cutajar, M. C., Mann, E., Mullen, P., Wei, F. T. Y., Hassan, H. A. B., & Yih, T. H. (2012). Child sexual abuse and subsequent offending and victimisation: A 45 year follow-up study. *Trends & Issues in Crime and Criminal Justice, 440*, 1–6. https://www.aic.gov.au/publications/tandi/tandi440

Olafson, E. (2011). Child sexual abuse: Demography, impact, and interventions. *Journal of Child & Adolescent Trauma, 4*(1), 8–21. https://doi.org/10.1080/19361521.2011.545811

Olafson, E., Corwin, D. L., & Summit, R. C. (1993). Modern history of child sexual abuse awareness: Cycles of discovery and suppression. *Child Abuse & Neglect, 17*(1), 7–24. https://doi.org/10.1016/0145-2134(93)90004-o

Pérez-González, A., & Pereda, N. (2015). Systematic review of the prevalence of suicidal ideation and behavior in minors who have been sexually abused. *Actas espanolas de psiquiatria, 43*(4), 149–158.

Radford, L., Allnock, D., & Hynes, P. (2015). *Preventing and responding to child sexual abuse and exploitation: Evidence review.* UNICEF.

Rafferty, Y. (2013). Child trafficking and commercial sexual exploitation: A review of promising prevention policies and programs. *The American Journal of Orthopsychiatry, 83*(4), 559–575. https://doi.org/10.1111/ajop.12056

Rafferty, Y. (2018). Mental health services as a vital component of psychosocial recovery for victims of child trafficking for commercial sexual exploitation. *The American Journal of Orthopsychiatry, 88*(3), 249–260. https://doi.org/10.1037/ort0000268

Rohde, P., Ichikawa, L., Simon, G. E., Ludman, E. J., Linde, J. A., Jeffery, R. W., & Operskalski, B. H. (2008). Associations of child sexual and physical abuse with obesity and depression in middle-aged women. *Child Abuse & Neglect, 32*, 878–887.

Sachs-Ericsson, N., Blazer, D., Plant, E. A., & Arnow, B. (2005). Childhood sexual and physical abuse and 1-year prevalence of medical problems in the National Comorbidity Survey. *Health Psychology, 24*, 32–40.

Schaefer, G. A., Mundt, I. A., Feelgood, S., Hupp, E., Neutze, J., Ahlers, C. J., Goecker, D., & Beier, K. (2010). Potential and dunkelfeld offenders: Two neglected target groups for prevention of child sexual abuse. *International Journal of Law and Psychiatry, 33*, 154–163. https://doi.org/10.1016/j.ijlp.2010.03.005

Sedlak, A. J., Mettenburg, J., Basena, M., Petta, I., McPherson, K., Greene, A., & Li, S. (2010). *Fourth National Incidence Study of child abuse and neglect (NIS–4): Report to congress, executive summary.* U.S. Department of Health and Human Services, Administration for Children and Families.

Shannon, D. (2008). Online sexual grooming in Sweden—Online and offline sex offences against children as described in Swedish police data. *Journal of Scandinavian Studies in Criminology and Crime Prevention, 9*(2), 160–180. https://doi.org/10.1080/14043850802450120

Shin, S., Hong, H., & Hazen, A. (2010). Childhood sexual abuse and adolescent substance use: A latent class analysis. *Drug and Alcohol Dependence, 109*(1–3), 226–235.

Siegel, J. A., & Williams, L. M. (2003). The relationship between child sexual abuse and female delinquency and crime: A prospective study. *Journal of Research in Crime and Delinquency, 40*(1), 71–94. https://doi.org/10.1177/0022427802239254

Simpson, T. L., & Miller, W. R. (2002). Concomitance between childhood sexual and physical abuse and substance use problems: A review. *Clinical Psychology Review, 22*, 27–77.

Smallbone, S., Marshall, W. L., & Wortley, R. (2008). *Preventing child sexual abuse: Evidence, policy and practice.* Willan Publishing.

Smith, D. K., Leve, L. D., & Chamberlain, P. (2006). Adolescent girls' offending and health-risking sexual behavior: The predictive role of trauma. *Child Maltreatment, 11*(4), 346–353. https://doi.org/10.1177/1077559506291950

Snyder, H. N. (2000). *Sexual assault of young children as reported to law enforcement: Victim, incident, and offender characteristics.* U.S. Department of Justice, Office of Justice Programs, Bureau of Justice Statistics. http://www.ojp.usdoj.gov/bjs/pub/pdf/saycrle.pdf

Spring, M. (2020, July 15). Wayfair: The false conspiracy about a furniture firm and child trafficking. *BBC News World.* https://www.bbc.com/news/world-53416247. Retrieved December 4, 2020.

Symons, K., Ponnet, K., Walrave, M., & Heirman, W. (2018). Sexting scripts in adolescent relationships: Is sexting becoming the norm? *New Media & Society, 20*(10), 3836–3857. https://doi.org/10.1177/1461444818761869

Tenbergen, G., Wittfoth, M., Frieling, H., Ponseti, J., Walter, M., Walter, H., Beier, K. M., Schiffer, B., & Kruger, T. H. (2015). The neurobiology and psychology of pedophilia: Recent advances and challenges. *Frontiers in Human Neuroscience, 9*, 344. https://doi.org/10.3389/fnhum.2015.00344

The Canadian Centre for Child Protection Inc. (2018). *Survivor's survey: Full report.* https://protectchildren.ca/pdfs/C3P_SurvivorsSurveyExecutiveSummary2017_en.pdf

The Refuge Circle of Care. (2020). Retrieved December 18, 2020, from https://therefugeaustin.org/circle-of-care

Thorn. (2020, October). *Decoding the language of child sexual exploitation: Acronyms to know.* https://www.thorn.org/blog/decoding-the-language-of-child-sexual-exploitation-acronyms-to-know/

Townsend, C., & Haviland, M. (2016). *The impact of child sexual abuse training for educators on reporting and victim outcomes: The Texas Initiative.* Darkness to Light. http://www.d2l.org/site/c.4dICIJOkGcISE/b.9358399/k.5FEC/Efficacy_of_Stewards.htm

Tyler, K. A., Whitbeck, L. B., Hoyt, D. R., & Cauce, A. M. (2004). Risk factors for sexual victimization among male and female homeless and runaway youth. *Journal of Interpersonal Violence, 19*, 503–520.

U.S. Burden of Disease Collaborators, Murray, C. J., Atkinson, C., Bhalla, K., Birbeck, G., Burstein, R., Chou, D., Dellavalle, R., Danaei, G., Ezzati, M., Fahimi, A., Flaxman, D., Foreman, Gabriel, S., Gakidou, E., Kassebaum, N., Khatibzadeh, S., Lim, S., Lipshultz, S. E., London, S., Lopez, MacIntyre, M. F., Mokdad, A. H., Moran, A., Moran, A. E., Mozaffarian, D., Murphy, T., Naghavi, M., Pope, C., Roberts, T., Salomon, J., Schwebel, D. C., Shahraz, S., Sleet, D. A., Murray, Abraham, J., Ali, M. K., Atkinson, C., Bartels, D. H., Bhalla, K., Birbeck, G., Burstein, R., Chen, H., Criqui, M. H., Dahodwala, Jarlais, Ding, E. L., Dorsey, E. R., Ebel, B. E., Ezzati, M., Fahami, Flaxman, S., Flaxman, A. D., Gonzalez-Medina, D., Grant, B., Hagan, H., Hoffman, H., Kassebaum, N., Khatibzadeh, S., Leasher, J. L., Lin, J., Lipshultz, S. E., Lozano, R., Lu, Y., Mallinger, L., McDermott, M. M., Micha, R., Miller, T. R., Mokdad, A. A., Mokdad, A. H., Mozaffarian, D., Naghavi, M., Narayan, K. M., Omer, S. B., Pelizzari, P. M., Phillips, D., Ranganathan, D., Rivara, F. P., Roberts, T., Sampson, U., Sanman, E., Sapkota, A., Schwebel, D. C., Sharaz, S., Shivakoti, R., Singh, G. M., Singh, D., Tavakkoli, M., Towbin, J. A., Wilkinson, J. D., Zabetian, A., Murray, Abraham, J., Ali, M. K., Alvardo, M., Atkinson, C., Baddour, L. M., Benjamin, E. J., Bhalla, K., Birbeck, G., Bolliger, I., Burstein, R., Carnahan, E., Chou, D., Chugh, S. S., Cohen, A., Colson, K. E., Cooper, L. T., Couser, W., Criqui, M. H., Dabhadkar, K. C., Dellavalle, R. P., Jarlais, Dicker, D., Dorsey, E. R., Duber, H., Ebel, B. E., Engell, R. E., Ezzati, M., Felson, D. T., Finucane, M. M., Flaxman, S., Flaxman, A. D., Fleming, T., Foreman, Forouzanfar, M. H., Freedman, G., Freeman, M. K., Gakidou, E., Gillum, R. F., Gonzalez-Medina, D., Gosselin, R., Gutierrez, H. R., Hagan, H., Havmoeller, R.,

Hoffman, H., Jacobsen, K. H., James, S. L., Jasrasaria, R., Jayarman, S., Johns, N., Kassebaum, N., Khatibzadeh, S., Lan, Q., Leasher, J. L., Lim, S., Lipshultz, S. E., London, S., Lopez, Lozano, R., Lu, Y., Mallinger, L., Meltzer, M., Mensah, G. A., Michaud, C., Miller, T. R., Mock, C., Moffitt, T. E., Mokdad, A. A., Mokdad, A. H., Moran, A., Naghavi, M., Narayan, K. M., Nelson, R. G., Olives, C., Omer, S. B., Ortblad, K., Ostro, B., Pelizzari, P. M., Phillips, D., Raju, M., Razavi, H., Ritz, B., Roberts, T., Sacco, R. L., Salomon, J., Sampson, U., Schwebel, D. C., Shahraz, S., Shibuya, K., Silberberg, D., Singh, J. A., Steenland, K., Taylor, J. A., Thurston, G. D., Vavilala, M. S., Vos, T., Wagner, G. R., Weinstock, M. A., Weisskopf, M. G., Wulf, S., & Murray. (2013). The state of US health, 1990–2010: Burden of diseases, injuries, and risk factors. *JAMA, 310*(6), 591–608.

UN General Assembly. (1989). Convention on the Rights of the Child. United Nations. *Treaty Series, 1577.* https://www.refworld.org/docid/3ae6b38f0.html

van Dam, C. (2001). *Identifying child molesters: Preventing child sexual abuse by recognizing the patterns of the offenders.* Haworth Maltreatment and Trauma Press/The Haworth Press, Inc.

Walsh, K., Zwi, K., Woolfenden, S., & Shlonsky, A. (2015). School-based education programs for the prevention of child sexual abuse: A cochrane systematic review and meta-analysis. *Research on Social Work Practice, 28.* https://doi.org/10.1177/1049731515619705

Wethington, H. R., Hahn, R. A., Fuqua-Whitley, D. S., Sipe, T. A., Crosby, A. E., Johnson, R. L., Liberman, A. M., Mościcki, E., Price, L. N., Tuma, F. K., Kalra, G., Chattopadhyay, S. K., & Task Force on Community Preventive Services. (2008). The effectiveness of interventions to reduce psychological harm from traumatic events among children and adolescents: A systematic review. *American Journal of Preventive Medicine, 35*(3), 287–313. https://doi.org/10.1016/j.amepre.2008.06.024

Whealin, J. (2007). *Child sexual abuse.* National Center for Post Traumatic Stress Disorder, US Department of Veterans Affairs.

White, J. (Host). (2020, October 14). How conspiracy theorists are disrupting efforts to fight human Trafficking. In *1A. WAMU/NPR.* https://www.npr.org/2020/10/12/923019289/how-conspiracy-theorists-are-disrupting-efforts-to-fight-human-trafficking

Williamson, C., & Prior, M. (2009). Domestic minor sex trafficking: A network of underground players in the Midwest. *Journal of Child & Adolescent Trauma, 2*(1), 46–61. https://doi.org/10.1080/19361520802702191

Wolak, J., Finkelhor, D., Mitchell, K. J., & Ybarra, M. L. (2008). Online "predators" and their victims: Myths, realities, and implications for prevention and treatment. *American Psychologist, 63*, 111–128.

Wolak, J., Finkelhor, D., Walsh, W., & Treitman, L. (2018). Sextortion of minors: Characteristics and dynamics. *Journal of Adolescent Health, 62*(1), 72–79.

Chapter 10
Relationship and Dating Violence in School-Aged Adolescents

Barbara Burcham, Mackenzie Leachman, and Virginia Luftman

Definition and Prevalence

Adolescence is a normal transitional phase of growth and development that falls between childhood and adulthood. The World Health Organization (WHO) sets this phase between the ages of 10 and 19 years. In many societies, however, adolescence is more narrowly equated with the time when physical changes appear that lead to adult physical maturity. The term adolescence also encompasses a broader definition that includes the psychological, social, and moral changes that occur.

Adolescence can be difficult terrain, as it is a time characterized by rapid physical development and deep emotional change. As adolescents begin to individuate and emotionally separate from parents/family, they can experience a sense of undefined status. They are faced with the increased need to make decisions, a myriad of social pressures, a search for self, and endless, often negative, comparisons with peers.

Adolescents, in a way, are "waking up" to the world. They begin to notice, evaluate, and question everything, most importantly themselves. A child who has been adopted might have accepted that as fact for 10 years and then at 12 years, the magnitude of "being adopted" becomes overwhelming and confusing. Domestic violence, alcoholism, and sexual abuse, while disturbing, might have been incorporated as their "norm," but in adolescence, these personal facets of their "self" are called into stark clarity when compared with the different circumstances of peers.

B. Burcham (✉)
Georgetown College, Georgetown, KY, USA
e-mail: Barbara_Burcham@georgetowncollege.edu

M. Leachman
Fayette County Public Schools, Lexington, KY, USA

V. Luftman
Department of Psychiatry, University of Kentucky, Lexington, KY, USA

© The Author(s), under exclusive license to Springer Nature Switzerland AG 2023
T. W. Miller (ed.), *School Violence and Primary Prevention*,
https://doi.org/10.1007/978-3-031-13134-9_10

Dating is very common in adolescence and can be a healthy and rewarding part of social skill development. Parents might know this theoretically, but it is still something with which they are uncomfortable. A large part of this is related to the fact that adolescence is when their "child" experiences a marked upsurge of sexual feelings and desires. Adolescence is hopefully a time when the individual begins the process of understanding and recognizing the importance of controlling these sexual urges.

While most dating relationships among adolescents are a healthy and positive part of their journey to adulthood, during which their self-esteem and self-confidence grow, some can be unhealthy and damaging (Sears et al., 2007), increasing the risks of negative behavior and health outcomes, specifically Teen Dating Violence (TDV).

Teen Dating and Violence

Violence between teens has been extensively studied and has been given different definitions and parameters (Follingstad & Ryan, 2013). Violence between teens in a dating relationship is referenced differently throughout the literature. It might be referenced as any of the following:

- Adolescent Relationship Abuse (ARA)
- Adolescent Dating Aggression (ADA)
- Adolescent Dating Violence (ADV) and
- Dating Violence (DV)

For consistency, throughout this chapter, we will be addressing this phenomenon as Teen Dating Violence (TDV). Where appropriate it will be delineated as Psychological TDV, Physical TDV, Sexual TDV, and Digital TDV. Teen dating violence will also be addressed in terms of teen dating violence victimization and teen dating violence perpetration. Historically, teen dating violence included physical violence, sexual violence, psychological aggression, and stalking (Breiding, 2014). Dating violence (DV) overall is defined as intimate partner violence between two individuals currently or formerly romantically involved (Moore et al., 2015). Teen dating violence can start with something innocent, such as teasing or flirting, but these can be a precursor to more overt and harmful types of psychological, physical, or sexual aggression.

Definition of TDV

A national survey on Teen Relationships and Intimate Violence (STRIV) for 12- to 18-year-olds provided the first nationally representative household survey that focused on teen dating violence (Taylor & Mumford, 2016). The sample consisted of 1804 completed surveys. For this survey, the following definitions were developed.

Psychological TDV

Psychological teen dating violence ranges from flirting, threats to end the relationship, jealous behavior, excessive tracking of the victim, hostile tones, and insulting behavior, to more serious psychological teen dating violence including maligning friends, spreading rumors, and trying to turn others against friends.

Physical TDV

Physical teen dating violence is defined as kicking, hitting, punching, scratching, bending fingers, slapping, pulling hair, threatening to hit, pushing, shoving, shaking, ridiculing, and destroying or threatening to destroy something valued by the victim. This could progress to more serious physical teen dating violence in the form of burning, choking, biting, threatening or using a gun or knife against the victim, or forcing sexual behavior.

Sexual TDV

Sexual teen dating violence encompasses threatening the victim in an attempt to have sex, touching the victim sexually, kissing against the victim's will, and forcing sexual behavior.

Prevalence of TDV

A national US survey in 2016 expanded this definition to Teen Dating Violence Victimization (TDVV) and found a very high level of prevalence. It was documented that 65.5% of teens experienced psychological abuse during dating, 17.5% physical violence, and 18.0% sexual abuse during their short lifetimes (Taylor & Mumford, 2016).

The Centers for Disease Control and Prevention (CDC) has found that 1 in 11 female and 1 in 15 male high school students report having experienced physical dating violence in the past year. Additionally, 1 in 9 female and 1 in 36 male high school students experienced sexual dating violence in the last year. It is reported that

9% of all high school students report being hit, slapped, or physically hurt on purpose in the past 12 months in 2011 (CDC, 2019a).

The CDC Youth Risk Behavior Survey (2018) reports varying percentages of youth who experience teen dating violence, based upon their background and orientation. For example, 20% of Native American youth and 19% of African American youth reported sexual dating violence in high school, while 16% of Latinx youth and 13% of Asian youth reported such violence. Among the general LGBTQA teen community, 16% reported sexual dating violence; 17% of bisexual teens and 12% of transgender teens reported sexual dating violence. West and Rose (2000) report that although there are research gaps regarding the implications and interventions among the youth of color, teen dating violence is all too common among African American adolescents.

Overall, 26% of adult women and 15% of adult men have been victims of sexual, physical, and/or stalking violence by an intimate partner in their lifetime. They first experienced these forms of violence between the ages of 11 and 17 years (CDC, 2019a). This data clearly shows that teen dating violence is something that occurs well before high school, at an alarming level, as middle school children have been found to experience teen dating violence at similar rates to older high school counterparts (Lormand et al., 2013).

Even though the level of teen dating violence is disturbing, it might in fact be an underestimate that does not reflect the true scope of the problem. While there have been National Surveys (Taylor & Mumford, 2016), a great majority of surveys are conducted in a school setting. The reticence of teens to report being abused is a limitation of getting accurate assessments of incidence. Moore et al. (2015) found that while 9% of high school students reported having been physically hurt by a boyfriend or girlfriend in the last 12 months, only 33% ever reported that they were in a violent relationship. This indicates that there is another 66% who are at risk of further victimization because they received no intervention for the abuse. The reasons postulated for why teens will not report their violent relationships to authorities might well lie in the fact that teachers and school counselors do not always identify TDV as a major health problem. They often lack specific training to deal and assist with TDV victims and perpetrators, as 90% of counselors and 88% of school nurses were found to have had no specific training in this area (Moore et al., 2015). As a result, the teen tends to turn to friends who are easily and readily available, but not developmentally mature enough to pursue resources to help. Surveys done in schools often will not include questions regarding sexual violence and stalking because school administrators are uncomfortable with these types of questions. They are concerned with the potential reactions of parents and this is especially true in the middle school population (Goldman et al., 2016). Surveys have been found to have inherent barriers to accuracy, as they use scales adapted from adult screening instruments used in interpersonal violence. This is problematic, as adults and teens have very different levels of concrete thinking, and their world views differ greatly (Goldman et al., 2016). In efforts to more clearly define TDV, some surveys have queried respondents by using language that might create a false negative response to questions regarding violence. Items such as, "Have you been thrown into furniture?" or "Have you been thrown into a wall?" could easily be given a "No" response by a teen when they in fact have been thrown on a bed or onto the ground (Follingstad & Ryan, 2013). Even though the statistics might, in fact, underestimate the actual level of TDV, it is still at a level sufficient to have prompted twenty-five states to introduce, or pass, dating violence prevention policies. These legislations are predicated on the statistics of more than two-thirds (69%) of 12- to 18-year-old respondents reporting current or recent TDV at some point in their relationship, demonstrating a significant prevalence of dating violence in the United States (Smith et al., 2015).

Characteristics of TDV Victims and Perpetrators

Due to the alarmingly high incidence of teen dating violence in adolescents and teens, often beginning in middle school, research has attempted to better understand the individual characteristics of the victims and perpetrators of teen dating violence.

While girls have traditionally been characterized as victims and boys as perpetrators, the statistics show a very different picture. Girls aged 15–18 years did report the highest rate of any TDV victimization (73%) and girls aged 12–14 years the lowest (53%). The most common form of TDV was psychological abuse. Almost 1 in 5 adolescents aged 12–18 years reported experiencing sexual abuse victimization (18%) and physical abuse victimization (18%). Girls aged 15–18 years, again, reported the highest levels of sexual (21%) victimization. However, boys aged 12–15 years reported the highest rates of physical abuse victimization (27%). More and more literature have found that while girls are at greater risk of victimization, they are also very likely to be perpetrators of physical TDV (Decker et al., 2014; Taylor & Mumford, 2016; Dimissie et al., 2018; Taquette & Monteiro, 2019). Girls aged 15–18 years reported the highest rate of any perpetration (66%) and girls aged 12–14 years the lowest (56%). Overall, the most common type of perpetration was psychological (62%), with other girls more likely to be the victims of psychological abuse (Karlsson et al., 2016). Boys aged 15–18 years reported the highest rates of perpetration of sexual abuse (15%), their victims being more likely to be female.

There was an observed significant overlap between victimization and perpetration, in that 58% of all respondents reported both, with a bivariate analysis yielding an overall figure of 84% of any teen dating violence victim also being a perpetrator of teen dating violence. This held across genders and ages, indicating the vast majority of teen dating violence victims are also perpetrators (Moore et al., 2015). Both boys and girls are victims and perpetrators of teen dating violence with girls being more inclined to be perpetrators of physical and psychological violence, especially after age 15, but then as they age they are at greater risk of sexual victimization (Ackard et al., 2007). Though violence toward girls is substantial, same-sex violence within a dating relationship, along with girls' violence toward boys, are also alarmingly prevalent (Levine, 2017).

Bullying

Adolescents first exert power through bullying behaviors in adolescence. Dominance and power over peers do not generally center on sex and gender but rather on personal psychology and situational factors such as appearance, gender identity, body parts, sexual orientation, or sexual identity. Bullying peaks earlier than sexual harassment and tends to decline, overall, during adolescence. It is generally during school transitions, such as from middle school to high school, that other aggressive behaviors, such as sexual harassment, begin to emerge (Cutbush et al., 2016). There has been found to be a significant link between bullying and teen dating violence, this being greater for physical teen dating violence. There appears to be a longitudinal link, in that evidence of bullying, over a period of time, strongly predicts future sexual harassment, in particular. This was not found to be gender-specific as it was documented in both boys and girls (Cutbush et al., 2016; Foshee et al., 2016; Debnam et al., 2016).

Interpersonal Family Violence Exposure

Family of origin and exposure to interpersonal violence (IPV) has been found to have a profound effect and to be a predictor of both victimization and perpetration of TDV. As many as 15% of adolescents who report a history of domestic violence, report TDV victimization, and 9% report perpetration of TDV (Foshee et al., 2016). The average length of exposure to domestic violence, in TDV victims and perpetrators, is 5 years, with the majority endorsing violence against mother by father or father figure. Witnessing mother-to-father or female-to-male violence has been found to also be a significant predictor of both physical and psychological TDV, especially in boys. However, witnessing male-to-female violence was found to be highly more predictive of psychological TDV. Psychological violence is more subtle than physical violence, and growing up with a physically abusive father figure and seeing the consequences of physical violence might cause a child to subconsciously reject this behavior. The child might then retain an inner hostility that would result in psychological perpetration within the dating relationship (Karlsson et al., 2016). Overall, both girls and boys are more accepting of female-perpetrated violence than male-perpetrated violence, possibly interpreting it as protective in a violent situation in which there is no physical equality (Karlsson et al., 2016).

Violence as a Norm

Exposure to intimate partner violence in the home that predicts teen dating violence seems to be associated with acceptance of aggression as a norm (Ludin et al., 2018). This is further perpetuated if the adolescent has previous experience as a witness or victim in an intimate relationship. The presence of violence in the adolescent's life appears to support attitudes that accept violence as a norm. These adolescents seem to be more susceptible to the use of control and coercion and have poorer social skills that might be needed to mediate this effect (Tapp & Moore, 2016; Shamu et al., 2016; Karlsson et al., 2016). Exposure to violence over a long period can contribute to stereotypical gender and dating beliefs. It has been found that adolescents with positive family relationships and strong gender equality messages engaged in less teen dating violence and were less likely to tolerate it in their own intimate relationships (Taquette & Monteiro, 2019). Safe, nurturing stable relationships have been found to actually interrupt the intergenerational cycle of violence (Latzman et al., 2018).

Gender Stereotypes and TDV

Gender stereotype research has shown that girls are found to prioritize romantic ideas of a dating relationship. They feel they should be sexually appealing but modest and should not be too sexually active. Conversely, boys feel they should be assertive and tend to prioritize sex over romantic attachment. This male gender belief can lead to greater aggression and more sexually coercive tactics. Internalization of these beliefs has a strong correlation to increased use of substances and delinquency. This greater acceptance of violence has been shown to correlate with lower self-esteem, and depression and anxiety (Reed et al., 2018; Ludin et al., 2018). A patriarchal society, often found in Hispanic countries and/or neighborhoods, in which men are more domineering and women are dominated, favors gender inequality and tends to endorse boys' perpetration of violence, especially if they are goaded by peers or feel threats to their virility (Taquette & Monteiro, 2019). Adolescents with strong family relationships that stress strong gender equality messages engaged in less teen dating violence (Taquette & Monteiro, 2019). Adolescents who endorse, "Most boys hit their girlfriends" or "Most girls hit their boyfriends," similarly report greater teen dating violence victimization and perpetration (Reyes et al., 2016). Reed et al. (2018) have found that internalization of negative gender beliefs correlates with increased use of substances, delinquency, and a greater acceptance of violence, lower self-esteem, higher depression, and lower self-efficacy in girls, all of which have been linked with increased teen dating violence.

Psychological Distress

Psychological distress has been postulated as having a causal role in the relationship between domestic violence (DV) and victimization in adolescent dating, as it may be related to a history of maltreatment in childhood, witnessing interfamilial violence, being the recipient of poor care provision by parents and/or feeling insecure in social settings. Often this distress is manifest in anxiety and depression that are themselves predictors of eventual teen dating violence. Having endured child sexual abuse or maltreatment has repeatedly been shown to significantly correlate with TDV. Youths with a history of child maltreatment, emotional, physical or sexual abuse, and neglect have been shown to report both engaging in, and being a victim of, teen dating violence (Cascardi & Jouriles, 2018; Haselschwerdt et al., 2019; Taquette & Monteiro, 2019; Dardis et al., 2015). Internalized symptoms such as anxiety, loneliness, and sadness have been linked with lower self-esteem which possibly leads to adolescents being less likely to resist when being victimized by teen dating violence. The youths dealing with these symptoms might display a demeanor and body language that makes them targets for perpetrators (Ludin et al., 2018). As discussed, exposure to violence in the home and witnessing teen dating violence at school can create an inner hostility that can result in TDV perpetration.

TDV and Substance Use

The use of alcohol has been repeatedly shown to be associated with teen dating violence. It is a high predictor and a pathway to violence in dating relationships. This finding has been found consistent across all grade levels, genders, races and nationalities (Shamu et al., 2016; Foshee et al., 2016; Dimissie et al., 2018; Lormand et al., 2013; Johnson et al., 2017). This is an increasing problem in both middle school and high school with Parker et al. (2017) finding that 32% of girls and 38% of boys reported the use of alcohol in the last 30 days.

With the easing of restrictions regarding marijuana use in several states, the use of marijuana has been examined in terms of a link to teen dating violence. Johnson et al. (2017) found that 23% of high school students have used marijuana in the past 30 days. There was found to be a 42% increase in the odds of perpetration of violence but there is discrepancy among researchers as to the severity of that violence. It does seem to be present but not to the same level as alcohol use, which holds true globally (Johnson et al., 2017). Parker and Debnam et al. (2016) found an association between marijuana use and teen dating violence victimization and perpetration; however, causality of marijuana use and teen dating violence has not been shown scientifically (Johnson et al., 2017).

Contextual Factors of TDV: Family, Neighborhood, School

Family context is a variable that is multi-faceted in terms of teen dating violence. Adolescents with good family relationships and strong gender equality messages engaged in less teen dating violence and were less likely to tolerate it when directed at them (Taquette & Monteiro, 2019). Parental monitoring also has been found to have a moderating effect, as there is less teen dating violence when the adolescent perceives that their parents are overseeing their behavior. This is evidenced in adolescents who positively endorse, "My parents tell me when I must come home" (Foshee et al., 2016). Mumford et al. (2016) identified three parenting profiles: positive parenting, strict/harsh parenting and strict/disengaged parenting and found that positive parenting, compared longitudinally with the other two styles, was significantly predictive of lower levels of TDV. While autonomy is often perceived as a positive attribute in teens, it has been shown that a greater autonomy, or lack of monitoring, is predictive of higher adolescent reports of perpetration. Reported "high levels' of autonomy," and/or the greater promotion of autonomy by the parent, have been shown to result in higher levels of physical aggression against dating partners. When the adolescent reports higher levels of autonomy, paired with greater parental warmth, this correlation dissolves and is not predictive of greater teen dating violence (Niolon et al., 2015a).

When the parent/child relationship was examined, specifically, it was found that the greater the quality of the relationship, as endorsed by the adolescent, the less likelihood of physical or sexual perpetration and lower rates of psychological teen dating violence (Taylor et al., 2017). This held true for both the father and the mother/child relationship.

The overall context of the family as supportive and encouraging, "My family cares about me," "My family wants me to go to college," "My family generally gets along," were predictive of lower TDV, both as victim and perpetrator. If the adolescent endorsed, "People in my family hit one another," or "People threaten or slap each other in my family," the converse was found to be true (Reyes et al., 2018). A positive, over-reaching value system such as "It is good to be honest" and "It is good to finish high school" were positive affirmations that correlated highly with lower TDV of any type.

While the context of family is apparently a strong predictor of both future teen dating violence victimization and perpetration of teen dating violence, there are other contextual factors that impact the adolescent. Adolescents spend time outside of their homes, predominantly in the school setting and/or within their neighborhoods, with peers and adults other than their parents.

Within the greater context of a neighborhood, if the adolescent feels that most of those who live and work in the neighborhood are "honest," "don't get into trouble," "finish high school," "go to college," there is a positive context that is predictive of less teen dating violence (Reyes et al., 2018). Adolescents who affirm that they live in violent neighborhoods, see violence often, i.e., "People where I live have violent arguments," "Most of those in my neighborhood never finished high school,"

"People where I live did not go to college," have a high correlation with higher levels of teen dating violence. When adolescents feel they live in a safer more supportive environment, "People in my neighborhood look out for one another," they report a high correlation with lower levels of teen dating violence. Lower parent education has been identified as having an association with increased odds of membership in high-risk profiles, significantly so in boys (Reyes et al., 2018). Youth in lower socioeconomic levels (SES) were at greater risk, as 25% of boys and girls in this category reported teen dating violence, whereas it was 20% in higher levels of parental education and socioeconomic level (Ackard et al., 2007; Dardis et al., 2015).

The variable of school context has definite implications in terms of prediction of teen dating violence. When adolescents are in a school setting that engenders a perception of safety and support, they are less likely to be in a teen dating violence situation and more likely to seek help if they are. School connectedness, and the feeling that school personnel are supportive, has been shown to have a protective effect in terms of teen dating violence (Parker et al., 2016). Boys, in particular, have shown increased odds of reporting that they are experiencing victimization if they have an increased perception of school safety (Parker et al., 2017). Adolescents who affirm that "My school feels like home" similarly are less likely to state that they are in a TDV situation (Taquette & Monteiro, 2019). The stigma of teen dating violence often precludes the adolescent from reporting or seeking help for a teen dating violence situation; however, a supportive environment that openly addresses the subject of teen dating violence ensures more reporting to authorities. Other school-related factors are size and overall discipline issues. Increased school size was associated with an increased level of teen violence victimization. Size is often associated with higher levels of violence and higher suspension rates and both of these variables were associated with higher teen dating violence (Parker et al., 2016).

In summary: "Emotion regulation deficits and pro-violence norms that result from exposure to family and school violence may be exacerbated for youth in high violence neighborhoods that reinforce antisocial norms and provide limited opportunities to learn self-regulatory skills" that could avert TDV (Reyes et al., 2018).

Digital TDV

Digital media and cell phone use, along with the many platforms of social media, have exploded in the past 5 years. In a 2012 study, 77% of adolescents owned a cell phone, and 80% of 12- to 18-year-olds had a social networking account such as Twitter. A majority of 12- to 18-year-olds use social media daily (Reed et al., 2018). Researchers have struggled with the use of digital media in the context of TDV, in terms of treating this as another form of teen dating violence or as its own entity. There is a lack of consensus about what defines electronic TDV, i.e., is it a separate entity that requires separate measurement or a technology that provides another means for perpetration. Goldman et al. (2016) found that adolescents view the area of their relationship that exists in the digital space as highly integrated in all aspects of their relationships and are unable to separate it, as they see it as all-inclusive. This finding indicates that questions regarding TDV must include the use and misuse of digital media. Previous studies have incorporated questions to measure electronic abuse but have been "project developed" and are not previously vetted or validated. While this area needs greater standardization, it is clear that this area of the adolescent experience is robust. One in four high school students affirm being a victim of "Digital Dating Violence" at some point in time and 29–46% admit to being perpetrators (Cutbush et al., 2016). The terminology used to assess this includes monitoring someone's activities and whereabouts, hostility, name-calling, and pressuring for sexual behavior (Reed et al., 2018). Digital TDV is seen in greater frequency in girls and it is postulated that girls are more likely to use less aggressive and more passive forms of abuse, such as digital psychological teen dating violence. Digital TDV is, similarly, more passive and less aggressive than the physical TDV, which is seen more in boys. Girls view digital TDV as less harmful and more acceptable than more overt teen dating violence (Reed et al., 2018). When high school boys and girls endorse negative gender stereotypes, they then use them to perpetrate digital TDV, through passive monitoring, as a means of exercising possessiveness and ensuring fidelity. Boys are more likely to use aggressive and sexually oriented pressuring and coercive tactics than girls, and girls have been found to be less likely to report any sexual coercion. Girls profess more distress over "sexting" and yet girls (9.2%) are more likely to send naked pictures when asked than boys (8%). Addressing these issues in terms of intervention can be difficult because, as reported, schools are uncomfortable with sexual content (Parker et al., 2017).

Impact of Intimate Partner Violence Among Teens

Thus, it is clear that teen dating violence is a prevalent public health issue and adversely impacts the physical and mental health of those involved (CDC, 2019a; Halpern et al., 2001; Silverman et al., 2004). Adolescent dating violence occurs across all economic, gender, racial, and social lines as it does not discriminate based on these issues, although it occurs at varying degrees in different populations (Surface et al., 2012; Bonds & Stoker, 2000). It is also important to note there is a significant overlap between victims and perpetrators, and perpetrators were often once victims themselves (Gomez, 2011). The familiar saying "hurt people hurt people" accurately describes what is happening when teen violence occurs. According to the work of Taylor and Mumford (2016), there is no homogenous group that can describe those teenagers involved in intimate partner violence, either as victims or as perpetrators.

There is a healthy range of dating behaviors that are designated by age-appropriate, safe, and respectful actions and most teens do not experience violence when dating (Eaton et al., 2007). Surface et al. (2012) describe a continuum of behaviors among teens who want to date ranging from healthy to playful, to non-mutual age inappropriate, to harassing, to abusive and violent behaviors. Sometimes when youth lack dating experience, have been desensitized to violence due to environmental factors, are unskilled at negotiating socially stressful situations, are underdeveloped in expressing their feelings or have not been taught the parameters of safe behaviors, the stage may be set for teen dating violence. Other youth may suffer from dysregulation punctuated by mental health issues that will impair their decision-making. Surface et al. (2012) suggest that these issues make teens more vulnerable to dating violence.

There is an unspoken or spoken social contract between two people when they move across the continuum from an innocent flirt to intimate interaction. Just like any contract, it can and should be terminated when either party says "stop." Often perpetrators report they wish they could have stopped on the first sign of their target saying "no," but they could not because that would strip them of power (T. Hockenbury, 2020, personal communication). Many times, teen dating violence, unlike adult intimate violence, is carried out in a public manner where there is a third party or many parties present. Although it is developmentally appropriate for teens to be in groups at school or at parties, if a girl hits a boy, the boy is more likely to hit back to save face if he is in a group (Eaton et al., 2007). During adolescence, peers have a huge influence on attitudes and behaviors as it relates to teen dating violence and the norms within a peer group have a significant impact on teen behavior. So, even though there is less power play in teens than adults, there is, among teens, a significant element of lesser developed coping skills as it relates to negotiating romantic relationships and their ability to express complex feelings (Fredland et al., 2005).

If a teen perpetrator has a belief system that they have the right to control their partner, their feelings of strength and power may be enhanced by engaging in physical aggressiveness. They may feel a loss of respect if their partner, their target, does not submit to their violent form of intimate behavior. If a teenager believes they are responsible for solving every problem in a relationship, they may fall into a pattern of seeing possessive jealousy, and acted out in aggression, as a form of romantic love (Surface et al., 2012).

These mindsets in teens can be seen in inappropriate jokes, gestures, sexual touching, grabbing, or pinching that is witnessed in school classrooms, restrooms, and hallways across America (Bonds & Stoker, 2000), but it can lead to more dangerous acting out according to Taquette and Monteiro (2019). This includes a plethora of problems including, but not limited to, posttraumatic stress, high anxiety, lowered self-esteem, increased suicide and homicide, depression, alcohol, and drug abuse, as well as high levels of having unprotected sex. The list is further expanded by others, including decreased physical and mental health (Howard et al., 2007), increased suicide attempts (Chiodo et al., 2012), engagement in risky sexual behaviors, unplanned pregnancy (Silverman et al., 2004), issues in unhealthy weight management (Ackard & Neumrk-Sztainer, 2002), and higher levels of adult relationship aggression (Berkowitz, 2010). Clearly, the stage is set for exacerbated mental health issues if a teen has been involved with TDV.

Case Studies

Three case studies, real-life examples that occurred in public high school settings, are reviewed in the next sections. All names and identifying details have been changed to protect the identity of those involved. These vignettes may be beneficial in group discussions with an emphasis on the lessons learned, as well as examining prevention and intervention initiatives.

Although teen dating violence is not an easy dynamic to understand, it often involves a power imbalance. As Susan Strauss (2000) indicates in "Bully Proofing Your School," sexual perpetration is not about sexual attraction, it is about the misuse and abuse of power. The acting out person does not feel as loved as they want to be and may feel inferior; just never good enough. They choose a person they think they might love, and that person just does not fill that deep emptiness. The feeling that their love interest leaves them with is one of feeling incomplete and that sparks anger and they are left feeling very much "less than." The person who does not love as much has more power and the one who wants to be loved feels inadequate and has to posture to feel more powerful. Feeling diminished is a terrible emotion and the power imbalance leads to anger and significant acting out.

The Case of Feeling Powerless

Let us review the case of Izzie and Patrick. Izzie is a smart capable young woman looking to be loved as is her boyfriend Patrick. Izzie is a 17-year-old female; she has a positive relationship with her teachers and earned a 25 on the ACT exam as a junior in high school. Although her grades were satisfactory, Izzie seemed distracted and disengaged in school on some days, according to her teachers. Izzie's parents are hardworking individuals employed at a local manufacturing plant. Her boyfriend of 2 years, Patrick, attends the alternative school; he had been placed there due to multiple violent outbursts at his school district. It was not part of his program to have regular access to counseling services at the alternative school. Patrick's father is incarcerated for assault and his mother is a waitress, with a strong work ethic. Izzie walked into the school psychologist's office one April morning, a support she sought out on an occasional basis, to talk about her mood swings and minor arguments with her boyfriend. However, this day was different. She asked if she could meet in the nurse's office where there was more privacy. This day she was crying as she turned her back to the psychologist and pulled her t-shirt up to reveal her back. Tears rolled down her face. On her back was carved, and revealed clearly in scar tissue, an extreme obscenity, and numerous other fresher cuts. Izzie and the psychologist sat on the floor in that examination room as Izzie emotionally vomited, stating her boyfriend had been carving on her back for at least 2 years to create physical pain to avoid the pain of anal sex. He demanded that method of sex for his pleasure and recently had started hitting her in addition to cutting her back. She was exhausted, felt unloved, powerless, and abused. She asked for help to get away from him. Izzie agreed to involve her parents, change schools, and engage in counseling. She is now a successful professional woman and reports she continues to see a therapist into her adult years. Izzie's relationship with school personnel, formed through positive prior interactions, helped her bridge the chasm from total despair and isolation to that of asking for help.

Lessons Learned and Interventions

There are several lessons learned from the case of Izzie and Patrick.

Lesson one: The importance of having mental health professionals at schools to provide support to the children.

Intervention one: Many schools have guidance counselors and some have school psychologists, school social workers, and nurses. Having a staff that is accessible and knowledgeable to support students who are in trouble makes a difference. School mental healthcare support personnel have to find ways to build relationships with youth with whom they are serving through a variety of activities including being present in the hallways at school, having informal conversations with students, attending events, learning the names of students, inviting students to be a part of school think tanks, etc. Izzie was able to reveal, in an authentic manner, the pain she was experiencing because she had an established, positive and confidential relationship with the school psychologist. Through this foundational connection, Izzie was able to redefine the relationship to one of abuse and make changes that would ultimately lead her to a life of peace and productivity. The school psychologist had the skills to facilitate an intervention involving the family of this young girl and had the networking to access immediate community-based psychological care.

Lesson two: There is also a lesson embedded in this case about the role of teachers working with children who are exhibiting atypical behavior in the classroom.

Intervention two: In the case of Izzie, she was viewed as most capable but was sometimes disengaged and restless. This was the platform for the teacher to approach Izzie and nudge her to see a preferred mental health person in the building. Teachers being aware and asking poignant questions to students can make an enormous difference in helping children access care.

Lesson three: As it relates to Patrick, it is important to pay attention to children who have violent acting out at school.

Intervention three: Students who act out are often being hurt physically or psychologically, setting the stage for intimate partner violence. Many people who engage in violent intimate behaviors express sincere sorrow after they are aggressive with their partner and beg them not to leave, explaining they will never re-abuse again (T. Hockenbury, 2020, personal communication). This speaks clearly to their need to be loved, accepted, and valued; to be worthy of love. An intervention that should not be lost in this case is exploring ways for school personnel and other adults to access care for the perpetrator rather than walking away from that student in a judgmental fashion. If this is not explored, then perpetration will likely continue.

The Case of Murder-Suicide

Next, let us examine the case of Corrie and Billy, which unfortunately had an extremely bad outcome. Corrie, a 17-year-old, athletic-looking, smart and spunky junior, was dating a young man, Billy, aged 19. Corrie's parents, a physician and a physical therapist, strongly disapproved of Corrie dating him. Billy lived with his uncle, had poor grades, and had skipped school regularly until he was the age he could formally drop out. Corrie was rebellious and told her school counselor she loved the fun that Billy brought to her life and she had no intention of leaving the relationship with Billy, even though she hesitantly admitted that he talked to her disrespectfully sometimes and had pushed her. Every time he was aggressive with her, he begged her to forgive him, which she did. The counselor had many sessions with Corrie discussing her feelings, Billy's actions, and the cycle of violence. Additionally, the counselor contacted social services on at least three occasions regarding concerns linked to suspected abuse and violence in Billy's home, however, nothing was ever confirmed. Corrie's parents and Billy's uncle were contacted on several occasions about Billy's aggressive actions toward Corrie. One day, Corrie's friends reported to a teacher that Billy talked Corrie into going on an out-of-state weekend trip; unfortunately, neither Corrie nor Billy ever came home. After 3 days of being missing and high levels of investigation, both of these young people were found dead in a hotel room in another state with a weapon along with empty bottles of alcohol and pills. Sadly, it was ruled a murder-suicide. Corrie was pregnant. Three lives were lost while families were dramatically changed forever. In this case, it is noteworthy that her friends, who saw/heard something, had said something at school and the appropriate steps were taken, but unfortunately, this did not change the outcome. Corrie's friends found out the three were dead while at school and extreme chaos ensued.

Lessons Learned and Interventions

Lesson one: Schools need a response plan in place when tragedy strikes, ensuring that school-based teams have adequate training in crisis response best practice.

Intervention one: Depending on several factors, including the likeability of either of the students, their history at the school, their involvement in school activities, etc., the outpouring of grief and disruption at school can be remarkable. If the school has a culturally and developmentally appropriate plan to assist the students in addressing their grief, it can aide them in managing their stress and can help the students learn how to use their existing coping skills in new and unfamiliar situations. Some students have persistent and significant lingering fears after a school-based trauma and may need to be referred for ongoing focused treatment. If school personnel are well-networked with mental healthcare professionals in the community, facilitation of student care can be optimized.

Lesson two: Adults working with youth sometimes have residual grief and trauma after the episode.

Intervention two: The adults involved with Corrie and Billy were making serious efforts to intervene with this couple. They were addressing the blazing red flags, yet there was a horrifically bad outcome. Often mental healthcare personnel and other school-based adults receive no care, not even the opportunity to formally process the situation. School personnel will need to find ways to take care of themselves, which means high-level self-care. This may look like asking for peer consultation, watching for under- or over-involvement with trauma cases, and pursuing balance in their lives. Additionally, school-based mental healthcare workers may want to get involved in trainings such as evidence-based intervention programs for trauma-affected youth which would increase confidence with the helping process.

Lesson three: This case also punctuates the need for educating young teens, perhaps even in middle school, on what physical, psychological, and sexual abuse looks like and what to do if indeed one finds themselves in that circumstance.

Intervention three: What Corrie described as "fun" led to death and serious grief for family and friends. What we want students to do, to know, must be taught to them explicitly. Schools may need to develop a relationship safety task force and explore developmentally correct and culturally sensitive methods to teach students how to care for themselves in this arena of sexual curiosity.

Lesson four: It is important to teach children to report, in a timely fashion, any events they witness that involve any kind of danger, particularly relationship violence.

Intervention four: Many times, students do not report things they see and hear because of the perceived and often real negative impact it may have on them. In this case, friends did report that Corrie and Billy had left the state, but the issue of immediacy was lost on them. It is important to educate our middle and high school students to report potential issues of danger to trusted adults and provide a mechanism for them to do so without social repercussions. This may consist of actually talking to an adult at school. It is important to teach students the difference between tattling and telling, setting up an anonymous phone tip/helpline, organizing a school safety team, and having an anonymous report form or a confidential and anonymous computer report form. Obviously, the student body must be taught how to use these mechanisms and confidentiality assurances reviewed.

The Case of Sexual Grooming

Next, let us review the case of Jake and Sean. Keep in mind that those who sexually act out in aggressive ways may have been previously hurt and have been the victim of intimate partner violence themselves. The perpetrator as well as the victim may well have limited coping skills to tolerate the frustration of not having their sexual desires met. Adolescents who perpetrate, or who are victims, may feel both helpless and incapable of finding ways of meeting their own needs.

Jake, a 14-year-old ninth grader, reported to a school social worker that he was unsure of his sexual identity. He indicated he had tried to talk to his parents, who shamed him regarding this revelation and said they were going to send him away to a military camp. Jake stopped talking about his sexual identity with his parents or any adults at school. He did begin "dating" an older man, Sean, age 20, who allowed Jake to smoke, access pornographic material, and consume alcohol, although he was under age. Sean urged Jake not to tell his parents he was allowing him to smoke and drink at his house. Both these young men reported they were in love. Soon they were engaged in intimate sexual behaviors and Jake grew more and more attached to Sean. Sean's slight initial touches were uncomfortable for Jake at first. The touching progressed to more intimate acts, and Jake did not stop it. He was embarrassed, felt that no one would believe him anyway and it did feel good, which made him feel guilty. Sean was effective at grooming Jake for anal perpetration and Jake tried to push down the feelings of shame. Jake experienced serious mental conflict and started feeling an inferno of confusion, as a result of the fear of losing Sean and the resultant loneliness; he just wanted to die. Jake's grades dropped and his mood became erratic and his parents became very concerned, asking the school for help.

Through investigation and many serious and frank discussions with Jake, he ultimately revealed the relationship had become controlling, abusive physically and verbally, and he wanted to "end it all" by completing suicide. It was learned that Sean, himself, had a long history of being abused by a relative.

With wraparound support from school personnel, a community therapist, and his parents, Jake was able to separate from the abusive dating partner, engage in counseling and begin the journey of healing. Neither Jake nor his parents were willing to involve law enforcement, due to fear of retaliation, and Sean was not willing to seek mental health support. Even so, the school psychologist made a report to Crimes Against Children with the local police department.

Lessons Learned and Interventions

Lesson One: In the case of Sean and Jake, we learn that it is important for adults to pay attention to the cues associated with inappropriate sexual contact. Mental health workers who are at least open to the hypothesis of sexual grooming (followed by sexual abuse), when a student's behavior changes and grades decline, can interrupt a psychologically and physically traumatic experience for youth.

Intervention One: When an adolescent is befriended by someone older than them, and an emotional connection is established, that is often a healthy, normal and a genuinely positive connection. However, sometimes the intent is to lower the younger person's inhibitions with the intent of sexual misconduct/abuse, and this leads to confusion and trauma. An embedded intervention in this vignette is the necessity of teaching children how to know who is safe in the world, how to act when one feels pleasure but shame, and how to report this conduct when being threatened not to tell.

Lesson two: Another lesson is to know how mental healthcare workers or other school staff should respond to reporting requirements of sexual misconduct when parents and students do not want to involve law enforcement.

Intervention two: Understanding the ethical and legal responsibilities linked with the concern of preventing future perpetration certainly drives mental health professionals to make reports consistent with their professional board obligations.

Lesson three: It is important for school personnel and parents to keep communication lines open so students will reveal their deepest fears.

Intervention three: Developmentally, teens prefer talking to teens rather than adults; however, it is essential to be involved in what is going on in the life of adolescents both at home and at school. Sometimes teens tune adults out, as they "ask too many direct questions" rather than observe and listen. Engaging in activities with teens, knowing their friendship group, validating their feelings, giving them opportunities to earn trust, and giving them explicit praise are some strategies to set the stage for open conversations.

Lesson four: Ensure that someone on the school support staff team is deeply knowledgeable about community resources.

Intervention four: The complexity of this case begs for knowledge and networking among school-based and community-based mental health professionals. Knowing about available community resources and then networking to facilitate high-level care are essential. Making sure that a variety of professionals are on school-based intervention teams can create a climate of sharing information and accessing care for students who are in significant need of mental health support.

These are three cases among the thousands that could be told, many filled with horrific pain, drugs, alcohol, sexually transmitted diseases (STDs), pregnancy, poor body image, dependency, family issues, dysregulation, disinhibition, and a sincere longing to belong. Each and every case of dating violence has an impact and in a vast majority of cases, the consequences are adverse, long-lasting, and in some cases dire.

Overall, it is urgent that schools do not tolerate or, even at some level, promote sexual harassment, sexual misconduct, or sexual abuse in any form. The historical thinking that males are expected to be aggressive and predatorial and females weak and submissive has added to the culture's acceptance of this patriarchal conceptualization of relationships. Any type of inappropriate behavior escalates when it is ignored or tolerated and this includes sexually inappropriate behavior (Bonds & Stoker, 2000). Schools need to have a plan that allows students to confidentially report concerns. They need to provide schoolwide training to staff and students on what this behavior looks like and what is going to happen if it occurs. They need to be sure that teachers and staff have knowledge of and access to the available community resources.

School-based Prevention and Intervention

Given the prevalence of TDV and the adverse immediate and long-lasting impact on teens, schools have a responsibility to embed prevention and intervention programs into the fabric of the school curriculum. School is the only agency that reaches all adolescents and can play a strategic role in teaching age-appropriate healthy and safe dating behaviors. In this way, students will know without question what TDV looks like and what to do if behaviors are consistent with definitions of TDV. The following is a review of current school violence prevention and intervention programs that illustrate best practices in the field.

Background

Currently, schools have begun to integrate mental health, social-emotional learning, and trauma-informed care practices as part of their schoolwide prevention programs. Schools have adopted a Multi-Tiered System of Supports (MTSS) to provide universal, targeted, and intensive interventions through the Response to Intervention Framework, Positive Behavior Interventions and Supports, Schoolwide Positive Discipline, Social Emotional Learning, Trauma-Informed Care for Educators and Interconnected Systems Framework (Fuchs et al., 2012; Durlak et al., 2011; Horner & Sugai, 2015). Several school-based curricula incorporate direct instruction on healthy relationships and violence prevention, which include empathy training, problem-solving strategies, conflict resolution skills, and skills for learning.

Universally, school-based initiatives provide a promising approach to assist in student's development in school and life. According to a meta-analysis of school-based interventions, studies affirm increased prosocial behaviors, decreased conduct and internalizing symptoms, and increased achievement. The largest effect size, which sustained significance 6 months post-intervention, included social-cognitive and affective skills consisting of emotion recognition, stress management, empathy, and problem-solving or decision-making skills (Durlak et al., 2011). The recommendations for mental health promotion and social and emotional learning (SEL) have been recommended with support from outcome studies from the Institute of Medicine and The Report of the Surgeon General's Conference on Children's Mental Health. At the federal level, bills have been written to promote academic and social and emotional learning. These recommendations are reflected in the reauthorization of the Elementary and Secondary Education Act. Several states have incorporated SEL skills as part of their student learning standards. For example, the Illinois State Board of Education adopted the Illinois Social and Emotional Learning Standards (https://www.isbe.net/sel), providing goals, age-appropriate benchmarks, and performance descriptors. Peskin et al. (2019) similarly recommend multilevel interventions to develop cognitive skills necessary for the formation of healthy dating relationships. Sohn and Davis (2018) recommend school professionals to identify healthy and unhealthy relationship behaviors in young adolescents, help young people navigate online and offline relationships with peers, and utilize everyday gestures that promote trauma-informed relationships with students.

State Legislation

In Ohio, House Bill 19 passed in 2009 mandated prevention programs in schools regarding dating violence. Specific details surrounding the mandate include the following:

- Education about violence in dating relationships in grades 7–12
- Age-appropriate instruction in dating violence prevention education, which shall include instruction in recognizing dating violence warning signs and characteristics of healthy relationships
- Updating of the harassment, intimidation, and bullying policy to include violence in dating relationships
- Identify specified staff members that are required to be trained about dating violence in dating relationships and every 5 years after initial in-service training
- Directs school boards to incorporate training in the prevention of dating violence into the in-service training required by current law for nurses, teachers, counselors, school psychologists, or administrators

Providing universal education over universal screening is recommended practice (Ohio Domestic Violence Network, 2012). Some research suggests adopting a screening approach if universal approaches may not be able to be adequately funded or provide the appropriate intervention dose. Incorporating prevention programs with students who are identified with risk factors might be one way to provide more targeted intervention support (Cohen et al., 2018). Other practices would include supporting approaches to be implemented early in schools, which include family and community education and support (Taquette & Monteiro, 2019).

There are 23 states that currently have laws that allow, urge, or require school boards to develop or include curriculum on teen dating violence. The Every Student Succeed Act supports prevention to provide for students' mental and behavioral health by integrating physical and psychological safety for schools, families, and communities. The Framework for Safe and Successful Schools supports school safety efforts by creating opportunities to provide prevention and intervention in efforts to prevent violence, including teen dating violence (Cowan et al., 2013).

Best Practices and Effective Strategies for Prevention and Intervention

Strategies recommended by the National Center for Injury Prevention and Control and the Centers for Disease Control and Prevention include teaching safe and healthy relationships skills, engaging influential adults and peers, disrupting the developmental pathways toward partner violence, creating protective environments, strengthening economic supports for families, and supporting survivors to increase safety and lessen harm (Niolon et al., 2017).

In addition, there is a need to create and strengthen awareness among adults in the school. Activating and empowering adults to reflect on their own attitudes toward such behaviors (threatening, harassing, controlling, or violent behavior) is not a normal part of growing up. Providing support for reflection and assisting staff in understanding their role in stopping or preventing the behavior is necessary. Explicit teaching in adult education that reviews definitions of dating violence and how dating violence is different from other types of peer violence is recommended. Providing information to support understanding and strategies to address dating violence to teachers, students and families can increase awareness and prevention. Training support for student support and specialized staff members is recommended (school psychologist, mental health specialist, school social worker, school counselor, administration, or another school-based mental health professional). Teachers should be encouraged to refer students to support staff if dating violence is suspected. The development of protocols regarding early identification, counseling services, and referrals to outside support services will support managing cases and reporting specific situations (Dimissie et al., 2018).

Research on interventions implemented on a college campus comparing traditional awareness and bystander education programs demonstrated improvements in attitudes. The bystander approach was more effective at changing attitudes, beliefs, efficacy, intentions, and self-reported bystander behaviors (Peterson et al., 2018).

Table 10.1 describes explicit approaches to implement the recommended strategies to prevent IPV.

Barriers to Services

Moore et al. (2015) found that 81.3% of school counselors and 86.4% of school nurses reported that there was a lack of protocol/procedures in place for screening and assisting adolescents in violent relationships. Ninety percent of school counselors and 88.1% of school nurses reported that training to assist victims of dating violence had not been provided within the last 2 years. School counselors and nurses included in the study reported that they felt it is not their responsibility to help survivors of dating violence or see dating violence as a major issue when compared with other health issues. The following barriers have been identified to prevent

Table 10.1 Preventing intimate partner violence

Strategy	Approach
Teach safe and healthy relationship skills	Social-emotional learning programs for youth Healthy relationship programs for couples
Engage influential adults and peers	Men and boys as allies in prevention Bystander empowerment and education Family-based programs
Disrupt the developmental pathways toward partner violence	Early childhood home visitation Preschool enrichment with family engagement Parenting skill and family relationship programs Treatment for at-risk children, youth, and families
Create protective environments	Improve school climate and safety Improve organizational policies and workplace climate Modify the physical and social environments of neighborhoods
Strengthen economic support for families	Strengthen household financial security Strengthen work-family supports
Support survivors to increase safety and lessen harms	Victim-centered services Housing programs First responder and civil legal protections Patient-centered approaches Treatment and support for survivors of IPV, including TDV

Source: Niolon et al. (2017); https://www.cdc.gov/violenceprevention/intimatepartnerviolence/prevention.html

adolescents from accessing services: stigma attached to dating violence, a preference for seeking informal sources of help, and a lack of protocols for screening, supporting, and responding when dating violence is reported or suspected. The US Preventive Services Task Force recommends that regardless of the reason for visit or diagnosis, all adolescents, 13 years and older, be screened for dating violence. Recommendations for school-based strategies include: development of policies and procedures to help adolescents who have been in a violent relationship, increased screening of adolescents for dating violence, screening students for dating violence to identify the prevalence within the student population to be able to provide assistance, and additional training and ongoing education for counselors and nurses to improve prevention efforts in school.

Programs and Resources

Several organizations provide information on evidence-based, school-based programs and curriculums: the CDC; the Collaborative for Academic, Social, and Emotional Learning (CASEL); Blueprints for Healthy Youth Development; National Association of School Psychologists; American School Counselor Association; and School Social Work Association of America. Several social-emotional learning, bullying, and violence prevention curriculums teach the skills recommended to prevent, intervene, and mitigate the effects of dating violence.

In addition to the list in Table 10.2, several social-emotional learning curriculums incorporate healthy relationships and healthy dating with direct instruction. Table 10.2 presents a description of sample programs described in the literature. This is not an exhaustive list. Many of these programs are free and have support available online.

Based on the review of literature and current school violence prevention and intervention programs that illustrate best practices in the field, the following practices are recommended to help providers support and prevent youth exposed to or experiencing dating violence:

1. Providers should familiarize themselves with state laws and regulations regarding teen dating violence. In states without laws/regulations, providers can advocate to include and adopt teen dating violence as part of school-based and community-based violence prevention policies of agencies and schools.
2. Agencies supporting young people should adopt protocols and policies for how to educate, identify and make referrals for support. Professional development for primary providers of youth in terms of education, interventions and supports available for youth experiencing teen dating violence is recommended.
3. Communities should consider identifying root cause factors that seem to be contributing to teen dating violence and point to system-level interventions. Activities to increase family and community awareness around teen dating violence are recommended.
4. The use of universal education including direct, explicit skills instruction related to healthy/unhealthy relationships and assertiveness skills is recommended. In addition, providing information on and strategies for bystander intervention and reporting. Universal education programs and social-emotional learning can provide a preventative approach to mitigating teen dating violence. Include definitions and examples of healthy, unhealthy, and abusive relationships. Include examples of different types of abuse that may occur: physical, emotional, sexual, or digital.
5. As a universal public health intervention, identify points of contact that provide opportunities to screen for teen dating violence beginning at age 13 years, similar to screening for trauma exposure and/or abuse.
6. Educating youth on how to seek help and assuring them that abuse is never their fault. Identifying a support system and encouraging them to talk to a friend, family member, or other trusted adult. Provide resources to connect to a healthcare professional to assist with support. If the person reports feeling like they are in danger or need immediate help, call 911. Providing the following helpline information:

   - National Teen Dating Abuse Helpline: 1-866-331-9474 or 1-866-331-8453 TTY
   - National Domestic Violence Hotline: 1-800 799-7233 or 1-800-787-3224 TTY
   - National Suicide Prevention Hotline: 1-800-273-8255
   - GLBT Talkline: 1-888-843-4564
   - GLBT Youth Talkline: 1-800-246-7743
   - Trans Lifeline: 1-877-565-8860

Table 10.2 Instructional programs and curriculums supporting healthy relationships and healthy dating

Resource	Description
Expect Respect (Ball et al., 2009) https://www.safeaustin.org/our-services/prevention-and-education/expect-respect/	A school-based program for preventing teen dating violence and promoting safe and healthy relationships in middle and high school and reduce emotional and physical victimization and perpetration
Safe Dates (Foshee & Langwick, 2010) https://youth.gov/content/safe-dates	A 10-session prevention dating abuse interactive curriculum educating youth about healthy and unhealthy relationships. Can be integrated into a larger school violence prevention model.
Positive Prevention Plus https://positivepreventionplus.com/	A comprehensive school-based prevention curriculum to improve students' communication and negotiation skills to assist with assertiveness, abstain from sexual intercourse, and use birth control effectively.
Me & You (Peskin et al., 2019) https://sph.uth.edu/research/centers/chppr/meandyouhealthy/MeYou-Parent-Newsletter-1-2-21-14-FINAL-BW.pdf	A technology-enhanced adolescent dating violence (DV) intervention to reduce DV perpetration and victimization among ethnic-minority early adolescent youths
Dating Matters: Strategies to Promote Healthy Teen Relationships (CDC, 2019b) https://vetoviolence.cdc.gov/apps/dating-matters-toolkit/explore-component#/	An evidence-based strategy and a community-driven approach to educate youth, parents, educators, schools, and neighborhoods about healthy relationships to stop dating violence before it starts. The focus is on healthy relationships and promotion of healthy lifestyle. Community-based programming is offered. School-based programming designed for students in the 6th, 7th, and 8th grades.
Break the Cycle	Support program for young people ages 12–24 years. The focus of this program is to build healthy relationships and create a culture without abuse.
Second Step www.secondstep.org	A social-emotional skills-based program with content related to bullying, problem-solving skills, emotion management, and empathy. Programs available for pre-K, K-5, and 6–8 grade students.
School-Connect: Optimizing the High School Experience https://school-connect.net/index.html	SEL 80-lesson curriculum designed to improve high school students' social, emotional, and academic skills and strengthen relationships among students and between students and teachers. Modules include: Creating a Supportive Learning Community, Developing Self-Awareness and Self-Management, Building Relationships and Resolving Conflicts & Preparing for College and the Workforce.
Voices: A Program of Self-Discovery and Empowerment for Girls [Covington, S.S., Covington K. and Covington, M. (2004, rev. 2017). Carson City, NV: Change Companies]	Empowerment program with a focus on self, connecting with others, healthy living, and future goals.

(continued)

Table 10.2 (continued)

Resource	Description
Coaching Boys into Men https://cvp.uni.edu/coaching-boys-men	A toolkit for high school coaches to assist in teaching young athletes about relationship abuse, respect, and personal responsibility. Education about healthy relationships, advocacy, and how to respond.
It's All One https://www.popcouncil.org/research/its-all-one-curriculum-guidelines-and-activities-for-a-unified-approach-to-	A curriculum that includes topics around sexual health, human rights, HIV, healthy relationships, communication skills, and advocating for rights. Available in English, French, Spanish, Chinese, Bangla, and Arabic.
Serving Teen Survivors (2018) National Sexual Violence Resource Center https://www.nsvrc.org/sites/default/files/publications/2018-12/Serving%20Teen%20Survivors%20A%20Manual%20for%20Advocates.pdf	A manual that provides information sheets on working with teen survivors, confidentiality and mandated reporting laws, the teen brain, and recent research.
FLASH https://kingcounty.gov/depts/health/locations/family-planning/education/FLASH/high-school.aspx	A science-based sexual health education curriculum designed to prevent pregnancy, STDs, and sexual violence. Includes a family component to create stronger support for students and encourages healthy decision-making through education and choice.
Green Dot https://alteristic.org/green-dot-institute/	A prevention program to increase positive bystander behavior, change social norms, and reduce sexual and other forms of interpersonal violence perpetration and victimization.
Violence Prevention Works (Respect Works) https://www.violencepreventionworks.org/public/respect_works.page	*Speak.Act.Change*: A 10-session service-learning kit that promotes positive youth development. *Ending Violence*: A 3-session curriculum that focuses on dating violence prevention from a law and justice perspective. Curriculum includes bystander intervention and skills to build healthy relationships. Spanish-language version available. *School Policy Kit*: Supports the process of creating policies and protocols to meet the concerns of teen dating violence.

Take-Home Messages

There are several take-home messages for school personnel when working with teens, based upon this literature review and the personal experiences of the authors. The first take-home message is the well-documented fact that teen dating violence (TDV) is a major factor in the lives of middle school and high school students. According to the CDC (2019a), 26% of females and 15% of males report sexual, physical, or stalking violence between the ages of 11 and 17 years. Youth of color and teens who are of gender minority are at the highest risk for sexual dating violence according to the 2018 CDC Youth Risk Behavior Survey. Many adolescents report psychological abuse in dating relationships, and one in four high school students report being a victim to digital dating violence and even more (29–46%) admit to being digital/electronic perpetrators. These numbers are most likely underestimations as teens turn to teens to discuss the issues, thus the numbers are not in data banks. Thus, it is important to know that teen dating violence is real and it would be irresponsible to not acknowledge it as such.

The second take-home message is that girls are just as likely to engage in teen violence as boys. While girls are most often characterized as being victims and males as perpetrators, that is not always the case. It is noteworthy that girls ages 15–18 years report the highest level of sexual victimization and boys ages 12–15 years report the highest level of physical relationship abuse victimization by girls. It appears that young girls perpetrate physical relationship abuse when they are in middle and early high school and then are at high risk for sexual victimization later in adolescence.

The third take-home message speaks to the significant overlap of victimization and perpetration. It is noteworthy that there is a significant overlap between victimization and perpetration in that the majority of perpetrators were also at one time victims (Moore et al., 2015). Overall, violence toward girls is substantial, same-sex violence is prevalent, and girls being violent toward boys is significant (Levine, 2017). Clearly, the traditional thought that only males are the aggressors is not bore out in the literature.

The fourth take-home message is that there are factors that seem predictive of teen dating violence including home exposure to intimate partner violence, being the victim of sexual abuse or maltreatment as a child, alcohol use, aggressive neighborhood climate, level of parent education, lower family SES, larger school sizes and the perceived lack of safety and support of school personnel. Issues associated with entrenched racism and poverty cannot be overlooked as contributing to youth engaging in or allowing dating violence into their lives. Taquette and Monteiro (2019) suggest that positive family relationships with strong gender equality messages are protective factors regarding the development of teen dating violence. Taylor et al. (2017) support this finding by indicating the greater the quality of the parent–child relationship, as viewed by the teen, the less the likelihood of teen dating violence of any kind.

Next, the adverse impact of teen dating violence is significant and long-lasting. Mental health issues include increased levels of anxiety, depression and other mood disorders, posttraumatic stress, suicidal and homicidal actions, low self-esteem, eating disorders, substance abuse, and increased levels of adult relationship aggression. Physical health issues include unplanned pregnancies, weight management issues, sleep issues, STDs, and increased levels of high-risk sexual behavior.

Last, it is important to note that school is the only agency that reaches all children and can play a strategic role in teaching healthy, safe dating behaviors. It is so interesting, as it relates to school, that 20% of teens with D's and F's have engaged in dating violence, while only 6% of those with A's have done so. Thus, helping students connect with and do well in school may well be a protective factor. Additionally, it is remarkable that 50% of those who report teen dating violence indicate the abuse took place on school grounds. Teens are social creatures, so often there is an audience for adolescent teen dating violence and the bystander research indicates that if you see something, you say something. Teens will talk to each other very often before they utilize other resources. It is important to educate students so they can help their friends (Henry & Zeytinoglu, 2012). There is an opportunity for schools to teach children what to do if they see someone hurting someone or being hurt.

Twenty-three states now allow, urge, or require schools to include information in the curriculum about teen dating violence. The Multi-Tiered System of Supports (MTSS) allows targeted interventions in schools, as issues arise, through the Response to Intervention Framework utilizing Positive Behavior Interventions and Supports (PBIS), schoolwide discipline plans, social-emotional learning initiatives, and trauma-informed care plans. There are several suggested programs with promise such as those from the CDC; the Collaborative for Academic, Social, and Emotional Learning (CASEL); Blueprints for Healthy Youth Development; the National Association of School Psychologists; the American School Counselor Association; and the School Social Work Association of America. There are barriers to providing support to teens adversely impacted by school dating violence. School personnel are typically not schooled in how to screen and respond to teen victims or perpetrators, many teens feel stigmatized and seek support from peers rather than adults, and adults at school may not even view teen dating violence as a major health issue. Training for school mental health personnel is generally lacking and data are not consistently reported.

In summary, it is clear that teen dating violence is not revealed in a nice homogenous package. While some factors increase the likelihood of teen dating violence (e.g., such as exposure to violence in the home, personal history of abuse, substance use, poor school or neighborhood context), all adolescents are adversely impacted if they are involved with dating violence, regardless of their gender identification, race, or economic status. It is important for school personnel and other adults to consider teen dating violence as a hypothesis when working with adolescents who are struggling academically and/or behaviorally and provide support, counseling, and safety planning as needed (Henry & Zeytinoglu, 2012). Students who are connected and valued by the school personnel, their families, and their peers will engage in less violent behavior. If students cannot connect and there are signs of consistent behavioral dysregulation, then accessing mental health care for them may well be necessary. A systematic, collaborative and strategic effort between schools and families shows promise in helping teens navigate the world of online and offline dating.

We do not have to be stuck in the framework of the past, ignoring the issues of teen dating violence. There are training programs available for providers, there is research to be understood, there are barriers to be overcome and there are prevention and intervention programs that show promise. Teen dating violence impacts not only the youth in our schools but also parents, caregivers, school personnel, friends, and the community at large. We can do harm by not treating teen dating violence as a major health issue, raising awareness and promoting healthy dating relationships among adolescents.

Bibliography

Ackard, D. M., Eisenberg, M. E., & Neumark-Sztainer, D. (2007). Long-term impact of adolescent dating violence on the behavioral and psychological health of male and female youth. *The Journal of Pediatrics, 15*(5), 476–481.

Ackard, D. M., & Neumrk-Sztainer, D. (2002). Date violence and date rape among adolescents: Associations with disordered eating behaviors and psychological health. *Child Abuse and Neglect, 26*, 455–473.

Ackard, D. M., Neumrk-Sztainer, D., & Hannan, P. (2003). Dating violence among a nationally representative sample of adolescent girls and boys: Associations with behavioral and mental health. *The Journal of Gender-Specific Medicine, 6*(3), 39–48.

Ayers, J., & Davies, S. (2011). Adolescent dating and intimate relationship violence: Issues and implications for school psychologist. *School Psychology Forum, 5*(1), 1–12.

Ball, B., Kerig, P. K., & Rosenbluth, B. (2009). "Like a family but better because you can actually trust each other": The expect respect dating violence prevention program for at-risk youth. *Health Promotion Practice, 10*, 45S–58S.

Berkowitz, A. D. (2010). Fostering healthy norms to prevent violence and abuse: The social norms approach. In K. Kaufman (Ed.), *The prevention of sexual violence: A practitioner's sourcebook* (pp. 147–171). NEARI Press.

Black, B. M., Chido, L. M., Preble, K. M., Weisz, A. N., Yoon, J. S., Delaney-Black, V., Kernsmith, P., & Lewandowski, L. (2015). Violence exposure and teen dating violence among African American youth. *Journal of Interpersonal Violence, 30*(12), 2174–2195.

Bonds, M., & Stoker, S. (2000). *Bully proofing your school* (p. 29). Sopris West, Inc.

Bradshaw, C. P., Pas, E. T., Debnam, K. J., & Lindstrom Johnson, S. (2015). A focus on implementation of Positive Behavioral Interventions and Supports (PBIS) in high schools: Associations with bullying and other indicators of school disorder. *School Psychology Review, 44*(4), 480–498. https://doi.org/10.17105/spr-15-0105.1

Breiding, M. J. (2014, September 5). Prevalence and characteristics of sexual violence, stalking and intimate partner violence victimization – National Intimate Partner and Sexual Violence Survey, US, 2011. *HHS Public Access MMWR Surveillance Summary, 63*(8), 1–18.

Brock, S. E., Nickerson, A. B., Louvar Reeves, M. A., Conolly, C. N., Jimerson, S. R., Pesce, R. C., & Lazzaro, B. R. (2016). *School crisis prevention and intervention: The PREPaRE model* (2nd ed.). National Association of School Psychologists.

Burns, M. K., Kanive, R., & Karich, A. C. (2014). Best practices implementing schoolbased teams within a multitiered system of support. In P. L. Harrison & A. Thomas (Eds.), *Best practices in school psychology*. Bethesda, MD.

Cascardi, M., & Jouriles, E. N. (2018). A study space analysis and narrative review of the trauma-informed mediators of dating violence. *Trauma, Violence and Abuse, 19*(3), 268–285.

CDC. (2006). Physical dating violence among high school students – United States, 2003. *MMWR, 55*(19);532–535. https://www.cdc.gov/mmwr/preview/mmwrhtml/mm5519a3.htm. Retrieved September, 2011.

CDC. (2018). *Youth risk behavior survey: Data summary and trends report 2007–2017*. https://www.cdc.gov/healthyyouth/data/yrbs/pdf/trendsreport.pdf

CDC. (2019a). *Preventing teen dating violence [Fact Sheet]*. https://www.cdc.gov/violenceprevention/pdf/tdv-factsheet.pdf. Retrieved April, 2022.

CDC. (2019b). *Dating matters toolkit: Strategies to promote healthy teen relationships.* https://vetoviolence.cdc.gov/apps/dating-matters-toolkit/. Retrieved April, 2022.

CDC. (2022). *Fast facts: Preventing teen dating violence.* https://www.cdc.gov/violenceprevention/intimatepartnerviolence/teendatingviolence/fastfact.html. Retrieved April, 2022.

Cha, S., Ihongbe, T. O., & Masho, S. W. (2016). Racial and gender differences in dating violence victimization and disordered eating among US high schools. *Journal of Women's Health, 25*(8), 791–800.

Chiodo, D., Crooks, C. V., Wolfe, D. A., McIsaac, C., Hughes, R., & Jaffe, P. G. (2012). Longitudinal prediction and concurrent functioning of adolescent girls demonstrating different profiles of dating violence and victimization. *Prevention Science, 13*, 350–359.

Cohen, J. R., Shorey, R. C., Menon, S. V., & Temple, J. (2018). Predicting teen dating violence perpetration. *Pediatrics, 141*(4), e20172790. https://doi.org/10.1542/peds.2017-2790

Cowan, K. C., Vaillancourt, K., Rossen, E., & Pollitt, K. (2013). *A framework for safe and successful schools [Brief].* National Association of School Psychologists.

Cutbush, S., Williams, J., & Miller, S. (2016). Teen dating violence, sexual harassment, and bullying among middle school students: Examining mediation and moderated mediation by gender. *Prevention Science, 17*, 1024–1033.

Dardis, C. M., Dixon, K. J., Edwards, K. M., & Turchik, J. A. (2015). An examination of the factors related to dating violence perpetration among young men and women and associated theoretical explanations: A review of the literature. *Trauma, Violence and Abuse, 16*(2), 136–152.

Debnam, K. J., Waasdorp, T. E., & Bradshaw, C. P. (2016). Examining the contemporaneous occurrence of bullying and teen dating violence victimization. *School Psychology Quarterly, 31*(1), 76–90.

Decker, M. R., Peitxmeier, S., Olumide, A., Acharya, R., Ojengbede, O., Coarrurubias, L., Gao, E., Cheng, Y., Delany-Moretlwe, S., & Brahmbhatt, H. (2014). Prevalence and health impact of intimate partner violence and non-partner sexual violence among female adolescents aged 15-19 years in vulnerable urban environments: A multi-country study. *Journal of Adolescent Health, 55*, S58–S67.

Dimissie, Z., Clayton, H. B., Vivolo-Kantor, A. M., & Estefan, L. F. (2018). Sexual teen dating violence victimization: Associations with sexual risk behaviors among US high school students. *Violence and Victims, 33*(5), 964–980.

Durlak, J. A., Weissberg, R. P., Dymnicki, A. B., Taylor, R. D., & Schellinger, K. B. (2011). The impact of enhancing students' social and emotional learning: A meta-analysis of school-based universal interventions. *Child Development, 82*, 405–432.

Eaton, D. K., Davis, K. S., Barrios, L., Brener, N. D., & Noonan, R. K. (2007). Associations of dating violence victimization with lifetime participation, co-occurrence, and early initiation of risk behaviors among U.S. high school students. *Journal of Interpersonal Violence, 22*(5), 585–602. https://doi.org/10.1177/0886260506298831

Fawson, P. R., Jones, T., & Younce, B. (2017). Teen dating violence: Predicting physical and sexual violence and mental health symptoms among heterosexual adolescent males. *Violence and Victims, 12*(5), 886–896.

Follingstad, D. R., & Ryan, K. M. (2013). Contemporary issues in the measurement of partner violence. *Sex Roles, 69*(3–4), 115–119.

Foshee, V., & Langwick, S. (2010). *SAFE dates: An adolescent dating violence prevention curriculum* (2nd ed.). Hazelden Foundation.

Foshee, V. A., Bauman, K. E., Ennett, S. T., Linder, G. F., Benefield, T., & Suchindran, C. (2004a). Assessing the long-term effects of the safe dates program and a booster in preventing and reducing adolescent dating violence victimization and perpetration. *American Journal of Public Health, 94*, 619–624. https://doi.org/10.2105/AJPH.94.4.619

Foshee, V. A., Benefield, T. S., Ennett, S. T., Bauman, K. E., & Suchindran, S. (2004b). Longitudinal predictors of serious physical and sexual dating violence victimization during adolescence. *Preventive Medicine, 39*, 1007–1016.

Foshee, V. A., Reyes, L. M., Tharp, A. T., Chang, L.-Y., Ennett, S. T., Simon, T. R., Latzman, N. E., & Suchindran, C. (2015). Shared longitudinal predictors of physical peer and dating violence. *Journal of Adolescent Health, 56*, 106–112.

Foshee, V. A., Reyes, H. L. M., Chen, M. S., Ennett, S. T., Basile, K. C., DeGue, S., Vivolo-Kantor, A. M., Moracco, K. E., & Bowling, J. M. (2016). Shared risk factors for the perpetuation of physical dating violence, bullying, and sexual harassment among adolescents exposed to domestic violence. *Journal of Youth and Adolescence, 45*, 672–686.

Fredland, N. M., Ricardo, I. B., Capbell, J. C., Sharps, P. W., Kub, J. K., & Yonas, M. (2005). The meaning of dating violence in the lives of middle school adolescents: A report of a focus group study. *Journal of School Violence, 4*, 95–114.

Fuchs, D., Fuchs, L. S., & Compton, D. L. (2012). Smart RTI: A next-generation approach to multilevel prevention. *Exceptional Children, 78*(3), 263–279. https://doi.org/10.1177/001440291207800301

Giordano, P. C., Soto, D. A., Manning, W. D., & Longmore, M. A. (2010). The characteristics of romantic relationships associated with teen violence. *Social Science Research, 39*, 863–874.

Goldman, A. W., Mulford, C. F., & Blachman-Demner, D. R. (2016). Advancing our approach to teen dating violence: A youth and professional defined framework of teen dating relationships. *Psychology of Violence, 6*(4), 497–508.

Gomez, A. M. (2011). Testing the cycle of violence hypothesis: Child abuse and adolescent dating violence as predictors of intimate partner violence in young adulthood. *Youth and Society, 43*, 171–192. https://doi.org/10.1177/0044118X09358313

Halpern, C. T., Oslak, S. G., Young, M. L., Martin, S. L., & Kupper, L. L. (2001). Partner violence among adolescents in opposite sex romantic relationships: Findings from the national longitudinal study of adolescent health. *American Journal of Public Health, 91*(10), 1679–1685.

Haselschwerdt, M. C., Savasak-Luxton, R., & Hlavaty, K. (2019). A methodological review and critique of the "intergenerational transmission of violence" literature. *Trauma Violence and Abuse, 20*(2), 168–182.

Henry, R. R., & Zeytinoglu, S. (2012). African Americans and teen dating violence. *The American Journal of Family Therapy, 40*, 20–22.

Horner, R. H., & Sugai, G. (2015). School-wide PBIS: An example of applied behavior analysis implemented at a scale of social importance. *Behavior Analysis in Practice, 8*(1), 80–85. https://doi.org/10.1007/s40617-015-0045-4

Hoss, L., Toews, M. L., Perez-Brena, N., Goodcase, E., & Feinberg, M. (2019). Parental factors as predictors of dating violence among latinx adolescent mothers. *Journal of Interpersonal Violence*, 1–18.

Howard, D. E., Wang, M. Q., & Yan, F. (2007). Psychosocial factors associated with reports of physical dating violence among U.S. adolescent females. *Adolescence, 42*(166), 311–324.

Johnson, R. M., LaValley, M., Shneider, K. E., Musci, R. J., Pettoruto, K., & Rothman, E. F. (2017). Marijuana use and physical dating violence among adolescents and emerging adults: A systematic review and meta-analysis. *Drug and Alcohol Dependence, 174*, 47–57.

Karlsson, M. E., Temple, J. R., Weston, R., & Le, V. D. (2016). Witnessing interparental violence and acceptance of dating violence as predictors for teen dating violence victimization. *Violence Against Women, 22*(5), 625–646.

Latzman, N. E., Vivolo-Kantor, A. M., Niolon, P. H., & Ghazarian, S. R. (2015). Predicting adolescent dating violence perpetration: Role of exposure to intimate partner violence and parenting practices. *American Journal of Preventive Medicine, 49*(3), 476–482.

Latzman, N. E., D'Inverno, A. S., Niolon, P. H., & Reidy, D. E. (2018). *Gender inequality and gender based violence* (pp. 283–314). ISBN 9780128117972.

Levine, E. (2017). Sexual violence among middle school students: The effects of gender and dating experience. *Journal of Interpersonal Violence, 32*(4), 2059–2082.

Lormand, D. K., Markham, C. M., Pekin, M. F., Buryd, T. L., Addy, R. C., Baumler, E., & Tortolero, S. R. (2013). Dating violence among urban minority middle school youth and associated sexual risk behavior and substance use. *Journal of Adolescent School Health, 83*(6), 415–421.

Ludin, S., Bottiani, J. H., Debnam, K., Orozco Solis, M. G., & Bradshaw, C. P. (2018). A cross-national comparison of risk factors for teen dating violence in Mexico and the United States. *Journal of Youth and Adolescence, 47*, 547–559.

Mahoney, M. (2020). Implementing evidence-based practices within multi-tiered systems of support to promote inclusive secondary classroom settings. *The Journal of Special Education Apprenticeship, 9*(1), 1–12.

McCurdy, B., Thomas, L., Truckenmiller, A., Rich, S., Hillis-Clark, P., & Lopez, J. C. (2016). School-wide positive behavioral interventions and supports for students with emotional and behavioral disorders. *Psychology in the Schools, 53*(4), 375–389.

Miller, E., Jones, K. A., & McCauley, H. L. (2018). Updates on adolescent dating and sexual violence prevention and intervention. *Current Opinion in Pediatrics, 30*(4), 466–471. https://doi.org/10.1097/MOP.0000000000000637

Miller, E., Jones, K. A., Ripper, L., Paglisotti, T., Mulbah, P., & Abebe, K. Z. (2020). An athletic coach-delivered middle school gender violence prevention program: A cluster randomized clinical trial. *Journal of the American Medical Association Pediatrics, 174*(3), 241–249. Advance online publication. https://doi.org/10.1001/jamapediatrics.2019.5217

Moore, A., Sargenton, K. M., Ferranti, D., & Gonzaea-Guarda, R. M. (2015). Adolescent dating violence: Supports and barriers in accessing services. *Journal of Community Health Nursing, 32*, 39–52.

Mumford, E. A., Liu, W., & Taylor, B. G. (2016). Parenting profiles and adolescent dating relationship abuse: Attitudes and experiences. *Journal of Youth and Adolescence, 45*(5), 959–972.

National Association of School Psychologists. (2015). *Dating violence: Prevalence, risk factors, consequences, and prevention. [Research summary]*. Author.

National Association of School Psychologists. (2018). *Framework for safe and successful schools: Considerations and action steps [Brief]*. National Association of School Psychologists.

Niolon, P. H., Kupermine, G. P., & Allen, J. P. (2015a). Autonomy and relatedness in mother-teen interactions as predictors of involvement in adolescent dating aggression. *Psychology of Violence, 5*(2), 133–143.

Niolon, P. H., Vivolo-Kantor, A., Latzman, N. E., Valle, L. A., Burton, T., Kuoh, H., Taylor, B., & Tharp, A. T. (2015b). Prevalence of teen dating violence and co-occurring risk factors among middle school youth in high risk urban communities. *Journal of Adolescent Health, 56*, S5–S13.

Niolon, P. H., Taylor, B. G., Latzman, N. E., Vivolo-Kantor, A. M., Valle, L. A., & Tharp, A. T. (2016). Lessons learned in evaluating a multisite, comprehensive teen dating violence prevention strategy: Design and challenges of the evaluation of dating matters: Strategies to promote healthy teen relationships. *Psychology of Violence, 6*(3), 452.

Niolon, P. H., Kearns, M., Dills, J., Rambo, K., Irving, S., Armstead, T., & Gilbert, L. (2017). *Preventing intimate partner violence across the lifespan: A technical package of programs, policies, and practices*. National Center for Injury Prevention and Control, Centers for Disease Control and Prevention. https://www.cdc.gov/violenceprevention/intimatepartnerviolence/prevention.html

Niolon, P. H., Vivolo-Kantor, A. M., Tracy, A. J., Latzman, N. E., Little, T. D., DeGue, S., Lang, K. M., Estefan, L. F., Ghazarian, S. R., McIntosh, W., Taylor, B., Johnson, L. L., Kuoh, H., Burton, T., Fortson, B., Mumford, E. A., Nelson, S. C., Joseph, H., Valle, L. A., & Tharp, A. T. (2019). An RCT of dating matters: Effects on teen dating violence and relationship behaviors. *American Journal of Preventive Medicine, 57*(1), 13–23. https://doi.org/10.1016/j.amepre.2019.02.022

Ohio Domestic Violence Network (ODVN). (2012). *Teen relationship violence: A resource guide for increasing safety*. https://www.odvn.org/wp-content/uploads/2020/05/Teen_Relationship_Resource_Guide_2012_Revised.pdf. Retrieved April, 2022.

Parker, E. M., Debnam, K., Pas, E. T., & Bradshaw, C. P. (2016). Exploring the link between alcohol and marijuana use and teen dating violence victimization among high school students: The influence of school context. *Health Education and Behavior, 43*(5), 528–536.

Parker, E. M., Johnson, S. L., Debnam, K. J., & Bradshaw, C. P. (2017). Teen dating violence among high school students: A multilevel analysis of school-level risk factors. *Journal of School Health, 87*(9), 696–704.

Peskin, M. F., Markham, C. M., Shegog, R., Baumler, E. R., Addy, R. C., Temple, J. R., Hernandez, B., Cuccaro, P. M., Thiel, M. A., Gabay, E. K., & Tortolero Emery, S. R. (2019). Adolescent dating violence prevention program for early adolescents: The me & you randomized controlled trial, 2014–2015. *American Journal of Public Health, 109*(10), 1419–1428. https://doi.org/10.2105/AJPH.2019.305218

Peterson, K., Sharps, P., Banyard, V., Powers, R., Kaukinen, C., Gross, D., Decker, M., Baatz, C., & Campbell, J. (2018). An evaluation of two dating violence prevention programs on a college campus. *Journal of Interpersonal Violence, 33*(23), 3630–3655.

Reed, L. A., Ward, L. M., Tolman, R. M., Lippman, J. R., & Seabrook, R. C. (2018). The association between stereotypical gender and dating beliefs and digital dating abuse perpetration in adolescent dating relationships. *Journal of Interpersonal Violence*, 1–25.

Reyes, H. L. M., Foshee, V. A., Niolon, P. H., Reidy, D. E., & Hall, J. E. (2016). Gender role attitudes and male adolescent dating violence perpetration: Normative beliefs as moderators. *Journal of Youth and Adolescence, 45*, 350–360.

Reyes, H. L. M., Foshee, V. A., Chen, M. S., & Ennett, S. T. (2017). Patterns of dating violence victimization and perpetration among Latino youth. *Journal of Youth and Adolescence, 46*, 1727–1742.

Reyes, H. L. M., Foshee, V. A., Markiewitz, N., Chen, M. S., & Ennett, S. T. (2018). Contextual risk profiles and trajectories of adolescent dating violence. *Prevention Science, 19*, 997–1007.

Sears, H. A., Byers, E. S., & Price, E. L. (2007). The co-occurrence of adolescent boys' and girls' use of psychologically, physically, and sexually abusive behaviours in their dating relationships. *Journal of Adolescence, 30*(3), 487–504.

Shamu, S., Gevers, A., Mahlangu, B. P., Jama Shai, P. N., Chirwa, E. D., & Jewkws, R. (2016). Prevalence and risk factors for intimate partner violence among grade 8 learners in urban South Africa: Baseline analysis from the Skhokho Supporting Success cluster randomized controlled trial. *International Health, 8*, 18–26.

Sianko, N., Kunkel, D., Thompson, M. P., Small, M. A., & McDonell, J. R. (2019). Trajectories of dating violence victimization and perpetration among rural adolescents. *Journal of Youth and Adolescence, 48*(12), 2360–2376. https://doi.org/10.1007/s10964-019-01132-w

Silverman, J. G., Raj, A., & Clements, K. (2004). Dating violence and associated sexual risk and pregnancies among adolescent girls in the United States. *Pediatrics, 114*, 220–225.

Smith, J., Mulford, C., Latzman, N. E., Tharp, A. T., Niolon, P. H., & Balckman-Demner, D. (2015). Taking stock of behavioral measures of adolescent dating violence. *Journal of Aggressive Maltreatment and Trauma, 24*(5), 674–692.

Sugai, G., & Horner, R. R. (2006). A promising approach for expanding and sustaining school-wide positive behavior support. *School Psychology Review, 35*(2), 245.

Surface, J., Stader, D., Graca, T., & Lowe, J. (2012). Adolescent dating violence: How should schools respond? *Journal of Inquiry and Action in Education, 4*(3), 27–43.

Sweeten, G., Larson, M., & Piquero, A. R. (2016). Predictors of emotional and physical dating violence in a sample of serious juvenile offenders. *Criminal Behavior and Mental Health, 26*, 263–277.

Tapp, J., & Moore, E. (2016). Risk assessments for dating violence in mid to late adolescence and early adulthood. *Criminal Behavior and Mental Health, 26*, 278–292.

Taquette, S. R., & Monteiro, D. L. M. (2019). Causes and consequences of adolescent dating violence: A systematic review. *Journal of Injury and Violence, 11*(2), 137–147.

Taylor, B., & Mumford, E. A. (2016). A national descriptive portrait of adolescent relationship abuse: Results from the national survey on teen relationships and intimate violence. *Journal of Interpersonal Violence, 31*(6), 963–988.

Taylor, B., Joseph, H., & Mumford, E. (2017). Romantic relationship characteristics and adolescent relationship abuse in a probability-based sample of youth. *Journal of Interpersonal Violence*, 1–29.

Thurston, I. B., & Howell, K. H. (2018). To screen or not to screen: Overreliance on risk without protective factors in violence research. *Pediatrics, 141*(4), e20180075.

US Department of Education. (2013). *Teen dating violence in the United States: A fact sheet for schools.* Retrieved July 27, 2020, from https://www2.ed.gov/about/offices/list/oese/oshs/teendatingviolence-factsheet.html

Vivolo-Kantor, A. M., Niolon, P. H., Estefan, L. F., Tracy, A. J., Latzman, N., Little, T. D., DeGue, S., Lang, K. M., & Le, V. D. (2019). Middle school effects of the Dating Matters® comprehensive approach on peer violence, bullying, and cyber-bullying: A cluster-randomized controlled trial. *Prevention Science*, advance online publication.

West, C. M., & Rose, S. (2000). Dating aggression among low income African American youth. *Violence Against Women, 6,* 470–494.

Whitten, E., Esteves, K. J., & Woodrow, A. (2019). *RTI success: Proven tools and strategies for schools and classrooms – updated and revised.* Free Spirit Publishing Inc.

Chapter 11
School Shootings and Clinical Management: Directions Toward Prevention

Thomas W. Miller

Introduction

Over the past decade, the Gun Violence Archive (2020), an online archive of gun violence incidents collected from over 7500 law enforcement, media, government, and commercial sources daily in an effort to provide near real-time data about the results of gun violence, reports that nearly 180 American schools experienced some form of school-related shooting. The Gun Violence Archive (2020) examined school shootings on K-12 campuses and found two sobering findings that school shootings are increasing, and that no type of community can feel safe in the light of vulnerable children under stress, the difficulties in gaining access to mental health services for children and families in need, the level of bullying in communities, and the availability of guns. This chapter examines theoretical considerations involving escape theory, the risk and protective factors for school violence, and case analyses of studies and discusses school shootings with fatal injuries involving others. Identifying at-risk and high-risk students is essential as a part of prevention of school violence. This chapter also examines clinical issues in understanding children who are at risk for committing lethal acts of violence in the school setting. Suggestions and recommendations, including recommendations provided by the National School Safety Center (2002) for school personnel, as well as steps to be taken in creating a safe school environment, are offered. A report on indicators of school crime and safety as reported by Irwin et al. (2021) provides the most recent data from a variety of sources, including national surveys of students, teachers, principals, and

T. W. Miller (✉)
Department of Psychiatry, College of Medicine, Department of Gerontology, College of Public Health, University of Kentucky, Lexington, KY, USA

Institute for Collaboration on Health, Intervention, and Policy, University of Connecticut, Storrs, CT, USA
e-mail: tom.miller@uconn.edu

T. W. Miller (ed.), *School Violence and Primary Prevention*,
https://doi.org/10.1007/978-3-031-13134-9_11

post-secondary institutions. Results noted that students of ages 12–18 years experienced 764,600 victimizations at school and 509,300 victimizations away from the school setting. Bullying-related incidents are sometimes a precursor to more serious forms of violence. In addition, about 22% of students of ages 12–18 years reported being bullied at school during the school year in 2019 (Irwin et al., 2021). The researchers found that "between 2009 and 2019, the percentage of students in grades 9–12 who reported carrying a weapon anywhere during the previous 30 days decreased (from 17% to 13%), as did the percentage of students who reported carrying a weapon on school property (decreased from 6% to 3%)" (Irwin et al., 2021). Realizing there are gradients and multiple forms of violence, these researchers further noted that the data revealed that in the 2019–2020 school year, "there were a total of 75 school shootings with casualties, including 27 school shootings with deaths and 48 school shootings with injuries only. In addition, there were 37 reported school shootings with no casualties in 2019–2020" (Irwin et al., 2021).

The intent of the chapter is to provide a current picture of the nature and information with respect to school-related shootings. In doing so these trends may be useful in the development of models for prevention intervention, beneficial to educational, medical, and healthcare professionals; law enforcement personnel; and school boards that oversee administratively and provide services to school-aged children. Since the school shooting at Sandy Hook Elementary School in 2012, the Gun Violence Archive (2020) reports that more than 400 children and school personnel have been victims in over 200 reported school shootings in the United States. More than 100 of these people were killed. This Sandy Hook Elementary School shooting gained worldwide attention and concern. These tragedies are as diverse as the United States, but the depth of trauma is hard to conceptualize. There is no standard definition for what qualifies as a school shooting in the United States nor is there a universally accepted database. Legislators have an important role in working with educators, teachers, and parents to address gun violence in the United States.

Congressional Efforts to Address School Violence

Efforts to address the challenges of school violence involving guns and school shootings have gained the attention of school administrators, teachers, parents, and legislators. The efforts of Nicole Hockley and Mark Barden with the Sandy Hook Promise (see Chap. 28) have been embraced by legislators with the EAGLES Act legislation. More specifically, the EAGLES Act (2021) is a legislation that would provide statutory authority for the National Threat Assessment Center (NTAC) within the US Department of Homeland Security to (1) identify individuals who are exhibiting pre-attack behavior; (2) assess whether the individual poses a threat; and (3) manage the threat. The NTAC was established in 1998 by the US Secret Service to conduct research on various types of targeted violence, including school shootings. Through its research, the NTAC found that most school shooters exhibited indicators of pre-attack behavior.

Access to guns and lethal weapons continues to be a serious problem with no federal legislation that closes the loopholes with respect to the sale of guns. Federal law only requires background checks when the gun salesperson is a licensed dealer. It fails to include unlicensed private sellers, providing access for online sales and at gun shows. These individuals are not required to perform background checks on the people to whom they sell guns and other lethal weapons. Congressional leaders need to address this issue and provide the passage of legislation requiring background checks that eliminate gun access to prohibited individuals. Lawmakers have passed legislation in some twenty states to date that require some form of check and monitoring. Much more needs to be done by lawmakers at the Federal level in providing legislation that would be standardized throughout the United States for the safety and security of children, school personnel, and communities.

This legislation would authorize the functions of the NTAC and expand their scope of practice to include the establishment of a national program on targeted school violence prevention. The Senate companion bill was introduced in 2018 by Senators Chuck Grassley (R-IA), Catherine Cortez Masto (D-Nev.), Marco Rubio (R-Fla.), Joe Manchin (D-W.Va.), Rick Scott (R-Fla.), Maggie Hassan (D-N.H.), and Susan Collins (R-ME.) who continue to need more support from fellow colleagues in both the House and the Senate of the United States Congress. Sen. Collins joined a bipartisan, bicameral group of lawmakers to reintroduce the EAGLES Act in 2021. As the bipartisan legislative initiative has gained support through the EAGLES Act of 2021, S. 391, NTAC's threat assessment operations have focused specifically on school safety.

This legislation, the EAGLES Act, which lawmakers have failed to pass in previous years, is named in honor of the mascot of Marjory Stoneman Douglas High School, where 14 students and 3 staff were killed during the February 2018 mass shooting. The legislation is inspired by the belief that no child should feel unsafe in the classroom, and it is imperative that legislators and law enforcement fully support such legislative action to ensure that schools are a safe learning environment for students, teachers, and staff. If this legislation were to be enacted, the act would expand the U.S. Secret Service's NTAC role and function in school violence prevention nationally, emphasizing the importance of "threat assessment."

Theory Applied to School Violence

Consider the contribution of escape theory (Baumeister, 1990; Heatherton & Baumeister, 1991), which postulates that peer victimization or bullying is driven by the desire to escape a state of painful self-awareness, characterized by inadequacy, negative affect, and low self-esteem. The emotions associated with this state of self-awareness are focused on the self-perceived failure to achieve acceptance among peers and are often based on rigid self-standards. According to the theory, certain individuals attempt to escape these negative self-perceptions and emotions by narrowing their consciousness to an immediate action, like bullying, which results in irrational cognitions that predominate over normal inhibitions against self-destructive behaviors. The psychological profile for bullies characterizes people who engage in escape behaviors. According to escape theory, the personality characteristics of bullies which predispose them to episodes of negative self-perceptions result in low self-esteem and high levels of self-awareness.

These risk factors set the stage for frequent episodes of acting out against others in the form of bullying accompanied by irrational thoughts which, in turn, activate the desire to escape. Frequent repetitions of this cycle create high levels of residual negative affect and irrational thinking. Children and adolescents who engage in escape behaviors on a regular basis tend to display more negative affect, irrational thinking, negative self-awareness, unrealistically high self-standards, and low self-esteem. This profile distinguishes both binge eaters and those with suicidal thoughts from normalcy. While there is a dearth of empirical research that has been done investigating escape theory and bullying behavior, there is reason to believe that escape theory has applicability to perpetrator motives in some school violence situations. Studies that have investigated aspects of escape theory have examined differing constellations of variables, with mixed findings (Beebe et al., 1995). While escape theory does not address how different "escape behaviors" emerge, it does aid in understanding risk factors that school personnel must be alert to in the school environment and that may result in violent behaviors.

The National School Safety Center (2019) offers a checklist (http://www.school-safety.us/media-resources/checklist-of-characteristics-of-youth-who-have-caused-school-associated-violent-deaths) derived from tracking school-associated violent deaths in the United States. After studying common characteristics of youngsters who have caused such deaths, the National School Safety Center has identified several behaviors which could indicate a youth's potential for harming himself/herself or others. Often present are a history of uncontrollable anger, name calling, and abusive language, resulting in serious disciplinary problems in school (National School Safety Center, 2002). The characteristics that emerge from the reported information can benefit educators, school administrators, teachers, and support staff in addressing the needs of children and adolescents confronted with various forms of harassment and abuse. More specifically this may be addressed and implemented through designed parent–teacher conferences that outline and identify for parents the triggers that indicate potential for accentuating undesirable behavior and result in more lethal forms of violence. School safety and law enforcement, along with in-class teachers and aides; guidance and counseling staff; school healthcare professionals, including nurses, school psychologists, and social workers; and maintenance staff, need to be a part of efforts to address the implementation of prevention strategies with parents of perpetrators and victims within the aggravated gun-related violence realm. Threat assessments should be a regular part of prevention interventions as well as providing standardized education and training for parents and parental caregivers.

When it comes to assessing the potential for more lethal forms of violence, including the use of knives and guns and other threats of school-related violence, school administrators are advised to take the following steps in creating a safe learning environment:

- Develop a safety plan and implement the plan.
- Inspect the premises on a regular and predictable basis.
- Identify areas that individual schools are not controlling.
- Direct students to supervised areas when they arrive at school.
- Identify and conduct routine inspections of secluded areas.
- Monitor and inspect hallways and restrooms between classes.
- Document all incidents and complaints and report them to law enforcement.

Risk Factors in the School Environment

It is important to realize that several of the risk factors that emerge in the school environment are symptomatic of other problems, such as learning disabilities, emotional problems, or a temporary difficulty in the family's situation (Parker et al., 1995; Dean & Range, 1996; West et al., 1993). In addition, more serious symptoms may be caused by major problems associated with family dysfunction, domestic violence, or substance abuse (Miller, 1998; Puka, 1994). Some of the following risk factors in the school environment are symptomatic of problems experienced outside of school. In school, children and adolescents may behave aggressively or violently toward other students and teachers in the classroom or on the playground. They may use money as a means of winning other students' approval and acceptance. They may disrupt the classroom by failing to attend to the tasks of the class, to stay in their seats, respond appropriately to the teacher, and to participate in appropriate classroom behavior. These are students who may vandalize school property and classroom materials, make sexual gestures toward other students and teachers, or perform poorly in academic work, regularly scoring low on tests and consistently failing to complete classroom and homework assignments. Often these students spend free time with older students who behave aggressively in and out of the classroom and fail to show self-respect or respect for others.

The benefits of case studies and the methodology associated with this form of learning is that it allows the learner to identify and relate to practicalities of the illustration and the facts presented in the case. Furthermore, it allows the learner to relate to the thoughts and behaviors of both victims and perpetrators in stressful encounters and social situations, which can provide clarity for those seeking to better conceptualize the encounter between victim and perpetrator and problem-solve based on the behavioral patterns observed. When it comes to the potential for escalation, as, for example, with gun or lethal forms of violence, there are behavioral indicators that detect and predict escalating levels of violent behavior. It is critical that there is some level of monitoring internet and other online communications. This should also include emails, text messages, and social media, and consider the nature of the language used in expressing and processing what victims and perpetrators are feeling. It is not uncommon for victims or perpetrators to slowly reveal their thinking through plans and intentions. Teachers, administrators, and parents, along with other peers at school or siblings in the home, can recognize certain early warning signs. In some situations, and for some youth, different combinations of events, behaviors, and emotions may lead to aggressive actions, both verbally and non-verbally, and result in violent behavior toward themselves or others (Veltkamp & Miller, 1994).

Case Examples

Post-incident committees and school districts in Michigan, Kentucky, Arkansas, Florida, Connecticut, Oregon, Colorado, Virginia, and Texas have experienced a strikingly similar pattern of behavior among perpetrators, all in rural communities. What does emerge are demographic, interpersonal, and family factors that demonstrate consistency across incidents. Critical data have been collected on several cases and are summarized in a sequential fashion for the Kentucky, Arkansas, Connecticut, Florida, Oregon, Colorado, Virginia, Michigan, and Texas events. The subsequent observations of teachers, parents, professionals, and peers are summarized. In addressing some of the clinical factors, there are clinical indicators that observers need to attend to in each case.

Kentucky: Heath High School

In the West Paducah, Kentucky case, a 14-year-old stole a .22 caliber pistol from a neighbor. The perpetrator came from a sound home with both parents in the home and an older sister who was described as bright and socially well accepted by peers. On December 1, 1997, the perpetrator brought firearms in a blanket to the school and told security that it was part of a school project. In his backpack was a loaded .22-caliber pistol. He rode to school that morning with his sister. He fired multiple rounds at a group that included his sister and her friends meeting for prayer that morning. Three female students died and five other students were wounded.

Arkansas: Westside Middle School

The Jonesboro, Arkansas, case from March 24, 1998 involved two adolescents aged 11 and 13 years. In this case, three firearms were used, and they were stolen from relatives. One set of parents was divorced, the other intact and at home. The younger of the two perpetrators asked to be excused from his class, pulled a fire alarm, and joined the older boy outside the school in a wooded area 100 yards away from the school's gym. As the students responded to the alarm to vacate the school, both boys opened fire and killed four students, a teacher, and wounded ten other students.

Connecticut: Sandy Hook Elementary School

The Newton, Connecticut case concerns the Sandy Hook Elementary School. The perpetrator was 20-year-old Adam Lanza who was seen at the Yale Child Study Center for clinical referral several times but was non-compliant. On December 14, 2012, Lanza killed his mother at their home before fatally shooting 20 first graders, six adult employees, and then himself at the school.

Florida: Marjory Stoneman Douglas High School

On February 14, 2018, Nikolas Cruz, a student expelled from Marjory Stoneman Douglas High School in Parkland, Florida, opened fire at the school, killing 17 students and staff and wounding several other students. This school shooting event is the deadliest known gun violence incident at a high school in the United States. As a result of this school shooting, the governor appointed a commission to investigate the shooting and requested school districts across the state policy and procedures for the prevention of future incidents of this nature.

Oregon: Thurston High School

The Springfield, Oregon case involved a 15-year-old who used a semiautomatic and two pistols. He, like the perpetrator in the Heath High School shooting in Kentucky, was described as a loner. Both parents are in the home, and like the Kentucky case, there is a bright older sister. The perpetrator was scheduled to appear at an expulsion hearing the day before the shooting, when he murdered his parents. On May 21, 1998, the date of the school shooting, he fired on classmates in the cafeteria, killing two and wounding 25 others. A group of students was able to subdue the perpetrator, ending the shooting spree. He was arrested and eventually convicted, currently in prison for a term of 111 years without parole.

Colorado: Columbine High School

The Littleton, Colorado case considered the first mass school shooting in the United States at that time, involved two young men 17 and 18 years of age. Both are from parent homes and in one case a brother is a well-recognized athlete. Access to guns in this case involved friends who purchased the weapons. On April 20, 1999, the perpetrators, both seniors at the school, murdered twelve students and one teacher. Ten students were killed in the school library, where the pair subsequently committed suicide. Twenty-one students and staff were injured by the gunshots. Another three students and staff were injured in their attempt to escape the gunfire. In addition, the perpetrators fired on security staff and exchanged gunfire with the police.

Virginia: Virginia Tech

In the Virginia Tech case, Cho Seung-Hui, a 23-year-old senior English major from Centreville, Virginia, who had a history of mental illness, acted out against others because of anger and hostility that may have been the product of bullying and humiliation. He was taking medication to combat depression and his recent behavior was troubling, including setting a fire in a dormitory and stalking women on campus. His anger led to the wounding and killing of fellow students and teachers at Virginia Tech on April 16, 2007. Bullying again became a critical marker in mass school shootings in the United States (Espelage & Swearer, 2004; Boxer et al., 2005; Edwards et al., 2005).

Michigan: Oxford High School

In the Oxford Township, Michigan case, the 15-year-old perpetrator was a student at the school and a victim of bullying episodes by other classmates. Used in the shooting was a semiautomatic handgun that had been purchased for him by his parents. On November 30, 2021, the perpetrator shot and killed four fellow students while wounding seven others including a teacher. On the day prior to the shooting, there were rumors that indicated there was a threat of a potential school shooting. Based on those threats, some students chose not to attend school on that day. After his arrest, the perpetrator was charged as an adult with twenty-four crimes, including murder and terrorism. His parents were charged with involuntary manslaughter for failing to secure the weapon used in this incident. The perpetrator and his parents remain in custody without bail and the school district was the subject of legal allegations for failing to protect the safety of the children and staff of this high school in a suburb of Detroit, Michigan.

Texas: Robb Elementary School

The Uvalde, Texas school shooting case occurred at Robb Elementary School on May 24, 2022. The perpetrator was 18-year-old Salvador Rolando Ramos, who shot and killed 19 fourth-grade students and two teachers while injuring 17 others in less than 90 minutes. The perpetrator gained access to the school after shooting his grandmother at her home. An avid user of social media platforms, the gunman posted his interests and intent on social media. For his 18th birthday, he bought two AR-15 style weapons that were used in this school shooting. He held the children and two teachers' hostage, before succumbing to his own death by a tactical unit at the school.

Discussion of Cases

Risk factors identifying critical issues that heighten the potential for adverse behavior in the group of young men that acted out with lethal consequences are identified. In addition to the risk factor noted, the presence of a psychiatric disorder or symptoms consistent with a psychiatric disorder must be addressed. In addressing the psychiatric stability of each of the cases, there is reason to believe that there are psychiatric markers in each instance. The Kentucky teen has been described as depressed, with erratic fears, but had not received psychiatric treatment. He pleaded guilty and mentally ill at the time of his arraignment. The Arkansas youth was described as an aggressive, impulsive, and bully type of youngster, with his older counterpart being described as a tough and mean-spirited individual. The Springfield, Oregon, case has similarities to the Kentucky case in that this youngster was also described as depressed, was on Ritalin then Prozac. Most notable is the fact that this adolescent was described as a loner and was known to torture animals. In the Virginia Tech case, the perpetrator was described as having mental illness and was a person who showed symptoms from early childhood.

In the case of the Sandy Hook Elementary School shooting where 26 individuals were murdered after the perpetrator Adam Lanza shot and killed his mother at their home, of note is that he shared with peers his struggles with anxiety and depression and had a long history of non-compliance with seeking and maintaining contact with the psychiatric services offered to him. The Robb Elementary School shooting had communality with Sandy Hook in that the perpetrator had poor self-esteem and internalized anger over time, planned his initial strike against a parent figure in his life, used and was influenced by social media, and posted warning signals of his intentions. He then chose an elementary school child population, used an AR-15 weapon, and envisioned this form of violence as a desperate final "cry for help." In both of these instances, there were risk factors evident to others but failure to report and follow up with such risk factors contributed to these senseless acts.

The Michigan case that was cited is unique for several reasons, the most significant of which includes the fact that school officials were held responsible for negligence in failing to recognize and address evident warning signs exhibited by the perpetrator and resulted in this school shooting incident. Some of the warning signs included the loss of a friend, the death of his pet dog, drawings of school shootings that were drawn by the perpetrator, and text messages that his parents, as well as school officials, failed to address. It is also unique because this perpetrator, who was a minor at the time, was judged to be competent and charged as an adult for the murders of four fellow students and wounding six other students and a teacher at the school. There is yet another reason which makes this case unique, that is, his parents were arrested and held without bond in this case. Previous cases of school shootings in the United States have not seen parents directly held responsible for the acts of their child or adolescent in a school shooting.

There are well-researched protective factors that may buffer against the likelihood of acting-out behavior through gun violence. These protective factors may serve to reduce the chances of this level of activity and lethality in these situations. Perpetrators with self-esteem issues, limited anger management skills, or confusion brought on by a dysfunctional family system often disclose their pathology through their behavior by using the availability of several platforms for social media. It is through the internet and texting as well that offers clues to one's thinking and plans often emerge. The need for acceptance and recognition with these individuals finds potential perpetrators employing such acts of violence through social media. They are eager to share their ideas with peers as their efforts in seeking peer acceptance. One of the adolescent perpetrators, the Kentucky teen, in the weeks before he shot and killed three classmates and injured five other students at Heath High School in 1997, revealed the behavior pattern that communicated his rage, his confusion, and his desire to strike out against others. These words and actions displayed elements of hostility and destructive behavior just a few weeks before his shooting rampage. The perpetrator told a fellow classmate in his school that he hated her and this was based on what he likely perceived as rejection on her part. She was a close friend of three of the eight victims whom the 14-year-old had been charged with shooting in the lobby of the high school. On another occasion, the perpetrator was seen wearing a large button onto which he had pasted pictures of one of his victims and her twin sister. Under their pictures, he had written the words: "Preps suck." This victim now lies partially paralyzed by one of the bullets fired in the shooting spree. In another instance, the perpetrator helped throw a chair into a bonfire attended by a number of Heath High School students, most of whom, like him, were members of the school band. After the chair went into the fire, he threw his bike in and talked about throwing a cat into the fire.

Hostility directed toward animals is a serious predicator of hostility directed toward humans. Another instance is the perpetrator had previously shown hostility toward another member of a school group, who was wounded in the shooting. Two students told others that the perpetrator had developed a crush on one of his victims, who died in the shooting. Peers revealed that it was no secret among students that he had a romantic interest in one of the victims. Peers said students in the victim's circle of friends knew the perpetrator had a crush on her, but that she might not have known about it.

Students thought he had asked the girl out once or twice, but she did not accept his invitation. A fellow sophomore and band member was the girl to whom the perpetrator said "I hate you" repeatedly during the prior 6 months leading up to the shooting. The adolescent perpetrator in more recent months to the shooting had seemed attracted to a group of older students who dressed "grunge." He would wear oversized "greasy" pants, tie-dyed T-shirts, and attention-getting symbols. Fellow students reported that the perpetrator often stood with some of his friends on the fringes of the student prayer group that gathered every morning before school in a ring to hold hands and pray. The perpetrator would often mock the group and bully its members.

Diagnostic and Clinical Issues

Essential in gaining an understanding of the psychopathology present with the case illustrations and the other school shooting incidents not included in this summary is the information provided in *The Diagnostic Manual and Statistical Manual of Mental Disorders, Fifth Edition (DSM-5)* of the American Psychiatric Association (2013). Clinical indicators of at-risk and high-risk students are summarized here, which are important for school personnel and others to have a general understanding of as they relate to the psychopathology noted in these cases. For the purposes of our discussion, the reader may benefit from the complete presentation of these indicators available through the DSM series. Published in March 2022, *The Diagnostic and Statistical Manual of Mental Disorders, Fifth Edition, Text Revision (DSM-5-TR)* retains the earlier version of categories but includes text revisions in wording and usage within the existing diagnostic categories. Therefore, these diagnostic factors provide a starting point for understanding how the mental health community envisions the presence of symptoms that indicate a level of psychopathology in those who possess such factors. What is offered here includes some of those diagnostic factors that should be considered in creating a diagnostic impression. They include but are not limited to the following consideration.

From the perspective of the diagnostic manual, the question is asked as to whether there is a "pervasive pattern of disregard for and violation of the rights of others occurring?" (American Psychiatric Association, 2013, 2022). In assessing whether this pattern of behavior is present, does this individual demonstrate first and foremost, a failure to conform to social norms with respect to lawful behaviors? This is measured by one's compliance with the laws of the society in which he/she presides, along with symptoms reflecting a pattern of dishonesty, irresponsibility, impulsivity, irritability, aggressiveness, assault, bullying, and reckless disregard for the safety of self or others, and someone who fails to sustain consistent work behavior or honor one's financial obligations. Where there exists this pervasive pattern of instability and disregard for respecting the law, then one may match the initial criteria for this diagnostic category. Greater detail and specificity is provided within the criteria outlined in the *DSM-5*.

Clinical Management and School Intervention

Educators and clinicians can be very helpful in consulting with school administrators and teachers and can play an effective role in limiting and mitigating the influence of problematic behavior, including violence. The effectiveness of such efforts depends on the level of communication among school personnel and the speed of their response: school personnel must be in constant communication with one another, each employee must have a clearly designated response role, and employees must respond rapidly to any threat of violence. The U.S. Secret Service National Threat Assessment Center (2019) suggests the following actions to limit violence in the schools: acknowledge the student's problem immediately and seek help from local health or mental healthcare professionals, police, and community resources; educate all school personnel about risk factors for both individuals and groups; establish an informed communication network with students; initiate a strict visitor/trespassers policy in the schools; monitor and control points of access to the school; work closely with local police and establish procedures to share information with them; and consider the use of cameras to monitor potential sites for socially deviant behavior.

Observing and confronting agitated and troubled students send an important indicator that should be addressed. There are several markers to consider when encountering these students. Observe thinking and behavior change; a troubled child's behavior is reflective of a sharp shift in thinking. Individuals who are troubled may show signs of anxiety and depression, irritability, and acting out. Monitor these individuals. Be truthful to these children and be realistic. They need to know that they can manage with help. Send simple and direct communication that identifies the problems and the expected behavior. Troubled individuals need to know that they can count on the adults in their lives to listen to them, support them, and care for them. School is a home away from home, a place for students to share their lives with others. When students are troubled, they need to share their thoughts and feelings with an adult. Students need to know that school has expectations and requirements that require discipline and will be a stable and supportive refuge. When talking to students, move to their level of understanding and use good eye contact. Use open-ended questions to solicit their thoughts and feelings. Know your own assumptions and beliefs about what is troubling the individual. Address "character development" in your class, which emphasizes respect of self, respect for others, and responsibilities we have to one another when there are threats of harm to self or others. Recognize the "teachable moment." The teachable moment occurs when an opportunity to teach students about respect and responsibility arises through events happening around them. Create that moment by using opportunities in the curriculum. Model thoughts and feelings to offer students an appropriate way of dealing with life's stressful events. Observe clinical warning signs indicating the need for professional help and advice from competent and licensed authorities immediately.

Clinical warning signs may include but are not limited to the following:

- Feelings of isolation and withdrawal from family and friends

- Difficulty with sleep, loss of appetite, and feelings of rejection
- Problems with strategies for coping with stress
- Internalized anger, irritability, and frustration
- Suicidal or homicidal ideation or intent
- Shifts from friends to more troubled peers
- Expressions of violent thoughts and acts
- Poor school performance and school attendance

A child or adolescent psychiatrist, clinical or school psychologist, school counselor, clinical social worker, nurse practitioner, or qualified member of the healthcare community can help the student and assist persons associated with the individual through the process or referral. Many individuals express anxiety and depression by acting out. This behavior usually varies depending on the person's age and developmental level. The person may become unusually loud and noisy, have temper outbursts, start fights, defy authority, or simply rebel against everything. Drawing again on escape theory, escape in fantasy or reality may show itself in getting poor grades, assuming a general "I don't care about anything" attitude, or even running away from home or school to seek support for this anxiety and depression.

Clinical Issues and Implications

Some students who are at high risk for acting-out behaviors fail to successfully negotiate adolescence, because the behaviors that predispose them to negative experiences are a function of failure to bond with home and family, school teachers, and peers. Egocentrism is crucial to the adolescent. Elkind (2004) defines egocentrism as the stage which adolescents differentiate between the thoughts of others and their own, but they do not differentiate between the objects of their thoughts and the objects of the thoughts of others. They think all others are personally concerned with them. Since adolescents feel peers are as concerned and admiring of they as they are, they construct, react, and play to an imaginary audience, constantly on stage, and may wear outlandish clothing, sass adults, or engage in other risk-taking behavior to please this perceived audience.

However, other adolescents have their own imaginary audiences they are performing for and are not that concerned with other peers. This explains the power of the peer group over the individual during early or middle adolescence and illustrates how easily the adolescent can misinterpret others' perceptions. Most of the cases saw themselves as an outcast with peers, a failure, lost all self-worth, self-love, and self-esteem. Although most were not a known troublemaker, they did exhibit a number of behaviors that got them the attention and, in some cases, the acceptance that they so desperately wanted from others, which to them, as Elkind points out in his theory, is quite real (Miller, 1996).

Deemed totally driven by a perceived lack of and need for acceptance, the perpetrator repeatedly told students something big would happen on a specific day at school for attention, but never intended to do anything. He had hoped if he showed the guns, he would have friends and be liked, but they kept ignoring him, he said.

He strove for approval in his family, continuously acting out the role of the good son. He printed information off the Internet to gain favor with friends. He and his friends regularly tried to disrupt the prayer group. They often talked about taking over the school with firearms, as a prank to get attention from peers. These issues of vulnerability and resilience have stimulated an interest in the identification of protective factors in the lives of adolescents—factors that, if present, diminish the likelihood of negative social outcomes that result in the violence we have witnessed in this decade.

Among the constellation of forces that influence adolescent risk behavior, the most fundamental are the social contexts in which adolescents are embedded, in the family, their school, and their peers. Adolescents' connection to these contexts shapes their risk behaviors and necessitates further study. Other researchers (Zager & Arbit, 1998) report that adolescents may know and experience more violence than parents are aware. Although most young people reported never having been the victim of violent behavior, 24.1% indicated they had been a victim of violent acts. Additionally, 12.4% of students indicated that they had carried a weapon during the previous 30 days. Taken within the family context, demographic factors and family variables explained relatively little of the variability in violence perpetration, 7% and 5% among younger and older students, respectively. Items associated with higher levels of violence for all students included household access to guns and a recent history of family suicide attempts or completions. Factors associated with somewhat lower levels of interpersonal violence included parental and family connectedness. In addition, higher parental expectations for school achievement were weakly associated with lower levels of violence among older adolescents. Of interest is the school context. School context accounted for 6%–7% of the variability in violence among students. Specifically, higher levels of school bonding were correlated with somewhat lower levels of violence.

Finally, individual characteristics accounted for 44% of the variability in violent behavior among 7th and 8th graders and 50% of the variability among 9th through 12th graders. Among both younger and older adolescents, involvement in violence was associated with having been a victim or witness to violence, frequency of carrying a weapon, involvement in deviant or antisocial behaviors, and involvement in selling marijuana or other drugs within the past year. Among younger students, interpersonal violence was associated with lower grade point average and higher perceived risk of failure in peer, parent, and teacher relationships (Centers for Disease Control and Prevention, 2003).

Recently, there has been interest in whether high or low self-esteem underlies violent behavior. McEvoy & Welker (2000) suggested that the most dangerous people are those who have a strong desire to regard themselves as superior beings. They conducted two studies in which they explored the connection between narcissism, negative interpersonal feedback, and aggression in 540 students. Narcissists were found to be emotionally invested in establishing their superiority, yet while they care passionately about being superior to others, they were not convinced that they have achieved this superiority. While high self-esteem entails thinking well of oneself, narcissism involves passionately wanting to think well of oneself. In both studies, narcissism and self-esteem were measured, and subjects were given an opportunity to act aggressively toward a neutral third party, someone who had bullied or insulted them, or toward someone who had praised them. Results found that the most aggressive respondents in both studies were narcissists who were attacking someone who had given them a bad evaluation. Narcissists were exceptionally aggressive toward anyone who attacked or offended them, yet when they received praise, their level of aggression was not out of the ordinary. In both studies, self-esteem was not related to aggression, suggesting that the relationship between self-esteem and aggressive behavior is small at best. Considering several school shootings, the authors of the study note that many schools are attempting to increase their students' self-esteem, which will probably have no effects on violent behavior. But excessive self-love, or narcissism, could actually increase violence in schools (McEvoy & Welker, 2000).

Clinical researchers (Miller, 1996; Taub, 2002) assert that people with high self-esteem are a heterogeneous group that may be more different than alike since high self-esteem can be an accurate recognition of one's positive traits, or it may be a highly doubtful sense of personal superiority that is not reality based. While some individuals with high self-esteem are largely unaffected by feedback, others may require frequent confirmation and validation of their favorable self-image by others. These researchers suggest that aggression by narcissists is an interpersonally meaningful and specific response to an ego threat. Narcissists mainly want to punish or defeat someone who has threatened their highly favorable views of themselves.

Critical to our knowledge of acts of violence in the schools is the realization that there is a contagious effect in society that provides the vulnerable perpetrator a model of aggression sometimes seen in the angry loner. Clinician researchers Zager and Arbit (1998) suggest that the following factors predict with high accuracy teens who are likely to commit crimes similar to those in West Paducah, Kentucky; Jonesboro, Arkansas; Littleton, Colorado; Oxford Township, Michigan; and Springfield, Oregon. Case in point are the similarities identified in the Robb Elementary School shooting in Uvalde, Texas and the Sandy Hook Elementary School shooting in Newtown, Connecticut almost a decade earlier. A child's odds of committing such crimes are doubled when the child comes from a family with a history of abuse, or if this child belongs to a gang or uses alcohol and drugs. The authors further contend that the odds are tripled when along with these factors, the child uses weapons, has arrest records, has a neurological disorder, is truant, and has other school-related problems. The cultural influences give clues to the possible motives and the resulting use of violence in the course of the patterns of behavior exhibited by each. All were loners, did not mix into the mainstream of the peer group, and some had strong emotions for a girl that had resulted in perceived rejection. Peers teased most if not all and with the exception of the Arkansas youth who was seen as a perpetrator who used bully tactics, all were assessed after the fact as victims of bullying. The Kentucky youth was called gay, and the Colorado youth at Columbine High School were both teased by athletes, labeled "faggots," and called "the trench coat Mafia." The perpetrator of the Parkland, Florida shooting gave evidence of a troubled student and had a record of numerous disciplinary problems, peer conflict situations, and poor academic success. The Uvalde, Texas school shooter has been described as a loner who was bullied and had a "fraught home life." The motive for a response is certainly possible in these clinical indicators. The cultural influence for each comes consistently from the contemporary portrayal of violence in music and motion pictures. It was *The Basketball Diaries* and video games, such as Doom and Quake in the Kentucky case, the music of Tupac Shakur along with the video game Mortal Kombat in the Arkansas case. In both the Oregon and the Colorado cases, the music of Marilyn Manson and Nirvana. And with the Colorado case, video games like Quake and Doom also have been documented. The influence of Hitler was also noted in the Colorado case although it is not clear the extent to which this influenced the perpetrators' thinking and behavior.

Recommendations

Violence in the schools is sometimes random but often premeditated by the perpetrator. The following recommendations should be considered in addressing the clinical management of school shootings.

- Train teachers and school officials on recognizing signs and symptoms, better control exposure of youth to violence in the media, voluntary self-control, character education, and anger management skills training.
- Become aware of the identity issues in a child's life. Rejection, anger, and poor conflict resolution skills are found in most perpetrators.
- Provide education and training for all teachers, students, and parents. It appears from such behavior that males, because of "inadequacy to feelings," find that power and control can be achieved primarily through violence.
- Anonymous tip lines should be considered in the schools.
- Stricter gun control legislation and advocacy are needed and access for children and adolescents should be monitored, restricted, and managed more effectively.

Understanding the spectrum of psychopathology offers clues to potential reasons for the aggressive nature of these young perpetrators toward their peers. Further research needs to address the role of narcissism and other personality disorders in addressing the etiology and subsequent acts of violence we have observed in children and adolescents who have come to employ lethal methods as they displace their anger, hatred, frustration, and despair on peers, parents, and other victims of school violence.

What Have We Learned from a Forensic Perspective?

The media presents the news of gun violence in the schools with urgency. The November 2021 school shooting at Oxford High School in Michigan presents several new issues including the role and responsibilities of parents and their providing access to guns. Here a student had shot and killed fellow students and teachers with a gun purchased by his father as a gift. Also in this case, the parents failed to recognize several warning signs, bought an underage child a gun, failed to secure its storage, defended the child when the school officials presented warning signs to them, and challenged school personnel when they attempted to involve the parents in addressing all identified warning signs. The child perpetrator, his parents, and the school system, including school officials, have all been the focus of legal issues.

The incidents identified as notable cases in this chapter are reflective of the need for improved prevention interventions, revised legal statutes, and guidelines that address gun violence at the local community level, the state level, and at national level. Events such as these cause one to reflect again on one's involvement as a forensic examiner. As our society attempts to deal with these episodes of gun violence in the school setting after the fact, our own efforts have been plagued with glitches. It reminded me of my experience with a senior faculty member at University of Kentucky Medical Center, during years past. Psychiatric house staff regularly had the opportunity to present the more difficult psychiatric cases from the hospital ward to this expert for his thoughts about evaluation and treatment. The recurring script was that as the house staff member would complete his/her case presentation, the consultant would respond, "Yes, but what is the question?"

From a forensic perspective, the most obvious questions that need to be answered after any of these school shootings involve violations of the norms, standards, and values of society along with the legal implications of these actions. There also is the extent to which law enforcement can anticipate and enforce gun-related laws that protect against violence associated with such events. Furthermore, assessing the perpetrator for competency to stand trial is critical. In the Heath High School shooting from December 1997, for example, two teams of professional experts were assembled for the purposes of determining the status of this defendant. Those on the side represented by the Commonwealth's Attorney Office included Elissa Benedek, MD, Child and Adolescent Psychiatrist—University of Michigan; William D. Weitzel, MD, General Psychiatry—University of Kentucky (co-author of this chapter from the first edition), and Charles C. Clark, PhD, an academic neuropsychologist at the University of Michigan. This team of professionals, who evaluated the defendant with the intent of presenting a report to the Commonwealth's Attorney, posed the relevant questions earlier. The Defense employed two clinicians: Diane Schetky, MD, Child and Adolescent Psychiatrist—University of Vermont College of Medicine at Maine Medical Center, and Dewey Cornell, MD, Academic neuropsychologist—University of Virginia Medical School. Dr. Schetky concluded for the defense that although the defendant had evidence of a dysthymia, traits of schizotypal personality disorder with borderline, and paranoid features, he did not lack responsibility for his acts during the event of December 1, 1997.

The diagnoses rendered by the Commonwealth Attorney's team (which incorporates the needed terminology) included the following: These conclusions were delivered in the format recommended by *The Diagnostic and Statistical Manual of Mental Disorders, Fourth Edition* (DSM-IV) (American Psychiatric Association, 1994), which provides the official vocabulary to be used by mental health clinicians. The defense team did not appear to adhere closely to this orientation, and so their data were more varying in quality, as they reached their opinions. These findings by these two independent and adversarial employed teams of professionals are remarkably similar, and yet both teams violated the DSM admonition, which stresses that it is inappropriate to describe an individual as having a personality disorder until that individual has reached the chronological age of at least 18 years. Further, it is the professional opinion of this author that this "over reaching," by both teams, highlights the restricted usefulness of DSM in our attempts to explain anything more than narrowly drafted questions, for example, with respect to competency and criminal responsibility. But, then again, these questions were the ones that were proposed, among many others that could be proposed, as we attempt to understand these awful events. In this case the original examiners were interested in finding differences on how the defendant told his story about his different experiences and feelings. The defense psychiatrist advocated publicly that the defendant had many of the features of a schizotypal personality disorder, and in addition suffers from a depression. This would first appear in his first year of junior high school. Then it would appear in the fall of 1997, just prior to the killings. The defense psychiatrist further implied that this was due to his rejection and the teasing in the school setting.

Future Directions

Violence and gun-related crime has blemished our communities. Whether we use as examples the Oxford High School shooting of 2021 or the massacres at Marjory Stoneman Douglas High School in 2018 and Robb Elementary School in 2022, our legislators, parents, families, educators, and healthcare professionals must come to terms with gun violence in our schools and in our communities. Consideration should be given to the following:

- All children and their parents must be assured that the school in which they attend is safe at all times because of prevention interventions that have been adopted and implemented.
- Use of timed locks throughout the school, metal detectors on the doors, along with gun safety programs that address early warning signs and what to do when they are recognized by children, parents, and community members.
- Established, regularly reviewed, and updated policies to monitor students' behavior and activities associated with risk factors for all forms of deviant behavior including gun violence. Require safe and secure gun storage.

- Legislation that has the best interest of the safety of children and school personnel that monitors and restricts the access to guns. Unfortunately, at this writing, legislators at the national level have failed to pass legislation that can end school-related violence involving gun violence and mass shootings.
- Parental and community involvement and support for proactive advocacy that can provide assurance for the safety of our children, our schools, and our communities.
- Legislation and background checks that eliminate gun access to prohibited individuals. To date federal law only requires background checks when the gun seller is a licensed dealer. Unlicensed private sellers, including sales at gun shows and online, do not require background checks.
- The gun industry must be held accountable and ensure there is adequate oversight over the marketing and sales of guns and ammunition in our communities.
- Evidence-based programs that provide community education on prevention interventions necessary to keep our communities safe from gun-related violence. An example of this is the standardized training programs provided by various organizations targeting violence prevention.
- Educating at-risk families about the use of "Extreme Risk Protection Orders (ERPOs)" that are intended to empower family members and law enforcement to have the support of the judicial system in preventing gun access and violence for at-risk individuals and families.

All this requires a committed partnership seeking serious solutions that involve our children, parents, school personnel and officials, healthcare professionals, legislators, school safety personnel, local and regional law enforcement, gun dealers, and our community membership if we are to achieve better control of the gun-related violence in our country.

Acknowledgments The authorship acknowledges the assistance of Officer Debbie Wagner, Fayette County Police Department; Kathleen Banas, M.L.S.; James Clark, PhD; Lane J. Veltkamp, MSW., ACSW, BCD; Tag Heister, M.L.S.; Deborah Kessler, M.L.S.; Katrina Scott, M.L.S.; and Jill Livingston, M.L.S. Library Services are acknowledged for their support and assistance in the completion of this manuscript.

References

American Psychiatric Association. (1994). *Diagnostic and statistical manual of mental disorders* (4th ed.). American Psychiatric Association.
American Psychiatric Association. (2013). *Diagnostic and statistical manual of mental disorders* (5th ed.). American Psychiatric Association.
American Psychiatric Association. (2022). *Diagnostic and statistical manual of mental disorders* (5th ed., Text Revision (DSM-5-TR)). American Psychiatric Association.
Baumeister, R. F. (1990). Suicide as escape from self. *Psychological Review, 97*, 90–113.
Beebe, D. W., Holmeck, G. N., Albright, J. S., Noga, K., & DeCastro, B. (1995). Identification of "binge-prone" women: An experimentally and psychometrically validated cluster analysis in a college population. *Addictive Behaviors, 20*, 451–462.

Boxer, P., Goldstein, S. E., Musher-Eizenman, D., Dubow, E. F., & Heretick, D. (2005). Developmental issues in school based aggression prevention. *The Journal of Primary Prevention, 26*(5), 383–400.

Centers for Disease Control and Prevention. Web-based Injury Statistics Query and Reporting System (WISQARS) [Online]. (2003). National Center for Injury Prevention and Control, Centers for Disease Control and Prevention (producer). Available at: http://www.cdc.gov/ncipc/wisquars. Accessed on 17 Feb 2003.

Dean, P. J., & Range, L. M. (1996). The escape theory of suicide and perfectionism in college students. *Death Studies, 20*, 415–424.

Edwards, D., Hunt, M., Meyers, J., Grogg, K., & Jarrett, O. (2005). Acceptability and student outcomes of a violence prevention curriculum. *The Journal of Primary Prevention, 26*(5), 401–418.

Elkind, D. (2004). The problem with constructivism. *The Educational Forum, 68*(4), 306–312.

Espelage, D. L., & Swearer, S. M. (Eds.). (2004). *Bullying in American schools: A social-ecological perspective on prevention and intervention.* Lawrence Erlbaum Associates Incorporated.

Gun Violence Archive. (2020). *Online archive of gun violence incidents and results of gun violence.* Available at: https://www.gunviolencearchive.org/

Heatherton, T. F., & Baumeister, R. F. (1991). Binge eating as escape from self-awareness. *Psychological Bulletin, 110*, 86–108.

Irwin, V., Wang, K., Cui, J., Zhang, J., & Thompson, A. (2021). *Report on indicators of school crime and safety: 2020 (NCES 2021-092/NCJ 300772).* National Center for Education Statistics, U.S. Department of Education, and Bureau of Justice Statistics, Office of Justice Programs, U.S. Department of Justice. Washington, DC. Retrieved April 8, 2022 from https://nces.ed.gov/pubsearch/pubsinfo.asp?pubid=2021092

McEvoy, A., & Welker, R. (2000). Antisocial behavior, academic failure, and school climate: A critical review. *Journal of Emotional and Behavioral Disorders, 8*, 130–141.

Miller, T. W. (1996). *Theory and assessment of stressful life events.* International Universities Press Incorporated.

Miller, T. W. (1998). *Children of trauma.* International Universities Press Incorporated.

National School Safety Center. (2002). *Understanding, preventing and responding to school bullying.* SKU: RP-UPRSB. http://www.schoolsafety.us/products/resource-papers

National School Safety Center. (2019). *Checklist of characteristics of youth who have caused school-associated violent deaths.* http://www.schoolsafety.us/media-resources/checklist-of-characteristics-of-youth-who-have-caused-school-associated-violent-deaths

Puka, B. (Ed.). (1994). *Fundamental research on moral development.* Garland Publishers.

Parker, G., Hadzi-Pavolvic, D., Greenwald, S., & Weissman, M. (1995). Low parental care as a risk factor to lifetime depression in a community sample. *Journal of Affective Disorders, 33*, 173–180.

Taub, J. (2002). Evaluation of the second step violence prevention program at a rural elementary school. *School Psychology Review, 31*, 186–201.

U.S. Secret Service National Threat Assessment Center (NTAC), U.S. Department of Homeland Security. (2019). *Protecting America's schools: A U.S. Secret Service analysis of targeted school violence.* https://www.secretservice.gov/sites/default/files/2020-04/Protecting_Americas_Schools.pdf

Veltkamp, L. J., & Miller, T. W. (1994). *Clinical handbook of child abuse and neglect.* International Universities Press.

West, M. L., Keller, A. E. R., Links, P., & Patrick, J. (1993). Borderline personality and attachment disorders. *Archives of General Psychiatry, 53*, 502–505.

Zager, R., & Arbit, J. (1998). School violence in rural areas. *American Psychological Association Monitor, 29*(8), 35–41. Washington, DC: American Psychological Association.

Chapter 12
Boundary Violations, Harassment, Abuse, and Exploitation in the School Setting

Thomas W. Miller

Introduction

Across all professions, there exists moral and ethical responsibility to maintain limits to the relationship with a student, patient, client, or recipient of services that are dictated by Codes of Ethics and guidelines for the profession that necessitate an awareness of the scope of practice of the professional and the terms of a relationship. The relationship between a teacher and a student is established solely with the purpose of providing the education and learning environment in which the student has entered in the school setting. In instances where this relationship deviates from its basic goal and objectives, it is considered a boundary violation. The guiding principles that apply in a professional relationship, whether that is within the school setting, a healthcare professional's office, or in the business world, include beneficence, autonomy, and nonmaleficence.

The consequences of any form of physical or psychological abuse may be understood by utilizing the trauma accommodation syndrome model. The trauma accommodation model applies to how human beings tend to process the trauma experienced, in this case an abusive situation. The initial stage is that of the abusive event or experience. The second stage is one of reexperiencing the abuse and this is often

Portions of this chapter appear in Miller, T. W., & Veltkamp, L. J. (1997). *Clinical Handbook of Adult Abuse and Exploitation*, published by International Universities Press, Inc.

T. W. Miller (✉)
Department of Psychiatry, College of Medicine, Department of Gerontology, College of Public Health, University of Kentucky, Lexington, KY, USA

Institute for Collaboration on Health, Intervention, and Policy, University of Connecticut, Storrs, CT, USA
e-mail: tom.miller@uconn.edu

realized by reliving the event along with the emotional and cognitive responses to that traumatizing event. The third stage is one marked by cognitive confusion and uncertainty about what to do and how to deal with this and future events with the anticipatory anxiety that comes with fearing future abuse. In the fourth stage, the abused individual begins to understand, accept, and prepare for an effective way to handle similar situations. In doing so, the individual gains confidence in having a plan should such an event reoccur. The fifth and final stage is one of accommodation and acceptance of the traumatic event and the individual has learned to understand a way to address events, like the one experienced, in the future (Miller, 1998).

Relationship boundaries establish the role and responsibilities for both the provider and the recipient of any service. Therefore, the cognitive awareness and employment of boundary limitations in a relationship are the responsibility of the provider and within the school setting this includes the educational professionals at all levels.

School and college personnel are in a very unique position of trust, authority, guidance, and influence in the lives of the students they serve. Their behaviors and interactions should be in the best interest of their students. Awareness and utilization of professional boundaries define expected and appropriate standards of behavior between faculty and students where power imbalances may occur within that relationship, and the boundaries serve to protect both the student and the teacher or faculty member (Younggren, 2002; Peterman et al., 2020; Seddighi et al., 2019; The Alliance for Child Protection in Humanitarian Action, 2020). The presence of a boundary between student and teacher recognizes the existence of unequals in this relationship, where the teacher possesses a position of authority, whereas the student is subservient to that authority. In such a relationship, the person in a position of authority is obliged to abide by appropriate standards of conduct.

Boundary violations may appear in several forms, such as physical violations that may include touching a student or other without their permission and examining personal belongings such as their phone or computer without their permission (Guthiel & Simon, 2002). Emotional boundary violations are another form that educators must develop an awareness for and may show themselves through patronizing behavior, favoritism, ridicule, bullying, or sarcasm. Then there are sexual boundary violations that often show themselves through gradients of change that may include touching a student inappropriately or without their permission; sharing of sexually explicit content through texting, internet, or other social media formats; romantic or sexually related activities; and advancing a means of engagement beyond the expected student–teacher relationship or violating norms, standards, and professional guidelines and codes of conduct.

Among the several examples of boundary violations identified, there are less well-recognized boundary violations that require our cognizance in today's world. For example, instances where school personnel have been utilizing students for their personal gain in trafficking drugs in the school setting is an example of exploitation. Conversely, incidents have occurred that involve using a teacher's position of authority to harm a student as a form of punishment for noncompliance with the wishes of the teacher. Professional organizations associated with education at all levels have developed standards for their educators and other professionals, who must develop an awareness of these standards, a willingness to abide by these standards, and protect the safety and security of children in the school setting.

Reviewing the Literature

Boundary violations have been the object of both researchers and educators with specific attention to ethical compliance with established guidelines. Within the educational setting there may be a range from verbal bullying to exploitation to sexual harassment, and sexual boundary violations have become the focus of exploitation and abuse experts as a serious concern (Olweus et al., 2019; Ostrov et al., 2015; Manfrin-Ledet et al., 2015; Younggren, 2002). Alpert and Steinberg (2017) examined the ethical codes of practice that govern several organizations over the last century. All recognize that sexual boundary violations are an exploitative process but without wide variation as to specificity with respect to what constitutes a boundary violation and the ethical codes of conduct that govern various professional groups including teachers, school officials, school counselors, and social workers.

The spectrum of sexual boundary violations ranges from sexually tainted jokes, unwanted sexual advances, and inappropriate educator–child relationships to sexual harassment. During the past two decades, many organizations have endorsed rules of ethical conduct that prohibit sexual contact between professionals and clients and advised members on the importance of setting sexual boundaries (American Medical Association, 2011; American Psychiatric Association, 2015; American Psychoanalytic Association, 2013; American Psychological Association, 1995).

Major efforts have also been made to clarify and prohibit sexual contact in the workplace, but those have only begun to reach the educational setting. There is a dearth of research on sexual harassment or contact in either setting. The purpose of this chapter is to elucidate the specific spectrum of sexual boundary violations that professionals must be aware of in the course of providing school-based services. It offers the reader an understanding of the triggers for potential sexual boundary violations, a perpetrator profile and victim profile, the exploitation of the victim in the school setting and the trauma accommodation syndrome, and a legal case which has signatures for school-based professionals. Clinician Gabbard (1991) suggested that violations of sexual boundaries between educators and students can occur when the perpetrator confuses his or her own need to be loved with the needs of the victim. The perpetrator fantasizes that love in and of itself may cure his or her psychopathology. The tendency for incestuous sexual experiences—based, perhaps, on the perpetrator's past—to be reenacted in the perpetrator–victim dyad, and the close link between incest and the desire to be helpful and parental, reflects the immaturity and psychopathology of the perpetrator.

Perpetrators often act out their anger and frustration through the sexual exploitation of others. Olarte (1991) identified characteristics of perpetrators who violate sexual boundaries in the school setting. Such perpetrators are often middle-aged, going through some type of personal distress or conflict, professionally isolated, likely to overvalue their professional capacity, unorthodox in their moral decision-making processes, likely to over-personalize the teacher–student relationship, and likely to ignore or deny any ethical responsibility to the victim, society, or to their professional code of conduct.

Teacher as Exploiter and Abuser

Case 1: Jeffrey Epstein

Early in his career, Jeffrey Epstein was a teacher at the Dalton School in New York City. He taught courses in both physics and mathematics. In that school setting, he was recognized by fellow faculty as having unusual and noncompliant behavior toward guarding against relationships with his students. To the contrary, he savored the opportunity to engage students, primarily girls, both in the classroom and beyond with emotionally and sexually explicit violations of the expected standards of the institution. He was known to be flamboyant in nature and violated openly the school's code of ethics and behavior. He violated the school dress code, as well, often wearing clothes unacceptable to the norms of the institution. Outside the classroom and the school, he was also known to attend student parties with the intent of exploiting young females in attendance. Early efforts on his part toward sexual exploitation and trafficking of young high school girls are believed to have started during this period in his life at the Dalton School. His exploitation and abuse of women continued in the years following his teaching and is the focus of a chapter in this volume authored by Annie Farmer (Chap. 9), once a victim and now a professional healthcare provider, addressing her experience with this perpetrator which focuses on sexual exploitation, abuse, and trafficking of school-aged children. Epstein subsequently became a registered sex offender. In July 2019, he was charged with federal sex trafficking involving dozens of minor girls who were exploited in both New York and Florida during 2002–2005 (U.S. Attorney's Office, Southern District of New York, 2019). In July 2020, Ghislaine Maxwell was arrested on similar charges as his recruiter and confidante for exploitation and abuse.

Case 2: Debra Lafave

As a young, popular school teacher in her twenties at Angelo L. Greco Middle School in Florida, Debra Lafave initiated inappropriate contact with a young adolescent student with whom she was attracted through inappropriate email, texting, and touching. As with exploitation and sexual boundary violations, there were gradients of change that advanced from verbal expressions of attractiveness to inappropriate touching with the student and then to more sexually explicit content, including rides in her car and the use of texting and social media formats for transmitting explicit nude pictures of herself to this male student. Text messages from this middle school teacher communicated sexually suggestive content and her desire to have a sexual relationship with him. In the course of these sexual boundary violation experiences in the school setting, she involved other students to observe and look out for her should someone approach the school area where these encounters with the student occurred. When the mother of the juvenile victim in this case found out about these inappropriate relations, she notified the police, which led to Lafave's arrest and conviction. During her trial, the teacher attributed her indiscretions to irregular mood swings, hypersexuality, and poor judgment, reflecting that she was aware of the boundary violations that she was committing at the time. She pleaded guilty to lewd or lascivious battery and was sentenced to 20 years in prison for these series of boundary violations in the school setting.

Recognizing Boundary Violations

School administrators, teachers, school counselors, and others recognize sexual boundary violations as a form of school violence. Sexual boundary violations are defined as a spectrum of activities that may include but not be limited to self-disclosure of information about one's life, one's family, one's experiences, or feelings—including positive and negative reactions to a student. In the school environment, accompanying a student to any destination outside the school or a school-sponsored activity may exceed boundary issues. Accepting or giving a gift can all be forms of moving beyond the boundary of one's professional school-related activities. All of these instances have been identified in civil and licensing board litigation cases as evidence of the existence of an inappropriate relationship between teacher and student (Brodsky, 1989; Miller & Veltkamp, 1989; Megana, 1990). Unfortunately, there is a dearth of research on sexual contact in the school setting.

Teachers, like other professionals, are often confronted with duality of role issues with their students. Sexual boundary violations have become an important focus in understanding the spectrum of abuse and a serious concern for the mental health profession (Brodsky, 1989; Olarte, 1991). Within the construct of sexual boundary violations are unwanted sexual discussion and advances, educator–child relationships, and issues related to sexual harassment.

The American Medical Association has reinforced the Hippocratic Oath with a specific rule stating "sexual contact between a physician and a patient is unethical because it violates the trust necessary in the physician-patient relationship".

Incidence and Prevalence Data

While major efforts to clarify and prohibit sexual contact in health-related and educational settings have been made, there are educators and clinicians who continue to engage in sexual or sexualized contact with their students and clients. In the health-care arena, some self-reporting surveys reveal that 7–12% of therapists have engaged in sexual relationships with at least one patient (Schoener et al., 1989). One study found that 80% of therapists reporting any sexual involvement with patients became intimate with the patient. One study regarding psychiatrists found that 65% have counseled at least one patient who has been sexually abused by a previous professional (Gartrell et al., 1987; Kluft, 1990).

Clinical studies indicate that up to 90% of clients who engage in sexual contact with their therapists were psychologically harmed as a result. There is clinical research (Cantrell et al., 1989) which argues that the resulting impact and injuries may include sexual dysfunction, anxiety disorder, psychiatric hospitalization, increased risk of suicide, dissociation, depression, internalization, and feelings of guilt, anger, shame, fear, confusion, hatred, and worthlessness (Pope, 1986). In addition, the abuse by a therapist may exacerbate the patient's presenting illness and may create new psychopathology, such as posttraumatic stress disorder in the client or student (Jorgenson, 1994). Among other issues, patients are vulnerable when they enter treatment. There is a significant power imbalance: the therapist over the patient. Often, patients lack self-esteem and are fearful. Sexual contact with clients constitutes misuse of the therapist's power and places the patient in a vulnerable/helpless position.

Prevalence data related to sexual boundary violations are vague and there is a dearth of studies in the school setting. Much of the data are derived from questionnaire surveys of clinician–client relationships requesting respondents to be honest and truthful about unethical behavior. Several national surveys have been completed, suggesting prevalence in the range of 12% among male therapists and 3% among female therapists (Kluft, 1990). The study which surveyed three major mental health professions, including psychiatry, clinical psychology, and clinical social work, found no differences among the mental health disciplines in the incidents of such sexual boundary violations. The professions have also made considerable efforts to understand the origins and process of sexual boundary crossings and violations. Elliott (1990), addressing the issue of abuse-related countertransference and the therapist as an abuse survivor, suggests that clinicians are even more likely than other professionals to have been sexually or physically abused and to have come from homes where substance abuse was a problem for parents. Unresolved child abuse issues can impede or interfere with therapeutic effectiveness with patients.

Boundary Violations and Transference

Sexual boundary violations are, perhaps, the most dangerous form of abuse-related countertransference. Boundary incursion by a person entrusted to be a therapeutic agent may not only revisit the abuse-related issues for the patient but also reinforce abuse-related trauma in the survivor client. Megana (1990), researching this area, has concluded that sexual abuse survivors who are sexually victimized again and again by their therapists suffer greater symptoms than cohorts who were molested as children but not during therapy.

Gabbard (1991) addressed the psychodynamics of such violations wherein perpetrators who transgressed sexual boundaries with victims show considerable confusion of their own needs with that of victims' needs or experience a sense of love. Most notable among these psychodynamic themes are confusion of one's own need to be loved with those of the victim, particularly when one is vulnerable due to personal problems; the fantasy that love in and of itself may by curative; the proneness of the perpetrator–victim dyad to reenact incestuous sexual involvement from the victim's past; the close linkage between wanting to be helpful and sexual involvement; and the tendency of some perpetrators to act out their hostility through sexual exploitation of the victim. In addition, the perpetrator may sexually exploit a victim simply because he or she wants to or because he or she has the opportunity. Whether unwanted discussion or advances, sexual boundary violations, or the medium of sexual harassment in the school setting, three main methodologies have been utilized to collect data on the characteristics of the perpetrator. Olarte (1991) identifies these data summaries as including the following:

1. Composites of the descriptions of such perpetrators based on their treatment
2. Profile descriptions of perpetrators extrapolated from research surveys that guarantee anonymity to the professional
3. A detailed classification and description of offenders based on voluntary evaluations of such offenders by national centers that specialize in the diagnosis and treatment of victims of physical and sexual abuse

Olarte (1991) reports that characteristics frequently seen include a young to middle-aged perpetrator, usually a male but with increased frequency of female perpetration, who is undergoing some type of personal distress, who was isolated professionally, who tends to overvalue his or her healing capacity, who is unorthodox about his or her therapeutic methods, who frequently personalizes the teacher–student relationship, and who ignores or denies his or her ethical responsibility to his or her victim.

Symptom Indicators of Boundary Violations

In some cases of sexual exploitation or sexual abuse, the victim will notice that a precursor to these behaviors may involve sexually suggestive or other inappropriate behaviors. Often these behaviors are confusing and subtle and can be identified by the student because they often feel uncomfortable. Examples of warning signs in educational settings may include the following:

1. Faculty, staff who tell sexually tainted jokes or stories
2. Giving the potential victim seductive looks and flirting
3. Discussing the staff member's personal sex life and details regarding intimate relationships to students
4. Sitting too close to students, showing affection, and inappropriate touching

In addition, other warning signals include the following:

1. A teacher giving a student special status by scheduling after-school appointments
2. Making out-of-school appointments
3. Using the victim as a confidant or for personal support
4. Giving or accepting gifts
5. Getting involved in giving money or offering substances of abuse to the student

A Classic Legal Case Brief

The case *Davis v. Monroe County Board of Education* (1999) involved a fifth grader in Monroe County, Georgia, who alleged that a male student harassed her eight times during a 6-month period. The harassment included attempts to touch the student's private areas, sex-related vulgarities, and sexually suggestive behavior. All of the alleged incidents occurred in the school setting.

The student reported the incidents to three teachers. She also reported the last incident to the principal, who allegedly had learned of one previous incident from a teacher. The teacher took only one remedial action—assigning the harasser to a different seat in the classroom—and the principal threatened disciplinary action.

After the last incident, the perpetrator was charged with sexual battery, to which he pleaded guilty. The female student alleged that she suffered mental anguish, that her grades dropped, and that she wrote a suicide note.

The female student's mother sued, claiming that the failure of school officials to prevent her daughter's sexual harassment violated Title IX. A Federal District Court in Georgia dismissed the lawsuit, and the Circuit Court of Appeals affirmed that decision. Both courts concluded that a school district is not liable under Title IX for failing to prevent student-on-student, or peer, sexual harassment. After the two lower courts dismissed the case, the family appealed to the US Supreme Court, which found that Title IX damages may be found against a school board in cases of student-on-student harassment where the school was deliberately indifferent to sexual harassment so severe, pervasive, and objectively offensive that the victim has deprived access to the school's educational opportunities and benefits. In that the Plaintiff won, they will maintain the right to return to District Court for a trial for their suit on its merits. The amendments to Title IX regulations since this judicial decision have specifically defined harassment as a form of discrimination and clarified grievance procedures at postsecondary institutions.

This case involving sexual harassment, which is another form of sexual boundary violation, is critically important to school districts across the country. For the first time, the high court ruled on the contentious issue of a school board's liability for student-on-student harassment. The ruling set a national standard. This case became the litmus test for sexual boundary violations and for many women's and children's rights advocates, who argue that children deserve protection from physical and verbal abuse at school—the same protections employees are afforded in the workplace setting. While most school boards and administrators acknowledge that sexual harassment is a growing concern, this topic was the focus of the 2021 Conference on Sexual Harassment at Schools, Colleges, and Universities that addressed sexual harassment in education (UC Berkeley School of Law, Berkeley Center for Comparative Equality and Anti-Discrimination, 2021). Sexual harassment in our schools, colleges, and universities were addressed with estimates of sexual harassment that were found to approach 50% in secondary schools and were even higher in colleges and universities.

Prevention/Intervention in the School Environment

With respect to boundary violations in the school setting, teachers must be vigilant, as must all school personnel, to the recognition of and prevention intervention for all boundary violations between staff and students (Manfrin-Ledet et al., 2015; Miller, 1998; Clark & Walker, 2012).

The following policy guidelines will help educators address the issues of sexual boundary violations in the school setting:

- Provide awareness training designed to help educators recognize sexual boundary violations, with special attention given to the psychological, legal, and medical needs of the student victim
- Establish policies and procedures that are designed to help administrators and staff monitor and manage sexual boundary issues, making sure that they include clearly defined reporting procedures
- Identify areas of potential risk within the school setting that encompass student–educator relationships
- Utilize multidisciplinary professionals in the form of an advisory board within the school system and community to address the effect of sexual boundary violations and evaluate monitoring policies and procedures

- Prepare incident reports and submit them to the Departments of Education and Health and Human Services, as well as other appropriate licensing agencies, as required by state law

For therapists and counselors seeking resources, fortunately there have been countless guides published in articles and books, helping clinicians carefully weigh the factors, values, and possibilities in trying to arrive at the best possible decision about whether entering into various kinds of relationships with a client makes clinical and ethical sense. In addition to the more general decision-making aids, there are resources for virtually every kind of specialty practice and context, e.g., a 3-level model for family therapists involved with religious communities to negotiate dual relationships. A decision-making model for social dual-role relationships has been developed and cited by Gottlieb for use in assessing and managing such a relationship (Gottlieb, 1993; Gottlieb et al., 2007).

Younggren (2002) examines boundary violations in an 8-step model, "Ethical Decision-making and Dual Relationships." There may, of course, be times—even with such helpful models—when therapists reach an impasse and are unsure of whether to enter a complex dual (or multiple) relationship or try an intervention that involves similar boundary issues.

Pope (1986) outlines ten steps that therapists may find useful in addressing such impasses and thinking through whether to begin the potential dual relationship or intervention. Pope confronts a diverse set of situations, each with its own shifting questions, demands, and responsibilities. Every clinician is unique in important ways. Ethics that are out of touch with the practical realities of clinical work and with the diversity and constantly changing nature of the therapeutic venture are useless (Pope, 1986). The value in using these scenarios and questions to consider nonsexual dual or multiple relationships and other forms of boundary crossings may be in direct proportion to the ability, to disclose responses that may be politically incorrect, "emotionally incorrect," or otherwise at odds with group norms or with what some might consider the "right" response (Pope, 1986).

The Processing of a Boundary Violation

The impact of victimization can be both short and/or long term based on a number of factors, including (1) the duration of the abuse or exploitation, (2) whether there was a use of threat or intimidation within the context of the abusive behavior, and (3) the degree to which the abusive behavior occurred. However, even the most minimal forms of sexual exploitation can cause substantial psychological damage to students. For example, many children will (1) feel a sense of shame; (2) feel guilty even though it is the educator's responsibility to prevent such exploitation; (3) have mixed feelings toward the educator, for example, betrayal, love, anger, or feeling protective; (4) feel isolated and empty; (5) feel unable to trust one's own feelings or to judge trustworthiness in other people; (6) fear that no one will believe them or understand what has happened or fear that others will find out; (7) have posttraumatic stress-related symptoms, including unexpressed rage, numbness, nightmares, obsessive thoughts, depression, suicidal thoughts, or flashbacks; and (8) have confusion about dependency, control, and power.

Perpetrator/Victim Profiles

Composites of perpetrators which emerge include individuals who show impaired reality testing and poor social judgment, sociopathy and narcissism, ignorance and naiveté, anxiety, depressive symptoms, and impulsiveness. Schoener et al. (1989) have identified psychiatric data received in the voluntary evaluation of offenders.

They classified sexually exploitative persons into clusters, based on their years of clinical experience rather than through systematic research. Their categories include the following:

1. Uninformed naive—these individuals lack knowledge of the expected ethical standards or lack understanding of professional boundaries and confuse personal and professional relationships.
2. Healthy or mildly neurotic—These perpetrators know the professional standards, actual contact with students tends to be limited or isolated, situational stressors foster a slow erosion of professional boundaries, and the perpetrators often show remorse.
3. Severely neurotic and socially isolated—These individuals have long-standing emotional problems, such as low self-esteem, depression, feelings of inadequacy, and social isolation.
4. Impulsive character disorder—These persons have long-standing problems with impulse control in many areas of their life, their judgment is poor, and they tend to abuse more than one victim.
5. Sociopath or narcissistic character disorder—These perpetrators have long-standing serious personal pathology that expresses itself in most aspects of their lives and these perpetrators manipulate victims and colleagues to protect themselves from their unethical behavior.
6. Psychotic or borderline personality—Impaired reality testing and poor social judgment of these perpetrators hinder their ability to apply their knowledge of ethical standards or a clinical understanding of professional boundaries.

Schoener et al. (1989) believe that the uninformed naive and the mildly neurotic have a good prognosis, while the last four have a poorer prognosis. The search for a perpetrator profile must take into consideration the realization that the perpetrator bears the burden of responsibility for his or her behavior, including ethical and legal considerations, a moral code, and constraints. Wohlberg (1990) has suggested that after an extensive literature review, there is little support for a single profile of patients involved in sexual boundary violations. Gender and age combinations provide a range of diagnostic categories for both parties. What does emerge is what is referred to as commonalities representing recurring themes encountered in working with both perpetrators and victims. The central commonality is the vulnerability factor noted in both the victim and the perpetrator.

Stone (1982), exploring the issue of vulnerability to sexual exploitation and sexual boundary violations, examined a sample of 46 females who had terminated with male therapists and who were divided by criteria into four groups. The groups included those who were sexually intimate, those who were sexually propositioned, those who were prematurely terminated, and those who successfully completed therapy. The study found that women who had been sexually involved with therapists had the strongest anxious attachment to significant others, while there were no significant differences realized between groups and the amount of ego strength.

In another study, Averill et al. (1989) developed a profile of the victim who might be commonly vulnerable to sexual relations with a perpetrator. These researchers suggest that the typical victim may include those individuals with borderline personality disorder who have complained of loneliness or emptiness in their lives. They are often seen in treatment as resistant or actively self-defeating.

These individuals tend to show a pattern of instability in interpersonal relations, in their self-concept, and are often impulsive. In assessing the issue of outcome with respect to perpetrators, the prognosis is more favorable if the perpetrator:

- Recognizes the problem
- Takes responsibility for the problem
- Enters into treatment
- Remains in treatment until behavior change occurs and avoids denial and/or projection

According to the *Diagnostic and Statistical Manual of Mental Disorders, Fifth Edition* (DSM–5) criteria (American Psychiatric Association, 2013), individuals sexually abused or exploited by professionals including educators may have transient stress-related paranoid ideation; inappropriate and intense anger; affective instability due to marked reactivity of mood; impulsivity in the areas of sex, spending, and substance abuse; identity disturbance and unstable self-image; associations with feelings of imagined abandonment; and a general pattern of unstable interpersonal relationships with alternating extremes of idealization and devaluation.

Borderline personality disorder features may also be present in the perpetrator. These features generally demonstrate a pattern of instability in interpersonal relationships, poor self-concept, and impulsivity, and may include some of the following features:

- Identity disturbance often marked by unstable self-concept or sense of self.
- A pattern of unstable and intense interpersonal relationships that are often marked by alternating extremes of devaluation and idealization.
- Impulsive behavior that tends to be potentially self-damaging and may include self-mutilating behavior and recurrent gestures of suicidal ideation and intent.
- Unstable affective mood and chronic feelings of emptiness.

- Inappropriate and intense anger and poor management of anger and resulting behavior.
- Stress-related paranoid ideation with frantic efforts to avoid real or imagined loss or abandonment.

Numerous authors have indicated a history of abuse in the life of these individuals, which may include previous sexual abuse. Herman et al. (1989) have suggested that abuse victims may learn seductive behavior as a medium by which they tend to relate and reinforce the relationship with the perpetrator. Similarly, other clinician researchers (Veltkamp & Miller, 1994; Veltkamp et al., 1994) have noted that individuals who experience abuse in childhood may be more likely to enter abusive situations in adulthood, resulting in poor adaptation to adult life and poor survivor skills.

There may also be clinical features which suggest the presence of a personality disorder and a history of abuse as comorbid factors. Herman et al. (1989) found that 68% of the victims of abuse were diagnosed as borderline and were also sexually abused as children. The authors note that this event may indeed play a critical causative role in the formation of symptoms and the vulnerability factor noted in sexual boundary violations. The dynamic of repetition compulsion is seen as critically important to understanding the dynamics of the sexual boundary violations from the victim's perspective.

What Are the Lessons Learned?

Examined in this chapter are critical factors in addressing sexual boundary violations in the school environment. Identified initially are the several triggers that serve to put at-risk teachers and students in the traps of sexual boundary violations ranging from sexually tainted jokes to discussing personal sexual lives with students.

The Jeffrey Epstein case has brought to light some of the most serious concerns that parents, schools, colleges, authorities, and legislators need to address regarding the safety of students and prevention of sexual abuse and trafficking. The recruitment and enticement of minors to travel and to engage in illegal sex acts and activities has become a significant concern and raised public awareness of human trafficking globally.

Specific victim and perpetrator features are reviewed with an emphasis on recognition and empowerment to address such symptoms when they are observed in the school environment. Sexual boundary violations as an exploitative process must be addressed through adherence to the ethical codes of conduct that govern various professional organizations (Alpert & Steinberg, 2017). Such codes of conduct have been found to differ substantially across professional organizations. Educators, administrators, and practitioners in schools are encouraged to address the need for improvements to the overall codes of conduct that guide ethical behavior in our schools with specific attention to relevance of guidelines to the school setting, its staff, and students. Finally, a series of suggestions and recommendations are offered to provide a prevention model for sexual boundary violations in the school setting.

Issues and Implications in the Educational Setting

Recognition and response to the issues related to sexual boundary violations by persons in educational settings require well-defined approaches to addressing the needs of both the victim and the perpetrator (The Alliance for Child Protection in Humanitarian Action, 2020; New Zealand Family Violence Clearinghouse, 2020). Suggested as essential guidelines in addressing sexual boundary violations in the schools include the following:

- Recognizing and interrupting the sexual boundary violations and addressing the legal and medical needs of the student
- Establishing policies and procedures that monitor and manage sexual boundary issues in the schools
- Identifying areas of potential risk within the school setting and all student–educator relationships
- Utilizing multidisciplinary professionals within the school system and in the community to address the impact and monitoring of sexual boundary violations and the evaluation of policy and procedures
- Preparing reports of incidents as required by state law and submitting appropriate reports to the Departments of Education and Health and Human Services and other appropriate licensing agencies, as mandated by law
- Providing follow-up and established guidelines for monitoring and assessing the effectiveness of current policies and procedures in the schools
- Engaging public policymakers and legislators to assure laws and regulations are in the best interests of the public, children, and their families

Acknowledgments The author wishes to acknowledge the assistance of Kathy Banner, MLS; Jill Livingston, MLS; Tagalie Heister, MLS; Jodie Smith; and Betty L. Downing, the Department of Psychiatry at the University of Kentucky, Linda Brown, Dale Dubina, Brenda Frommer, and Rhonda T. Edwards, MS, for their assistance in the preparation of this manuscript.

References

Alliance for Child Protection in Humanitarian Action. (2020). *Technical note: Protection of children during the coronavirus pandemic*. Available at: https://alliancecpha.org/en/COVD19

Alpert, J. L., & Steinberg, A. L. (2017). Sexual boundary violations: A century of violations and a time to analyze. *Psychoanalytic Psychology, 34*(2), 144–150. https://doi.org/10.1037/pap0000094

American Medical Association. (2011). The Council on Ethical and Judicial Affairs, American Medical Association, "Sexual misconduct in the practice of medicine". *Journal of the American Medical Association, 266,* 25–38.

American Psychiatric Association. (2013). *Diagnostic and statistical manual of mental disorders* (5th ed.). American Psychiatric Association. https://doi.org/10.1176/appi. books.9780890425596

American Psychiatric Association. (2015). *Principles of medical ethics and annotations especially applicable to psychiatry.* American Psychiatric Association.

American Psychoanalytic Association. (2013). *Principles of ethics for psychoanalysis and provisions for implementation of the principles of ethics for psychoanalysis.* American Psychoanalytic Association.

American Psychological Association. (1995). *Ethical principles of psychologists.* American Psychological Association.

Averill, S. C., Beale, D., & Benfer, B. (1989). Preventing staff-patient sexual relationships. *Bulletin of the Menninger Clinic, 53*(2), 384–393.

Brodsky, A. M. (1989). Sex between patient and therapist: Psychology's data and response. In G. O. Gabbard (Ed.), *Sexual exploitation in professional relationships* (pp. 15–25). American Psychiatric Press.

Cantrell, K., Harmon, J., Olarte, S., Philstein, J., & Lacilio, T. (1989). Psychiatrists-patient sexual contact: Results of a National Survey, #1, Prevalence. *American Journal of Psychiatry, 143*(2), 1126–1131.

Clark, J., & Walker, R. (2012). Research ethics in victimization studies: Widening the lens. *Violence Against Women, 17*(12), 1489–1508.

Davis v. Monroe County Board of Education, (97-843) 526 U.S. 629 (1999). 120 F 3rd 1390. Argued January 12, 1999—Decided May 24, 1999 (97–843).

Elliott, D. M. (1990). *The effects of childhood sexual abuse on adult functioning in a national sample of professional women* (Unpublished doctoral dissertation). Biola University, Rose Mead School of Professional Psychology, Los Angeles, CA.

Gabbard, G. O. (1991). Psychodynamics of sexual boundary violations. *Psychiatric Annals, 21*(4), 651–655.

Gartrell, N., Herman, J., Olarte, S., Feldstein, M., & Localio, R. (1987). Reported practices of psychiatrists who knew of sexual misconduct by colleagues. *American Journal of Orthopsychiatry, 57*(3), 287–289.

Gottlieb, M. C. (1993). Avoiding exploitive dual relationships: A decision-making model. *Psychotherapy: Theory, Research, Practice, Training, 30*(1), 41–48. https://doi. org/10.1037/0033-3204.30.1.41

Gottlieb, M. C., Robinson, K., & Younggren, J. N. (2007). Multiple relations in supervision: Guidance for administrators, supervisors, and students. *Professional Psychology Research and Practice, 38*(3), 241–247. https://doi.org/10.1037/0735-7028.38.3.241

Guthiel, T. G., & Simon, R. I. (2002). Nonsexual boundary crossings and boundary violations: The ethical dimension. *Psychiatry Clinician North America, 2002*(25), 585–592.

Herman, J. L., Perry, J. C., & Van der Kolk, B. A. (1989). Childhood trauma in borderline personality disorder. *The American Journal of Psychiatry, 146*(2), 490–495.

Jorgenson, L. M. (1994). Sexual boundary violations. *Treatment Today, 6*(2), 18–24.

Kluft, R. P. (Ed.). (1990). *Incest-related syndromes of adult psychopathology* (pp. 263–288). American Psychiatric Press.

Manfrin-Ledet, L., Porche, D. J., & Eymard, A. S. (2015, June). Professional boundary violations: A literature review. *Home Healthc Now, 33*(6), 326–332. https://doi.org/10.1097/ NHH.0000000000000249

Megana, D. (1990). *The impact of client therapist sexual intimacy and child sexual abuse on psychosocial and psychological functioning* (Unpublished doctoral dissertation). University of California, Los Angeles, CA.

Miller, T. W. (1998). *Children of trauma: Stressful life events and their effects on children and adolescents* (Stress and health series. Monograph 8). International Universities Press, Inc.

Miller, T. W., & Veltkamp, L. J. (1989). The adult non-survivor of child abuse. *Journal of the Kentucky Medical Association, 87*(3), 120–124.

New Zealand Family Violence Clearinghouse (NZFVC). (2020). *Preventing and responding to family, Whānau and Sexual Violence during COVID-19*. Available at https://nzfvc.org.nz/COVID-19/preventing-responding-violence-COVID-19

Olweus, D., Limber, S. P., & Breivik, K. (2019). Addressing specific forms of bullying: A large scale evaluation of the Olweus Bullying Prevention Program. *International Journal of Bullying Prevention, 1*, 70–84. https://doi.org/10.1007/s42380-019-00009-7

Ostrov, J. M., Godleski, S. A., Kamper-DeMarco, K. E., Blakely-McClure, S. J., & Celenza, L. (2015). Replication and extension of the early childhood friendship project: Effects of physical and relational bullying. *School Psychology Review, 44*, 445–463. https://doi.org/10.17105/spr-15-0048.1

Olarte, S. W. (1991). Characteristics of therapists who become involved in sexual boundary violations. *Psychiatric Annals, 21*, 657–660.

Pope, K. S. (1986). Research and laws regarding therapist-patient sexual involvement: Implications for therapists. *American Journal of Psychotherapy, 40*, 564.

Peterman, A., Potts, A., O'Donnell, M., Thompson, K., Shah, N., Oertelt-Prigione, S., & Gelder, N. V. (2020). *Pandemics and violence against women and children*. Center for Global Development. Available at: https://www.cgdev.org/publication/pandemics-andviolence-against-women-and-children

Seddighi, H., Salmani, I., Javadi, M. H., & Seddighi, S. (2019). Child abuse in natural disasters and conflicts: A systematic review. *Trauma, Violence & Abuse*, 1524838019835973. Available at: https://doi.org/10.1177/1524838019835973

Schoener, G., Milgram, J., Gonsiorek, E., Luepker, J., & Conroe, D. (1989). Psychotherapists' sexual involvement with clients: Intervention and prevention. *Journal of Psychotherapy, 142*(3), 1181–1189.

Stone, L. B. (1982). A study of the relationship amongst anxious attachment, ego functioning and female patients' vulnerabilities to sexual involvement with male psychotherapists. California School of Professional Psychology, Los Angeles, CA, 1980. Doctoral dissertation. *Dissertation Abstracts International, 42*, 789B.

UC Berkeley School of Law, Berkeley Center for Comparative Equality and Anti-Discrimination. (2021, January 29). *Sexual harassment at schools, colleges, and universities: A global perspective [Conference]*. Available at: https://www.law.berkeley.edu/event/sexual-harassment-at-schools-colleges-and-universities-a-global-perspective/2021-01-29/

U.S. Attorney's Office, Southern District of New York. (2019, July 8). *Jeffrey Epstein charged in Manhattan Federal Court with sex trafficking of minors [Press Release]*. U.S. Department of Justice. https://www.justice.gov/usao-sdny/pr/jeffrey-epstein-charged-manhattan-federal-court-sex-trafficking-minors

Veltkamp, L. J., & Miller, T. W. (1994). *Clinical handbook of child abuse and neglect*. International Universities Press Inc.

Veltkamp, L. J., Miller, T. W., & Silman, M. (1994). Adult non-survivors: A failure to cope with victims of child abuse. *Child Psychiatry and Human Development, 24*(4), 231–243.

Wohlberg, J. (1990, February 10). *The psychology of therapist sexual misconduct. Panel discussion: Psychological aspects of therapist sexual abuse*. Presented at the Boston Psychoanalytic Society and Institute.

Younggren, J. (2002). Dual relationships; personal and professional boundaries among rural social workers. *British Journal of Social Work, 185*, 38–46.

Chapter 13
Harassment, Abuse, and Violence on the College Campus

Thomas W. Miller and Barbara Burcham

Introduction

College is a living laboratory for college-aged individuals for emotional and social learning along with intellectual learning. It is in many ways a rite of passage. For most students it is a time to envision the identity of each individual. The social and emotional learning is priceless. The American Institutes for Research (2022), one of the world's largest behavioral and social science research and evaluation organizations, has shown that students engaged in college have a variety of social experiences on several levels from the formal learning experiences with other students and faculty to the social interactions of Greek life. Self-awareness is a part of the emotional development that should blossom during this experience. It is a time when self-awareness develops, and this helps the student grow up and develop into a mature and independent adult. And while for most, that rite of passage is toward social and emotional maturity, for others there emerges an underdevelopment that shows itself through various forms of school-related violence.

Peer relationships and subsequent acceptance by other individuals and group members becomes critically important for each individual on the college campus. It is often referred to as one's popularity, which translates to how much other students like their classmates. From a socio-psychological perspective the degree to which one achieves peer acceptance is the measure to which they realize a sense of

T. W. Miller (✉)
Department of Psychiatry, College of Medicine, Department of Gerontology, College of Public Health, University of Kentucky, Lexington, KY, USA

Institute for Collaboration on Health, Intervention, and Policy, University of Connecticut, Storrs, CT, USA
e-mail: tom.miller@uconn.edu

B. Burcham
Georgetown College, Lexington, KY, USA

© The Author(s), under exclusive license to Springer Nature Switzerland AG 2023
T. W. Miller (ed.), *School Violence and Primary Prevention*,
https://doi.org/10.1007/978-3-031-13134-9_13

belonging within the college community. That sense of belongingness can weigh heavily and play a critical role in one's adaptation and involvement in both the academic and social aspects leading to success within the college and university community. When this process of peer acceptance is delayed, impaired, or fails to materialize, the results may lead to various forms of bullying, harassment, abuse, exploitation, or other forms of campus-related violence.

Educators, practitioners, and researchers have addressed the presence of bullying, a form of violence, on campus (Alberti, 2011; Allanson et al., 2015; Miller, 2008; Miller & Veltkamp 1998; Miller et al., 2005; Miller, Veltkamp, Kraus, 2005; Nickerson et al., 2019; Nickerson & Orrange-Torchia, 2015). Where bullying is present on campus, it may take several forms (Olweus, 1993, 2022). Among the most common forms of bullying that may occur on campus may be found through individual incident or in more organized experiences as through activities associated with hazing by some organizations, fraternities, or sororities on campus. On today's campus, bullying most commonly takes the form of verbal, non-verbal, and cyber abuse and harassment. They may be direct or indirect in nature. Verbal forms of bullying on campus can be recognized as verbal insults, intimidation, or the use of abusive language, while non-verbal bullying may involve pushing, shoving, hitting or physical or psychological traumatization to the person. Cyber bullying uses an electronic or digital technology as the medium of choice including but not limited to text, chat, or a social media platform to transmit harassing and abusive content toward the victim.

In addressing the college and university environment, the American Institutes for Research (2022) reveals that there is a collaboration between academic and social growth when one becomes a part of the college community. When an individual fails to experience early learning developmental characteristics such as a strong sense of self, independence, and emotional and social growth, their thinking and behavior resort to bully-type behavior in their encounters on the college campus.

Presentation of Violence

While efforts to increase awareness of various forms of violence is showing progress as a result of media attention and training programs related to bullying, exploitation, abuse, and harassment on campus, college-related forms of violence among college students remain a seriously neglected public health issue (Espelage, 2014; Espelage et al., 2013; Finkelhor, 2013; Nocentini & Menesini, 2016; Noltemeyer et al., 2019; Olweus et al., 2019). While college-related violence can take several forms, with advances realized in today's technology, the presence of bullying on campus has new dimensions. The students who bully may use several forms of behavior that do not treat their fellow students with dignity and respect. They use a myriad of behaviors that include verbal bullying, ridicule, stalking, complicity, retaliation, inappropriate amorous relationships, sexual and gender-based harassment, sexual assault, sexual exploitation, and intimate partner-related violence experiences.

The contemporary college campus is witness to various forms of harassment, bullying, discrimination, abuse, and exploitation which have emerged with technological change. Through on-campus education and training, more college students are being encouraged to develop an awareness of this twenty-first century phenomenon (Miller, 2016).

The *National Network of Schools in Partnership* (2020) advocates nationally against all forms of violence on campuses across our country. Women of ages 18–24 years are three to four times more likely than women in all other age groups to experience sexual violence (Sinozich & Langton, 2014), and most survivors do not report the incident to law enforcement. This chapter introduces the latest policy guidelines and development led by the US Department of Education's Office for Civil Rights (OCR) within the context of college-related violence and suggests prevention and intervention initiatives to address these issues.

The Civil Rights of College Students

The US Department of Education's Office for Civil Rights (OCR) has led the effort to formalize the content and detail the necessary terms of guidelines linked to violence at colleges and universities, including scope and content. OCR issued, during August 2020, needed guidelines that aid college and university communities in formulating the necessary directives that address various forms of school-related violence on college campuses. In doing so, educational institutions now have the toolbox for formulating their own policy that addresses various forms of bullying, discrimination, misconduct, harassment, and relationship violence in today's world (US Department of Education, Office for Civil Rights, 2021).

With these revised guidelines, the OCR has included a new definition of Prohibited Conduct, "Title IX Sexual Harassment." Incidents falling under this definition of Title IX Sexual Harassment will be investigated pursuant to updated investigation procedures as required by the new federal Title IX regulations. Also, the Campus Sexual Violence Elimination Act, known as the Campus SaVE Act, requires colleges to be transparent regarding sexual violence on college campuses, guarantees rights for victims of sexual violence, provides accommodations and support for students, and ensures there are protocols for impartial disciplinary procedures in matters related to sexual misconduct.

Definitions of Campus-Related Violence

Provided in the US Department of Education's Office for Civil Rights (OCR) guidelines (2021) are groups within key categories of identified campus violence. Let's examine these categories of violence on campus. The initial form of violence examined by the OCR in the document is what is referred to as discriminatory harassment which is discrimination based on a legally protected right resulting in the failure to assure reasonable accommodation, consistent with state and federal law, to persons with disabilities. Beyond this it examines various forms of harassment.

Under consideration here are three forms of harassment that may occur on the college or university campus. These include what are referred to as "discriminatory harassment," "hostile environment harassment," and "sexual and gender-based harassment." Compliant colleges and universities have designed and implemented necessary guidelines that address these forms of harassment on campus. This author is grateful to his home institution for sharing their "University of Connecticut Policy Against Discrimination, Harassment, and Related Interpersonal Violence" as one model that may serve as a reference for the reader.[1] Their guidelines provide a definition and scope of each of these three forms of harassment.

Discriminatory harassment is understood to occur when such harassment is realized through "verbal, physical, electronic, or other conduct based upon an individual's race, color, ethnicity, religious creed, age, sex, marital status, national origin, ancestry, sexual orientation, genetic information, physical or mental disabilities" (University of Connecticut, 2020). Attention is drawn to what may be included under the term mental disabilities which for a student could include an intellectual or learning disability. A history of military service and "veteran status, prior conviction of a crime, workplace hazards to reproductive systems, gender identity or expression, or membership in other protected classes set forth in state or federal law that interferes with that individual's educational or employment opportunities" are covered under this terminology (University of Connecticut, 2020). Such conduct is a violation of this guideline and an indication of a hostile environment. A *hostile environment harassment* is viewed as a situation where "discriminatory harassment is so persistent or pervasive that it unreasonably interferes with, limits, deprives, or alters the conditions for education" to occur (University of Connecticut, 2020). The reader is encouraged to visit the entire document for terms and conditions affecting one's understanding of discriminatory harassment.

With respect to sexual- and gender-related harassment, the policy and guidelines are defined in this manner. Sexual or gender-based harassment, which is a category covered in the new OCR policy as a form of campus-related violence, is very important as students develop new relationships on campus. *"Sexual harassment*

---

[1] Parts of this chapter published previously in: University of Connecticut (2020). Used with permission.

is unwelcome conduct of a sexual nature. This may include, but is not limited to, unwanted sexual advances, requests for sexual favors, inappropriate touching, acts of sexual violence, or other unwanted conduct of a sexual nature, whether verbal, non-verbal, graphic, physical, written, [cyber] or otherwise. Such conduct is a violation of this policy when the conditions for Hostile Environment Harassment or Quid Pro Quo Harassment are present, as defined above" (University of Connecticut, 2020).

By definition, *"gender-based harassment* includes harassment based on gender, sexual orientation, gender identity, or gender expression, which may include acts of aggression, intimidation, or hostility, whether verbal or non-verbal, graphic, physical, written or otherwise, even if the acts do not involve conduct of a sexual nature. Such conduct is a violation of this policy when the conditions for hostile environment harassment or Quid Pro Quo harassment are present, as defined" earlier (University of Connecticut, 2020).

Title IX defines sexual harassment as "conduct that occurs on the basis of sex in a [college or] university based educational program or activity" (US Department of Education, Office for Civil Rights, 2021) and that satisfies one or more of the following conditions:

- An employee of the college such as a faculty member, graduate assistant, or staff member who conditions the provision of a benefit, or service on an individual's participation in unwelcome sexual conduct, thus a quid pro quo situation.
- Unwelcome conduct determined by a reasonable person to be so severe, pervasive, and objectively offensive that it effectively denies a person equal access to an education program or activity, thus a hostile environment.
- Sexual assault or "dating violence," "domestic violence," or "stalking" as defined by the Violence Against Women Act (US Department of Education, Office for Civil Rights, 2021).

Within the context of these noted conditions, one must understand sexual assault. Sexual assault consists of the following terms: (1) Sexual contact and/or (2) Sexual intercourse that occurs without (3) Consent. In addressing the conditions under which sexual assault occurs, the revised 2020 OCR policy, published in 2021, explains that "consent" cannot be given if any of the following conditions are present including any form of force, coercion, or incapacitation. The term "force" refers to verbal or physical acts to gain sexual access. "Coercion" is verbal or physical pressure to initiate sexual activity. "Incapacitation" refers to a state of mind where an individual is judged to be incapable of making rational decision. "Sexual contact" involves inappropriate touching for the purpose of obtaining sexual gratification. "Sexual intercourse" is any sexual penetration. "Consent" is an "understandable exchange of affirmative words or actions, which indicate a willingness to participate in mutually agreed upon sexual activity. Consent must be informed, freely and actively given" (University of Connecticut, 2020). A more robust discussion of these terms, specific examples, and indicators of each term are available in the formal OCR document (US Department of Education, Office for Civil Rights, 2021).

Defining Exploitation Within the College Experience

According to the Rape, Abuse, and Incest National Network (RAINN) (2022), the Campus Sexual Violence Elimination Act, better known as the Campus SaVE Act, requires colleges to be transparent regarding crimes of sexual violations on campuses that receive any type of federal funding. Colleges must guarantee the rights for victims of sexual violence and provide appropriate accommodations and support. They must also provide campus-wide sexual violence prevention and educational programming and have protocols for impartial disciplinary procedures.

Sexual exploitation tends to involve the taking advantage of the sexuality and attractiveness of a person for some form of personal gain. The use of sexual exploitation as realized in the case of Jeffrey Epstein and Ghislaine Maxwell, where young women were solicited for providing sexual favors for money, has exemplified the issues related to exploitation and sexual trafficking. The OCR guidelines identify several situations where a person is judged to be exploited or abused because of their sex and/or gender identity for personal gain or gratification of the perpetrator. Such situations may include compromising and sexual-specific images through photographs or video images with the intent to circulate or actually post such images without consent through cyber technology, live streaming, or social media. There are further indicators of exploitative actions that include fetish behaviors, voyeurism, prostitution, exposing another to a sexually transmitted infection, or forcing students into viewing or participating in illegal sexual activities.

The College Setting and Intimate Partner Violence

Sexual assault, stalking, and/or physical assault includes any act of violence or threatened act of violence that occurs between individuals who are involved or have been involved in a sexual, dating, spousal, domestic, or other intimate relationship. The term "intimate partner violence" usually denotes the need to establish a power base by the perpetrator toward the victim. It may be preceded by stalking. College and university campuses have witnessed stalking as a form of violence. While stalking may show itself differently, it often consists of repeated and unwanted advances that create emotional stress and anxiety for the victim of stalking. It is evidenced by harassing behavior on the part of the perpetrator and may be in person or through various forms of cyber communication (US Department of Education, Office for Civil Rights, 2021).

Retaliation and Campus Violence

With any form of campus violence, the reporting of such events can lead to various forms of retaliation by the perpetrator toward the victim. Retaliation involves an adverse action taken against a person for making a good faith report of any unwanted or abusive form of violence on campus. Non-acceptance of or non-compliance with the advances of a perpetrator may result in some form of retaliation that is usually based in the anger and frustration experienced by the perpetrator as evidenced by coercive and intimidating forms of harassment.

Adverse Impact of College-Related Amorous Relationships

The 2020 OCR guidelines address and define "amorous relationships" that are campus related as "intimate, sexual, and/or any other type of amorous encounter or relationship, whether casual or serious, short-term or long-term" (US Department of Education, Office for Civil Rights, 2021). Exploitation and potential abuse concerns involving university faculty and staff toward a student may qualify as an amorous relationship which could result in serious personal and professional risk for censure by the university. University guidelines and codes of conduct require faculty and staff to be vigilant toward the nature and intent of their relationships with students. In much the same way, graduate assistants who are hired to assist, serve, or supervise other students, whether in the classroom or a research laboratory, need to develop an awareness of the same guidelines and avoid any potentially exploitative behavior or abuse. Where there may be a pre-existing relationship that could be described as amorous in nature with a person who has now become a student, such a relationship should be disclosed to the Office of Institutional Equity by the faculty and staff who possess such a position of authority (US Department of Education, Office for Civil Rights, 2021).

Summarizing the Case of Campus-Related Violence

The college and university setting is a social psychological, interpersonal living laboratory for young adults. The contemporary college campus, including its fraternities and sororities, is witness to various forms of harassment, bullying, and abuse that are recognized as serious social problems. Stalking, inappropriate amorous relationships, sexual and gender-based harassment, sexual assault, sexual exploitation, and intimate partner-related violence experiences are reported at universities and colleges globally.

The Centers for Disease Control and Prevention and the US Department of Education identify bullying as aggressive behavior on the part of the perpetrator that is unwelcomed by the victim. They further indicate that such behavior within this context may be direct and indirect and can be characterized as physical, verbal, relational/social or involves damage to property related to the victim (CDC, 2021).

Bullying and harassment of students with disabilities has been recognized as a very serious concern. The US Department of Health and Human Services (n.d.) addresses issues related to bullying individuals with special needs and has noted that students with disabilities are as likely or perhaps are more likely to experience some form of bullying, harassment, and sexual misconduct. On their "Stopbullying. gov" website, they provide several resources, including Federal Civil Rights laws relating to youth with disabilities. In addition, there are prevention intervention strategies that can have a positive effect on reducing the incidence and prevalence of such activities experienced by students with disabilities.

Skills Development for Prevention and Intervention

Several respected efforts to address school-based interventions to reduce dating and sexual violence have been recognized in the research literature (De La Rue et al., 2014). Public health professionals and the range of counseling and therapeutic professionals on campus need to explore programs cited by these authors that have provided evidence-based results for reducing dating-related and sexual forms of violence on campus (van Starrenburg et al., 2013; Williams, 2014; Williford et al., 2012; Yeager et al., 2015). Healthcare professionals providing campus services should recognize the strengths of all students including those with disabilities and provide them with modeled verbal response patterns that empower these students to develop the necessary skills and ability to respond to perpetrators in harassing, exploitative and abusing situations. It may go without saying, but prior to beginning any campus-wide or school-wide prevention or intervention initiative, the provider should review state laws and regulations linked to teen/dating violence and know how and where to make referrals for those students who need individualized support. Critical skills are important in guiding victims and victimizers in developing self-awareness and an understanding as to why sexual violence and bullying behaviors may be occurring. Across the several models that have been generated are such core components as recognizing warning signs, developing the skills to respond, and learning personalized strategies that empower victims of harassment and abuse with resiliency, self-efficacy, and competencies needed to address their perpetrator. Educational and healthcare staff must be creative and flexible with each individual and foster the strengths and comfort levels of the individual. In some situations, the best prevention intervention for the victim is to recognize when it may be best to ignore bullying behavior, avoid situations where bullying might occur, engage bystanders or peers who are supportive with an encounter, or leave a potential bullying encounter in favor of safety and support.

In addition to group interventions, some educators suggest implementing school-wide initiatives such as those described by Bonds and Stoker (2000) in "Bully

Proofing Your School." They suggest implementing a school-wide bully proofing program. Although this is most commonly used in middle and high school settings, it could be adapted for use in a college setting. Their suggested program is designed as a systemic, comprehensive initiative with a commitment to intolerance for bullying. The focus is to develop a prosocial school climate. This is completed by systematically teaching skills and strategies that decrease victimization and show how to take a stand for others while developing a caring majority. The desired outcome is to develop a sense of community within a school where everyone feels safe and respected.

One more point to consider when developing prevention and intervention practices in a campus setting is the issue of trauma. Other chapters in this book (e.g., Chap. 10) explicitly discuss how sexual violence and bullying at school can be traumatic and create long-lasting mental and physical issues. Often, students carry a lot of baggage linked to violence in their backgrounds to school including reoccurring partner violence, discrimination, and bullying. Thus, when providing group-based or school-wide initiatives, always be aware of this invisible subset of students who may be triggered by the process and be in need of trauma-informed interventions such as trauma-focused cognitive behavioral therapy, cognitive restructuring therapy, stress inoculation therapy, EMDR (Eye Movement Desensitization and Reprocessing), or other forms of psychological first aid.

Suggested Resources for Prevention Interventions on Campus

There are several helpful resources which provide research-based curricula that may be useful for college counseling center providers wishing to provide campus-wide social emotional learning experiences and bullying and violence prevention programs that may restore a climate of safety for students seeking guidance in how to address harassment, bullying, or other forms of abuse in the college environment. Examples of these programs include, but are not limited to:

- "Expect Respect," a program of the SAFE Alliance, works to promote healthy dating relationships and prevent violence and abuse among teens. They provide innovative, research-based trainings and collaborate with schools and other organizations that serve youth. Their website is: https://www.expectrespectaustin.org/
- "SAFE dates" is an evidence-based program to prevent dating violence. It provides a curriculum that educates youth on how to identify and prevent intimate partner violence. The program is available through Hazelden Betty Ford Foundation and their website is https://www.hazelden.org/web/public/safe-dates.page
- The "Positive Prevention Plus" sexual health education curriculum, developed by Kim Clark and Christine Ridley, originated in California with the collaboration of staff representing the nursing and public health education professionals. The initiative provides comprehensive evidence-based sexual health and

pregnancy prevention curriculum for young adults. Their website is https://www. positivepreventionplus.com
- Campus-based healthcare providers are also encouraged to examine the work of Professor Dorothy Espelage (2014) and her discussion of "ecological theory" in attempting to apply and implement individualized campus intervention strategies addressing youth bullying, aggression, and victimization.

These prevention intervention resources should assist on-campus providers to gain a better understanding of evidence-based models that have good applicability and move from theory to practice in addressing violence prevention and successful interventions for use on our university and college campuses.

Individual Importance of Responding if You Are Aware

Being aware and responding to sexual misconduct if you are a student or an employee on a college campus is important as these behaviors have physical, psychological, and social health consequences for the victim. Some behaviors violate the law as in the case of sexual violations and rape and if reported, result in criminal and/or civil actions against the person responsible for the misconduct. Other forms of sexual misconduct and harassment may appear as with verbal insults and intimidation. When students, faculty, and staff on college campuses are made aware through designed models of education and training, the ability to recognize these warning signs associated with sexual violence and sexual misconduct is likely to impact the incidence and prevalence of such violence on campus through a decline in their presence. Failure to understand, recognize, and know how to respond to observed peer violence results in a campus climate of acceptance for unwanted discrimination and violent behavior.

Witnessing behaviors that appear dangerous and include a person of any gender being bullied, harassed, or violated requires competency and immediate action that should include some form of reporting of the incident, such as calling campus security and/or local law enforcement, as well as contacting the Title IX office on campus. Awareness of these inappropriate and unwanted behaviors by a bystander intervention often works best if victims or bystanders can enlist the involvement and the support of others when acts of bullying, harassment, or abuse are present. In these situations, it may be helpful to the victim if a bystander were able to provide the victim with contact information for counseling and mental health services on campus.

Being aware of and understanding what sexual harassment, exploitation, sexual misconduct, and abuse are provides students with the opportunity to intervene more effectively for the victim of abuse on campus. Universities and colleges have an obligation to educate students on all forms of violence such as bullying, sexual assault, dating violence, and stalking behavior. For the informed student on campus, it is important to know campus-specific reporting guidelines. The Campus SaVE

Act and Title IX are federal regulations that guarantee rights for victims of sexual violence on college campuses in the United States. It is always helpful if a bystander is an effective listener and is willing to report any form of campus-related violence, holding perpetrators accountable, and contributing to safe and civil college and university environments (Wilson-Simmons et al., 2006).

Concluding Thoughts and Take-Home Messages

In this chapter, topics examined include various forms of campus-related violence, a range of developmental issues faced by college and university level students, the civil rights of students as defined by the US Department of Education's Office for Civil Rights (OCR) within the context of college-related violence, evidence-based resources, and suggested prevention and interventions addressing violence associated with campus life. What has been learned from this recent initiative of the OCR (US Department of Education, Office for Civil Rights, 2021) is that each college and university has now had an opportunity to generate guidelines which address the presence and the prevention of all forms of identified campus violence as evidenced in their official policy statement. In addition, the civil rights of college students are explored as gender-based harassment, sexual harassment, intimate partner violence, and skills development for prevention intervention.

Provided are directions for the future that provide a framework for colleges and universities to create and uphold in a campus-wide public health policy, a policy similar to the University of Connecticut (2020) *Policy Against Discrimination, Harassment, and Related Interpersonal Violence.* Such a document "prohibits discrimination, as well as discriminatory harassment, sexual assault, sexual exploitation, intimate partner violence, stalking, sexual or gender-based harassment, [bullying,] complicity in the commission of any act prohibited by [university-created] policy, retaliation against a person for the good faith reporting of any of these forms of conduct or participation in any investigation or proceeding under this policy…These forms of prohibited conduct are unlawful and undermine the mission and values of our academic community. In addition, engagement in or pursuit of inappropriate amorous relationships with employees in positions of authority can undermine the University's mission when those in positions of authority abuse or appear to abuse their authority" (University of Connecticut, 2020).

College and university programs must be committed to the prevention of violence on their campuses and of all prohibited conduct through regular and ongoing education and awareness programs for all constituents. Undergraduate and graduate students and all employees should receive primary prevention and awareness programming as part of their orientation each year. College/university administration should make every effort to provide the necessary training, education, and awareness programs to faculty, students, and staff to ensure a broad understanding of their policy on discrimination, harassment, and related interpersonal violence and the topics and issues related to maintaining an education and employment environment on campus that is free from harassment, exploitation, and discrimination.

Acknowledgments Acknowledged are the guidance, support, institutional policies, and resources at the University of Connecticut's Institute for Collaboration on Health, Intervention and Policy. The authors also wish to acknowledge the contributions of several colleagues, including Janet Saier, M.S.; Jill Livingstone, M.L.S.; and Kathleen Banner, M.L.S., and thank them for their assistance in the completion of this chapter.

References

Alberti, J. M. (2011). *Guiding philosophy for the Dr. Jean M Alberti Center for the Prevention of Bullying Abuse and School Violence*. University at Buffalo.

Allanson, P. B., Lester, R. R., & Notar, C. E. (2015). A history of bullying. *International Journal of Education and Social Science, 2*, 31–36. http://www.ijessnet.com/uploades/volumes/1576145463.pdf

American Institutes for Research. (2022). *About AIR: Mission focused, evidence driven* [Internet]. https://www.air.org/about

Bonds, M., & Stoker, S. (2000). *Bully proofing your school*. Sopris West, Inc.

CDC. (2021). *Violence prevention – Fast fact: Preventing bullying*. https://www.cdc.gov/violenceprevention/youthviolence/bullyingresearch/fastfact.html

De La Rue, L., Polanin, J., Espelage, D., & Pigott, T. (2014). School-based interventions to reduce dating and sexual violence: A systematic review. *Campbell Systematic Reviews, 10*(7), 5–104. https://doi.org/10.4073/csr.2014.7

Espelage, D. L. (2014). Ecological theory: Preventing youth bullying, aggression, and victimization. *Theory Into Practice, 53*(4), 257–264. https://doi.org/10.1080/00405841.2014.947216

Espelage, D. L., Low, S., Rao, M. A., Hong, J. S., & Little, T. D. (2013). Family violence, bullying, fighting, and substance use among adolescents: A longitudinal transactional model. *Journal of Research on Adolescence, 24*, 337–349. https://doi.org/10.1111/jorg.12060

Finkelhor, D. (2013). *Trends in bullying and peer victimization*. Crimes against Children Research Center, University of New Hampshire. Available at: http://www.unh.edu/ccrc/pdf/CV280_Bullying%20%26%20Peer%20Victimization%20Bulletin_1-23-13_with%20toby%20edits.pdf

Miller, T. W. (2008). *School violence and primary prevention*. Springer. https://doi.org/10.1007/978-0-387-77119-9

Miller, T. W., & Veltkamp, L. J. (1998). *Clinical Handbook of Adult Exploitation and Abuse*. Madison Connecticut: International Universities Press Inc.

Miller, T. W., Holcomb, T. F., & York, C. (2005). Camp as a Cohort in Character Development: Strategies in Prevention Education. *Kentucky Counseling Association Journal, 24*(4), 24–34.

Miller, T. W., Veltkamp, L. J., & Kraus, R. F. (2005). Character education as a prevention strategy in school related violence. *The Journal of Primary Prevention, 26*(5), 455–467.

Miller, T. W. (2016). Coping with life transitions. In J. Norcross, G. Vanderboos, et al. (Eds.), *APA handbook of clinical psychology* (Vol. IV, p. 21). American Psychological Association Press Inc.

Nickerson, A. B., Fredrick, S. S., Allen, K. P., & Jenkins, L. N. (2019). Social emotional learning (SEL) practices in schools: Effects on perceptions of bullying victimization. *Journal of School Psychology, 73*, 74–88. https://doi.org/10.1016/j.jsp.2019.03.002

Nickerson, A. B., & Orrange-Torchia, T. (2015). The mental health impact of bullying. In P. Goldblum, D. Espelage, J. Chu, & B. Bongar (Eds.), *The challenges of youth bullying and suicide* (pp. 39–49). Oxford University Press.

Nocentini, A., & Menesini, E. (2016). KiVa anti-bullying program in Italy: Evidence of effectiveness in a randomized controlled trial. *Prevention Science, 17,* 1012–1023. https://doi.org/10.1007/s11121-016-0690-z

Noltemeyer, A., Palmer, K., James, A. G., & Wiechman, S. (2019). School-Wide Positive Behavioral Interventions and Supports (SW-PBIS): A synthesis of existing research. *International Journal of School and Educational Psychology, 7,* 253–262. https://doi.org/10.1080/21683603.2018.1425169

Olweus, D. (1993). *Bullying at school: What we know and what we can do.* Blackwell.

Olweus, D., Limber, S. P., & Breivik, K. (2019). Addressing specific forms of bullying: A large scale evaluation of the Olweus Bullying Prevention Program. *International Journal of Bullying Prevention, 1,* 70–84. https://doi.org/10.1007/s42380-019-00009-7

Olweus, R. (2022) Examining the Effectiveness of School-Bullying Intervention. Available at: https://doi.org/10.1007/s42380-019-0007-4

Rape, Abuse & Incest National Network (RAINN). (2022). *Campus SaVE Act* [Internet]. https://www.rainn.org/articles/campus-save-act

Sinozich, S., & Langton, L. (2014). *Special report: Rape and sexual assault victimization among college-age females, 1995–2013.* NCJ 248471. U.S. Department of Justice, Office of Justice Programs, Bureau of Justice Statistics. https://bjs.ojp.gov/content/pub/pdf/rsavcaf9513.pdf

U.S. Department of Education, Office for Civil Rights. (2021). *Enforcement of title IX with respect to discrimination based on sexual orientation and gender identity in light of Bostock v. Clayton County.* Available at: https://www2.ed.gov/about/offices/list/ocr/frontpage/faq/rr/policyguidance/index.html

U.S. Department of Health and Human Services. (n.d.). *Bullying and youth with disabilities and special health needs* [Internet]. StopBullying.Gov. Available at: https://www.stopbullying.gov/bullying/special-needs

University of Connecticut. (2020). *Policy against discrimination, harassment, and related interpersonal violence.* Available at: https://policy.uconn.edu/wp-content/uploads/sites/243/2021/08/Policy-Against-Discrimination-with-Title-IX-Regulatory-Updates-Approved-by-Cabinet-on-7.20.20-Technical-8.16.2021.pdf

van Starrenburg, M. L. A., Kuijpers, R. C. W. N., Hutschemaekers, G. J. M., & Engels, R. C. M. E. (2013). Effectiveness and underlying mechanisms of a group-based cognitive behavioral therapy-based indicative prevention program for children with elevated anxiety levels. *BMC Psychiatry, 13,* 183. https://doi.org/10.1186/1471-244X-13-183

Williams, B. D. (2014). *Federal efforts on bullying in schools.* Master's thesis. John Hopkins University.

Williford, A., Boulton, A., Noland, B., Little, T. D., Antti, K., & Salmivalli, C. (2012). Effects of the KiVa anti-bullying program on adolescents' depression, anxiety, and perception of peers. *Journal of Abnormal Child Psychology, 40,* 289–300. https://doi.org/10.1007/s10802-011-9562-y

Wilson-Simmons, R., Dash, K., Tehranifar, P., O'Donnell, L., & Stueve, A. (2006). What can student bystanders do to prevent school violence? *Journal of School Violence, 5*(1), 43–62. https://doi.org/10.1300/J202v05n01_04

Yeager, D. S., Fong, C., Lee, H. Y., & Espelage, D. (2015). Declines in efficacy or anti-bullying programs among older adolescents: Theory and a three-level meta-analysis. *Journal of Applied Developmental Psychology, 37,* 36–51. https://doi.org/10.1016/j.appdev.2014.11.00

Part III
Key Personnel in Addressing Violence in the Schools

Chapter 14
The Role of School District Superintendent in School Violence and Prevention: Softening Schools While Hardening Buildings

Matthew D. Thompson

Introduction

As a school or district administrator, there really is no such thing as downtime or completely disconnecting. This is even more true as a school district superintendent. You are on call 24-hours-a-day, 7-days-a-week. During those times when you are not physically present in the schools or the district, your mind is always drifting back towards the district. This creates a bit of a mindset where superintendents often find themselves waiting for the other shoe to drop, anticipating the next phone call, or expecting the inevitable text message or email regarding something going on in the district. In addition, since our schools and districts are a microcosm of the society and community in which we exist, all of the issues that exist around us are found in our schools. Issues of race, sexuality, bullying, stress, depression, and many others are exacerbated under the constant microscope of social media and the limits of teenage and adolescent brains that have not fully developed yet. The part of the brain that controls instincts such as fear, hunger, and pleasure is hyperactive during adolescence, while the part that is in charge of self-control, planning, and self-awareness is still developing (Merrill, 2019). The result is schools full of students who are facing adult issues and concepts while dealing with confusing emotions and thoughts. Is it any wonder why our students sometimes act out in ways that exhibit the extremes of society, such as taking crazy risks and engaging in dangerous behavior and violent outbursts (Steinberg, 2014)? Is it any wonder why a school district superintendent is always a bit on edge when out of the district? Both of these rhetorical questions will be addressed in the following anecdote.

M. D. Thompson (✉)
Montgomery County Schools, Mt. Sterling, KY, USA
e-mail: matthew.thompson@montgomery.kyschools.us

Fight Week

Driving back from a meeting out of district on a Tuesday afternoon the week before Thanksgiving, my cell phone rang. Glancing at the phone I saw it was my deputy superintendent who was back in the district while I was gone. When I answered, he told me he wanted to give me a heads up regarding a couple of fights that had occurred at the high school. There had been one fight that morning following two fights the previous day and he had seen a few comments on social media regarding "fight week" in the school. In a school of almost 1500 students, while certainly not common, it is not unheard of to have a few altercations that become physical between students. Three fights in 2 days was more than we had experienced in quite some time, yet it certainly was not indicative of anything more than heighted tensions and poor decision making by the students involved.

Upon returning to the district later that afternoon, I discussed the situation with the high school administrators and saw that they had reset behavioral expectations across the school and had limited the time available for students to congregate and linger in the hallways during class change. Common areas within the building where students liked to gather in groups (large hallway intersections, foyers, cafeteria, etc.) had increased supervision and safety protocols were reinforced. Things were under control and I was able to share that with our local newspaper when the editor inquired about a rumor there had been 12 fights in 2 days at the high school. During my tenure as superintendent, our district has been successful in creating an honest, accurate, and transparent reputation in our community. Our parents understand that we are going to be honest with them, provide them with accurate information, and provide transparency in all areas in which we are able. As I became aware of the exaggerated information taking social media by storm, I drafted and recorded the following message to our students, staff, and families and sent it out through our telephone calling service:

> Student and staff safety is always our number one priority. We are aware of numerous social media posts and comments referencing a large number of fights over the past two days at Montgomery County High School. These posts and comments do not contain accurate information and exaggerate the number of events occurring. The truth is that there were far fewer incidents than referenced on social media and the vast majority of our students engaged in appropriate behavior. In the few cases, each situation was investigated, students involved were given due process and MCHS administration used the Code of Conduct to determine appropriate consequences. Administration and staff have increased supervision and are proactively addressing the matter with students. Our administrators investigate every situation that is reported and we encourage any parent with concerns about their child to share them with the appropriate administrators. We encourage our parents to be aware of what your children are posting on social media and when you see something concerning to reach out to us.

However, even with sending the message out, the rumor of an exorbitant amount of fights was soon to take wing more fully on social media where it would soar and expand and take on mythical size over the next few days.

I spent most of the next day, Wednesday, at the high school helping out in any way I could so that I could tell any who asked that I had personally observed the climate and could vouch that things were very calm. Wednesday went very smooth until the very end of the day when two students engaged in a verbal altercation. By Wednesday evening, however, the story that had emerged on social media, fueled by adult instigators on Facebook and a video montage of the same few fights viewed from different angles making it seem as if there were dozens, was that fighting was out of control at the high school and that the administration was not doing anything about it. By Thursday morning I had two television station reporters calling my office asking for on-camera interviews, low student attendance because parents were nervous to send their children to school and social media posts calling for the removal of all the high school administrators (who were doing a great job keeping things moving smoothly at the school). After explaining to the reporters that "fight week" was not a real thing, the number of fights were greatly exaggerated, and that all the attention was making things incredibly worse, I saw the full ramifications of the social media and news attention when I arrived at the high school that morning. The tension could be felt as soon as I walked through the doors. There was the buzz of anxiety moving in an undercurrent throughout the common areas of the school. Students talked in small groups but looked up quickly any time a loud noise or rapid movement caught their attention. Staff supervised closely but did not seem to be able to draw the students into easy conversations like normal. Everyone was on edge, including me and the high school administrators. I met again with the administrators and discussed their conversation with the student council group the previous day where they had asked the student leaders to help engage their peers in calming the situation. That meeting had gone well and since there had been no major incidents yesterday we held off on a plan to meet with the different grade levels in class-wide meetings. Yet the tensions increased throughout the day and after two more issues during lunch, one of which involved the same few students as earlier in the week, we quickly reengaged our plan to meet with the entire student population in separate grade level meetings in the auditorium.

On Friday, after spending three full, consecutive days at the high school, speaking with all the students, and devoting hours to phone conversations with parents discussing their questions and concerns, it was obvious that I needed to take control of the message more fully in the community. There was so much exaggeration and misinformation out there that I needed to provide an absolute accurate account of what exactly had occurred. Earlier in the week, when the video montages had first emerged making it appear that there would dozens of fights, the high school administration and I had begun to counter the misinformation with an accurate number. However, upon further review, we realized that the same students had engaged in multiple fights and that the total number of students engaged in physical altercations was a significantly lower number than what was being portrayed over social media and in the news. After speaking with our students in the class meetings we also realized that the largest majority of our students were embarrassed by the behavior of a very small number of their peers. These facts became the basis of my message to our students, staff, families, and community. On Friday afternoon I sent the following letter (Fig. 14.1) out to our families, staff, and key community contacts over the telephone call system, email, and social media.

The weekend came and went and we entered the short week of Thanksgiving but the tension had passed and our high school was back to its normal level of calmness. Looking back in retrospect, it is easy to see ways in which we may have been able to handle the situation better and quicker. However, it is also easy to see that the relationships we built with our students, staff, families, and community along with strong behavioral expectations and safety protocols allowed us to successfully contain what could have been a complete disaster. It is vital that all leaders within a school district create a climate and expectations for these things to occur; however, as superintendent, it is even more important to ensure that I am leading by example. I have to be the one to build relationships, not only with administrators, teachers, and staff but also with students even though I may not be in their building every single day. The conversations I had with students, some of whom I had never met before, during fight week were some of the most beneficial one I had ever had. I was able to listen to their concerns, share thoughts, and build the foundation for future conversations that will, ultimately, benefit our schools and districts. I have to be the one to help establish the strong procedures and expectations for behavior. When the high school administration met with students to reset expectations for behavior, I was there in the auditorium providing occasional input. The students were able to see that expectations for behavior were consistent from not only the school but also the district. When questions were raised by the students, families, and community, I

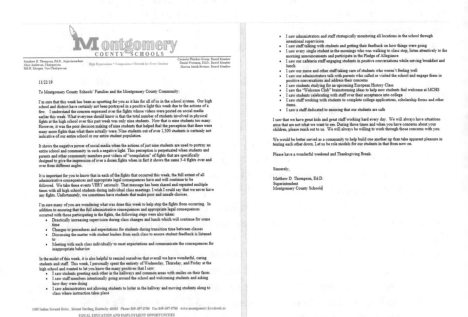

Fig. 14.1 Letter to parents and community about fights at the high school. (Used with permission)

was able to provide accurate, timely, and transparent communication with all involved to help calm the waters.

The above anecdote provides information that can be used to establish an appropriate framework for further elaboration regarding two main ways in which school districts are successfully and proactively preventing large-scale violence: (1) Softening schools while (2) Hardening buildings.

The School Safety and Resiliency Act: Softening Schools and Hardening Buildings

In January 2019, in response to the shooting at Marshall County High School in western Kentucky that left two students dead, the Kentucky Legislature passed the School Safety and Resiliency Act. A work of bipartisan, collaborative efforts between state legislators and all school stakeholders, it was designated as Senate Bill 1; identifying it as the first bill considered and reflecting the intent of it being the top priority during the short 30-day legislative session. The School Safety and Resiliency Act is truly a landmark piece of legislation as it includes a comprehensive approach to school safety. It established a State School Safety Marshall position while also establishing best practices for training and protocols. However, it also took the unique approach to legislate the need for intervention and mental health services for students. In essence, the new law established a balanced approach to school safety that softened schools (i.e., focusing on relationship building, mental health services, increased training on diversity, bias awareness training, trauma-informed actions, and de-escalation strategies, and increasing the number of mental health professionals in school buildings) while at the same time hardening the school buildings (i.e., mandating the locking and closing of all classroom doors while students are present, mandating specific security features in entryways of school buildings, and establishing regular monitoring of the adherence to safety protocols from the State Safety Marshall's office) (Loftus & McLaren, 2019). This balanced approach was lauded across the state as a major accomplishment in identifying true barriers to student and staff safety and confident faith existed that when the legislature established the biennial budget in the 2020 legislative session that funds would help make the full implementation of the School Safety and Resiliency Act a reality.

Softening Schools

The concept of softening schools is based on the belief that by making schools more accessible to, welcoming of, and supportive for students and families, we provide multiple opportunities for our students to feel connected to the school community in which they attend. Blum (2005) suggests that most cases of school violence do not occur with students who feel connected to their school they. The 2013 report, A Framework for Safe and Successful Schools, released by the national organizations representing school counselors, school psychologists, school social workers, elementary school principals, secondary school principals, and school resource officers, lists as its top three "best practices for creating safe and successful schools" (A Framework, 2013, p. 1):

1. Fully integrate learning supports (e.g., behavioral, mental health, and social services), instruction, and school management within a comprehensive, cohesive approach that facilitates multidisciplinary collaboration.
2. Implement multitiered systems of support (MTSS) that encompass prevention, wellness promotion, and interventions that increase with intensity based on student need, and that promote close school-community collaboration.
3. Improve access to school-based mental health supports by ensuring adequate staffing levels in terms of school-employed mental health professionals who are trained to infuse prevention and intervention services into the learning process and to help integrate services provided through school-community partnerships into existing school initiatives.

Creating a school environment that supports students comprehensively helps the students feel connected to the school community as a whole and provides a way to seek and/or receive assistance in ways ranging from the physical (e.g., clothing and food) to the educational (e.g., tutoring and instructional interventions) to the psychological (e.g., counseling and mental health services). As a school superintendent, one of the most important things I can do is establish the culture, climate, and expectations that ensure a welcoming environment for our students. Let us take a look at some of the specific ways in which school districts can soften schools to better support students and proactively stop school violence.

Relationship Building

Building relationships are the key to every interaction with students. As the well-known quote often attributed to Theodore Roosevelt (among others) states, "People don't care how much you know until they know how much you care." Our students do not have any reason to listen to us, follow our directions, or answer our questions other than that is what most of their parents and society expect them to do. However, once we establish a personal connection and bond with our students, indicate that we are interested in them as individuals and prove that we care about them, their work, and their future, there is much more motivation for them to contribute to the relationship in the form of instructional engagement and work. Establishing a culture in a school district where relationship building is a priority is important and does not occur without appropriate examples. The superintendent and district and school administrators model this expectation in our interactions with both staff and students. Examples of ways in which to model relationship building with students include the following:

- Learning names: It can often be a challenge for superintendents and other district level administrators to learn the names of students when not in the buildings on a daily basis. Yet it helps remember that since most students know who I am, due to my role as superintendent, I must try to learn their names and find out a little about them. This tends to be easier with students who are involved in a lot of activities. I often learn students' names by listening to the announcer at athletic events or by talking with extracurricular sponsors about the students on their teams/clubs. These topics also give me wonderful and numerous opportunities to engage and connect with students by discussing the game the previous night in which they hit two doubles or the academic team competition in which they answered three straight questions correctly. However, even though it is a bit more difficult, it is even more important to do so with students who may not be involved in activities as much. During the difficult week at the high school I specifically went up to students who I did not know and who seemed to live on the periphery of things and engaged them in conversation. My conversation with one student, who I had often seen and who appeared to always display a frown, resulted in the realization that we both liked the same television show offered me the opportunity to touch base with him throughout the rest of the school year. It is impossible to underestimate the relationship building power of calling a student by his or her name.
- Celebrating milestones and achievements: As superintendent one of my favorite activities is celebrating the achievements of our students. Our kids are truly amazing in what they are able to accomplish. At the beginning of our monthly school board meetings, we routinely recognize students and staff who have accomplished wonderful things. Calling them each by name, asking them to come to the front of the room to receive a certificate, and then taking their picture in front of their family and friends is a fantastic way to build relationships around an event that everyone will remember for some time. During the COVID-19 pandemic, I also began creating a weekly video message for our students, staff, families, and community in order to communicate face-to-face with a larger number of people and help explain complex plans and decisions. This video message also provided an opportunity to celebrate our students and staff in ways I had been unable to do so previously. For example, I was able to celebrate specific students' achievements by name and using pictures from events in which they participated. Our students have really seemed to enjoy this added touch this year.
- Increasing student voice: One of the best ways to build relationships with students as a superintendent is to give them voice in what goes on in the school and district. This can be done by creating a student advisory group and meeting with them regularly and by providing opportunities for students to provide feedback and their thoughts on issues which impact them through surveys and other techniques. When, as a district, we began to review our return to in-person instruction during the COVID-19 pandemic and were looking at a timeline to possibly increase the amount of in-person instruction for students, we sent a survey to our students asking them for their thoughts and feedback. Our administrative team

and Board of Education took those comments to heart when creating a revised plan.

Implicit Bias Training

The Kirwan Institute for the Study of Race and Ethnicity at The Ohio State University defines implicit bias as the attitudes or stereotypes that affect our understanding, actions, and decisions in an unconscious manner. During the spring and summer of 2020 as our nation was forced to raise its level of awareness to the racial tensions across the country, I made a concerted effort to do the same in my school district and community. Through numerous conversations with staff members, students, parents, and key community members, I came to the realization that our school district was not doing everything it could to address implicit bias in our schools. The personal social media posts of two recent graduates described the struggles with racism they had faced silently while in our schools. Determined to have our district become a change agent within our community, I was able to work with a regional trainer to provide implicit bias training first for all our district and school administrators and then for the staff in each of our schools. By becoming aware of, acknowledging, and reflecting upon our unconscious biases, we begin to create an environment, culture, and climate that is more supportive of all our students, especially those most in danger of becoming marginalized and isolated. This is one of the key ways in which we can help our students, who may not feel connected to our schools, begin to realize that we truly care about them and, while we may not always understand everything they are going through, are willing to make changes that help them feel safer and more supported.

Bullying Prevention

An average of 14% of students report being bullied in schools (Luxenberg et al., 2019). Students who are bullied are more likely to suffer from anxiety and depression (Cook et al., 2010; Klomek et al., 2007; Olweus, 1993), while those participate in bullying are more likely to engage in vandalization of property and drop out of school (Arcadepani et al., 2019; Haynie et al., 2001; Olweus, 2011). Our district, through the financial support of the Kentucky Department of Education (KDE), began to implement a comprehensive approach to bullying prevention 2 years ago through training and implementation of the Olweus Bullying Prevention Program (OBPP). This program includes school wide, classroom, individual, and community components and is focused on long-term change creating a safe and positive school climate. We established training teams in each of our schools and provided them with the tools to implement OBPP with their students, empowering students to no longer be bystanders as bullying behaviors occur. As superintendent, it is important to establish sustainable structures that are implemented with fidelity. Providing the support, resources, and training for systemic change using scientific research-based materials, like Olweus, is crucial to implementing sustainable strategies.

Identification of At-Risk Students Combined with Naming and Claiming

Even with training to identify implicit bias and the implementation of bullying prevention programs, students in danger of falling through the cracks still exist. Schools and districts must have procedures in place to identify students who are "at-risk." Our district administrators work with our schools to develop Student Assistance Teams (SATs) that meet regularly to review student specific data such as attendance, academic progress, and behavior as well as other information regarding issues outside of school. Students may be identified as at-risk because of academic grades and lack of progress, school attendance and truancy, behavior and discipline records, and other situations outside school such as a death in the family or the incarceration of a parent. Once students are identified as at-risk, however, a process must be in place to "name and claim" them where an individual plan is developed and specific staff members are assigned to mentor the student and implement the intervention plan. Combining the SAT and "name and claim" structures with Trauma-Informed Care training for school counselors and staff provides a multi-faceted approach in which we recognize the many variables that impact our students and their overall mental health. Often, students' negative behaviors in schools stem from types of trauma they have experienced outside of school (Hickman & Higgins, 2019). How we react and respond, as educators, must be with the understanding that most of our students have experienced some form of trauma in their lives. Creating a culture where we appropriately respect, understand, and respond to trauma at all levels of schooling can make the difference for our students and their subsequent responses. From the at-risk student perspective, it is much harder to fade away, disappear, and remain disconnected with school when an adult is building a relationship with you and checking up on your progress daily.

These are just a few of the many ways in which superintendents, district and school administrators, teachers, and other school staff can "soften" our schools and make them a more inclusive, supportive, and safe environment for our students. This in turn results in students feeling more connected and thus decreasing the possibility of school violence. However, unfortunately, softening schools is not enough. We must also strengthen our safety protocols and the safety of our school facilities in order to proactively prevent situations from occurring involving those who want to do harm to our students. This is often referred to as "hardening" our buildings and facilities.

Hardening Buildings

The sad truth, however, is that while softening schools may help make our students feel more connected with and supported by the school and staff there is still a need to strengthen the safety protocols and procedures throughout the school community. This often occurs through the establishment and implementation of emergency plans and by physically changing the actual building facility to make it more difficult to enter without permission. Unfortunately, previous examples of school shootings have shown a need to make schools more secure while not making them less inviting. Hardening buildings cannot be the only approach taken; however, it is an important part of a comprehensive plan to prevent school violence.

Emergency Plans

Planning for certain types of events is paramount to being successful when and if those events occur. Examples of emergency plans and protocols include the following:

- Lockdown drills: In the event of an intruder in the building, students and staff need to understand the procedures for when and how to lockdown for all areas within the building and how to proceed after the initial alarm is sounded. In Kentucky we are required to practice lockdown drills multiple times per year. While practicing lockdown drills may initially be frightening to some children it is a necessary piece to a fully equipped emergency plan.
- Evacuation drills: The need to evacuate a school building may occur for multiple reasons. Fire, earthquake and intruders may all be reasons why students and staff need to know the best way in which to exit a building quickly. Once outside, it is also important to know where to go to gather and what the reunification procedures are.
- Locking classroom doors during instruction: In the event of needing to quickly implement lockdown procedures, staff and students may not be able to take the time necessary to lock and close classroom doors. As a result, Kentucky law requires classroom doors to be closed and locked at all times when students and staff are inside.

Facility Changes

Changing the facilities involves many newer approaches to school building design that have never had to be considered before. While we often think of additions such as metal detectors as a way to make the buildings safer, there are, in fact, many other kinds of facility changes that help secure the buildings. Collaborating with local law enforcement agencies and conducting a facility audit of your schools provides excellent information on specific areas that can be addressed. Examples of facility changes that may be considered include the following:

- Blocking entrances: We want our schools to be as inviting as possible. This includes making the front entrances noticeable and accessible with large sidewalks and entryways where students and parents may gather in groups. Sinking metal bollards or placing large planters with soil and flowers (a much more welcoming picture) at key locations in front of these sidewalk and entryway areas prevents anyone from using a vehicle as a ramming device or weapon without hiding the entryway from sight and making it appear uninviting.
- Locked entrances with cameras and intercoms: All entrances to school should be secure at all times. The use of outside cameras and intercoms allow visitors to receive a warm welcome while viewing them and asking them kindly to identify themselves before allowing them entrance into the building.
- Security vestibules: A safety vestibule is a front foyer that visitors enter after being admitted in through the front entrance. Doors into the front office or hallways from the vestibule are locked and visitors must again be granted access to enter further into the building. This allows school staff to once more view, monitor, and made decisions regarding visitors before granting them access to any other part of the school.

Other facility changes may include security cameras and additional types of door and entryway hardware.

Conclusion

The safety of our students and staff is always the number one priority of any school district. Yet, in keeping everyone safe we cannot create such an unwelcoming and inhospitable environment that our students cannot learn. By balancing the softening of our schools with the hardening of our buildings we provide a multifaceted approach to protecting our students and staff physically, mentally, emotionally, and academically.

References

A Framework for Safe and Successful Schools. (2013). *Resource document.* National Association of School Psychologists. https://www.nasponline.org/schoolsafetyframework. Accessed 4 Oct 2020.

Arcadepani, F. B., Eskenazi, D. Y., Fidalgo, T. M., & Hong, J. S. (2019, May 2). An exploration of the link between bullying perpetration and substance use: A review of the literature. *Trauma, Violence, & Abuse, 22*(1), 207–214.

Blum, R. W. (2005). A case for school connectedness. *Educational Leadership, 62*(7), 16–20.

Cook, C. R., Williams, K. R., Guerra, N. G., Kim, T. E., & Sadek, S. (2010). Predictors of bullying and victimization in childhood and adolescence: A meta-analytic investigation. *School Psychology Quarterly, 25*(2), 65–83.

Haynie, C. L., Nansel, T., Eitel, P., Crump, A. D., Saylor, K., Yu, K., & Simons-Morton, B. (2001). Bullies, victims, and bully/victims: Distinct groups of at-risk youth. *Journal of Early Adolescence, 21*(1), 29–49.

Hickman, J., & Higgins, K. (2019). 10 simple steps for reducing toxic stress in the classroom. *Education Week, 39*(14), 19.

Klomek, A. B., Marrocco, F., Kleinman, M., Schonfeld, L. S., & Gould, M. S. (2007). Bullying, depression, and suicidality in adolescents. *Journal of the American Academy of Child and Adolescent Psychiatry, 46*(1), 40–49.

Loftus, T., & McLaren, M. (2019, January 7). School safety bill will deal with counselors, security – But not guns. *Courier Journal.* https://www.courier-journal.com/story/news/politics/2019/01/07/school-safety-response-expected-during-kentucky-legislative-session/2482323002/. Accessed 4 Oct 2020.

Luxenberg, H., Limber, S. P., & Olweus, D. (2019). *Bullying in U.S. schools: 2019 status report.* https://olweus.sites.clemson.edu/documents/Status%20Report_2019.pdf. Accessed 4 Oct 2020.

Merrill, S. (2019). Decoding the teenage brain (in 3 charts). In *Edutopia.* Available via https://www.edutopia.org/article/decoding-teenage-brain-3-charts. Accessed 3 Oct 2020.

Olweus, D. (1993). *Bullying at school: What we know and what we can do.* Blackwell.

Olweus, D. (2011). Bullying at school and later criminality: Findings from three Swedish community samples of males. *Criminal Behavior and Mental Health, 21,* 151–156.

Steinberg, L. (2014). *Age of opportunity: Lessons from the new science of adolescence.* Houghton Mifflin Harcourt.

Chapter 15
Role of Law Enforcement in School Violence Prevention Through Positive Intervention and Relationship Building

Christopher S. Barrier

Introduction

Students in the school environment who exhibit disruptive or violent behavior can take on many forms, and the measures taken to reduce the number of incidents have been applied from many different angles—some with success and others without success. The purpose of this chapter will be to examine the role of the law enforcement officer in the school setting to reduce violent incidents in schools. We will examine a historical overview of the function that law enforcement has played in this over time and how that role within the schools has evolved into the modern school environment. What began as a rather primitive approach to policing juveniles in schools has grown into a much more intentional method, supported by education and experience that is conducive to a better learning climate and culture for students in schools. This chapter will further discuss, from the law enforcement practitioner point of view, approaches that have been used nationally as well as in states like Kentucky, which have yielded favorable results in the reduction of violent incidents in schools.

Understanding the Problem

According to the National Center for Education Statistics during the 2015–2016 school year, 79% of public schools recorded that one or more incidents of violence, theft, or other crimes had taken place, amounting to 1.4 million crimes. This

C. S. Barrier (✉)
Montgomery County School District Police Department, Montgomery County Public Schools, Mount Sterling, KY, USA
e-mail: chris.barrier@montgomery.kyschools.us

translates to a rate of 28 crimes per 1000 students (NCES, 2019). Because of this alarming rate of increase in reported crime in schools, many schools have placed law enforcement officers in schools to help combat school violence. But understanding school violence on a larger scope is critical to understanding how to prevent violent acts in schools. School violence may take any of the following forms: physical violence (typically student-on-student), psychological violence (bullying/harassment), sexual violence (typically sexual harassment but could encompass rape), and weapons-related offenses. What has been learned over time, however, is that the placement of law enforcement in schools alone is not a significant deterrent to such violent acts. It takes more than the officer presence. This article will emphasize how positive intervention and relationship building between the student and the officer can help reduce the number of violent acts that result in law enforcement action in schools. In my nearly 20 years as a law enforcement officer, it has been my experience that the best tool afforded to me was not one found on my duty belt but rather the positive rapport and relationships that were developed with those I serve. That idea was further cemented in 2008 as I transitioned from law enforcement in a small local municipality in Central Kentucky to a school-based law enforcement agency in that same community. Many times over it has been proven that, through the development of those relationships, I have seen a reduction in crime data statistics in our school as well as a reduction in the recidivism (the tendency of a person to reoffend) rates among juvenile offenders.

A Closer Look at the Numbers

In an effort to more clearly define the problem, look at how crime data statistics helps steer the working of law enforcement officers in schools to reduce the number of reported crime in the school setting. Nearly 80% of our public schools are now reporting to law enforcement that a crime has occurred in their school building. As such, 68% of the reported crime was an act of violence as reported by the NCES study and is illustrated in Fig. 15.1.

While it has been acknowledged that violence has been occurring in schools for some time, and arguments can be made that the presence of law enforcement officers in schools might inadvertently assist in driving up student encounters with law enforcement, data shows that, when done correctly, law enforcement in schools can actually help drive down the number of arrests in schools. This is critically important as we look more closely at data related to reported crime numbers and recidivism in the next two sections. It is worth noting again that the success of the SRO (School Resource Officer) program hinges on the ability of the law enforcement in the SRO program to build long-term, meaningful relationships with students.

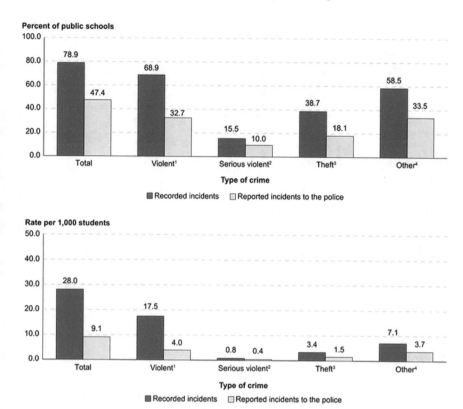

Fig. 15.1 US Department of Education, National Center for Education Statistics (2019)

Crime Data

The following chart is data pulled from the Montgomery County School District Police Department, which shows a statistically significant decrease in the number of reported criminal incidents in a 9-year test sample (current year data not yet available). Specifically, the data shows a consistent decline in reported criminal offenses reported from the 2012–2013 school year forward (Fig. 15.2). We feel the decline is due to intentional actions taken after the Sandy Hook Elementary Shooting in Newtown, Connecticut, where 28 lives were lost as a result of that school shooting. In an effort to ensure that our district would not be a victim of a copycat occurrence, the district made the decision to increase the presence of law enforcement officers from two to five and strategically placed them in schools throughout all levels of learning, including elementary schools.

In addition, during the test sample provided, a significant decrease in the number of physically violent assaults was observed. The reduction in number of assaults, which was cut 50% during this test sample, has led to a much safer school learning environment for all of the students in the district. Based on the data and our

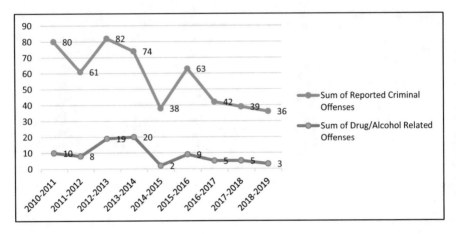

Fig. 15.2 Montgomery County Schools annualized crime data report 2019 (Barrier, 2019)

experience, we feel that the right decision was made at the right time to ensure safety to all students, staff, and stakeholders in the school district.

Recidivism

The concept of recidivism rates, and the importance of the reduction in that rate, is crucial in understanding the numbers and the overall impact it has on the life of the student, particularly post-graduation. National recidivism rates for juveniles do not exist, but state studies have shown that re-arrest rates for youth within 1 year of release from an institution average 55%, while reincarceration and reconfinement rates during the same timeframe average 24% (Snyder & Sickmund, 2006). Other studies show that once a child enters the criminal justice system, there can be as high as a 70% likelihood that he/she will reoffend. With that in mind, there must be a calculated focus on the part of law enforcement to arrest and adjudicate youthful offenders only as a last resort or when it is critical to the safety of self and others. Another factor to consider when juveniles are placed into custody is how it impacts demographic groups differently, and certainly disproportionately, across all states. Most juveniles (54%) in residential facilities are ages 16–17, and the vast majority are male (85%) and racial or ethnic minorities (69%), including black, Hispanic, and American Indian (Sickmund et al., 2017). While these numbers are not solely the result of encounters from law enforcement officers in schools, many of the arrest encounters are initiated at the school level. This is why there is a moral imperative on the part of law enforcement or SROs to maintain a high level of understanding how the decisions that are made in the moment, at the school level, can have a lasting effect on youthful offenders. For example, if Officer A is not duty or ethically bound to affect an arrest for a crime which is reported to them, that said officer must weigh the impact both on the overall climate/culture of the school, the safety therein, and most importantly the well-being of the child involved. Allowing the school district administrators to handle an offender who could be legally charged with a crime will instantaneously cultivate a relationship of trust if a relationship was not previously forged. Additionally, keeping the child out of the criminal justice system, without the knowledge of the child, ultimately ensures that the "risk of recidivism" is not a factor. Through exercising appropriate discretion, the SRO has the potential to alter the pathway a young person may take in life. Unlike in the previous segment on reported crime data, an officer's relationship to the student and the use of sound judgement can have immediate and life-altering consequences. It literally is that critical, and that is why relationships are the foundational building block for every successful SRO program. In the ensuing discussion, we will explore the methods by which SROs use education and experience to employ deliberate tactics to reduce school violence.

Methods

During the 1950s, law enforcement became cognizant of the need to protect students and staff in schools. In the early years only a small number of districts employed the practice of placing officers in schools, but this practice became much more commonplace in the 1970s. For instance, in Kentucky, Fayette County (Lexington), which is the second largest school district in the state, began their police department with 21 sworn officers. In an interview conducted with Lieutenant Tracy Day of the Fayette County School District Police Department, Day detailed how their agency has grown to 64 sworn officers with a specific focus of addressing school safety in a holistic manner (T. Day, May 18, 2018, personal communication). Again, they used the department's training and experience to make necessary changes in the safety model for the students and staff they protect. Day went on to say that the 64 officers in the district have the responsibility of policing over 42,000 students over 69 educational settings. Fayette County Public Schools (2018) adopted a comprehensive 10-point comprehensive safety investment plan in 2018 which covered several critical areas for school safety. Some of the areas addressed were as follows:

- Additional officers
- Additional mental health providers
- Facility upgrades
- Metal detectors

The 10-point safety investment plan can be viewed in its entirety at the Fayette County Public Schools webpage (https://www.fcps.net/cms/lib/KY01807169/Centricity/Domain/4/2018-19/safety_points.pdf).

While Fayette county is a metropolitan school environment and may not be necessarily reflective of every school in the country, it does a splendid job of acknowledging that the most critical first step to ensuring a quality SRO program begins with the people you employ in the agency.

Selection and Training

While it may be a shared vision among the school district and the law enforcement agency regarding which direction they wish to steer the SRO program, in order for there to be sustained success, there must be both careful selection of the SRO and high levels of proper training. It is imperative that both prerequisites are accounted for in the selection of the SRO. Following the School Shooting deaths of two students in Benton, Kentucky, on January 23, 2018, State Senator Max Wise and State Representative Bam Carney began the daunting task of ensuring, among other things, that SROs in Kentucky would be among the most qualified and well-trained SROs in the nation. The bi-partisan legislative initiative, officially titled, The School Safety and Resiliency Act of 2019, requires officers in Kentucky to complete 120 hours of SRO training in three phases over three consecutive years, as well as meet the state required Police Officer Professional Standards (POPS) training (LRC School Safety and Resiliency Act, 2019). It is often said there is no state in the nation that has more stringent training/selection requirements placed on SROs for the purpose of servicing youth in schools. According to Bill Eckler, Supervisor of the School Resource Officer Training SECTION at the Department of Criminal Justice Training, "SRO training now includes new topics such as working with special-needs students, mental health awareness and trauma-informed action. Firearms and defensive tactics refresher training will also be included" (Eckler, 2020). These are just a few of the training standards now utilized in Kentucky that are quickly becoming the nationwide standard to guarantee SROs have the appropriate foundation to be effective SROs in their school community. Let us dive a little deeper into the details of the SRO training that directly impacts the students in schools.

SRO Triad

The single best example that I can think of to illustrate the function the SRO serves in the school setting is defined by the National Association of School Resource Officers (NASRO). NASRO teaches that SROs typically serve as one of three roles best laid out in the SRO Triad Model, the elements of which are laid out as follows (NASRO, 2012):

- Law Enforcement Officer
- Informal Counselor
- Teacher

When used appropriately, the triad shows how SROs can have the greatest impact on the students that they serve. With such a program, the officer represents much more to the students and staff in the building than the "cop in the school." The SRO program reflects a whole community commitment to ensure that our schools are safe and secure learning environments.

The SRO should be viewed as a trusted resource for the school community. As such, the SRO fulfills three key roles by using a triad approach. First, and most naturally, the SRO acts as a law enforcement officer. Second, the SRO acts as a trusted informal counselor who can build healthy relationships and educate students about law-related issues. As a law enforcement officer, the primary purpose, obviously, is to safeguard the students/staff of the education institution. As an informal counselor, the officer provides resource guidance to students, parents, teachers, and staff and acts as a link to support services both inside and outside the school. This is the area that occupies much of the SRO's time and adds great value to those the SRO serves in that trust and relationships are fostered through this role. Here, the foundation is laid for the success of the SRO program and the backbone by which the image of the officer will be shaped in the mind of the student—*it is about relationships*. Lastly, as a law-related educator, the officer will share special law enforcement expertise by presentations in the classroom to promote a better understanding of our laws. Furthermore, the SRO also serves as positive role model for the students on campus during school hours and off campus at extracurricular activities. For example, for 15 years I have coached at various levels and sports within the district. Currently serving as an Asst. Football coach gives me the opportunity to develop relationships with students I ordinarily may not have had the chance to reach inside a school setting. SROs must be properly selected, highly trained, and equipped with a road map for how to positively intervene in the life of a young person. Now we can explore how the suitable placement of the SRO plays a part in how successful the SRO program can be in reducing school violence.

Suitable Placement

It is known that even when an SRO is properly selected and highly trained in the various aspects of how to be an effective SRO, finding suitable placement within the organization is hugely important to the success of the program. Let us take a look at a "real-world" example[1] of this:

Scenario: Officer White, having served 30 years as a military veteran, state police officer, and military police trainer, came to work to serve as an SRO in our agency. Given his unique set of circumstances, the decision was made to assign him to the oversight of the elementary schools in the district. Immediately, he began to make his impact known by addressing some infrastructure security shortfalls at his school. He determined a more efficient way to

---

[1] All names and other personal identifiers have been changed to protect privacy and confidentiality.

alleviate traffic flow concerns in the community. The impact that Officer White was having on the community school was both welcomed and appreciated by those in the community. But his impact was felt much greater inside the walls of the school. Officer White took on a student to mentor during his time at the school. Little Johnny only had negative reflections of the police because his only encounters with law enforcement were when the police would respond to his home during domestic squabbles his parents were engaged in or if the police pulled his dad over for a traffic violation. Generally, those types of encounters embed negative thoughts and emotions in the impressionable minds of young people, particularly if the encounter results in an arrest or some type of punitive action. But Officer White was not going to allow preconceived notions about who and what police officers were to impact how he treated Johnny. He just continued to mentor Johnny with positive reinforcement gestures like back pats and head taps when he saw Johnny hold the door to the cafeteria. He gave him peppermints when Johnny got out of the car in the mornings after breaks from school since he didn't know if his Christmas vacation was joy filled or sorrow stricken. Officer White continued to build a relationship with Johnny.

Johnny's story is not unique by any stretch, but one has to wonder how the relationship developed between Johnny and Officer White may have helped to shift the worldview of what Johnny saw in the police. Are the police people I can trust and rely on in times of need, or are they someone to cause hurt and pain in my home? The impact that SROs can have on the developing mind of a young person can literally change a generation of mindsets. This is why early intervention with students is critically important. If you allow a child to formulate their own opinions through early childhood and adolescence, there is a strong likelihood it will not be a positive viewpoint. In truth, most encounters with law enforcement can have negative outcomes. As a law enforcement executive, I made the decision to place Officer White in a community elementary school, not necessarily because of the visible crime deterrence he presented but to help form a favorable impression of law enforcement during the formative years of a young person's life. As expected, the relationships that he was able to form there have produced great dividends.

Law Enforcement Issues in School Environment

The function of the SRO in the school setting is certainly one that does not come without immense sacrifice from stakeholders in the community. When a local municipality and local school district decide to work together in an effort to commit an officer(s) to the school, a series of events has to first take place.

Memorandums of Understanding

Community leaders and school leaders must first agree to terms on how the officer in the school will work with the district in a formal agreement called a memorandum of understanding or agreement (MOU or MOA). These agreements are legally binding process orders that set guidelines and protocols for how the officers carry out their daily functions in the schools. MOU and MOA contracts typically also address areas such as pay and fringe benefits for both parties as well as hours of operations. Because schools are no longer 7 am to 4 pm places of business, the contract agreement will also spell out how the law enforcement services will provide coverages in after hour events and special occasions.

Goal Setting

Another such issue that could possibly arise with an SRO program is differences in opinions of various stakeholders. All stakeholders must work together to determine goals for the SRO program. Any differences in opinions must be discussed prior to engagement with students so that all parties adhere to the agreed upon norms. Differences in philosophy and operational tactics may still exist, but the newly created team/partnership must work toward common goals that are identified and agreed upon by both parties. Philosophical differences primarily exist in the form of cultural differences between police agencies and schools. The climate and culture in schools should provide a nurturing environment where students can learn in a loving environment. This culture does not naturally occur in a police department setting, so the SRO must learn this new climate and all parties must work to find common ground from which to build their relationship. Operational obstacles may include dual assignments for the officer, lack of relevant training options, or lack of opportunities for engagement with students. All of these are logical precursors for why an SRO program may not experience its full level of success.

Barriers to Relationships

School partnerships with law enforcement often experience their greatest failures during their infancy, when the relationships between police and schools as well as SRO and students are not properly fostered. Both relationships matter equally. The administrative relationship matters because there must be commitment to the SRO program. It takes enormous commitment from the school staff to welcome into their bubble, or comfort zone if you will, a police presence into the school. This may not be easy for teachers/staff to accept but is necessary from a safety standpoint. Relationships must be built on trust and mutual understanding so that each are there to serve the greater good of the student. Second, and certainly most importantly, is the relationship of the student and SRO. As mentioned earlier in the chapter, I discussed the idea of fostering "long-term, meaningful relationships." The relationships must be long term and meaningful and function together to be successful. For example, it is possible for an SRO to have a meaningful relationship that is not long term. Conversely, it is possible to have a long-term relationship that is not meaningful. Each scenario does not provide for optimal results. The SRO must work to achieve both simultaneously for best results.

Another obstacle to building critical relationships is how inconsistent police departments can be in their ability to place a particular SRO in the school setting for an extended period of time. For most agencies, an SRO is on assignment to schools for just a few years. The SRO is typically a "high flyer" and destined for promotion or placement in another area the department has a greater need. Because of this, you often might see a revolving door of officers. On the opposite end of that spectrum is the officer who is "Retired on Duty" or placed in the schools because of a disciplinary sanction against the officer. These are all ill-advised operational tactics, which can ultimately cause the dissolution of the program in its entirety. If the common goal is to have a program where the SRO is to build long-term, meaningful relationships with students and have a consistently productive program for the community stakeholders, I can think of no better reason than to put the very best candidates possible in the school with the most valuable resources—our students.

Education Programs

Education programs are often viewed as essential parts of school district safety models. School administrators feel better that some types of prevention strategies are implemented to help give students an educational foundation for why they should not use or abuse substances. The problem is these programs often lack quantifiable data that suggests they actually work. The biggest example of this is the DARE campaign of the 1980s and 1990s. Even as a young child I can remember sitting in elementary class and having an instructor take us through the course. The DARE program was created by the Los Angeles Police Department in the early 1980s, and it immediately became hugely popular in school districts across the country. And rightfully so, again, administrators were happy to have a program designed to teach kids it was socially acceptable to say no. But data did not support the program's efficacy: "Despite this fanfare, data indicate that the program does little or nothing to combat substance use in youth. A meta-analysis (mathematical review) in 2009 of 20 controlled studies by statisticians Wei Pan, then at the University of Cincinnati, and Haiyan Bai of the University of Central Florida revealed that teens enrolled in the program were just as likely to use drugs as were those who received no intervention" (Lilienfeld & Arkowitz, 2014). This data, while focused specifically on DARE, is not unique to this program alone. The fact is there is little to no data that suggests any social education program in schools has been effective in curtailing the use or abuse of substances among students in schools. This is why I advocate so strongly for the presence of SROs in schools and believe that the positive relationship building with students, which leads to positive mentorship opportunities, is much more effective than educational programs. I believe that there is a place for programs like DARE or others in the educational setting so that students will at least be making informed decisions but would argue that positive interventions with SROs and other role models are more effective in deterring substance abuse and ultimately reducing crime in schools.

The Value Is in the SRO

Across the landscape of the various models used to reduce crimes in schools and keep students/staff safe in schools, one common thread emerges. The value is in the SRO. I have long believed that school safety is a focused application of three critical areas of emphasis: policies/procedures, infrastructure, and personnel management. The particular climate/culture of a community will ultimately determine how much of each ingredient is appropriate for a given community. I like to call it the "appetite for safety." Each community has a different appetite based on certain demands for levels of safety. Some prefer the school to have enhanced physical security measures with cameras and safety vestibules and others to have robust safety protocols. Infrastructure can be upgraded and improved continually, and policies/procedures can be reviewed often, yet one truth remains. Nothing will ever be able to replace the properly selected and highly trained SRO. Further, there has never been a school shooting where a SRO was present "inside" the school, and there has never been loss of life of a stakeholder once engaged by law enforcement. What does that tell us? The SRO is the single greatest deterrent to violent criminal behavior in schools. That fact cannot be changed by the presence of cameras and protocols for active threats. SROs save lives and keep people safe in schools.

Aside from the visible deterrence, SROs have the ability to discern human tendencies and make daily threat assessment determinations. Because they are in the schools, building long-term, meaningful relationships with students, SROs have been able to thwart violent acts countless times. The relationship with students and staff is the basis for everything good that the SRO can bring to the climate and culture in a school building.

Conclusion and Recommendations

In nearly 20 years as a law enforcement practitioner, I have had the good fortune of spending a considerable amount of my career in a school building—12 years to be exact. During that time, countless students who I may have never imagined finding their path to success in life have accomplished wonderful achievements. Some are bankers and business owners and healthcare workers. And I am thankful for the opportunity to have been able to serve these young people and hopefully had some kind of impact on their paths in life. There is no way for me to determine if my role as the school SRO made a major impact on the decision of a student to commit a serious violent act or not, but years of data has shown that the processes we have put in place have reduced crime in the school. This is not because we arrest more and not because we treat kids like prisoners in school, but because we treat every student with respect and dignity and focus on developing relationships and positive interventions to help steer students in the right direction. Thankfully for us in Montgomery County, Kentucky, it has worked incredibly well, and I am confident that, when applied appropriately elsewhere, schools will see the same success. The focus must remain that everything is about relationships. Hopefully in this chapter, I have helped to give a little glimpse into the life of an SRO and provoked a healthy thought pattern for how to view SROs in schools and their impact on the climate and culture in schools.

Recommendations as lessons learned from working in the school environment include the following:

1. *Take the time to know the people you serve with.* You may know their name but not their story. You may know their actions, but do you know where they come from?
2. *Be intentional – Do not focus on the data.* The data is the reward for the intentional behaviors used to make the difference in the life of the young person. This is true in both education and law enforcement alike.
3. *Be persistent* – Do not let organizational or societal influences stand in the way of doing what is best for kids. Always do the right thing for the child.

Being an SRO has been the enjoyment of my life and no question the duty call for my life's work. But that would be an empty call if it were not for the relationships that have been made over the years. The intrinsic value of watching students succeed and knowing that in some small way our relationship played a factor in that success is simply priceless.

References

Barrier, C. (2019). *Montgomery County School district police annualized crime data report 2019.*
Eckler, B. (2020). *School resource officer training.* https://www.docjt.ky.gov/school-resource-officer
Fayette County Public Schools. (2018). *Fayette County Public Schools comprehensive 10-point safety investment plan.* https://www.fcps.net/cms/lib/KY01807169/Centricity/Domain/4/2018-19/safety_points.pdf
Institute of Education Sciences, National Center for Education Statistics. (2019). *Fast facts: school crime.* https://nces.ed.gov/fastfacts/display.asp?id=49
Lilienfeld, S. O., & Arkowitz, H. (2014, January 1). Why "just say no" doesn't work – A popular program for preventing teen drug use does not help. Here's what does. *Scientific American.* https://www.scientificamerican.com/article/why-just-say-no-doesnt-work/
National Association of School Resource Officers (NASRO). (2012). *To protect & educate: The school resource officer and the prevention of violence in schools.* https://www.nasro.org/clientuploads/resources/NASRO-Protect-and-Educate.pdf
Sickmund, M., Sladky, T. J., Kang, W., & Puzzanchera, C. (2017). *Easy access to the census of Juveniles in residential placement.* National Center for Juvenile Justice. http://www.ojjdp.gov/ojstatbb/ezacjrp

Snyder, H. N., & Sickmund, M. (2006). *Juvenile offenders and victims: 2006 national report.* U.S. Department of Justice, Office of Justice Programs, Office of Juvenile Justice and Delinquency Prevention. https://www.ojjdp.gov/ojstatbb/nr2006/downloads/nr2006.pdf

Wise, M., & Carney, B. (2019). *School Safety and Resiliency Act 2019.* https://apps.legislature.ky.gov/recorddocuments/bill/19RS/sb1/bill.pdf

Chapter 16
Toward Understanding Classroom Socialization: Teacher Roles in Peer Victimization

Jina Yoon, Chunyan Yang, and Marie L. Tanaka

The context of school has been recognized as one of the most critical settings that affect peer victimization. Defined as "safe (emotionally and physically), engaging, collaborative (between teachers, students, and parents), and respectful," positive school climate is linked to less peer victimization (Gottfredson et al., 2005), whereas students are less likely to report peer victimization when they perceive school climate to tolerate peer victimization (Unnever & Cornell, 2004). Meta-analyses have indicated that the whole school approach is associated with the most positive impact on peer victimization (Ttofi & Farrington, 2011; Vreeman & Carroll, 2007). Given that the school is an important developmental context for social competencies, and that peer victimization often takes place in schools, identifying specific sources and mechanisms of influences on peer victimization provides particular insight into prevention and intervention efforts. Within the school context, peers have been also recognized as a strong influence on peer victimization. Research on peer relations and victimization continues to inform us that various participatory roles of peers are a strong force (e.g., Salmivalli et al., 2011). Peers' bystander behaviors or behaviors supportive of bullies are likely to perpetuate a cycle of peer victimization, which provides a strong rationale for prevention and intervention programs that target peer groups. This line of research has broadened the focus of peer victimization from an individual approach (e.g., working with bullies and victims) to an ecological approach (e.g., school-wide bullying prevention, upstander training), especially gaining more nuanced understanding of specific characteristics of the school context.

J. Yoon (✉) · M. L. Tanaka
Department of Disability and Psychoeducational Studies, College of Education, University of Arizona, Tucson, AZ, USA
e-mail: jinayoon@arizona.edu

C. Yang
Graduate School of Education, University of California, Berkeley, Berkeley, CA, USA

T. W. Miller (ed.), *School Violence and Primary Prevention*,
https://doi.org/10.1007/978-3-031-13134-9_16

373

Classroom contexts are important for understanding students' peer victimization experiences and their adjustment outcomes. To a large extent, classroom compositions and social climate determine whom children are exposed to and interact with throughout the school day (Leadbeater & Hoglund, 2006), thus impacting their interactional qualities. A recent study found that victim's distress as measured by depression was lower in middle school classrooms where class-level bully-related defending (e.g., standing up to bullying) was higher, whereas the same effect was not observed for class-level victim-related defending (e.g., comforting) (Yun & Juvonen, 2020). This robust finding further supports the importance of classroom climate and its protective effect for victims. Similarly, Gage et al. (2014) found that adult support in school was associated with less peer victimization; high-risk students reported less peer victimization when they attended schools where adults were perceived as trustworthy, respectful, and caring and that students' respect for racial diversity was associated with less victimization in elementary schools. In addition to the direct influence on students' victimization risks, classroom contexts also impact the magnitude of the association between peer victimization and students' adjustment outcomes. For example, Gini et al. (2020) found that the student victims in classrooms with lower levels of victimization were more likely to report somatic problems. This finding highlights the effects of class norms on victims' adjustment and the importance of addressing the possible risks for those who continue to be victimized.

Meanwhile, many researchers have noted that the role of teachers has been less explored in the prevention and intervention efforts to reduce peer victimization. Yoon and Bauman (2014) argued that teachers are "a critical but overlooked component of bullying prevention and intervention" (p. 308). Valle et al. (2020) noted in a systemic review of literature that all school-based programs included teachers, yet studies rarely examined teacher reports. Although teachers are often responsible for implementing anti-bullying programming, factors that affect their implementation are not well known. Swift et al. (2017) found in a U.S. sample of 4th and 5th grade teachers that professional burnout level was associated with program dosage; teachers experiencing more burnout were less likely to implement the KiVa program. In the first edition of this handbook, we presented existing evidence for critical roles that teachers play in the dynamics of victimization and highlighted these roles in specific areas of prevention and intervention (Yoon & Barton, 2008). Since the first edition of this handbook, there has been increasing interest in how teachers play a pivotal role in the prevention and intervention of peer victimization. Researchers have also examined various aspects of teacher influences in peer victimization and broader peer relationships. In this chapter, we present a review of existing data that document how teachers may affect peer victimization and the experiences for bullies, victims, and other students who are engaged in various roles in peer dynamics. Based on the review, we discuss practical implications for prevention and intervention as well as future research directions.

Current Conceptual Frameworks

To conceptualize the roles of teachers in students' experiences of peer victimization, we draw from several theories and models. Grusec and Hastings (2015) suggest that teachers are one of the key socializing agents who communicate relevant values and rules. Wentzel (2003) further elaborates on the socializing processes and proposes that teachers not only directly influence students' social behavior via modeling, providing advice, and informing but also indirectly by communicating goals and expectations and by providing experiences through which these goals and expectations are learned and internalized. The goal framing theory (Lindenberg, as cited in Veenstra et al., 2014) further suggests that significant adults such as teachers are agents who activate goals and norms when addressing specific situations. When applied to peer victimization, the goal framing theory underscores the extent to which teachers address peer victimization incidents and activate relevant goals and norms (e.g., anti-bullying) to promote prosocial behaviors and prevent future peer victimization.

Another theoretical approach attempts to explain how teachers influence the classroom peer ecology. With a metaphor of the "invisible hand," Farmer et al. (2018) argue that (1) teachers affect social dynamics—the interactions and relationships they have with students "collectively set the tone for how peers interact with each other" (p. 179) and (2) teachers' awareness and knowledge of naturally occurring social dynamics in the classroom (teacher attunement) guide their efforts to facilitate students' social experiences (e.g., specific grouping strategies, seating assignments, disciplinary practices, and other methods that affect students' social experiences [Farmer et al., 2010; Gest et al., 2014]). Similarly, Rodkin and Gest (2011) proposed a construct of network-related teaching as a way to explain teacher influences on peer ecology, which includes social status managing, social network management, aggression/bullying management, and peer ecology knowledge.

These theoretical approaches together highlight several points. First, teachers as socializing agents have tremendous influences on peer victimization. Second, their ongoing and consistent pattern of socializing students through rules and routines serves an important social context that have implications for students' experiences of peer victimization. Third, teachers should be considered as a target of prevention and intervention, just as we focus on peer behaviors, such as bystander behaviors that deter or perpetuate peer victimization. Fourth, these theoretical approaches all recognize the importance of teacher–student interactions. Inherent to these interactions is the interpersonal context between teachers and students. We argue that the relationship quality cannot be ignored when we attempt to understand how teachers promote and facilitate the internalization of social goals and expectations. Next, we offer a review of existing evidence on how teachers may influence peer victimization and their implications for practice.

Mechanisms of Teacher Influences on Peer Victimization

Teacher Responses to Peer Victimization

Consistent with the notion of socializing agents, researchers have examined various ways that teachers may socialize their students, affecting the way students interact with one another. One area of research has examined how teachers respond to victimization incidents. According to the goal framing theory, victimization incidents serve as opportunities for teachers to activate the norms and goals that denounce peer victimization and encourage prosocial behaviors. Thus, teachers' handling of peer victimization contributes to students' perceived norms and goals in classrooms and schools. Although the way teachers address victimization incidents may reflect broader classroom management, we argue that teachers' handling of victimization incidents may be salient socializing experiences closely tied to the experiences of perpetrators, victims, and other students in the classroom.

Extant evidence suggests that teacher responses to victimization incidents significantly vary, ranging from ignoring, disciplining perpetrators, involving classroom-level intervention to involving other adults such as principals, parents, and counselors (Yoon et al., 2016). Although we have limited evidence linking various strategies used by teachers to levels of victimization, the following general themes have emerged: (1) teachers' inaction is associated with high levels of peer victimization (Marachi et al., 2007); (2) teachers' attempts to stop victimization are related to low levels of perpetration (Mucherah et al., 2018); (3) relying on reprimanding the perpetrators (i.e., a punitive approach) is not associated with less victimization (Troop-Gordon 2015; Wachs et al., 2019); (4) perpetrators are more likely to stop when teachers communicate victim's feelings and their own disapproval for victimization (Garandeau et al., 2016); and (5) long-term reduction of peer victimization is associated with teachers' supportive-individual strategies (e.g., talking to involved students, emotionally supporting them) and supportive-cooperative strategies (e.g., working with all students in class, cooperating with others, taking actions at class/school level [Wachs et al., 2019]). Little is known about how specific teacher responses to peer victimization affect bystanders, defenders, and other students; however, we can speculate that teachers' strategies to deter and prevent victimization will encourage other students to defend victims and report victimization incidents. Emerging evidence suggests that teachers' handling of bullying incidents influences students' social cognition, which is hypothesized to affect their behaviors. Demol et al. (2020, 2021) found that when students were presented with vignettes where teachers actively responded to a bullying incident (e.g., correcting the bully and comforting the victim), they were more willing to report bullying, less likely to expect pro-bullying behaviors, and more likely to expect defending behaviors in the classroom.

Given the importance of effective handling of peer victimization by teachers, many researchers have proposed training programs and professional development for teachers and pre-service teachers (e.g., Oldenburg et al., 2016; Yoon et al., 2016).

However, a few available data indicate that the extent to which these trainings lead to changes in teachers' practice is questionable. For example, Yoon & Bauman (2014) found no differences in teacher responses to a hypothetical bullying scenario whether they were previously trained in bullying responses or not. In a systematic review of the whole school anti-bullying programs, Valle et al. (2020) found that most programs have a component that involve teachers (e.g., training or information materials), but its impact on teachers (or teachers' perspective of its impact on students) is rarely examined. Thus, we need not only to evaluate teacher training but also to identify critical components of trainings that will lead to significant improvement in teachers' handling of peer victimization.

Several challenging issues have been noted in teachers' ability to respond to victimization incidents. Overall, teachers are lacking in their knowledge about bullying, skills and self-efficacy, and attitude toward victimization (Bradshaw et al., 2011; Troop-Gordon & Ladd, 2014; Wachs et al., 2019), all of which are likely to influence the way teachers respond to an incident. Even in a high-quality program such as KiVa, teachers are unsure of what bullying is (Oldenburg et al., 2015); they do not feel they have adequate skills to address peer victimization (Bradshaw et al., 2011). In a qualitative study of Dutch teachers, van Verseveld et al. (2020) found four areas of challenges when addressing peer victimization: identifying bullying that teachers do not witness, evaluating its seriousness, addressing more chronic and pervasive aggression, and working with parents to reduce bullying. These challenges were particularly noticeable among those with less teaching experiences (1–5 years). Consistent with other studies, these findings suggest a significant need for specific training and support for teachers.

Teacher–Student Relationships and Peer Victimization

Quality relationships between teachers and students are widely recognized as a critical relational context for positive youth development (Pianta et al., 2008; Rimm-Kaufman et al., 2014; Merritt et al., 2012). Consistent with the theoretical framework above, we argue that the teacher–student relationship (TSR) is a critical relational context of socializing experiences provided by teachers. Evidence suggests that TSRs characterized as caring, warm, and supportive have been linked to positive peer relationship and less victimization (Gregory et al., 2010; Richard et al., 2012) and more defending (Jungert et al., 2016). Schwab and Rossman (2020) found in a sample of secondary school students in Austria TSRs predicted later peer integration, or the extent to which students are connected to others as measured by friendship in class.

Studies have found that TSRs may serve as a protective factor, mitigating the negative impact of peer victimization. Sulkowski and Simmons (2018) found that positive TSRs as reported by students moderated the effects of peer victimization on psychosocial distress in a sample of high school students. Similarly, Davidson and Demaray (2007) found that middle school students' perceived social support from teachers buffered victims from the effects of peer victimization on internalizing and externalizing problems. In addition to the protective role, TSRs may also facilitate the process of students' social cognition. In a recent study of a Swedish sample of early adolescents, Iotti et al. (2020) found that close TSRs were positively related to autonomous motivation (e.g., "because I like to help other people" or "because I think it is important to help people who are treated badly") and negatively related to extrinsic motivation to defend victims (e.g., "to become popular"). One explanation for these findings is that close and warm relationships with teachers may motivate students to defend victims and also facilitate their internalization of rules and values. While day-to-day interactions and classroom experiences may establish, communicate, and enforce rules and expectations, teachers' warm and close relationships with students may serve as an important motivational context for cultivating and internalizing the values and beliefs that discourage bullying and promote defending.

In summary, these studies have indicated that TSRs are an important area of intervention and prevention of peer victimization. Given the association between autonomous motivation and greater defending, efforts to enhance TSRs may be beneficial to prevent peer victimization for all students, particularly bystanders. Although developing positive TSRs is considered an important aspect of intervention, we also caution that teacher liking toward specific students may backfire. In a study by Hendrickx et al. (2016), teacher support for specific students was associated with peer disliking, illustrating a complex interaction between peer relationships TSRs, potentially influenced by individual student and teacher characteristics and classroom-level characteristics. Importance of TSRs further challenges us to examine classroom processes of teacher practices and interactions with students.

Teacher Practices and Peer Victimization

Consistent with the concept of socializing agents, we posit that teachers' daily interactions with students and the entire class in the context of instruction and class management serve as "social experiences" that communicate the rules and expectations while forming classroom-level norms about peer relations (e.g., peer victimization and defending). The question of overall positive teacher practices that promote positive peer relations and classroom climate is particularly important because it focuses on preventing victimization and promoting positive peer interactions. With respect to teachers' general classroom management, Casas et al. (2015) found that positive teacher management (e.g., teachers' personal involvement in activities, teacher support to students) was related to less victimization. In a sample of 4th to 6th graders in Norway, Roland and Galloway (2002) found that teachers' management (e.g., caring, teaching, monitoring, and intervention) was directly related to less victimization but also indirectly related via its impact on social dimensions of the class such as norms about peer relations and teacher authorities. Surprisingly, little attention has been paid to the overall classroom management and its impact on how students treat and interact with each other, particularly related to peer victimization. Future studies should shed light on various domains of class-room management that are particularly robust for positive peer relations.

One particular aspect of classroom management is the social management of students, as suggested by Farmer et al. (2010) and Rodkin and Gest (2011). Although not all teachers believe they are responsible for helping students develop peer rela-tionships and facilitating their social adaptation (Gest et al., 2014), many instruc-tional and non-instructional strategies that they already use are likely to impact students' individual peer relationships and the overall classroom social network. A few extant studies indicate that teachers' direct approach to manage students' social experiences promote more positive classroom-level ecology. For example, in a study of elementary classrooms, Rodkin and Gest (2011) found that strategies such as separating students with behavior problems were related to having students with more liking nominations, denser friendship networks, and a less hierarchical social structure among girls. When teachers publicly recognize successful performance of students in low performing groups and stress their multiple abilities, there were more friendships reported by students in class (Cohen & Lotan, 1995). Rodkin and Gest (2011) further suggest that teachers' use of cooperative learning groups (e.g., reading groups) should be intentionally planned so that certain social dynamics (e.g., disruptive clique) can be considered to minimize behavioral problems and promote social integration of students. Examples include teachers' strategic group-ing of victims not in the same group with bullies, or teachers' intentional separation of students from a disruptive clique. Teachers' intentional strategies to minimize social hierarchy and promote social integration of students should be part of broader prevention efforts to promote positive classroom climates. In a recent study of 48 elementary classrooms (Grades 3–5), Pan et al. (2020) found that children with social dominance goals are more likely to bully others in a classroom with strong inequality in social status, suggesting that the classroom social dynamics should be carefully evaluated and considered for addressing peer victimization.

Considering the multiple layers of peer relations and differing peer status in a classroom, teachers' accurate knowledge of these peer affiliations and structure is critical for successful social management. While teachers' awareness of students' social dynamics is limited (Hoffman et al., 2015), studies have documented that the awareness is associated with several positive classroom characteristics. For exam-ple, teachers who are attuned to peer affiliations have strong anti-bullying norms in their classes (Neal et al., 2011) and their students report a greater sense of belong-ingness and willingness to defend others (Farmer et al., 2010). Marucci et al. (2018) found that teachers' awareness of students' peer liking and disliking and other social behaviors (measured by peer nominations) varied, with less awareness of negative characteristics (disliking, aggression, and risk behaviors) and greater awareness in smaller classes. Hoffman et al., (2015) found that teachers' general knowledge of peer groups (group membership) was related to greater popularity, whereas teach-ers' precise knowledge of students' individual ties was related to greater centrality, a measure of students' interpersonal connections in the classrooms. Teacher training on peer relationships, social structures, and affiliation, with a primary focus on sup-porting students' social adjustment, is promising. For example, a randomized control trial by Hamm et al. (2011) found that a professional development program led to significant improvement in teacher attunement, and students whose teachers were more attuned to peer group affiliations reported improved perceptions of social environment in schools. Overall, these studies highlight the importance of teacher attunement but do not demonstrate that the awareness leads to appropriate social management strategies. Future studies should examine not only how teacher attunement is related to social management but also what specific social management strategies are available and deemed effective for certain social dynamics.

With respect to how teacher-student interactions contribute to the peer relations, several lines of research have demonstrated that teachers' attitudes and behaviors toward specific students may shape the underlying social hierarchy of classroom and peer groups. Hughes et al. (2001) found that teacher liking predicted peer acceptance over time in a sample of aggressive children and argued that both teacher support for and conflict with certain students may serve as a social referent for peer relationships; "classmates make inferences about children's attributes and likeability based, in part, on their observations of teacher-student interactions" (p. 289). That is, through their daily interactions with students, teachers influence the way their peers perceive these students while communicating certain levels of teacher liking and disliking. Similarly, Mikami et al. (2010) argue that teacher interactions with a specific student result in "differential values" (p. 126) for the student, which serves as a basis for peer evaluation of the student. Further supporting the notion of teachers as a social referent, Hendrickx et al. (2016) found that when students indicated more conflicts between teachers and specific students, they reported more disliking for each other and more aggression in their classrooms.

One powerful mechanism of teacher influences may be through emotional tones that are embedded in these exchanges and communications between teachers and students. For example, when a teacher's negative interactions with a particular student are pervasive and repetitive, the interactions will elicit negative affect among peers, creating affective biases toward the student, which may also increase the vulnerability of the student for peer difficulties. In contrast, teachers' positive attention of a rejected student in class (e.g., praise) may improve peer perceptions of the student (White et al., 1996).

Minoritized Students' Classroom Context and Peer Victimization

Minoritized students in terms of race, ethnicity, sexual orientation, gender identity, immigration status, religion, and disability are particularly vulnerable to peer victimization (Bucchianeri et al., 2016; Mitchell et al., 2014; Zhang et al., 2016). Jones et al. (2018) found in a sample of US adolescents (10–20 years) that about 17% experienced at least one biased-based incident. More alarming is that these incidents involve multiple perpetrators and multiple episodes, suggesting more traumatic, chronic distress for some minoritized students. Many have highlighted the supportive role of teachers for LGBTQ youth (Greytak et al., 2013; Yoon et al.,

2020). However, we have not found a substantial discussion on the ways that teachers' interactions with racial minority students or how un/biased practices are likely to contribute to peer relationships beyond academic achievement and other school adjustment outcomes. We posit that as socializing agents, teachers' biased, negative interactions with minoritized students make a significant contribution to a peer ecology that reflects a hierarchy of power and privileges, thus making minoritized students particularly vulnerable for peer victimization.

The broader education literature has long documented racialized classroom practices (e.g., Minor, 2014; Weiner, 2016). Disproportionate disciplinary action for black males in particular has been reflected through decades of research (Carter et al., 2017). Casteel (1998) found that Black students—particularly boys—received more negative interactions from their White teachers than their White peers did and that White peers were more likely to receive frequent praise, positive feedback, and more clues or help. This pattern of differential treatment, particularly when enacted between White teachers and Black students, seems to start as early as kindergarten (Downey & Pribesh, 2004). In a study using nationally representative data across four decades, Quinn and Stewart (2019) found that White educators held more negative racial stereotypes of African American students and purported being more socially distant from minoritized students. Tenenbaum and Ruck (2007) found that teachers overall had more positive expectations for White students compared to their ethnic-minoritized peers. Even more troubling is how White teachers may be entirely unaware of their own biases and stereotypes (Warikoo et al., 2016).

In a recent study on prospective teachers' abilities to accurately recognize facial emotions, Halberstadt et al. (2020) found that teachers more often perceived Black boys as angry compared to White boys. The ability to accurately recognize Black girls' facial expressions and emotions were also half that of those of White girls. Such (mis)interpretations of student emotions and behaviors have serious implications for how teachers interact with and respond to students. For example, Splett et al. (2018) found that teachers rated behavioral and emotional risk of Black and male students higher, indicating how measures of universal screening may be more characteristic of such biases over actual reflections of students' behaviors and adjustment. In a review of quantitative literature examining teacher–student racial matching in the classroom, Redding (2019) found that teachers' race was a significant factor in their differentiated ratings and perceptions of externalizing problem behaviors in Black and Latinx students; when Black and Latinx students shared the same race or ethnicity as their teacher, they received fewer and less frequent ratings of fighting, being disruptive, and being argumentative. Further, White teachers are more likely to punish Black students with office discipline referrals and suspensions when compared to Black teachers who teach Black students (Lindsay & Hart, 2017).

In summary, the extant literature indicates biased patterns of perception and misunderstanding of racial minority students among teachers, which leads to negative interactions between students and teachers. Not surprisingly, minoritized students report the highest rates of unfair treatment by teachers (Niwa et al., 2014; Seaton et al., 2008). Weiner (2016) argues that through these racialized mechanisms of negative interactions and low expectations, minority students become "disproportionately disparaged, disciplined, and silenced" (p. 1351). This is especially concerning given the increasingly diverse student population coupled with a stagnantly and predominantly white, female educator population (National Center for Education Statistics [NCES], 2020a, b). Of relevance to this chapter is the extent to which these negative interactions contribute to students' peer relations and class ecology. Consistent with the notion of teachers as social referents aforementioned, we argue that teachers' biased interactions with and their negative affect toward minoritized students in the classroom contribute to the social structure of the classroom, where bias-based victimizations are sanctioned by teachers (authority figures) and these students' social standings are further reinforced by ongoing processes of negative teacher–student interactions.

Adult social support in school is particularly important for racially minoritized students in predicting fighting and violent behaviors (James et al., 2020). The more supported racially minoritized students felt by adults, the less likely they were to fight in school, particularly when there were more perceived injustices. Using data from Canada, Larochette et al. (2010) also found that there were significant interactions between school support and teacher diversity in racial bullying; students reported less racial bullying to a greater degree when there was more teacher diversity than just with school support alone. In addition to providing support and learning opportunities to discuss race, teachers' instructional strategies in the classroom have been shown to reduce racial discipline gaps. Teachers who used instructional strategies that facilitated higher-level thinking skills, problem solving, and metacognition were significantly associated with more equitable and infrequent use of disciplinary referrals (Gregory et al., 2016).

Consistent with the role of socializing agents, of particular importance is teacher practices that demonstrate and communicate the strong commitment to diversity, equity, and respect, which in turn is likely to promote positive peer relations. Supporting this argument, Gage et al. (2014) found that teachers' respect for diversity and student differences (e.g., racial diversity) predicted within-class decreases in victimization and that there was less aggression in middle school classrooms when students participated in rulemaking and teachers cultivated cultural sensitivity (Reis et al., 2007). We believe this is another important area of prevention and intervention effort in peer victimization; how do we create classroom experiences with equity, respect, sensitivity at the forefront? What specific strategies do teachers utilize to create positive classroom contexts characterized by more egalitarian relationships, less hierarchy, and greater respect for all students? How do teachers' self-awareness and insight into their own biases and perceptions of students contribute to classroom ecologies?

Teacher's Role in Social Emotional Learning

In recent years, an increasing body of research has recognized the importance of social and emotional learning (SEL) in promoting students' learning and development (Durlak et al., 2011). Researchers and policymakers have also called for leveraging SEL to prevent bullying and other forms of school violence. Social and emotional learning is an integral part of education and human development. It is defined as "the process through which all young people and adults acquire and apply the knowledge, skills, and attitudes to develop healthy identities, manage emotions, and achieve personal and collective goals, feel and show empathy for others, establish and maintain supportive relationships, and make responsible and caring decisions." (Collaborative for Academic, Social, and Emotional Learning [CASEL], n.d.). The school-wide SEL approach "defines the entire school community as the unit of change and aims to integrate SEL into daily interactions and practices at multiple setting levels in the school using collaborative efforts that include all staff, teachers, families, and children" (Oberle et al., 2016, p. 278). The school-wide SEL approach emphasizes not only the improvement of students' SEL competencies but also the simultaneous establishment of a caring, safe, and positive school climate (CASEL, 2005; Devaney et al., 2006). Improving students' SEL competencies must be a collective responsibility, shared by all the students and adults in the building and reinforced by school-wide practices (Smith & Low, 2013). Also, it is crucial to establish a positive school climate and provide students with the opportunity to connect with others, to learn and emulate behaviors they come to value, and to interact socially with peers to further learn, practice, and refine SEL skills (Catalano et al., 2004; Yang et al., 2018). The positive impact of school-wide SEL on students' development, learning, and engagement in schools has been well documented (Yang et al., 2018). In particular, recent studies have indicated that the two integrated dimensions of school-wide SEL approach are associated with reduced bullying and cyberbullying victimization incidents among students across elementary, middle, and high schools (Yang et al., 2020, 2021).

Within the school-wide SEL framework, we argue that teachers play critical roles in preventing bullying and other forms of school violence in schools by functioning as an active agent in improving individuals' SEL competencies through high-quality instruction, professional development, and role modeling, and by promoting positive school climate. Our argument is grounded in the Prosocial Classroom Model (Jennings & Greenberg, 2009), which argues that teachers' social-emotional competencies and well-being influence how effectively they manage students' problematic behaviors in the classroom and school settings, build relationships with students, and implement SEL programs and restorative justice practices. These factors also contribute to the healthy classroom and school climate, which provide the essential social-ecological contexts for reducing bullying incidents and school violence and increased students' academic and SEL success (Jennings & Greenberg, 2009).

To date, an array of SEL frameworks has emerged from the literature to depict critical dimensions of social-emotional competencies in the school-wide SEL framework (Jones & Bouffard, 2012; Zins et al., 2004). While there is a lack of consensus depicting the key social-emotional competencies of teachers, some important competencies have been discussed in the empirical literature, such as social awareness, self-beliefs, self-management, and social relationships. For example, studies found that teachers with a stronger sense of social awareness about others were more likely to understand the emotions of students, parents, and other staff members in the schools and recognize others' perspectives that may differ from their own (Buettner et al., 2016; Jennings & Greenberg, 2009). Such skills could help them negotiate positive solutions when managing students' aggressive behaviors and peer victimization. In contrast, the lack of social awareness among teachers could lead to misguided interpretations of another's intention and communication that can perpetuate negative interaction cycles between students and teachers or among students (Schussler et al., 2010, 2015).

Self-beliefs also play an important role in teachers' implementation of bullying prevention. In a study based on 556 teachers in Germany, researchers found that teachers with high self-efficacy beliefs are 1.5 times more likely to intervene immediately than teachers with average self-efficacy beliefs (Fischer & Bilz, 2019). These findings were independent of gender and of work experience. The importance of teachers' self-beliefs in bullying prevention was evidenced among not only in-service teachers but also pre-service teachers. For example, based on a mixed group of in-service and pre-service teachers, Garner (2017) found that the self-confidence of both in-service and pre-service teachers in managing bullying incidents was positively associated with their beliefs and confidence in the bullying victims to develop an appropriate response to their peers with the proper adult support. Moreover, teachers' positive representations of relationships were negatively related to dismissive peer victimization-related beliefs and their reports of positive emotional expressiveness were negatively related to normative, assertive, avoidance, and dismissive victimization-related beliefs. In contrast, teachers' reports of negative emotional expressiveness were negatively related to avoidant victimization-related beliefs and prosocial peer beliefs. The competence in regulating and managing emotions may also help teachers focus on student needs and maintain constructive engagement during emotionally charged situations rather than focus on their own frustrations and disengage from the interaction or respond negatively (Brackett et al., 2010). Furthermore, teachers with positive prosocial values and skills have more sources of social support to help them cope with the stress triggered by the conflicts and challenging behavioral problems among students (Spilt et al., 2011).

Similar to SEL, another important school-based preventative approach to bullying and school violence is that of character education. Character education is defined as "an explicit learning process from which students in a school community understand, accept, and act on ethical values such as respect for others, justice, civic virtue and citizenship, and responsibility for self and others" (U.S. Department of Education, 2005). Although character education and SEL are sometimes used interchangeably, they are not exactly the same (Gulbrandson, 2016). One important difference is that developing morally responsible youth is considered as a defining feature of character education, but not of SEL (Gulbrandson, 2016). Despite the different defining features, both character education and SEL approaches emphasize the important role of teachers in creating a positive and safe school community and teaching core characters traits (Pearson & Nicholson, 2000) and SEL competencies (Schonert-Reichl, 2019) effectively and authentically. Both positive school climate and instructional support for developing core competencies and characters are key dimensions to consider in school-wide bullying prevention efforts (Yang et al., 2021).

Utility of Existing Instructional Opportunities

A significant challenge in any school-based intervention is that schools face pressure for academic achievement and there are many competing demands. Because of the challenges, new programs or initiatives are often not fully implemented nor sustained over time. One promising approach is to utilize existing curricula and learning activities in school as a way to promote empathy, kindness, and other prosocial behaviors and prevent peer victimization. In addition to the interpersonal socialization process between teachers and students and among students, daily instructional activities and learning experiences are part of the socialization. Although not explored extensively, the academic socialization presents a potential area of prevention. With a goal of promoting positive peer relations and condemning victimization, teachers can intentionally utilize these instructional activities and facilitate students' internalization of classroom values and goals. For example, as a content area, social studies draws upon historical and current events/issues in many disciplines (e.g., history, economics, geography). The National Council for the Social Studies (2013) states that the area of social studies is to cultivate engaged citizenship and concerns for the rights and welfare of others. Several researchers have further noted that the subject of social studies offers critical opportunities to explore issues of power, equity, and oppression and cultivate students' concerns for the rights and welfare of others (Ladson-Billings, 2003; Loewen, 2007). Meanwhile, social studies scholars have also noted that the social studies often focus on facts and information, with little to no emphasis on the interpersonal aspects of the subject. In fact, teachers often avoid having difficult conversations in the classroom and rarely discuss possible implications for interpersonal relationships (e.g., the way students treat each other) (Smith et al., 2018).

Another area that has gained more attention is literacy as a tool for prevention. Bibliotherapy has been a tool for addressing stressful life events and coping strategies for children (Flanaga et al., 2013). Although empirical research on addressing bullying experiences is limited, several studies have documented potential benefits of using storybooks to address bullying in young children. Freeman (2014) implemented a 12-week program that involved reading storybooks with a bullying theme, followed by discussions and activities. Children ages 4–6 improved their knowledge about bullying (as measured by accurate awareness of bully characteristics) and how to respond to a bully from pre- to post-intervention. Targeting elementary school students, Wang and her colleagues found a 5-week classroom-wide intervention using storybooks to be effective in (1) increasing teacher-reported prosocial behavior and students' report of social-emotional assets (e.g., emotional knowledge, empathy, coping, and problem solving) (Wang et al., 2015) and (2) decreasing victimization and moral disengagement (Wang & Goldberg, 2017). These programs were implemented and facilitated by non-school personnel (e.g., researchers), thus presenting challenges for sustainability, and little is known about how effective teachers' specific approaches using instructional activities were effective, and if they were, what specific impacts this approach has on peer victimization and peer ecology in the classroom. This is a critical area of future study, considering that instructional activities and learning experiences are part of teachers' socialization of students toward positive peer relations.

Key Points of Practical Implications and Future Directions

Despite the relatively little attention in the literature, existing studies indicate teachers' critical role in peer relations including peer victimization. This review has provided strong theoretical and empirical rationales of examining teachers' socialization and interactions with students, suggesting several important implications for practice. Given the overwhelming evidence of teacher influences on peer relations, we must re-conceptualize the role of teachers to consider various processes that influence peer victimization and shape peer ecology, as outlined in this review, and more importantly evaluate how their influence on students' peer relations can be utilized in the current school-wide programs.

It is clear that a special attention to classroom-level socialization is needed as a part of broader intervention and prevention efforts, specifically how teachers are developing and maintaining relationships with students and how they socialize students around positive peer relations through daily activities. Some socialization experiences are related to addressing peer victimization directly (e.g., how teachers handle incidents or using existing instructional opportunities to instill anti-bullying attitudes/values) and other socialization may be more preventive (e.g., teachers' effort to promote positive peer relations and teacher-student relationships). These experiences cover a wide range of classroom interactions and processes. The approach to work with teachers is likely to benefit the whole class, not just those involved in peer victimization, offering opportunities to understand and address classroom processes, and social climate. It will be interesting to investigate the extent to which the existing anti-bullying programs influence teachers' classroom-level socializations; we speculate that the effectiveness of programs will be moderated by teachers' specific attempts to promote positive peer relations and prevent peer victimization.

This review has also highlighted that teachers should have accurate understanding of peer relationships and dynamics that are involved in peer victimization. A simple approach of punishing bullies is not effective for long-term changes (e.g., Wachs et al., 2019). Effective handling of peer victimization will require an approach that involves a thorough assessment of a particular incident and underlying social dynamics and resources such as a problem-solving approach. Solutions generated from this approach are likely to have ecological validity, allowing to develop specific strategies that fit the situation, reflecting the complexity of peer victimization.

Despite the promising utility of data-driven decision making and network-related teaching (Rodkin & Gest, 2011), current literature offers little practical guidance on specific processes and strategies to collect and interpret relevant data, including resources and tools. For example, social network analyses provide useful information about individual students' relationships and classroom-level peer ecology, but they require statistical expertise to interpret student data, resulting in limited access to this tool. Future research studies should further examine how classroom data can be used to guide teachers' effort in addressing peer relations and what strategies are effective to reduce peer victimization and increase prosocial behaviors in the classroom context. A school-wide monitoring system of students' well-being and social networks, as well as class climate, can provide regular data that can guide teachers (e.g., Bloomsights). However, we need longitudinal studies that examine the effects of teacher interventions/strategies on student outcomes, such as peer relations, social isolation, and peer victimization; for example, direct evidence that links specific interventions and strategies to less hierarchical social networks and more cohesive classroom climate is much needed.

Several implications for teacher training and professional development emerged from this review. They must target not only the foundational knowledge about peer victimization (e.g., prevalence and negative consequences) but also a broader perspective of classroom processes, peer ecology, and group dynamics management. In Shuman's domains of professional knowledge necessary for effective teaching (1987), teachers' knowledge of educational contexts (e.g., classroom groups, communities, and cultures) specifically addresses the importance of understanding social dynamics and developing positive learning environments. Future work should examine how teachers' knowledge of social dynamics and peer relations can be used and integrated into effective classroom management. In addition to recognize the positive influence of classroom and school climate on bullying prevention, it is important for teachers to be aware that bullying victims might face higher risk of maladjustment when they perceive their classroom or school's climate is changing to a positive direction and they are still suffering from bullying (Gini et al., 2020; Yang et al., 2018). Thus, teacher training and professional development should also emphasize on improving teachers' skills in improving school's bullying reporting systems and facilitating confidential discourse among victimized students to help them process their negative experience, develop more objective perception of social context, and empower them to seek for social support. Moreover, considering the key roles that teachers play in school-wide SEL and existing anti-bullying programs, of particular importance is a consideration of how training programs and professional development opportunities enhance teachers' knowledge but also facilitate skill development and consistent implementation of these skills.

References

Brackett, M. A., Palomera, R., Mojsa-Kaja, J., Reyes, M. R., & Salovey, P. (2010). Emotion-regulation ability, burnout, and job satisfaction among British secondary-school teachers. *Psychology in the Schools, 47*(4), 417. https://doi.org/10.1002/pits.20478

Bradshaw, C. P., Wassdorp, T. E., & O'Brennan, L. M. (2011). *Findings from the National Education Association's nationwide study of bullying: Teachers' and education support professionals' perspectives* (pp. 1–42). National Education Association.

Bucchianeri, M. M., Gower, A. L., McMorris, B. J., & Eisenberg, M. E. (2016). Youth experiences with multiple types of prejudice-based harassment. *Journal of Adolescence, 51*, 68–75.

Buettner, C. K., Jeon, L., Hur, E., & Garcia, R. E. (2016). Teachers' social–emotional capacity: Factors associated with teachers' responsiveness and professional commitment. *Early Education and Development, 27*, 1018–1039. https://doi.org/10.1080/10409289.2016.1168227

Carter, P. L., Skiba, R., Arredondo, M. I., & Pollock, M. (2017). You can't fix what you don't look at: Acknowledging race in addressing racial discipline disparities. *Urban Education, 52*(2), 207–235.

Casas, J. A., Ortega-Ruiz, R., & Del Rey, R. (2015). Bullying: The impact of teacher management and trait emotional intelligence. *British Journal of Educational Psychology, 85*(3), 407–442. https://doi.org/10.1111/bjep.12082

CASEL. (n.d.). *What is social and emotional learning?* Retrieved March 2, 2022, from https://drc.casel.org/what-is-sel/

Casteel, C. A. (1998). Teacher-student interactions and race in integrated classrooms. *The Journal of Educational Research, 92*(2), 115–129. https://doi.org/10.1080/00220679809597583

Catalano, R. F., Oesterle, S., Fleming, C. B., & Hawkins, J. D. (2004). The importance of bonding to school for healthy development: Findings from the social development research group. *Journal of School Health, 74*, 252–261. https://doi.org/10.1111/j.1746-1561.2004.tb08281.x

Cohen, E. G., & Lotan, R. A. (1995). Producing equal-status interaction in the heterogeneous classroom. *American Educational Research Journal, 32*, 99–120.

Collaborative for Academic, Social, and Emotional Learning (CASEL). (2005). *Safe and sound: An educational leader's guide to evidence-based social and emotional learning programs—Illinois edition.* Author.

Davidson, L. M., & Demaray, M. K. (2007). Social support as a moderator between victimization and internalizing-externalizing distress from bullying. *School Psychology Review, 36*, 383–405.

Demol, K., Verschueren, K., Salmivalli, C., & Colpin, H. (2020). Perceived teacher responses to bullying influence students' social cognitions. *Frontiers in Psychology, 11*, 3363. https://doi.org/10.3389/fpsyg.2020.592582

Demol, K., Verschueren, K., Jame, M., Lazard, C., & Colpin, H. (2021). Student attitudes and perceptions of teacher responses to bullying: An experimental vignette study. *European Journal of Developmental Psychology.* https://doi.org/10.1080/17405629.2021.1896492

Devaney, E., O'Brien, M. U., Resnik, H., Keister, S., & Weissberg, R. P. (2006). *Sustainable schoolwide social and emotional learning (SEL): Implementation guide and toolkit.* CASEL.

Downey, D. B., & Pribesh, S. (2004). When race matters: Teachers' evaluations of students' classroom behavior. *Sociology of Education, 77*, 267–282.

Durlak, J. A., Dymnicki, A. B., Taylor, R. D., Weissberg, R. P., & Schellinger, K. B. (2011). The impact of enhancing students' social and emotional learning: A meta-analysis of school-based universal interventions. *Child Development, 82*(1), 405–432.

Farmer, T. W., Hall, C. M., Petrin, R., Hamm, J. V., & Dadisman, K. (2010). Evaluating the impact of a multicomponent intervention model on teachers' awareness of social networks at the beginning of middle school in rural communities. *School Psychology Quarterly, 25*(2), 94.

Farmer, T. W., Dawes, M., Hamm, J. V., Lee, D., Mehtaji, M., Hoffman, A. S., & Brooks, D. S. (2018). Classroom social dynamics management: Why the invisible hand of the teacher matters for special education. *Remedial and Special Education, 39*(3), 177–192. https://doi.org/10.1177/0741932517718359

Fischer, S. M., & Bilz, L. (2019). Teachers' self-efficacy in bullying interventions and their probability of intervention. *Psychology in the Schools, 56*, 751–764. https://doi.org/10.1002/pits.22229

Flanaga, K. S., Vanden Hoek, K. K., Shelton, A., Kelly, S. L., Morrison, C. M., & Young, A. M. (2013). Coping with bullying: What answers does children's literature provide? *School Psychology International, 34*, 694–706. https://doi.org/10.1177/0143034313479691

Freeman, G. G. (2014). The implementation of character education and children's literature to teach bullying characteristics and prevention strategies to preschool children: An action research project. *Early Childhood Education Journal, 42*, 305–316. https://doi.org/10.1007/s10643-013-0614-5

Gage, N. A., Prykanowski, D. A., & Larson, A. (2014). School climate and bullying victimization: A latent class growth model analysis. *School Psychology Quarterly, 29*, 256–271.

Garandeau, C. F., Vartio, A., Poskiparta, E., & Salmivalli, C. (2016). School bullies' intention to change behaviour following teacher interventions: Effects of empathy arousal, condemning of bullying, and blaming of the perpetrator. *Prevention Science, 17*(8), 1034–1043. https://doi.org/10.1007/s11121-016-0712-x

Garner, P. W. (2017). The role of teachers' social-emotional competence in their beliefs about peer victimization. *Journal of Applied School Psychology, 33*, 288–308. https://doi.org/10.1080/15377903.2017.1292976

Gest, S. D., Madill, R. A., Zadzora, K. M., Miller, A. M., & Rodkin, P. C. (2014). Teacher management of elementary classroom social dynamics: Associations with changes in student adjustment. *Journal of Emotional and Behavioral Disorders, 22*(2), 107–118. https://doi.org/10.1177/1063426613512677

Gini, G., Holt, M., Pozzoli, T., & Marino, C. (2020). Victimization and somatic problems: The role of class victimization levels. *Journal of School Health, 90*, 39–46. https://doi.org/10.1111/josh.12844

Gottfredson, G. D., Gottfredson, D. C., Payne, A. A., & Gottfredson, N. C. (2005). School climate predictors of school disorder: Results from a national study of delinquency prevention in schools. *Journal of Research in Crime and Delinquency, 42*, 412–444. https://doi.org/10.1177/0022427804271931

Gregory et. al. (2010) Data_Information_and_Knowledge_a_candid_and_pragmatic_discussion

Gregory, A., Hafen, C. A., Ruzek, E., Mikami, A. Y., Allen, J. P., & Pianta, R. C. (2016). Closing the racial discipline gap in classrooms by changing teacher practice. *School Psychology Review, 45*(2), 171–191.

Greytak, E. A., Kosciw, J. G., & Boesen, M. J. (2013). Educating the educator: Creating supportive school personnel through professional development. *Journal of School Violence, 12*, 80–97. https://doi.org/10.1080/15388220.2012.731586

Grusec, J. E., & Hastings, P. D. (2015). *Handbook of socialization: Theory and research* (2nd ed.). Guilford Press.

Gulbrandson, K. (2016). *Character education and SEL: What you should know*. Retrieved from https://www.cfchildren.org/blog/2018/07/character-education-and-sel-what-you-should-know/

Halberstadt, A. G., Cooke, A. N., Garner, P. W., Hughes, S. A., Oertwig, D., & Neupert, S. D. (2020). Racialized emotion recognition accuracy and anger bias of children's faces. *Emotion*, Advance online publication. https://doi.org/10.1037/emo0000756

Hamm, J. V., Farmer, T. W., Dadisman, K., Gravelle, M., & Murray, A. R. (2011). Teachers' attunement to students' peer group affiliations as a source of improved student experiences of the school social-affective context following the middle school transition. *Journal of Applied Developmental Psychology, 32*(5), 267–277. https://doi.org/10.1016/j.appdev.2010.06.003

Hendrickx, M. M. H. G., Mainhard, M. T., Boor-Klip, H. J., Cillessen, A. H. M., & Brekelmans, M. (2016). Social dynamics in the classroom: Teacher support and conflict and the peer ecology. *Teaching and Teacher Education, 53*, 30–40. https://doi.org/10.1016/j.tate.2015.10.004

Hoffman, A. S., Hamm, J. V., & Farmer, T. W. (2015). Teacher attunement: Supporting early elementary students' social integration and status. *Journal of Applied Developmental Psychology, 39*, 14–23. https://doi.org/10.1016/j.appdev.2015.04.007

Hughes, J. N., Cavell, T. A., & Willson, V. (2001). Further support for the developmental significance of the quality of the teacher-student relationship. *Journal of School Psychology, 39*, 289–301.

Iotti, N. O., Thornberg, R., Longobardi, C., & Jungert, T. (2020). Early adolescents' emotional and behavioural difficulties, student–teacher relationships, and motivation to defend in bullying incidents. *Child & Youth Care Forum, 49*, 59–75. https://doi.org/10.1007/s10566-019-09519-3

James, K., Watts, S. J., & Evans, S. Z. (2020). Fairness, social support, and school violence: Racial differences in the likelihood of fighting at school. *Crime and Delinquency, 66*(12), 1655–1677. https://doi.org/10.1177/0011128719890269

Jennings, P. A., & Greenberg, M. T. (2009). The Prosocial Classroom: Teacher social and emotional competence in relation to student and classroom outcomes. *Review of Educational Research, 7*, 491–525. https://doi.org/10.3102/0034654308325693

Jones, S. M., & Bouffard, S. M. (2012). Social and emotional learning in schools: From programs to strategies and commentaries. *Social Policy Report, 26*(4), 1–33. https://doi.org/10.1002/j.2379-3988.2012.tb00073.x

Jones, L. M., Mitchell, K. J., Turner, H. A., & Ybarra, M. L. (2018). Characteristics of bias-based harassment incidents reported by a national sample of U.S. adolescents. *Journal of Adolescent, 65*, 50–60. https://doi.org/10.1016/j.adolescence.2018.02.013

Jungert, T., Piroddi, B., & Thornberg, R. (2016). Early adolescents' motivations to defend victims in school bullying and their perceptions of student–teacher relationships: A self-determination theory approach. *Journal of Adolescence, 53*, 75–90. https://doi.org/10.1016/j.adolescence.2016.09.001

Ladson-Billings, G. (2003). Lies my teacher still tells: Developing a critical race perspective toward the social studies. In Ladson-Billings (Ed.), *Critical race theory perspectives on the social studies: The profession, policies, and curriculum* (pp. 1–11). Information Age Publishing.

Larochette, A., Murphy, A. N., & Craig, W. M. (2010). Racial bullying and victimization in Canadian school-aged children: Individual and school level effects. *School Psychology Interventional, 31*(4), 389–408. https://doi.org/10.1177/0143034310377150

Leadbeater, B., & Hoglund, W. (2006). Changing the social contexts of peer victimization. *Journal of the Canadian Academy of Child and Adolescent Psychiatry, 15*(1), 21–26.

Lindsay, C. A., & Hart, C. M. D. (2017). Exposure to sam-race teachers and student disciplinary outcomes for black students in North Carolina. *Educational Evaluation and Policy Analysis, 39*(3), 485–510.

Loewen, J. W. (2007). *Lies my teacher told me: Everything your American history textbook got wrong*. Touchstone.

Marachi, R., Astor, R. A., & Benbenishty, R. (2007). Effects of teacher avoidance of school policies on student victimization. *School Psychology International, 28*, 501–518.

Marucci, E., Oldenburg, B., & Barrera, D. (2018). Do teachers know their students? Examining teacher attunement in secondary schools. *School Psychology International, 39*(4), 416–432. https://doi.org/10.1177/0143034318786536

Merritt, E. G., Wanless, S. B., Rimm-Kaufman, S. E., Cameron, C., & Peugh, J. L. (2012). The contribution of teachers' emotional support to children's social behaviors and self-regulatory skills in first grade. *School Psychology Review, 41*(2), 141–159.

Mikami, A. Y., Lerner, M. D., & Lun, J. (2010). Social context influences on children's rejection by their peers. *Child Development Perspectives, 4*(2), 123–130. https://doi.org/10.1111/j.1750-8606.2010.00130.x

Minor, E. C. (2014). Racial differences in teacher perception of student ability. *Teachers College Record, 116*(100303), 1–21.

Mitchell, K. J., Ybarra, M. L., & Korchmaros, J. D. (2014). Sexual harassment among adolescents of different sexual orientations and gender identities. *Child Abuse & Neglect, 38*(2), 280–295.

Mucherah, W., Finch, H., White, T., & Thomas, K. (2018). The relationship of school climate, teacher defending and friends on students' perceptions of bullying in high school. *Journal of Adolescence, 62*, 128–139. https://doi.org/10.1016/j.adolescence.2017.11.012

National Center for Education Statistics. (2020a). *Characteristics of public school teachers*. The Condition of Education. https://nces.ed.gov/programs/coe/indicator_clr.asp

National Center for Education Statistics. (2020b). *Racial/ethnic enrollment in public schools*. The Condition of Education. https://nces.ed.gov/programs/coe/indicator_cge.asp

National Council for the Social Studies. (2013). Revitalizing civic learning in our schools. http://www.socialstudies.org/positions/revitalizing_civic_learning.

Neal, J. W., Cappella, E., Wagner, C., & Atkins, M. S. (2011). Seeing eye to eye: Predicting teacher–student agreement on classroom social networks. *Social Development, 20*(2), 376–393. https://doi.org/10.1111/j.1467-9507.2010.00582.x

Niwa, E. Y., Way, N., & Hughes, D. L. (2014). Trajectories of ethnic-racial discrimination among ethnically diverse early adolescents: Associations with psychological and social adjustment. *Child Development, 85*, 2339–2354. https://doi.org/10.1111/cdev.12310

Oberle, E., Domitrovich, C. E., Meyers, D. C., & Weissberg, R. P. (2016). Establishing systemic social and emotional learning approaches in schools: A framework for schoolwide implementation. *Cambridge Journal of Education, 46*, 277–297. https://doi.org/10.1080/0305764X.2015.1125450

Oldenburg, B., van Duijn, M., Sentse, M., Huitsing, G., van der Ploeg, R., Salmivalli, C., & Veenstra, R. (2015). Teacher characteristics and peer victimization in elementary schools: A classroom-level perspective. *Journal of Abnormal Child Psychology, 43*(1), 33–44.

Oldenburg, B., Bosman, R., & Veenstra, R. (2016). Are elementary school teachers prepared to tackle bullying? A pilot study. *School Psychology International, 37*(1), 64–72.

Pan, B., Zhang, L., Ji, L., Garandeau, C. F., Salmivallie, C., & Zhang, W. (2020). Classroom status hierarchy moderates the association between social dominance goals and bullying behavior in middle childhood and early adolescence. *Journal of Youth Adolescence, 49*, 2285–2297. https://doi.org/10.1007/s10964-020-01285-z

Pearson, Q. M., & Nicholson, J. I. (2000). Comprehensive character education in the elementary school: Strategies for administrators, teachers, and counselors. *Journal of Humanistic Counseling, Education and Development, 38*(4), 243–251.

Pianta, R. C., Belsky, J., Vandergrift, N., Houts, R., & Morrison, F. J. (2008). Classroom effects on children's achievement trajectories in elementary school. *American Educational Research Journal, 45*(2), 365–397. https://doi.org/10.3102/0002831207308230

Quinn, D. M., & Stewart, A. M. (2019). Examining the racial attitudes of white PreK-12 educators. *The Elementary School Journal, 120*(2). https://doi.org/10.1086/705899

Redding, C. (2019). A teacher like me: A review of the effect of student-teacher racial/ethnic matching on teacher perceptions of students and student academic and behavioral outcomes. *Review of Educational Research, 89*(4), 499–535. https://doi.org/10.3102/0034654319853545

Richard, J. F., Schneider, B. H., & Mallet, P. (2012). Revisiting the whole-school approach to bullying: Really looking at the whole school. *School Psychology International, 33*(3), 263–284.

Reis, J., Trockel, M., & Mulhall, P. (2007). Individual and school predictors of middle school aggression. *Youth Society, 38*, 322–347. https://doi.org/10.1177/0044118X06287688

Rimm-Kaufman, S. E., Larsen, R. A., Baroody, A. E., Curby, T. W., Ko, M., Thomas, J. B., & DeCoster, J. (2014). Efficacy of the responsive classroom approach results from a 3-year, longitudinal randomized controlled trial. *American Educational Research Journal, 20*(10), 1–37. https://doi.org/10.3102/0002831214523821

Rodkin, P. C., & Gest, S. D. (2011). Teaching practices, classroom peer ecologies, and bullying behaviors among schoolchildren. In D. L. Espelage & S. M. Swearer (Eds.), *Bullying in North American schools* (2nd ed., pp. 75–90). Routledge.

Roland, E., & Galloway, D. (2002). Classroom influences on bullying. *Educational Research, 44*(3), 299–312.

Salmivalli, C., Voeten, M., & Poskiparta, E. (2011). Bystanders matter: Associations between reinforcing, defending, and the frequency of bullying behavior in classrooms. *Journal of Clinical Child & Adolescent Psychology, 40*, 668–676. https://doi.org/10.1080/15374416.2011.597090

Schonert-Reichl, K. A. (2019). Advancements in the landscape of social and emotional learning and emerging topics on the horizon. *Educational Psychologist, 54*(3), 222–232.

Schussler, D. L., Stooksberry, L. M., & Bercaw, L. A. (2010). Understanding teacher candidate dispositions: Reflecting to build self-awareness. *Journal of Teacher Education, 61*, 350–363. https://doi.org/10.1177/0022487110371377

Schussler, D. L., Jennings, P. A., Sharp, J. E., & Frank, J. L. (2015). Improving teacher awareness and wellbeing through CARE: A qualitative analysis of the underlying mechanisms. *Mindfulness, 7*(1), 130–142. https://doi.org/10.1007/s12671-015-0422

Schwab, S., & Rossmann, P. (2020). Peer integration, teacher student relationships and the associations with depressive symptoms in secondary school students with and without special needs. *Educational Studies, 46*(3), 302–315. https://doi.org/10.1080/03055698.2019.1584852

Seaton, E. K., Caldwell, C. H., Sellers, R. M., & Jackson, J. S. (2008). The prevalence of perceived discrimination among African American and Caribbean black youth. *Developmental Psychology, 44*, 1288–1297. https://doi.org/10.1037/a0012747

Smith, B. H., & Low, S. (2013). The role of social-emotional learning in bullying prevention efforts. *Theory Into Practice, 52*(4), 280–287. https://doi.org/10.1080/00405841.2013.829731

Smith, W., Iurino, C., & Yoon, J. (2018, February). *Bullying and the social studies: A synthesis of research.* Paper presented at the annual meeting of the American Educational Research Association, New York.

Spilt, J.L., Koomen, H.M.Y. & Thijs, J.T. (2011). Teacher Wellbeing: The Importance of Teacher–Student Relationships. Educational Psychology Review, 23, 457–477. https://doi.org/10.1007/s10648-011-9170-y.

Splett, J. W., Smith-Millman, M., Raborn, A., Brann, K. L., Flaspohler, P. D., & Maras, M. A. (2018). Student, teacher, and classroom predictors of between-teacher variants of students' teacher-rated behavior. *School Psychology Quarterly, 33*(3), 460–468. https://doi.org/10.1037/spq0000241

Sulkowski, M. L., & Simmons, J. (2018). The protective role of teacher-student relationships against peer victimization and psychosocial distress. *Psychology in the Schools, 55*, 137–150. https://doi.org/10.1002/pits.22086

Swift, L. E., Hubbard, J. A., Bookhout, M. K., Grassetti, S. N., Smith, M. A., & Morrow, M. T. (2017). Teacher factors contributing to dosage of the KiVa anti-bullying program. *Journal of School Psychology, 65*, 102–115. https://doi.org/10.1016/j.jsp.2017.07.005

Tenenbaum, H. R., & Ruck, M. D. (2007). Are teachers' expectations different for racial minority than for European American students? A meta-analysis. *A meta-analysis. Journal of Educational Psychology, 99*(2), 253–273. https://doi.org/10.1037/0022-0663.99.2.253

Troop-Gordon, W., & Ladd, G. W. (2014). Teachers' victimization-related beliefs and strategies: Associations with students' aggressive behavior and peer victimization. *Journal of Abnormal Child Psychology.* https://doi.org/10.1007/s10802-013-9840-y

Troop-Gordon, W. (2015). The role of the classroom teacher in the lives of children victimized by peers. *Child Development Perspectives, 9*(1), 55–60. https://doi.org/10.1111/cdep.12106

Ttofi, M. M., & Farrington, D. P. (2011). Effectiveness of school-based programs to reduce bullying: A systematic and meta-analytic review. *Journal of Experimental Criminology, 7*, 27–56. https://doi.org/10.1007/s11292-010-9109-1

U.S. Department of Education. (2005). *Character education . . . Our shared responsibility* [Brochure]. Retrieved from https://www2.ed.gov/admins/lead/character/brochure.html

Unnever, J. D., & Cornell, D. G. (2004). Middle school victims of bullying: Who reports being bullied? *Aggressive Behavior, 30*(5), 373–388. https://doi.org/10.1002/ab.20030

Valle, J. E., Williams, L. C. A., & Stelko-Pereira, A. C. (2020). Whole-school antibullying interventions: A systematic review of 20 years of publications. *Psychology in the Schools, 57*, 868–883. https://doi.org/10.1002/pits.22377

van Verseveld, M. D., Fekkes, M., Fukkink, R. G., & Oostdam, R. J. (2020). Teachers' experiences with difficult bullying situations in the school: An explorative study. The Journal of Early Adolescence, 41, 43-690272431620939193.

Veenstra, R., Lindenberg, S., Huitsing, G., Sainio, M., & Salmivalli, C. (2014). The role of teachers in bullying: The relation between antibullying attitudes, efficacy, and efforts to reduce bullying. *Journal of Educational Psychology, 106*(4), 1135–1143. https://doi.org/10.1037/a0036110

Vreeman, R. C., & Carroll, A. E. (2007). A systematic review of school-based interventions to prevent bullying. *Archives of Pediatrics & Adolescent Medicine, 161*(1), 78–88.

Wachs, S., Bilz, L., Niproschke, S., & Schubarth, W. (2019). Bullying intervention in schools: A multilevel analysis of teachers' success in handling bullying from the students' perspective. *The Journal of Early Adolescence, 39*(5), 642–668. https://doi.org/10.1177/0272431618780423

Wang, C., Couch, L., Rodriguez, G. R., & Lee, C. (2015). The Bullying Literature Project: Using children's literature to promote prosocial behavior and social-emotional outcomes among elementary school students. *Contemporary School Psychology, 19*(4), 320–329. https://doi.org/10.1007/s40688-015-0064-8

Wang, C., & Goldberg, T. S. (2017). Using children's literature to decrease moral disengagement and victimization among elementary school students. *Psychology in the Schools, 54*, 918–931. https://doi.org/10.1002/pits.22042

Warikoo, N., Sinclair, S., Fei, J., & Jacoby-Senghor, D. (2016). Examining racial bias in education: A new approach. *Educational Researcher, 45*, 508–514.

Weiner, M. F. (2016). Racialized classroom practices in a diverse Amsterdam primary school: The silencing, disparagement, and discipline of students of color. *Race, Ethnicity, and Education, 19*(6), 1351–1367. https://doi.org/10.1080/13613324.2016.1195352

Wentzel, K. R. (2003). Motivating students to behave in socially constructive ways. *Theory Into Practice, 42*, 319–326. https://doi.org/10.1207/s15430421tip4204_9

White, K. J., Sherman, M. D., & Jones, K. (1996). Children's perceptions of behavior problem peers: Effects of teacher feedback and peer reputed status. *Journal of School Psychology, 34*, 53–72. https://doi.org/10.1016/0022-4405(95)00025-9

Yang, C., Sharkey, J. D., Reed, L. A., Chen, C., & Dowdy, E. (2018). Bullying victimization and student engagement in elementary, middle, and high schools: Moderating role of school climate. *School Psychology Quarterly, 33*(1), 54–64. https://doi.org/10.1037/spq0000250

Yang, C., Chan, M.-K., & Ma, T.-L. (2020). School-wide social emotional learning (sel) and bullying victimization: Moderating role of school climate in elementary, middle, and high schools. *Journal of School Psychology, 82*, 49–69. https://doi.org/10.1016/j.jsp.2020.08.002

Yang, C., Chen, C., Lin, X., & Chan, M.-K. (2021). School-wide social emotional learning and cyberbullying victimization among middle and high school students: Moderating role of school climate. *School Psychology, 36*(2), 75–85. https://doi.org/10.1037/spq0000423

Yoon, J., & Barton, E. (2008). The role of teachers in school violence and bullying prevention. In T. Miller (Ed.), *School violence primary prevention* (pp. 249–275). Springer.

Yoon, J., & Bauman, S. (2014). Teachers: A critical but overlooked component of bullying prevention and intervention. *Theory Into Practice, 53*, 308–314. https://doi.org/10.1080/00405841.2014.947226

Yoon, J., Sulkowski, M. L., & Bauman, S. A. (2016). Teachers' responses to bullying incidents: Effects of teacher characteristics and contexts. *Journal of School Violence, 15*(1), 91–113.

Yoon, J., Bauman, S., & Corcoran, C. (2020). Role of adults in prevention and intervention of peer victimization. In L. Rosen, S. Scott, & S. Kim (Eds.), *Bullying in my eyes: Understanding the vantage point of the bully, victim, and bystander* (pp. 179–212). Palgrave Macmillan.

Yun, H. Y., & Juvonen, J. (2020). Navigating the healthy context paradox: Identifying classroom characteristics that improve the psychological adjustment of bullying victims. *Journal of Youth and Adolescence, 49*, 2203–2213. https://doi.org/10.1007/S10964-020-01300-3

Zhang, A., Musu-Gillette, L., & Oudekerk, B. A. (2016). *Indicators of school crime and safety: 2015* (NCES 2016–079/NCJ 249758). National Center for Education Statistics, U.S. Department of Education and Bureau of Justice Statistics, Office of Justice Programs, U.S. Department of Justice.

Zins, J. E., Bloodworth, M. R., Weissberg, R. P., & Walberg, H. J. (2004). The scientific base linking emotional learning to student success and academic outcomes. In J. E. Zins, R. P. Weissberg, M. C. Wang, & H. J. Walberg (Eds.), *Building academic success on social and emotional learning: What does the research say?* (pp. 3–22). Teachers College Press.

Chapter 17
The Psychiatrist's Role After a School Shooting: The Emergency Room and Beyond

Praveen R. Kambam and Elissa P. Benedek

Introduction

Although violent crime in the United States has generally trended downwards since peaking in the early- to mid-1990s, gun violence overall remains a significant problem. During the 2011 to 2018 time period, homicide due to firearm has been the third leading cause of death among people aged 15–24 and among the top five causes of death among people aged five to 24 (CDC, 2020a). School shooting perpetrators demonstrate significant heterogeneity, with various offender characteristics, motives, and background (Holland et al., 2019).

In the absence of official national statistics for shootings occurring in educational institutions, estimates vary depending on the definitions and methodology used. According to an analysis drawing from news articles, open-source databases, law enforcement reports, and calls to schools and police departments by *The Washington Post*, there has been an average of 10 school shootings per year from 1999 through early 2018 (Cox & Rich, 2018). Black and Hispanic students were disproportionately affected by campus gun violence. *The Washington Post*'s ongoing database indicates that there was a substantial uptick in the number of shootings during 2018 and 2019, with a decrease in 2020 (likely due to COVID-19 pandemic-related school changes). The analysis excluded colleges and universities, after-hours

P. R. Kambam (✉)
Court-Based Mental Health Programs, Division of Forensic Psychiatry, Los Angeles County Department of Mental Health, Los Angeles, CA, USA

Department of Psychiatry and Biobehavioral Sciences, The David Geffen School of Medicine at UCLA, UCLA Semel Institute for Neuroscience and Human Behavior, Los Angeles, CA, USA
e-mail: pkambam@g.ucla.edu

E. P. Benedek
Department of Psychiatry, University of Michigan, Ann Arbor, MI, USA

© The Author(s), under exclusive license to Springer Nature Switzerland AG 2023
T. W. Miller (ed.), *School Violence and Primary Prevention*,
https://doi.org/10.1007/978-3-031-13134-9_17

incidents, accidental discharges that caused no injuries, and suicides. According to a CNN analysis of news reports between January 1, 2009 to May 21, 2018, there were 288 school shootings during that time period (Grabow & Rose, 2018). This higher number than indicated by *The Washington Post* database is likely due to CNN's more inclusive criteria (e.g., including kindergarten through the college/university level and vocational schools). Other more comprehensive datasets from Everytown for Gun Safety and Gun Violence Archive indicate significantly higher numbers of school shootings in about the past decade compared to what both CNN and *The Washington Post* reported. Taken together, even with the varying methodology, figures from CNN and *The Washington Post* are likely an underestimation of the true extent of the school shooting problem in this country.

Even though school shootings are relatively low base rate events, the salience of such incidents, especially multiple victim incidents, in the public consciousness has increased. Prior to the COVID-19 pandemic, the public and media increasingly focused on school shootings (and mass shootings generally); it is likely that when schools return to more traditional in-person learning as the pandemic ends (and unfortunately new school shooting incidents begin occurring), this focus will once again return. School shootings can be uniquely disturbing because they may be perceived as occurring unexpectedly, without warning, in a routine place associated with safety: an educational institution. The lethality of individual events (with more victims per incident in recent years) also capture the public's and media's attention. Survivors may come from nearly every race, religion, or socioeconomic background. What is more, ripple effects from the incidents extend well beyond the immediate vicinity, tearing at the very fabric of a community's sense of safety and security, and are amplified by media coverage.

In addition to gun violence generally, school shootings should also be understood in the broader context of overall school violence. In the CDC's nationwide Youth Risk Behavior Survey (YRBS), the percentage of high school students reporting they had carried a weapon (such as a gun, knife, or club) at school during the 30 days before the survey showed a decreasing trend from 2011 to 2019, mirroring a decreasing trend in the percentage of high school students who reported they had carried a weapon generally (CDC, 2020b). However, the percentage of students reporting they did not go to school because of safety concerns increased in the past few years. Additionally, the percentage of high school students reporting they were threatened or injured by a weapon on school property held relatively steady from 2011 to 2019, with a slight decrease between 2015 and 2017. Students who identified as "American Indian or Alaska Native" and "Multiple race" reported disproportionately higher prevalence of such threats or injuries.

Other authors have examined the factors contributing to trends in school violence, described changes in the school environment and the contemporary school community, detailed biological and social causes of school violence, and discussed threat assessment and prevention considerations. In this chapter, after presenting a hypothetical case example, we will discuss the multifaceted role of the emergency room psychiatrist in the aftermath of an incident involving a school shooting.

Case Example

JM, a 16-year-old boy, brought a duffle bag of guns to a suburban school on a Monday morning. He brought the loaded duffel bag into a school assembly, attended by 9th through 12th grade students. He quickly began discharging a firearm towards targets in a seemingly indiscriminate fashion. His gunfire killed one teacher, who tried to intervene, and three students; six other students were wounded. School administrators called local police, who began to surround the assembly building. When JM began to turn his weapon towards himself, a school resource officer was able to tackle him from behind and subdue him.

Police officers took JM into custody and brought him to a mid-sized hospital emergency room in handcuffs. JM's actions terrified the adolescents in the suburban high school, their parents, and the community at large. Depictions of the carnage, speculations about JM's motives, and descriptions of his life history flooded the media. In the hours to weeks that followed this tragedy, other adolescents were seen by the emergency room – some wounded physically and others emotionally. They were followed by a group of concerned parents, administrators, and the media. The emergency room psychiatrist played an important role in this complex situation.

Emergent Assessment and Interventions

Confidentiality

In the acute emergency situation, it is important for the psychiatrist to not forget issues related to confidentiality with which the physician may be confronted in an assessment of a perpetrator of a school shooting. At the outset of the interview, the psychiatrist should provide an explanation of the purpose of the assessment. During the assessment, the perpetrator may disclose significant information and then ask that it be withheld from the police and other law enforcement officials. Such information may be related to the violence itself, other psychiatric problems of the youth, such as substance abuse and prior family violence, or other issues. The youth should be made aware of the psychiatrist's legal obligations under State law and mandatory reporting, such as duty to warn if additional violence is intended (Sankaran & Macbeth, 2009).

Limits of confidentiality and related legal obligations of the clinician should also be discussed before any information is sought from collateral sources, such as victims, family members, other adolescents, and school officials (Simon, 2001). Additionally, students and their families should be informed of what information may be disclosed to other interested parties, such as police and media, before their disclosure during an interview.

With respect to the medical record, the emergency room psychiatrist should also recognize that his or her records of the assessment may later be subpoenaed and become a legal document, not protected by the doctor–patient relationship. The press and law enforcement may understand issues of confidentiality intellectually, but they may unwittingly or wittingly attempt to elicit health information that the psychiatrist typically protects as confidential.

In emergency medical care, sufficient information is vital to making sound clinical decisions. Psychiatrists should remember emergency exceptions to privacy laws/rules such as the Health Insurance Portability and Accountability Act (HIPAA) and recognize that HIPAA is not intended to interfere with a patient's care. In emergency situations, the HIPAA Privacy Rule allows disclosures as necessary to treat patients and to persons in imminent danger. It should be noted that HIPAA defers to state law with respect to minors' protected health information (HIPAA, 1996).

The Violent Youth

When assessing a youth brought in after a significant incident of violent behavior, the emergency room psychiatrist's first concern must be for personal safety, staff safety, and safety of the youth. The clinician must decide the best setting in which to interview the youth. In many situations, the youth may be interviewed alone in a room with an open door. When a clinician probes the youth about the violent act in question, the youth's response can include defensiveness, triggering of vivid recollections and emotions, and even increased violence. Clinicians may position themselves between a patient and the open door, in case escape is necessary. The clinician should not feel omnipotent, despite the viewpoints that others may have that a psychiatrist has magical powers and is able to calm all patients and stop their aggression. The physician or staff member should respect the possibility that he or she can become a target of aggression from the youth (Borum, 2009).

The emergency room doctor's task is to obtain a history of the recent event from the patient as efficiently as possible. A calm, non-provocative, non-judgmental, and non-confrontational approach is usually a sound initial strategy. The psychiatrist may first listen to the patient's perspective of the events and subsequent consequences, with an ear toward potential for additional violence to himself or herself as well as to others. The clinician may employ typical assessment strategies such as a chain analysis or antecedent-behavior-consequence root cause analysis of the incident. Many perpetrators may have experienced a narcissistic injury, either acutely or chronically, and this may be a point of inquiry with which to gain rapport.

Although risk factors for school shootings may seem, at first glance, less relevant after an incident has already occurred, these factors may serve as potential areas of intervention to consider for a post-incident treatment plan. These risk factors include individual factors, family factors, school and peer factors, societal and environmental, and situational factors and attack-related behaviors (Verlinden et al., 2000). Of note, some perpetrators of mass shootings experience suicidality and expect to die during their incidents of mass violence; the emergency psychiatrist should also inquire about this possibility in a youth perpetrator. Ultimately, the emergency room psychiatrist's role is to obtain the patient's view of the incident in question, including relevant antecedents and social context, and decide on an emergent treatment plan, which may include in-patient hospitalization or simply the return of the violent youth to the attending law enforcement officers with a recommendation for psychopharmacology (Borum, 2009; Barzman & Findling, 2009).

Youth Witnesses

Amid the chaos and stress of the emergency room milieu, it is easy to forget the youth who have witnessed the violent act and may follow the patient into the emergency room or be seen later for psychological or general medical symptoms. The psychiatric sequelae after a mass shooting can be significant and varied (Lowe & Galea, 2017). As described earlier in the hypothetical case, many of the adolescents in the assembly auditorium were in lethal danger had the student firing his gun turned on them. Other adolescents who observed the incident likely felt at risk of harm, and many may have been questioned as witnesses by the authorities and potentially by news media. Some youth may have discussed the violent plans of the perpetrator with him before the acts occurred, and these youth may have feelings related to what they believe they should or could have done. Should these young people present to the emergency room, they should be assessed for the potential for acute and eventual chronic stress problems. The emergency room psychiatrist's role is also to listen to their stories in a non-critical and non-judgmental fashion, evaluate the symptoms they describe, and suggest future treatment plans. Such treatment may include psychotherapeutic interventions, psychopharmacology, mental health care from a school health counselor, or psychoeducation about acute reactions and monitoring for further worsening.

Family

The emergency room psychiatrist may also have the role of interviewing the family of the young perpetrator in the emergency room. It is important to assess the family as a unit and to attempt to predict how the family will respond to this crisis. Will they be able to provide support to the youth or will their response be one of rejection, anger, anxiety, or depression? Depending on procedural and pragmatic considerations, the emergency room psychiatrist may choose to delegate this role to a social worker or another mental health worker. After assessing the parents, a decision about emergency treatment, be it psychopharmacology or referral, can be made. Parents may be open to receiving the emergency assessment when viewed as an initiation of a treatment process.

Forensic-Related Considerations

The emergency room psychiatrist may be asked to conduct an additional forensic evaluation. It may be tempting to acquiesce; however, the clinician should remember that the role of the treating psychiatrist (emergency room psychiatrist) and the forensic evaluator differ. Before deciding to agree, it is important for the physician to remember the risks of this dual-role conflict (Strasburger et al., 1997). There are ethical guidelines dissuading the treating psychiatrist from acting as the expert witness. Information may be disclosed in the initial emergency situation under the assumption of a doctor–patient relationship, not a forensic assessment. As such, the emergency room psychiatrist will have at his or her disposal confidential information that is not necessary, appropriate, or relevant to the forensic evaluation.

The emergency room doctor may be asked to evaluate a youth, after the immediate consultation in the emergency room, for risk for future violence. In such instances, a more complete evaluation and risk assessment for violence is indicated (Borum, 2009). A more extensive evaluation would include inquiry into topics, including current status of risk factors for violence, including individual factors, environmental/external factors, and present situational factors. It would include an evaluation of the severity, frequency, and chronicity of past violence and antisocial behaviors as well as an evaluation of the youth's violent thoughts, plan, and fantasy about family, friends, or peers. Questions may focus around future dispositional options, such as whether current violent ideation, threats, or acting-out behaviors need to be managed in a detention center or an inpatient psychiatric facility.

If the emergency room physician is asked to do a more complete forensic evaluation, it is generally advisable to decline, even though attorneys, courts, and family may attempt to sway the doctor, suggesting that the emergency room doctor knows the youth, has seen him/her in an acute situation, and is familiar with all the parties involved. However, referral to an independent forensic evaluator is prudent.

In some situations, the emergency room psychiatrist may be called to testify in future court proceeding in the role of a treater (fact witness). When this occurs, it is advisable to discuss the content of the testimony that the attorney requests, the extent and limitations of the testimony, and the actual time required for the testimony (Kambam & Bendek, 2009). The emergency room doctor may be able to answer some questions related to observations, diagnosis, and treatment even without completing a forensic evaluation. It may be tempting to hypothesize and address questions better directed to a forensic evaluator and outside of one's role, scope of assessment, and area of expertise and knowledge; however, this should be avoided. Attorneys involved may be adept at persuasion, and they may overtly or covertly attempt to coerce or seduce a clinician into an expression of opinions outside of the role of the treating psychiatrist.

The Aftermath

The role of the psychiatrist is not limited to evaluation, treatment, and referral in the emergency room. The clinician may also have a longer-term role in the broader community. As such, the psychiatrist may serve as a subject matter expert or become involved in longer-term consultations to schools, community agencies, parent groups, and the media.

School Personnel

In the aftermath of a mass shooting in an educational institution, uncertainty grips the school community about how such a terrible event could have occurred. The salience of the incident alters risk perception of these low base rate events and fears that many other schools in the community are at significant risk for similar incidents increases. Additionally, there is an increase in fears that there are significant numbers of other disturbed youth at risk for similar violence in the community who have not been identified by parents, teachers, and administrators.

The psychiatrist has a role in evaluating and managing acute distress and shock that may comprise the initial response of school personnel to a violent incident. The psychiatrist can provide information to school personnel about how to talk with the children and adolescents about what happened and how to help students cope with fears for their own safety.

The psychiatrist can share information about how traumatic experiences in the school may affect classrooms and school systems (e.g., classroom cohesion or disintegration, liaisons with law enforcement, etc.). Normal psychological response to a traumatic experience is typically not a detailed part of a teacher's standard curriculum or advanced training, and the difference between a normal emotional reaction to stress, i.e., coping, and a psychiatric or psychological disorder is not always intuitive. A message of hope to school personnel is that the majority of children do fairly well emotionally after a crisis and do not go on to develop psychiatric disorders. However, some students will need further support and may experience problematic symptoms and disorders, and school personnel may need to help such students connect with professional resources.

Teachers may be reassured that techniques that they are already familiar with may work well with students. Such techniques as empathic listening, validation of feelings, dispelling unrealistic fears and concerns about violence, and instilling reasonable hope can be useful after potential traumatic events. Opportunities for debriefings and allowing students to discuss at their own pace can be helpful and offer students opportunities for sharing information and talking about their fears, worries, and concerns in a safe setting.

Rather than only providing psychoeducation to teachers on how to assist students, it is critical for the psychiatrist to provide school personnel themselves with adequate support and attention to their own experiences, losses, ongoing distress, and reactivity to reminders of the tragedy. The psychiatrist may be one of the first people to candidly discuss acute grief reactions with administrators and school officials. The very school personnel whom students rely upon to help normalize the return to school may themselves be grieving and experiencing trauma stress responses (Rowan, 2001). They must have adequate guarantees of confidentiality so that they can take advantage of treatment offered, without having to worry that their teaching careers will be adversely affected by seeking help. When they have this assurance, they can in turn help impacted students and families.

When a child or adolescent has faced a violent situation, it is helpful for the youth to have empathic, supportive, normalizing, and affirmative contact with adult role models. Teachers need to know that while demonstrating empathy and understanding is helpful, they should avoid losing control or overreacting because it may send the unintended message that they cannot handle or be trusted with information that students may give them. Although some teachers may feel a temptation to withdraw from students because of their own potential reactions, withdrawal by such teachers may create problematic role models for the students. Teachers should also understand that they may be looked to as a trusted source of information by the students and that when faced with difficult questions, it is perfectly acceptable to say, "I'm not sure. I will find out for you."

Students

Not surprisingly, school shootings and mass shootings can have significant negative impacts on the mental health of students, including grief, trauma-related symptoms, depressive symptoms, substance use, behavioral disturbances, and maladaptive coping strategies. The good news is that most mass shooting survivors experience only short-term reactions or are resilient; however, about 12 percent report persistent posttraumatic stress disorder (Miron et al., 2014). A review of school shootings internationally found that greater proximity to the attack, direct exposure to the incident (versus learning about it), and being acquainted with deceased victims were associated with more severe mental health difficulties (Lowe & Galea, 2017). Furthermore, prior trauma exposure and lower levels of pre-incident functioning predisposed survivors to poorer long-term mental health outcomes. A meta-analysis found that those who were directly exposed to the shooting (those who were injured themselves or witnessed another person get shot) and those who perceived that their own lives were in danger are at increased risk of developing longer-term posttraumatic stress disorder symptoms and other mental health symptoms than those who were farther from the shooting or hiding nearby (Wilson, 2014).

The ability of students to be resilient appears to also be related to having social support (particularly within their families) and active coping strategies. Research suggests that it is helpful for survivors of incidents of mass violence to have support available to them and to feel connected to their communities. In a study examining college women after the Virginia Tech shooting, interpersonal and intrapersonal resource (e.g., hope, intimacy) gain or loss predicted greater or lower levels of psychological distress after the shooting, respectively. Social support and active coping (e.g., vs. self-blame) with the shooting predicted resource gain (Littleton et al., 2009).

In a Substance Abuse and Mental Health Services Administration bulletin (SAMHSA, 2017), stages of health after mass violence events were divided into three stages: acute (immediately afterward), intermediate (days to weeks afterward), and long-term (months afterward). During the acute period, survivors may experience shock, disbelief, and denial – the clinician may help normalize feelings and educate about support resources. There are psychological first aid and field operations guides that may be helpful for the clinician (Brymer et al., 2012; Berkowitz et al., 2010). Additionally, pragmatic concerns such as the possibility that medical, funeral, and mental health treatment costs might be covered by the US Department of Justice's Office for Victims of Crimes may be discussed.

In the intermediate phase, impacted students may experience feelings of fear and anger, sleep disturbances, depression, attention difficulties, and cognitive distortions related to risk perception, security, and fairness in the world. Evidence-based trauma interventions such as Cognitive Behavioral Intervention for Trauma in Schools (CBITS) teach coping tools (such as breathing and writing exercises to help manage distress), teach how to rebuild and enhance social connections and community supports, and encourage participation in positive activities.

In the long-term period, students may experience adjustment difficulties and relapse of previous difficulties. Other students may be resilient and experience post-traumatic growth, turning their grief into advocacy. During this phase, the clinician should observe and assess for the development of mental health disorders from untreated reactions. It is important for the clinician to convey that not everyone will recover at the same rate, that recovery is process not a discrete event, that symptoms are treatable, and that exposure to a traumatic event does not have to define who one is for the rest of one's life.

First Responders and Medical Staff

The emergency room psychiatrist should note that school shootings can affect the very personnel who are crisis responders and care for the people impacted. First responders may have witnessed carnage and medical staff may have been confronted with its immediate aftermath. The clinician should be mindful that often their suffering is overlooked. Just as with survivors and onlookers of the event, first responders and medical staff experience a variety of responses – both normative and sometimes problematic.

Community at Large

After an incident of mass violence, the community members who were not directly involved may request consultations from mental health professionals to understand and deal with their own feelings and reactions after a tragic event. This consultation may be in the form of a request for an office visit, a presentation/talk, or educational materials and resources. Again, it is important for the psychiatrist to normalize the transient reactions to a traumatic event, including sleep, appetite, and energy disturbances, as well as brief problems with memory, cognition, and sadness. Educating the community helps allay fears that these common reactions are signs that they are "going crazy" or necessarily have an impending mental illness.

The psychiatrist may be called upon to speak at community or school meetings. These forums should be viewed as opportunities for providing accurate information regarding incidence and risk probabilities of school shootings, psychoeducation, normalization of common reactions, and warnings about indications of more problematic reactions. Because information about more problematic reactions, such as posttraumatic stress disorder, may be inquired about, it may serve the psychiatrist well to have patient education documents available to be distributed. Online resources from organizational websites, such as the American Academy of Child & Adolescent Psychiatry's (www.aacap.org) "Facts for Families," can be conveniently downloaded and printed.

News Media

In the previous edition of this chapter, drawing from evidence related to suicide contagion, we made the case for imitative violence related to school shootings. Today, potential contagion effects related to media coverage of mass shootings is commonly discussed, and several studies have noted temporal clustering of mass shooting incidents. An analysis using a mathematical model of media coverage of school shooters and mass killings found that after a previous school shooting or mass killing involving firearms, there was, on average, a 13-day period of increased likelihood of another related incident (Towers et al., 2015). This crescendo–decrescendo pattern is similar to the pattern seen in the temporal relationship between news media coverage and suicides (Gould et al., 2003).

Several theoretical perspectives can be used to explain an imitative school shooting phenomenon. Common explanations rely on the learning of behaviors through observation and modeling and stem from social learning theory (Bandura, 1977). A close-fitting explanation views imitative school violence in the context of behavioral contagion theory (Wheeler, 1966). Here, a similar behavior spreads between people and groups, and certain factors may serve to modulate an approach-avoidance conflict in a particular behavior. Media or public attention may serve as an inadvertent reward associated with the observed behavior. Many attackers have stated that they were fame-seeking through their mass shootings, with some perpetrators even contacting media prior to or during their acts of violence to ensure media coverage (Lankford & Madfis, 2018). Media coverage may, in this manner, make an imitative school shooting more likely by reducing the avoidance gradient.

In consulting with news media after a school shooting, the psychiatrist has a potentially powerful role in educating the media regarding responsible coverage after a school shooting. A focus should be on shaping the characteristics of media coverage after an incident (a potentially modifiable risk factor for future imitative school shootings). The psychiatrist may reference various recommendations regarding media coverage of mass shootings that center around efforts to minimize identification with the perpetrator and avoid inadvertently bestowing fame and notoriety on the perpetrator (Follman, 2015; Lankford & Madfis, 2018). Key recommendations are as follows: (1) focus on victims, survivors, and others who took action to end the incidents; (2) do not put the perpetrator's name in a headline. (3) Avoid/minimize use of the perpetrator's name; (4) avoid/minimize use of pictures of the perpetrator. (5) Do not fixate on the number of fatalities; (6) avoid publicizing videos and manifestos from the perpetrator except when clearly valuable to the reporting; and (7) do not use names, photos, or likenesses of past perpetrators (Kambam et al., 2020).

The psychiatrist may receive interview requests by media outlets. These interviews represent a unique opportunity to educate the public on mental health topics, normalize help resources and treatment interventions, and help destigmatize mental illness, particularly regarding public/media misconceptions related to the association between violence and mental illness (Kambam et al., 2020). However, before responding, in addition to factors related to risk of contagion, the psychiatrist should be mindful of ethical considerations such as confidentiality and "The Goldwater Rule" when making public statements (American Psychiatric Association, 2013). Because continual news coverage of the shooting has the potential to impact the healing process of the affected community and may result in unintended adverse effects in viewers, a psychiatrist being interviewed may consider highlighting available help resources. In more recent years, typical news media narratives after mass shooting incidents attempt to find an oversimplified "cause" of the shooting, primarily focusing on either violent media content, clinical mental illness, or guns. The psychiatrist may also address misconceptions regarding a predictive "school shooter profile" and risk probability of mass school shootings, contextualizing them in overall school homicides, societal gun violence, and the like. The clinician accepting interview requests should be familiar with research in these areas and avoid oversimplifying factors that may lead an individual to commit a mass school shooting.

Conclusion

After a school shooting incident, the emergency room psychiatrist may be asked to fulfill an array of assessment, treatment, educational, and consultative roles for a variety of audiences including perpetrators, witnesses, communities, and news media. Such clinicians can play an important role in the healing and treatment processes of all parties involved and help minimize risk for future imitative shootings. These demands may require skills and knowledge not routinely used by an emergency room psychiatrist; the clinician would be served well to become familiar with the special implications beyond the routine emergency room case, from confidentiality to potential media impacts, and to understand his/her limitations with respect to the various demands that may be imposed.

References

American Psychiatric Association. (2013). *The principles of medical ethics: With annotations especially applicable to psychiatry*. https://www.psychiatry.org/File%20Library/Psychiatrists/Practice/Ethics/principles-medical-ethics.pdf. Accessed 15 Oct 2020.

Bandura, A. (1977). *Social learning theory*. General Learning Press.

Barzman, D. H., & Findling, R. F. (2009). Pharmacological treatment of pathological aggression in children. *International Review of Psychiatry, 20*, 151–157.

Berkowitz, S., Bryant, R., Brymer, M., Hamblen, J., Jacobs, A., Layne, C., Macy, R., Osofsky, H., Pynoos, R., Ruzek, J., Steinberg, A., Vernberg, E., & Watson, P. (2010). *Skills for psychological recovery: Field operations guide*. The National Center for PTSD & the National Child Traumatic Stress Network. https://www.nctsn.org/resources/skills-for-psychological-recovery. Accessed 15 Oct 2020.

Borum, R. (2009). Assessing violence risk in youth. In E. P. Benedek, P. Ash, & C. L. Scott (Eds.), *Principles and practice of child and adolescent forensic mental health* (pp. 279–292). American Psychiatric Publishing.

Brymer, M., Taylor, M., Escudero, P., Jacobs, A., Kronenberg, M., Macy, R., Mock, L., Payne, L., Pynoos, R., & Vogel, J. (2012). *Psychological first aid for schools: Field operations guide* (2nd ed.). National Child Traumatic Stress Network. https://www.nctsn.org/resources/psychological-first-aid-pfa-field-operations-guide-2nd-edition. Accessed 15 Oct 2020.

Centers for Disease Control and Prevention. (2020a). *Fatal injury data*. Web-based Injury Statistics Query and Reporting System (WISQARS), National Center for Injury Prevention and Control. http://www.cdc.gov/injury/wisqars/index.html. Accessed 15 Oct 2020.

Centers for Disease Control and Prevention. (2020b). *YRBSS data*. Youth Risk Behavior Surveillance System. https://www.cdc.gov/healthyyouth/data/yrbs. Accessed 15 Oct 2020.

Cox, J. W., & Rich, S. (2018). What happens to children who survive school shootings in America? *The Washington Post*. https://www.washingtonpost.com/classic-apps/what-happens-to-children-who-survive-school-shootings-in-america/2018/03/21/63046682-264f-11e8-874b-d517e912f125_story.html. Accessed 15 Oct 2020.

Follman, M. (2015). How the media inspires mass shooters. *Mother Jones*. https://www.motherjones.com/politics/2015/10/media-inspires-massshooters-copycats/. Accessed 15 Oct 2020.

Gould, M., Jamieson, P., & Romer, D. (2003). Media contagion and suicide among the young. *American Behavioral Scientist, 46*, 1269–1284.

Grabow, C., & Rose, L. (2018). The US has had 57 times as many school shootings as the other major industrialized nations combined. *CNN.* https://www.cnn.com/2018/05/21/us/school-shooting-us-versus-world-trnd/index.html. Accessed 15 Oct 2020.

Gun Violence Archive. https://www.gunviolencearchive.org/query/d7f40509-9969-441a-ad30-2307f6129f3c. Accessed 15 Oct 2020.

Health Insurance Portability and Accountability Act of 1996 (HIPAA), Pub. L. No. 104-191, 110 Stat. 1936 (codified as amended in scattered sections of 18, 26, 29, and 42 U.S.C.). https://www.hhs.gov/sites/default/files/ocr/privacy/hipaa/understanding/special/emergency/hipaa-privacy-emergency-situations.pdf. Accessed 15 Oct 2020.

Holland, K. M., Hall, J. E., Wang, J., Gaylor, E. M., Johnson, L. L., Shelby, D., & Simon, T. R. (2019). Characteristics of school-associated youth homicides—United States, 1994–2018. *Morbidity and Mortality Weekly Report, 68*(3), 53–60.

Kambam, P., & Bendek, E. P. (2009). Testifying: The expert witness in court. In E. P. Benedek, P. Ash, & C. L. Scott (Eds.), *Principles and practice of child and adolescent forensic mental health* (pp. 41–53). American Psychiatric Publishing.

Kambam, P. R., Pozios, V. K., Bond, K. L., & Ostermeyer, B. K. (2020). The influence of media related to mass shootings. *Psychiatric Annals, 50*(9), 393–398.

Lankford, A., & Madfis, E. (2018). Don't name them, don't show them, but report everything else: A pragmatic proposal for denying mass killers the attention they seek and deterring future offenders. *The American Behavioral Scientist, 62*(2), 260–279.

Littleton, H. L., Axsom, D., & Grills-Taquechel, A. E. (2009). Adjustment following the mass shooting at Virginia Tech: The roles of resource loss and gain. *Psychological Trauma: Theory, Research, Practice, and Policy, 1*(3), 206–219.

Lowe, S. R., & Galea, S. (2017). The mental health consequences of mass shootings. *Trauma, Violence, & Abuse, 18*(1), 62–82.

Miron, L. R., Orcutt, H. K., & Kumpula, M. J. (2014). Differential predictors of transient stress versus posttraumatic stress disorder: Evaluating risk following targeted mass violence. *Behavior Therapy, 45*(6), 791–805.

Rowan, B. (2001). Coping with school violence: An eyewitness account. In M. Shaffi & S. Shaffi (Eds.), *School violence assessment, management, prevention* (pp. 117–128). American Psychiatric Press.

SAMHSA. (2017). Disaster Technical Assistance Center Supplemental Research Bulletin: Mass Violence and Behavioral Health. https://www.samhsa.gov/sites/default/files/dtac/srb-mass-violence-behavioral-health.pdf. Accessed 15 Oct 2020.

Sankaran, V. S., & Macbeth, J. E. (2009). Legal issues in the treatment of minors. In E. P. Benedek, P. Ash, & C. L. Scott (Eds.), *Principles and practice of child and adolescent forensic mental health* (pp. 109–130). American Psychiatric Publishing.

Simon, R. I. (2001). Duty to foresee, forewarn, and protect against violent behavior. In M. Shaffi & S. Shaffi (Eds.), *School violence assessment, management, prevention* (pp. 201–215). American Psychiatric Press.

Strasburger, L. H., Gutheil, T. G., & Brodsky, A. (1997). On wearing two hats: Role conflict in serving as both psychotherapist and expert witness. *American Journal of Psychiatry, 154*, 448–456.

Towers, S., Gomez-Lievano, A., Khan, M., et al. (2015). Contagion in mass killing and school shootings. *PLoS One, 10*(7), e0117259.

Verlinden, S., Hersen, M., & Thomas, J. (2000). Risk factors in school shootings. *Clinical Psychology Review, 20*(1), 3–56.

Wheeler, L. (1966). Toward a theory of behavioral contagion. *Psychological Review, 73*, 179–192.

Wilson, L. C. (2014). Mass shootings: A meta-analysis of the dose-response relationship. *Journal of Traumatic Stress, 27*(6), 631–638.

Chapter 18
Preventing Violence Through Coordinated Responses to Classroom Disruption

Amy L. Murphy and Brian Van Brunt

The concept of classroom management and effective crisis de-escalation has been written about for decades in the fields of education and psychology. We know that students learn best in a classroom environment that is encouraging, safe, and creates a milieu of shared goals and a sense of community (Barton et al., 1998; Jones, 1996; Weissberg et al., 2003). Previous research and training typically ranged from finding more interactive ways to engage students, setting clear expectations on behavior at the outset of class and teaching tips and tricks to de-escalate crises as they occur. While these approaches can be cobbled together, a better methodology is the creation of single, seamless process that combines the best of these approaches and provides the best opportunities to manage conflict, improve learning outcomes, and get out in front of disruptive and dangerous behaviors in the classroom.

A supportive, violence-free classroom has a positive impact on the learning environment and reduces instructor stress, compassion fatigue, and burnout (Mcmahon et al., 2014; Musu-Gillette et al., 2017). It helps the students focus on learning the material, developing a sense of shared partnership with their peers, and allows the teacher and district to achieve learning objectives. Reducing disruptive behavior in the classroom leans into the concept of the broken window theory. By taking steps to prevent the smaller disruptions in classroom and training to intervene with low-level behaviors, we reduce the larger risk of violence in the educational setting (Musu-Gillette et al., 2017).

Understanding the roots of behaviors and classroom disruption must be the first step in preventing these escalations in the classroom. Students can behave badly in

A. L. Murphy (✉)
Department of Curriculum and Instruction, Angelo State University, San Angelo, TX, USA
e-mail: Amy.murphy@angelo.edu

B. Van Brunt
Creative Director, D-Prep, New Orleans, LA, USA
e-mail: brian@vanbrunts.com

T. W. Miller (ed.), *School Violence and Primary Prevention*,
https://doi.org/10.1007/978-3-031-13134-9_18

409

the classroom due to many reasons, including a mental illness or medication and counseling changes, the impact of social emotional learning (SEL) factors, food insecurity, trauma events, developmental delays, lack of preparation for participating in a classroom environment, and poor parenting resulting in difficulty with students responding to rules, boundaries, and authority. These often build upon each other and can lead to frustrations, lack of preparation toward a positive classroom environment, and reactive interventions that escalate rather than de-escalate behavior. Even the observation of a single aggressive behavior in the classroom can contribute to feelings of fear for students and impact their learning and academic progress (Akiba, 2010; Musu-Gillette et al., 2017). Barton et al. (1998) also confirm the link between order in the classroom and academic achievement. The importance of safe classroom climates and the adoption of programs to decrease the escalation of crises in the classroom remains a priority for K-12 and postsecondary educational institutions.

The Collaborative for Academic, Social, and Emotional Learning (CASEL, www.casel.org) promotes integrated academic, social, and emotional learning for all students. Social Emotional Learning (SEL) is the process of infusing our academic instruction with the understanding that emotions, empathy, feelings, attitudes toward others, and the development of positive relationships lead to better academic outcomes. They stress the development of self-awareness, self-management, social awareness, relationship skills, and responsible decision-making. Overall, this process can be described as teaching students to understand their own strengths and limitations and how they can manage their emotions, encouraging perspective-taking, balancing the place of self within a community, and improving how critical decisions are made in a constructive and respectful manner. By investing in this process, we help students behave better by addressing the root causes of many of the underlying contributing factors to disruptive behavior.

In the remainder of this chapter, we offer a three-tiered process of (1) investing in the development and growth of an engaging and supportive classroom with clear expectations for behavior and proactive skill building, (2) learning to apply the skills of crisis de-escalation during an active disruption, and (3) coordinating with the campus collaborative and multidisciplinary Behavioral Intervention Team (BIT) or Positive Intervention and Behavior Supports (PBIS) team. This three-tiered process is outlined in Fig. 18.1.

Tier One

Teachers spend a great deal of time and energy preparing for the beginning of the school year. They create lesson plans with creative learning activities for the various standards covered in their courses while also designing, organizing, and decorating their physical classroom to complement these lessons. Safety in the classroom also begins during this early time period as teachers plan for the overall instructional environment, classroom processes and structures, and how they will connect and

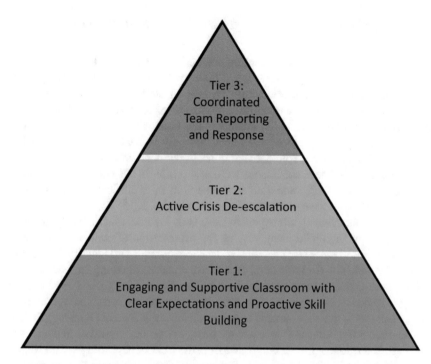

Fig. 18.1 Three-tier model for violence prevention in schools

build rapport with students. These concepts have been covered throughout the literature on teaching practices and classroom management but here, we highlight the clear connection to managing classroom disruption and preventing the escalation of violent incidents. The first tier of a coordinated approach to violence prevention in the classroom is creating an engaging and supportive classroom environment where expectations about behaviors are clear, and anti-violence skills and attitudes are intentionally taught to students.

It is easier to prevent fires than to try to stop them once they are blazing. School violence is also better prevented prior to the escalation of violent behavior. This first tier focuses on just this type of primary prevention: creating a classroom environment where violence is less likely to occur and cultivating protective factors in the class population to defend against elements that may insight or motivate violence.

Tier 1 of violence prevention in the classroom incorporates four concepts:

1. Providing engaging content with an authentic presence.
2. Involving students in establishing clear class expectations and standards.
3. Incorporating skill training for students.
4. Fostering a positive school culture.

Providing Engaging Content with an Authentic Presence

One of the best practices for preventing outbursts and crisis incidents in the classroom is "simply" being a good teacher, adopting proven instructional strategies and showing the class your authentic nature. By keeping students engaged in the course content and building positive relationships with students, teachers build in a protective bubble around the classroom making it less conducive to aggression and violence (Jones, 1996). This does not mean that only bad teachers experience bad behavior. However, it is a foundational concept that students engaged with meaningful, creative, and relevant lessons have less reason to act out. This also means using good learning differentiation for those with different learning preferences, including those who have experienced trauma (Crosby, 2015).

Common engagement strategies for teachers include incorporating physical movement, showing enthusiasm, varying the presentation of content, and making lessons relevant to students. Specifically, teachers monitor and identify disengaged students by watching for indicators, such as eye contact, following directions, interactions, note-taking. They also consider the overall class engagement level and use strategies to boost class energy levels, such as movement and breaks as well as using quick visual tools and assessments to gauge student engagement (Marzano, 2019).

The successful educator is seen as being authentic, positive, and genuine (Gatongi, 2007; Jones, 1996). This draws from the work of psychologist Carl Rogers called the Person Centered Approach. Rogers calls for genuineness, acceptance, and a deep understanding of the feelings of others as foundational characteristics for relationships, and in this case, it is applied to the teacher–student relationship as well. Part of showing an authentic presence means showing unconditional positive regard and building an expectation of mutual respect (Babkie, 2006; Dufrene et al., 2014). The teacher acts as a facilitator for the students where students help construct their own learning experiences by connecting learning problems to real life and providing ongoing feedback about the learning experience.

Setting Classroom Expectations and Behavioral Standards

When teachers facilitate the creation of classroom expectations with their students and clearly community, the expectations for classroom processes, behavior, and interactions, students will more often than not rise to the standards established. Classroom management regularly includes a discussion of well-communicated classroom expectations as an important element for preventing crisis and helping respond to them when they arise (Babkie, 2006; Meyers, 2003; Swick, 1985). School administrators can support what occurs in the classroom as well as beyond the classroom by having consistent community standards aligned with other school processes and policies (Emmer & Stough, 2001; Crosby, 2015).

Setting classroom and behavior standards is not a one-and-done process. It should occur at multiple points in the course of a school year and relate to a variety of contexts. Students and parents should be involved early and often in understanding the school environment and how individual behavior impacts the overall community as well as the learning experience. In addition to broader discussions of expectations and standards, this can include anticipating potential areas of conflict where students need to understand how to participate with civility, such as discussing difficult topics and an awareness of how outside factors can impact a current classroom experience (Landis, 2008; Simonsen & Myers, 2015). Broken window theory has been applied to this setting as well (Kelling & Wilson, 1982). In this framework, the prevention of minor infractions establishes a culture of order and rule which discourages broader misconduct. Effective teachers also use positive social attention, praise, and appropriate consequences to help students understand appropriate behaviors (Dufrene et al., 2014; Marzano, 2007). Finally, when this means creating up as necessary on behaviors that venture outside expectations and making appropriate referrals for discipline, counseling, or academic support (Ali & Gracey, 2013; Crosby, 2015).

Skill Training for Students

Another important aspect of preventing crisis and escalating behaviors is helping students learn attitudes, skills, and behaviors that enhance a student's ability to connect in healthy ways and to build positive relationships. Examples include developing ample social skills, incorporating character education, and promoting growth in SEL area (Couvillon et al., 2010; Crosby, 2015; Demirdag, 2015; Fourthun & McCombie, 2010). These types of strategies help students become part of the solution so that they can understand their behaviors, monitor their reactions, and contribute positively to others in these areas (Gonzalez, 2014). Meyers (2003) specifically discusses the importance of helping students with their social interactions, managing their emotions, and developing increased impulse control, frustration tolerance, and communication skills. Other strategies can focus on the development of empathy or compassion. When a person employs empathic thoughts and feelings, it pushes back against more concerning behaviors, such as the objectification or depersonalization of others.

Social emotional learning can be incorporated in a variety of ways within formal lessons as well as other school activities. Dr. Nay (2004) offers an example with the five "S" intensifiers related to anger and aggressive behavior. While this list of intensifiers is often out of a teacher's direct control, understanding how students' overall wellness, sleep, eating, stress, and substance use all can exacerbate their existing problems and lead to escalating disruptive behavior. In the same way a gardener ensures they have the right soil, sunlight, water, and nutrients for their plants, addressing anger intensifiers in the classroom and within the home environment can be useful to support the creation of a successful foundation in the first tier.

Consider for a minute how a teacher can be informed by anger intensifiers and proactively avoid activities or interactions that may be catalysts for student frustrations and anger (Nay, 2004):

- *Sleep*: Teachers may notice patterns of behavior associated with disruptions in sleep and should be attentive to comments the student makes about staying up too late or difficulty getting rest.
- *Sustenance*: Beyond meeting basic sustenance needs, poor eating or exercise habits can contribute to a student's ability to manage reactions.
- *Sickness*: Teachers should recognize that students who are sick or recovering from illness have less means for withstanding frustrations.
- *Substance Use and Abuse*: Alcohol, prescription drugs, and other illegal drugs have the potential to influence impulse control, and teachers can also watch for intake of caffeine and energy drinks as potentially problematic.
- *Stress*: While everyone has different stressors, of particular note here is cumulative stress, multiple stressors building up over time. Students dealing with divorce, school or family transitions, or financial concerns, for example, may be prone to distraction in the classroom and feel irritated by the impact of stress on their productivity and happiness.

Anger intensifiers also provide teachers with proactive ways to create healthy classrooms by incorporating these topics into educational lessons when appropriate, such as stress management, healthy eating, relaxation, and mindfulness strategies.

Foster a Positive School Culture

Each of the elements listed up to this point or important on their own and within individual classrooms, but they are more effective when they are weaved throughout the school community by leaders in messaging, policies, and initiatives. By doing so, this helps foster a positive culture and climate where mutual respect, positive group dynamics, inclusion and cultural competence, and student involvement are valued and showcased (Babkie, 2006; Emmer & Stough, 2001; Sorcinelli, 1994). A positive culture or climate in the classroom and throughout the school proactively considers opportunities to create positive trends and identify issues of concern. What are the norms, practices, and dominant paradigms of thinking and knowing that shape behaviors in the school community (Kuh & Whitt, 1988)? When these are acknowledged, understood, and recognized, it allows for intentional efforts to enhance or improve problematic aspects of the climate.

The school and classroom community should also incorporate cultural competencies, such as avoiding bias that leads to potential assumptions about behaviors, stereotypes, microaggressions, and discrimination as well as recognizing the influence of cultural diversity on the student experience (Brown, 2012; Crosby, 2015). This can be enhanced by fostering civil discourse, creating shared experiences, using cooperative learning activities, and promoting individual responsibility

(Guthrie, 2002). A positive school and classroom climate prioritizes and values the involvement and leadership of students throughout this process by encouraging feedback, reflection, and communication. When students are part of the development of these important classroom and school characteristics, it increases buy-in, but for our purposes, it also gives those who are frustrated and grieved alternatives to be heard instead of feeling as though the only option for change is violence.

Tier Two

Once the foundational work of preparing the classroom gestalt is completed, there will be a reduction in the number of disruptive and potentially dangerous behaviors that disrupt the learning environment. While we would like to think this first tier, done well, would eradicate all classroom behavior issues, that level of success is unlikely. Despite our best efforts, this first preventative tier will not always be successful. When preventive efforts fall short, educators should have the ability to de-escalate a crisis.

To respond to this problem, today's teachers must have access to the most effective crisis de-escalation techniques, in order to minimize the impact of disruptive behavior (Couvillon et al., 2010; Fourthun & McCombie, 2010; Manning & Bucher, 2013). These interventions must be timely, appropriate, and effective in order to be applied successfully. It may be fair to consider crisis de-escalation skills, like tools in a toolbox used for building a deck; it is equally appropriate and important to prepare, measure, level, and plan to be successful in the project. Jumping into classroom management without a plan or knowledge of the challenges is like starting to build a deck with all the right tools, but without any organization or process.

If we remain with this analogy, the advice to measure and level the ground prior to building a deck would mimic the following list when attempting to manage a crisis or disruptive behavior: (1) adopt a stance of equanimity and composure in the face of chaos and crisis, (2) avoid shaming or embarrassment as approaches to correct behavior, (3) stay solution focused and address the acute crisis in the moment, (4) leave the larger corrective actions for a time when the student is calm, and (5) ensure supportive resources are in place for the teacher and student alike during follow-up and aftercare (Van Brunt & Lewis, 2014).

Teachers who are successful at crisis de-escalation maintain calm, cool, and collected demeanors as well as a solid collection of tools to draw from for various crisis events. While each teacher will have a different approach to crisis, all must be grounded in the foundational principles of crisis de-escalation. They understand how a small disruption can lead to a larger escalation and are keenly aware of crisis antecedents and how they act as a catalyst to the crisis. They know each student and scenario has a unique keystone required to effectively redirect and reduce the disruption. When applied correctly, these techniques support a healthy classroom environment, promote student learning, and protect students and teachers physically and emotionally from the escalation of violence (Van Brunt & Murphy, 2017). The right technique, applied to the right situation with right level of experience and skill, is the overall goal.

Teachers who are successful at crisis de-escalation *adopt a stance of equanimity* in the face of chaos and crisis have a better capability of drawing from the full range of their training and skills to address the situation (Murphy & Van Brunt, 2018a). While difficult at times, approaching a student with respect and patience is essential. When the teacher is calm, cool, and collected with a disruptive student or during a crisis event, the management of the crisis is extremely effective and results in thoughtful consideration and growth within the student. There is also the need to recognize and prepare for escalation toward imminent danger. This requires the shift from a crisis de-escalation mode to an emergency mode. As students become increasingly upset, they often display a pattern of consistent behaviors and observable characteristics that teachers should develop a familiarity with to better identify a potentially violent episode in the school. This recognition and strategies for high-intensity situations (Marzano, 2007) include actions, such as planning for safety and action, physical restraint, monitoring, dismissing the class, and police involvement.

In terms of what research tells us works with taking down the temperature of a crisis or disruptive event, using one-on-one conversations that employ *helping and counseling skills*, such as active listening, reflection, reframing, and in some cases the use of humor, has been proven effective. Techniques, such as *motivational interviewing* (Miller & Rollnick, 2002) and *transtheoretical change theory* (Prochaska et al., 1994) offer understanding and insight in terms of how change occurs over time and how to work with those students who are resistant to change or double down on concerning behaviors. These blend well *with solution-focused techniques* that look toward the future, away from what was and toward what can be (Murphy & Van Brunt, 2018a). This means viewing a crisis as an opportunity and helping students identify their choices in behavior, encouraging critical thinking and personal responsibility. These are further explained in Table 18.1.

While space is limited in this chapter, we want to highlight two of these concepts for the reader to assist them in having some practical application. We will discuss Motivational Interviewing and Transtheoretical Change Theory.

Motivational Interviewing (MI) or Motivational Enhancement Therapy (MET) was developed by Miller and Rollnick (2002). While it was designed to help students change addictive behaviors, we have found their approach is useful for teachers improving the way they handle defensive, argumentative, and entitled behaviors from students. In each case, the core element of the individual being unwilling to change their behavior creates an opportunity for this off-brand usage. MI is a proactive approach to working with those who do not yet see they have a problem with their behavior or aren't ready to move in a new direction. The heart of this approach centers on five key concepts that are useful to see applied in a teacher/student conflict dynamic. These concepts are not part of any hierarchy, but rather used organically as the situation dictates. When applying these techniques, we want to mention the importance of following classroom boundaries and then finding opportunities for one-to-one conversations. If the student is breaking a clear classroom expectation or there is not a chance to use these techniques alone, they may not be the most

Table 18.1 Crisis de-escalation techniques (Murphy & Van Brunt, 2018b)

Description	Application
Equanimity and Patience: Those who display an ability to approach stressful situations with a sense of balance, calm, and level-headedness are more successful in their outcomes	Take a moment to breath and collect your thoughts prior to engaging in a conflict resolution intervention
Counseling Skills: Basic counseling skills are useful in re-directing concerning behaviors and help students feel heard and understood. By using techniques, such as active listening, simple and summary reflection, and narrative reframing, this will help the teacher more effectively reach their goals	While there is a temptation to respond immediately to classroom disruptions, it is useful to address the conflict first by engaging the student and listening to their perspective. This often takes the proverbial "wind out of their sails" and allows for an easier transition to a calm and more effective learning posture
Motivational Interviewing: These techniques are useful when addressing conflict in the classroom. They should be seen as a collection of interventions rather than a progressive hierarchy of engagement. MI tools include expressing empathy, developing discrepancy, avoiding argumentation, rolling with resistance, and supporting self-efficacy	Each of these approaches are tried and true, effective methods at de-escalating a crisis and helping re-direct the student back to their core learning goals. As mentioned, these should be seen as tools that are deployed for the behavior at hand, rather than any kind of progressive movement through levels or stages
Transtheoretical Change Theory: This approach to changes outlines the process of change through five central stages: They include pre-contemplation, contemplation, preparation, action, and maintenance/relapse	Ensure you have an understanding of what stage of change a student is at prior to using a particular intervention. For example, a student unaware that their behavior will impact their grades will not be motivated by an appeal to academic achievement or failure
Graduated Actions: Successful classroom management techniques require a staged and hierarchical approach to discipline. Simply stated, any corrective actions should be directly in measure with the severity and history of the behavior being exhibited. We want to ensure any intervention matches the assessment of behavioral concern	There are times in the classroom where the teacher becomes upset and the "punishment doesn't fit the crime." The heart of graduated actions is the creation of a fair and equitable system of assessment and intervention based on the severity and history of the behavior in question

effective tool for the job. In the following list, each of the five key motivational interviewing concepts are applied as a de-escalation technique for teachers (Miller & Rollnick, 2002):

- *Express empathy* as an opportunity to connect with the student's frustration. A teacher could say, "I've felt this way before when I am angry. I've gotten so angry at times I raised my voice and even stomped my foot."
- *Avoid argumentation* to not continue the cycle of escalation with additional debate. Imagine, for a moment, a student arguing about a poor grade on a test. One response might focus on all the opportunities a student had to study or better prepare for the exam. Instead, to avoid argumentation, a teacher could ask an

open-ended question such as, "what area of the test did you feel you struggled the most with?"

- *Rolling with resistance* is helpful when the student is resistant to change or defensive. Teachers often want to persuade or offer correction. Reflection is a better strategy here where the teacher can demonstrate understanding by saying, "It sounds like you want to perform better on the test, but you don't think you can."
- *Developing discrepancy* can help highlight when a student's behaviors are not in alignment with overall goals. A teacher might say, "you want to make more friends in the class, but you do not want to work with other students on the group project."
- *Support self-efficacy* by catching the student when behavior is positive and use praise or encouragement to help the student know you appreciate and acknowledge the actions.

Transtheoretical Change Theory offers a useful construct to better understand how each of us approaches change. Whether the charge is related to losing weight, exercising more, learning how to control our anger when we disagree with someone, communicating more effectively, reducing video game time, or quitting smoking, we all go through the same process of change. Transtheoretical Change Theory was developed by Prochaska et al. (1994). Their book, *Changing for Good*, offers an excellent overview of this process. These change concepts are universally helpful when looking to answer the question, "Why is it so hard for students to stop engaging in the same bad behaviors over and over again?"

When we look at changing our behavior, it is helpful to understand there are five phases of change that most of us move our way through as we strive to reach that behavioral goal. The speed at which we move through the change, and with how much effort, is different for each of us, but there is a consistency in how we shift from staged to stage. One practical example that may be useful for you as you look at this section would be to recall something that you have changed about yourself in the past. For example, this could be working out more at the gym, reading more books, quitting smoking, or trying to eat healthier. As you review the stages below, think about which stage of change you moved through when you changed your behavior. This may help you connect more easily with how your students may approach their own change in relationship to classroom management.

- *Pre-contemplation*: Here, the student lacks awareness their behavior needs to change and, as a result, they have taken no steps to consider or plan how to change. The instructor's role at this point is to help the student begin to make a connection between why their current behaviors are not serving them well. Engage the student with questions and allow them to explore the concept without bringing in your opinion. Help them see how their behavior may be impacting their social connections, long-term goals, and academic progress. Avoid any direct advice to the student and be aware they will not consider change until they see why it will be advantageous to them moving forward.

- *Contemplation*: This is a frequent place for most students to start at when a teacher addresses their behavior. They likely have thought about change and may even considered how to go about putting these thoughts into action. They are experiencing some tension and discomfort in their current situation and wish things were different. The challenge here is while they would like things to be different, they are not yet ready to take the steps to bring about that change. The teacher should seek to motivate and encourage them to explore how their current behaviors is impacting their life and help them find ways to plan to change their behavior. The teacher encourages exploration and helps move them closer to an action step. In the contemplation stage, we are less concerned about the *how* of this plan, but instead focused on the *why* they should want to engage in new behaviors.
- *Preparation for Action*: The student is aware of their behavior and is willing to take the steps needed bring about change and new outcomes. When the teacher helps develop plans with the student, the goals should be focused, short term, and revised to ensure their success. Plans should be operationalized, measurable, and simple to monitor to determine progress or failure. The teacher is in a position of assisting with problem solving, helping the student develop up with new ways to address their problems and develop plans that are robust and have a higher likelihood of working.
- *Action*: Here is where the person looking to change brings their ideas to reality. As they move forward, they will be successful or unsuccessful. If they are successful, they keep moving forward with their plan. If they are unsuccessful, they will need to adjust their plan and identify the ways they need to overcoming existing obstacles to their growth. When working with this student, consider ways to help them work through new strategies to problem solve, encourage, and inspire them to continue their process of change and brainstorm ways to overcome future obstacles.
- *Maintenance and Relapse Prevention*: If the change is going well, it is supported and the task for the teacher becomes continued encouragement and identifying any areas in that can be shored up in the future to prevent a potential relapse. Plans that are successful are the ones that are continually adapted to ensure they work with the stated goal. Any change that occurred needs to be supported and nurtured to ensure that it continues to grow and develop moving forward.

While these techniques and approaches have a proven track record of change in K-12 and college and university teaching, it is important to work collaboratively with your school Behavioral Intervention Team (BIT) or Positive Intervention and Behavior Supports (PBIS) group. In the final tier, we discuss how to ensure change can occur by making use of additional supports and resources in the community. As teachers are on the front line of student behavioral observation, they become the most critical element in preventing more dangerous and violent behavior from occurring at the school. They do this by sharing concerns with these teams early and often, providing essential data for the BIT or PBIS to successfully intervene in future escalations.

Tier Three

The prevention of violence includes early identification of concerns, using research informed assessments to better understand the nature of the risk, and the connection to resources and relationships to promote thriving in all aspects of life. An individual teacher can support these efforts, but they cannot and should not try to do all of this on their own. Behavioral Intervention Teams (BITs), CARE Teams, and/or Threat Assessment Teams (TATs) can provide this centralized effort for schools. This type of team effort is recognized nationally as a research-based, best practice for the prevention of violence by entities, such as the United States Secret Service (National Threat Assessment Center, 2018). The third tier advocates for classroom instructors to see their role as a part of a systemic, coordinated crisis and violence prevention response by reporting early concerns to a centralized team for review, assessment, and resource support.

Educators confronted with difficult and challenging scenarios involving potential risk of violence can turn to their campus team for support and assistance. In this section, we will discuss the advantages of using a team approach for violence prevention and explain the differences in Behavioral Intervention Teams (BITs) or CARE Teams and Threat Assessment Teams (TATs). Then, we will further detail the purpose and functions of each and how they are a critical piece of how educators identify and respond to concerns. We also describe other concepts of targeted violence and threat assessment important for educators to understand for violence prevention and early reporting of concerns.

Team Approach to Risk

There are a variety of reasons to report an incident of concern to a team and not try to respond and manage in isolation. Teachers can feel very isolated in their classroom management efforts, and it can hinder their likelihood of reporting low-level concerns or asking for help. This can limit the opportunities for collaboration with others in the school community. When done well, classroom management efforts are in sync with disciplinary interventions, mental health support, threat assessment, and on-going behavioral interventions and referrals. This also allows for appropriate involvement of parents, law enforcement, or other resources as needed for the situation. Some of the advantages of connecting classroom concerns with a centralized team are as follows:

- Connecting disparate pieces of information gathered from various parts of the school.
- Reduction of bias in decision-making.
- Inclusion of diverse professional expertise in responding to incidents.
- Coordinated resource referrals and on-going case management.
- Team processes grounded in research and best practice.

When teachers respond to a threat of violence in isolation, they miss the opportunity to gather more comprehensive information from others across the school community, and they miss out on a collaborative approach to the response and management of the concern. Think of the many individuals and agencies interacting with members of your school community. How many nuggets of information do we gather each day with those we work with and serve? This data can exist in isolation if there are not systems in place to intentionally compile information together to create a more complete picture of the context in which a situation occurs. A multidisciplinary team with the capacity to gather reports from across the school and then seek other related data from various pockets is just such a system. This type of team can also provide an objective risk assessment and create a response, intervention, and management plan for those involved. When schools do not promote a centralized reporting team, they risk the silo effect where "different domains of behavior are never linked together or synthesized to develop a comprehensive picture of the subject of concern, conduct further investigation, identify other warning behaviors, and actively risk-manage the case" (Meloy et al., 2011, p. 19). This keeps information compartmentalized within various departments and prevents the school from adopting at wider, more expansive view of data collection, analysis, and interventions. A better approach is making use of multidisciplinary BITs that can provide a 360-degree view of at-risk situations and develop better-informed, collaborative strategies for intervention. A team-based approach reduces isolated communication and combines efforts and experience to make the school a safer place.

Finally, when we individually review a distressing or disturbing incident, we are also influenced by our own individual experiences, perceptions, and bias. To fully understand potentially escalating behavior on the pathway to violence, it is critical to review the contextual information from more than one perspective. A key element of violence prevention and threat assessment involves evaluating how the individual responds to their environment and if there is an action imperative to address their frustrations, anger, and dissatisfaction through violence (Turner & Gelles, 2003). As O'Toole wrote in 2000, "In general, people do not switch instantly from nonviolence to violence. Nonviolent people do not 'snap' or decide on the spur of the moment to meet a problem by using violence. Instead, the path toward violence is an evolutionary one, with signposts along the way" (O'Toole, 2000, p. 7). With a collaborative team-based approach, more information is gathered instead of following an initial emotional response. The team provides a more balanced and complete view of information related to situations of concern especially when combined with objective, research-based assessment tools and followed by coordinated interventions.

Types of Teams

The Federal Bureau of Investigation (FBI), Department of Education and Secret Service launched studies and reports after the Columbine school shooting in April 1999 to study and prevent targeted violence (O'Toole, 2000; Vossekuil et al., 2000, 2002). Additional research and studies occurred after the Virginia Tech University shooting in 2006 (Virginia Tech Review Panel, 2007). Much of this built on what was already developed following the U.S. Post Office shootings in the 1980s. One of their recommendations related to the formation of centralized teams to provide early alert and threat assessment capabilities. The National Behavioral Intervention Team Association (www.NaBITA.org) was formed in 2007 to train and implement teams grounded in these recommendations.

The terms Behavioral Intervention Team (BIT), CARE Team, and Threat Assessment Team (TAT) are sometimes used interchangeably, but it is important to understand the historical evolution of each type of team and the typical scope of functionality of each. Prior to the 1990s, violent crimes occurred and law enforcement investigated following the crime. As the nature of crime evolved, the Secret Service and other law enforcement agencies began to conduct investigations based on threats and behaviors of individuals that could harm others in order to prevent targeted violence (Borum et al., 1999). This activity was called "threat assessment." Targeted violence is a process of thinking and includes attack-related behaviors all stemming from various interactions among the person of concern, their experiences, and the potential target for violence. With these principles in mind, threat assessment developed as "a fact-based method of assessment/ investigation that does not rely on profiles, but focuses on an individual's patterns of thinking and behavior to determine whether, and to what extent, they are moving toward an attack" (Borum et al., 1999, p. 335). Threat Assessment Teams are often focused on determining if an individual can safely continue in a specific environment or if the behavior has crossed a threshold requiring criminal action or hospitalization. Thus, teams are often coordinated via law enforcement or security units.

Behavioral Intervention Teams (BITs) or CARE Teams, in comparison, developed following incidents of targeted violence in closed communities of schools and workplaces. A school is considered a closed community because we interact with a regularly occurring population either because of their enrollment in courses or employment at the school. This closed community lends itself to the expanded scope of behavioral intervention compared to threat assessment which begins with an intentional cultivation of reporting from the community about behaviors of concern. BITs educate about the types of behaviors to report and how to report to a centralized reporting mechanism (Van Brunt, 2014). As we discussed earlier, this helps to eliminate silos of information that are not connected when a culture of reporting and collaboration does not exist. While the initial crisis or classroom disruption may be addressed, teachers should share information with the BIT to pass on these critical puzzle pieces to help administrators address the broader issues. The term CARE Team has evolved into popularity more recently to help highlight the preventative, nonpunitive focus of the team's work (NaBITA, 2018b). These teams offer something different from a "one and done" approach to threat and violence risk management by instead focusing on longer term, collaborative interventions that remain in place until the risk has been reduced. BITs are not punitive in their approach, but rather preventative and focused on connecting those at risk to resources and moving them from the pathway of violence to social integration and support.

Operations of a BIT

BITs are "small groups of school officials who meet regularly to collect and review concerning information about at-risk community members and develop plans to assist them" (NaBITA, 2018a, p. 4). These teams are made up of 5–7 professionals from school guidance and counseling, psychological services, school resource officers, disability, and 504 accommodation support and student discipline. There are typically three phases of BIT operations: (1) Gather Data, (2) Rubric/Analysis, and (3) Intervention (Van Brunt, 2014). The first phase entails collection of data at the student, campus, district, and even community level. The team actively solicits reports of concern from throughout the school community and uses trends in the data to identify issues in the community. Then, the group applies an objective risk rubric and violence risk or threat assessment. Once the level of risk is defined, the team deploys coordinated interventions in collaboration with other school efforts, such as 504 plans, positive behavioral supports, comprehensive school counseling programs, and Individualized Educational Plans (IEPs) while involving other resources and individuals as appropriate. The three phases continue as the situation evolves with additional data gathered as the interventions are deployed and the level of risk is adjusted accordingly.

The overall membership and operations of a BIT will vary from school to school and district to district. Some school districts will have one centralized BIT for the entire school community, and others will have a team located on each school campus. The typical team membership will include the following:

- *Team Chair* – BITs should have a designated chair to lead the group, coordinate operations, and plan for the long-term support and development of the team (Schiemann et al., 2019). In K-12, this is usually a principal or senior district administrator.
- *Mental Healthcare Expertise* – The role of this position is to help the team understand behaviors from a mental health lens and assist with the coordination of referrals and resources related to counseling and other mental health treatment. A school counselor or director of counseling will typically participate with the team in this capacity. Teams may also use the services of a licensed school psychologist to help with more advanced mental health care and treatment support.

- *Student Discipline or Conduct* – Coordination with a progressive and educational discipline process is important. This position in K-12 is usually an Assistant Principal responsible for discipline.
- *Law Enforcement* – The position of a school resource officer or a sworn law enforcement officer provides expertise on criminal offenses and processes.
- *504/Special Education Coordinator* – This member can coordinate processes related to individual education plans (IEPs), arrange for various accommodations, and consult with the team on disability-related issues.
- *Other Members* – The team may expand their membership based on the characteristics of the school or they may incorporate liaisons from other areas as needed for different cases. Examples include Title IX Coordinators or school nurses. Many teams are beginning to use case manager positions to support the work of the team by monitoring and coordinating access to care and resources for various cases.

With behavioral intervention, there is an intentional effort to seek reporting on concerns well before the nature of the threat becomes more direct or specific. This early level of risk is where you see concerns identified as developing when someone is experiencing situational stressors but generally demonstrating coping skills, for example, a teacher might overhear a student talking about financial challenges and stressors at home. BITs could also be notified about mild perspectives where there is no threat of violence. This might occur when a teacher talks with a student disgruntled about grading of a recent assignment who has strong ideas about why they know better than the teacher. Although incidents, such as these, do not appear to be high risk, BITs should take the opportunity to engage with each student, both to prevent the situation from escalating and to offer the student support and resources. BITs can be effective in preventing an elevated threat from emerging with this type of early intervention and support for students. If the BIT is not notified until higher risk levels, it loses this opportunity and is left with fewer and more severe intervention options, such as serious disciplinary action or law enforcement involvement.

While BITs should maintain a prevention-based philosophy, when a threat arises, they are able to perform a threat assessment (Van Brunt, 2014). Every incident that comes before the BIT is evaluated using an objective, research-based risk rubric to determine the level of risk present. Following a vague, conditional, or direct threat, a violence risk assessment is used. These assessments are not used to predict school violence or profile students based on their characteristics, but to determine the risk to the community using contextual questions about the nature of the threat, using computer-aided models, and balancing risk and protective factors to determine the likelihood of dangerousness. After the BIT has analyzed the concern, they can then identify corresponding interventions to mitigate the risks specific to the situation. These can include coordinated referrals to other resources, involvement of family or parents, referrals to disciplinary or conduct processes, case management efforts, and even additional advanced assessment to consider other mental health or violence-related risks.

This collaborative intervention plan is designed to manage and reduce the risk of violence. However, threat management is not just about the initial deployment of interventions but is a long-term process of managing the concern. This may include ongoing monitoring, scheduled interactions, managed referrals for mental health, academic, or personal support, temporary or permanent separation from the school community, and encouraging the expansion of protective factors similar to the early skill building discussed in Tier 1. Risk management also involves safety planning with any individuals who were targeted or otherwise impacted by the incident. While the team coordinates these efforts, they may involve the reporting teacher or others to help support the implementation of the threat management plan.

Risk Factors for Targeted Violence

Finally, educators should understand the two primary types of violence in order to better recognize threats and concerns. The two primary types of violence are affective and predatory violence (Meloy et al., 2014). Affective violence is more reactionary and does not include the planning of predatory violence. Affective violence is driven by adrenaline, more primal and instinctive, similar to fight or flight instincts. An example might be a fight that breaks out in the school hallway related to derogatory comments being made. On the other hand, predatory or targeted violence is much more strategic, planful, and intent driven. Targeted violence is mission or goal driven with a focused attack. Because of this planning and focus, it gives educators an opportunity to identify warning signs related to the plotting occurring as a plan develops.

Tier 3 outlines the clear advantage of a teacher collaborating with a centralized team for review, assessment, and resource identification when concerns arise. Moving forward, it can be helpful for educators to have a foundational understanding of targeted violence risk factors to be aware of in their interactions with students. Lists are always a little dangerous because they run the risk of leaving out important concepts or give the perception of being all inclusive, but we also know the power of a list for training purposes. Here, we describe ten general concepts identified based on research of more than 90 incidents of violence in schools (Van Brunt, 2015). Teachers and other educators should see this as a helpful starting place for concepts to attend to related to targeted violence as well as helpful in understanding the nature of this type of violent behavior. Table 18.2 identifies examples of red flags to report to a BIT or administrator for future investigation (Van Brunt & Murphy, 2018).

Classroom management is a concept emphasized in teacher training and development, but it is often not clearly connected to the prevention of school violence. Teachers find themselves addressing concerns in isolation. The three-tiered approach described in this chapter suggests to consider first the context in which violence is most likely to occur and to focus on establishing a positive, inclusive classroom, and school environment with clear expectations and opportunities for growth. Then,

Table 18.2 Examples of red flags concerns

Behavior	Description	Example
"Leakage" of planned attack	Leakage is communication about an intent to do harm (Meloy & O'Toole, 2011). In almost every targeted attack and mass shooting, the attacker shares their plans with others before implementation	A student draws in class a picture of a gunman firing bullets into a crowded hallway
Catalyst events	In past attacks, a key factor related to moving the student forward on the pathway to violence is a catalyst event or significant life change that further de-stabilizes their life and moves them toward an escalation of violence	A student is injured and removed from the football team. For the student, their entire identify was the team and they become depressed, frustrated, and angry. Their grades begin to slip and they fail a class
Unrequited romantic relationships	The loss, perceived or actual, of an important dating relationship can lead a student prone to injustice or grievance collecting to become despondent, desperate, and enraged	A student is rejected and embarrassed by a girl that he took a month to work up the courage to ask out on a date. He becomes enraged at the disrespect she showed him
Manifestos	In almost every mass shooting, the student creates communication describing their pain, frustration, or reasons for their desire to kill themselves or harm others	A student posts on Facebook that they "want to burn the entire school to the ground so that no one will be able to ignore their pain any longer. It will be everyone's pain"
Socially isolated	Here a student is alone and isolated, despite a desire to relate to others. They exist in an echo chamber of their own negative thoughts and feel increasingly hopeless and trapped	A student sits alone at lunch each day has few friends and does not belong to any club or sports team. They play video games for 10–12 h each night, but even here, they are playing alone and not interacting with others
Bullying behaviors	Teasing, both by the person doing the teasing and those being teased, is a risk factor for future violence. Teasing shows a lack of empathy to others pain and experience and for those who are teased, this bullying can lead to suicidal thoughts, dips in academic performance and further social isolation	A student is picked on in the classroom and teased about their clothes. The teasing evolves to giving them a nickname "Stinky Pete" and it catches on as a hashtag on social media
Hopeless, depressed, or suicidal	A student experiences intense hopeless in finding a positive future and struggles to focus on academics, make friends, or invest in school. The depression may become so painful they see their only way out as killing themselves	A student struggles with depression after his parents' divorce. They begin to isolate, lose friends, and fail academically. They post on social media "maybe the only way out is it just kill myself. I'm tired of waking up every day knowing that this day will be the worst in my life"

when aggression or threatening behavior occurs, the approach trains teachers, administrators, and staff in technical crisis de-escalation skills, so they are ready to respond confidently and safely to incidents. Finally, it adopts a centralized BIT team to receive reports, provide objective risk assessments, and coordinate interventions and referrals. These three-tiers work together to prevent violence before it occurs and to keep it from escalating when concerns arise. One tier without the others is not effective. The sole use of crisis de-escalation training does not consider repetitive behaviors or information available from others in the school community to help understand the whole perspective of the angry student. A centralized team without the other corresponding initiatives misses out on the prevention issues before they develop. The three-tiers provide the greatest opportunity not only for the prevention of school violence but also the identification of students who sincerely need support and resources to be more successful.

References

Ali, A. M. & Gracey, D. (2013). Dealing with student disruptive behavior in the classroom – A case example of the coordination between faculty and assistant dean for academics. *Issues in Informing Science and Information Technology, 10,* 1–15.

Akiba, M. (2010). What predicts fear of school violence among U.S. adolescents? *Teachers College Record, 112*(1), 68–102.

Babkie, A. M. (2006). Be proactive in managing classroom behavior. *Intervention in School & Clinic, 41*(3), 184–187.

Barton, P. E., Coley, R. J., & Wenglinsky, H. (1998). *Order in the classroom: Violence, discipline, and student achievement.* Policy Information Report. Policy Information Center. Educational Testing Service.

Borum, R., Fein, R., Bossekuil, B., & Berglund, J. (1999). Threat assessment: Defining an approach for evaluating risk of targeted violence. *Behavioral Sciences & the Law, 17,* 323–337.

Brown, G. (2012). Student disruption in a global college classroom: Multicultural issues as predisposing factors. *ABNF Journal, 23*(3), 63–69.

Couvillon, M., Peterson, R. L., Ryan, J. B., Scheruermann, B., & Stegall, J. (2010). A review of crisis intervention training programs for schools. *Teaching Exceptional Children, 42*(5), 6–17.

Crosby, S. D. (2015). An ecological perspective on emerging trauma-informed teaching practices. *Children & Schools, 37*(4), 223-230. https://doi.org/10.1093/cs/cdv027

Demirdag, S. (2015). Classroom management and students' self-esteem: Creating positive classrooms. *Educational Research and Reviews, 10*(2), 191–197.

Dufrene, B. A., Lestremau, L. & Zoder-Martell, K. (2014). Direct behavioral consultation: Effects on teachers' praise and student disruptive behavior. *Psychology in the Schools, 51*(6), 567–580.

Emmer, E.T. & Stough, L.M. (2001). Classroom management: A critical part of educational psychology, with implications for teacher education. *Educational Psychologist, 36*(2), 103–112.

Fourthun, L. F., & McCombie, J. W. (2010). The efficacy of crisis intervention training for educators: A preliminary study from the United States. *Professional Development in Education, 37,* 39–54.

Gatongi, F. (2007). Person-centered approach in schools: Is it the answer to disruptive behavior in our classrooms. *Counselling Psychology Quarterly, 2,* 205–211.

Gonzalez, J. (2014, July 29). Managing misbehavior in the college classroom. Cult of Pedagogy. https://www.cultofpedagogy.com/misbehavior-college-classroom/

Guthrie, P. M. (2002). *School-based practices and programs that promote safe and drug-free schools. CASE/CCBD Mini-Library Series on Safe, Drug-Free, and Effective Schools.* Council for Children with Behavioral Disorders and Council of Administrators of Special Education.

Jones, V. (1996). Classroom management. In J. Sikula (Ed.), *Handbook of research on teacher education* (2nd ed., pp. 503–521). Simon & Schuster.

Kelling, G. L. & Wilson, J. Q. (1982). Broken windows: The police and neighborhoods. *The Atlantic Monthly, 249*(3), 29–38.

Kuh, G. D., & Whitt, E. J. (1988). *The invisible tapestry. Culture in American colleges and universities* (ASHE-ERIC Higher Education, 1). Office of Educational Research and Improvement.

Landis, K. (2008). *Start talking: A handbook for engaging difficult dialogues in higher education.* University of Alaska Press.

Manning, M. L., & Bucher, K. T. (2013). *Classroom management: Models, applications and cases* (3rd ed.). Pearson.

Marzano, R. (2007). *The art and science of teaching: A comprehensive framework for effective instruction.* Association for Supervision & Curriculum Development.

Marzano, R. (2019). *The handbook for the new art and science of teaching.* Solution Tree.

Meyers, S. A. (2003). Strategies to prevent and reduce conflict in college classrooms. *College Teaching, 51*(3), 94–98.

Mcmahon, S., Martinez, A., Espelage, D., Rose, C., Reddy, L., Lane, K., Anderman, E., Reynolds, C. R., Jones, A., & Brown, V. (2014). Violence directed against teachers: Results from a national survey. *Psychology in the Schools, 51.* https://doi.org/10.1002/pits.21777

Meloy, J., & O'Toole, M. (2011). The concept of leakage in threat assessment. *Behavioral Sciences and the Law.* Advance online publication.

Meloy, J., Hoffmann, J., Guldimann, A., & James, D. (2011). The role of warning behaviors in threat assessment: An exploration and suggested typology. *Behavioral Sciences & the Law, 30*(3), 256–279.

Meloy, J. R., Hart, S., & Hoffman, J. (2014). Threat assessment and management. In J. R. Meloy & J. Hoffman (Eds.), *The international handbook of threat assessment* (p. 5). Oxford University Press.

Miller, W., & Rollnick, S. (2002). *Motivational interviewing: Preparing people for change* (2nd ed.). The Guilford Press.

Murphy, A., & Van Brunt, B. (2018a). Addressing dangerous behavior in the classroom. *Educational Leadership, 76*(1). Retrieved from www.ascd.org.

Murphy, A., & Van Brunt, B. (2018b). *A review of crisis de-escalation techniques for K-12 and higher education instructors.* Paper presented at the Southern Educational Research Association in New Orleans.

Musu-Gillette, L., Zhang, A., Wang, K., Zhang, J., & Ouderkerk, B. A. (2017). *Indicators of school crime and safety: 2016* (NCES 2017-064/NCJ 250650). National Center for Education Statistics, U.S. Department of Education, and Bureau of Justice Statistics, Office of Justice Programs, U.S. Department of Justice.

National Association of Behavioral Intervention Team (NaBITA). (2018a). *NaBITA standards for behavioral intervention teams.* National Behavioral Intervention Team Association.

National Association of Behavioral Intervention Team (NaBITA). (2018b). *2018 NaBITA survey summary of findings.* National Behavioral Intervention Team Association.

National Threat Assessment Center. (2018). *Enhancing school safety using a threat assessment model: An operational guide for preventing targeted school violence.* U.S. Secret Service, Department of Homeland Security.

Nay, R. (2004). *Taking charge of anger.* Guilford Press.

O'Toole, M. E. (2000). *The school shooter: A threat assessment perspective.* National Center for the Analysis of Violent Crime, Federal Bureau of Investigation.

Prochaska, J., Norcross, J., & DiClemente, C. (1994). *Changing for good.* Harper Collins.

Schiemann, M., Murphy, A., Fitch, P., Molnar, J., Woodly, E., Schuster, S., Sokolow, B., & Van Brunt, B. (2019). *Leadership of the behavioral intervention team.* National Behavioral Intervention Team Association (NaBITA).

Simonsen, B. & Myers, D. (2015). *Classwide positive behavior interventions and supports: A guide to proactive classroom management.* Guilford Press.

Sorcinelli, M. D. (1994). Dealing with troublesome behaviors in the classroom. In K. W. Prichard & R. M. Sawyer (Eds.), *Handbook of college teaching: Theory and applications* (pp. 365–373). Greenwood Press.

Swick, K. J. (1985). *Disruptive student behavior in the classroom.* (2nd ed.). National Education Association.

Tech Review Panel. (2007). *Mass Shootings at Virginia Tech: Report of the review panel presented to Governor Kaine, Commonwealth of Virginia.* Governor's Office. Retrieved on March 28, 2018, from https://governor.virginia.gov/media/3772/fullreport.pdf

Turner, J., & Gelles, M. (2003). *Threat assessment: A risk management approach.* Routledge.

Van Brunt, B. (Ed.). (2014). *The book on behavioral intervention teams (BIT)* (2nd ed.). National Behavioral Intervention Team Association (NaBITA).

Van Brunt, B. (2015). *Harm to others: The assessment and treatment of dangerousness.* American Counseling Association.

Van Brunt, B., & Lewis, W. (2014). *A faculty guide to disruptive and dangerous behavior in the classroom.* Routledge.

Van Brunt, B., & Murphy, A. (2017). *A staff guide to addressing disruptive and dangerous behavior on campus.* Routledge.

Van Brunt, B., & Murphy, A. (2018). Coordinate to curb student violence. *Educational Leadership, 76*(2). Retrieved from www.ascd.org

Vossekuil, B., Reddy, M., Fein, R., Borum, R., & Modzeleski, M. (2000). *USSS safe school initiative: An interim report on the prevention of targeted violence in schools.* US Secret Service, National Threat Assessment Center.

Vossekuil, B., Fein, R., Reddy, M., Borum, R., & Modzeleski, W. (2002). *The final report and findings of the safe school initiative: Implications for the prevention of school attacks in the United States.* Retrieved on March 28, 2018, from www.secretservice.gov/ntac/ssi_fi nal_report.pdf

Weissberg, R. P., Kumpfer, K., & Seligman, M. E. P. (2003). Prevention for children and youth that works: An introduction. *American Psychologist, 58*, 425–432.

Part IV
Prevention Interventions for School-Related Violence

Chapter 19
Public Health Approach to Gun Violence Prevention in Connecticut's Youth

Susan Logan

Introduction

Violence takes many forms, affecting people of all ages, genders, and socio-demographics and is currently of epidemic proportions. One may immediately think of violence as assault, murder, terrorism, or some other type of criminal or deviant behavior toward others. This is referred to as interpersonal violence. Physical and sexual abuse and maltreatment of others, such as children and the elderly, fall within this type of violence. Another type of violence is self-directed violence which refers to self-harm, suicide attempts, and suicide. In Connecticut, the ratio of suicide to homicide is 3.5:1, making suicide a much more common form of deadly violence in Connecticut than death due to interpersonal violence. The ratio of suicide to homicide is similar across the United States. Among 32 states studied, which includes Connecticut, the majority (62.3%) of deaths were suicides, followed by homicides (24.9%), and deaths of undetermined intent (10.8%) (Ertl et al., 2019).

The World Health Organization (WHO) has a compendium of youth violence-related studies conducted internationally and in the United States (Burrows et al., 2018). The organization described the major consequences and risk factors of interpersonal youth violence. According to the WHO (World Health Organization [WHO], n.d.), the primary consequences of violence range from health problems to social and behavioral problems. Interpersonal violence is a contributor to mental and neurological disorders and poor general health. It also leads to externalizing behavior problems, i.e., "acting out," and subsequent perpetration of violence. Thus, there is a far-reaching impact of violence for both victims and perpetrators, and it extends across the lifespan. It is important and necessary to try to determine the

S. Logan (✉)
Injury and Violence Surveillance Unit, Community, Family Health and Prevention Section, Connecticut Department of Public Health, Hartford, CT, USA
e-mail: Susan.Logan@ct.gov

© The Author(s), under exclusive license to Springer Nature Switzerland AG 2023
T. W. Miller (ed.), *School Violence and Primary Prevention*,
https://doi.org/10.1007/978-3-031-13134-9_19

causes and risk factors of violence and address these causes and factors to prevent it whenever possible.

The Public Health Approach For many years, public health epidemiologists, sociologists, and behavioral scientists have been using field-specific scientific methodologies to study violence and injury and the impact on society. Since the early 1990s, the federal Centers for Disease Control and Prevention (CDC) has recommended that the public health approach be utilized to study and prevent violence and injury (Centers for Disease Control and Prevention [CDC], n.d.). This approach has been successfully utilized in understanding and preventing infectious and chronic diseases on the population level and has been shown to be an effective method to target, reduce, and eliminate violence in our communities.

The Public Health Approach. The public health approach is a systematic four-step process which starts with defining the problem, which in this case is violence (CDC, n.d.). In the second step, the public health practitioner is to identify risk factors that are associated with violence and injury, such as low socioeconomic status, repeated exposure to violence in the home, and addiction to alcohol and drugs. Protective factors are also identified which help promote resiliency and emotional well-being, such as strong family connections, a commitment to school and high educational aspirations, and active parental involvement. The third step in the public health approach is to develop prevention strategies that aim to reduce the risk factors and enhance the protective factors within the study population and evaluate the strategies for effectiveness and successful outcomes. Finally, effective evidence-based prevention strategies are to be adopted and implemented on a larger scale to impact those at the highest risk of perpetration or victimization.

The injury and violence prevention field has started to put into practice this concept that violence can be addressed and reduced using the public health approach. In 2018, the American Public Health Association released a policy statement asserting that the public health approach was essential to monitoring, understanding, and preventing violence in the United States (American Public Health Association [APHA], 2018, November 13). The CDC's website has much information on reducing violence in general, including youth violence, while using the public health approach (CDC, n.d.).

Facts About Nonfatal and Fatal Violence In the United States, injuries due to violence increased from 2014 through 2017 in all age groups combined, but fell slightly in 2018 (CDC Web-based Injury Statistics Query and Reporting System [WISQARS], Nonfatal Injury Reports, n.d.). In youth less than 25 years of age, who are the primary focus of this chapter, it was the children 5–9 years of age whose rates continued to increase through 2018 (from 2016). The age-adjusted rate per 100,000 US population showed that about 150 nonfatal violent injuries per 100,000 US population occurred in this 5- to 9-year-old age group per year, but the highest rate of nonfatal violent injuries occurred in the 20- to 24-year-olds, ranging from 1,500 to 1,600 per 100,000 US population per year. The next highest rates of violent injuries were in the 15- to 19-year-olds (1,300 per 100,000) and in the 10- to 14-year-olds (500 per 100,000).

Although nonfatal violent injuries in the United States were on the rise until about 2017, the mortality rate in Connecticut did not significantly trend in either direction between 2015 and 2017 (Injury and Violence Surveillance Unit [IVSU], 2019). According to Connecticut data during this period, an average rate of 14.8 per 100,000 Connecticut residents of all ages died by violent death per year (IVSU, 2019).

The locations and situations of violence are numerous and complex. Interpersonal and self-directed violence occur in our homes, schools, places of worship, workplaces, and in other public spaces. Violence in school-age youth is an everyday occurrence within and outside school grounds and some of this violence can lead to serious injury and even death. Bullying, including electronic bullying, is prevalent on school campuses, as well as physical fights and intimidation. The WHO reported that about 15.8% of youth in the United States have experienced bullying in the past year and up to 23% of youth have experienced bullying in their lifetime (WHO, 2017). Bullying and intimidation can lead to feeling unsafe at school and contribute to school absenteeism and lower grades. The Connecticut School Health Survey (CSHS), also known nationally as the Youth Risk Behavior Survey (YRBS), indicated that in 2019, 7.1% of students in grades 9 through 12 felt unsafe at school or on their way to or from school on at least 1 day during the 30 days before they were surveyed, and this percentage has increased significantly over the last 10 years (Connecticut Department of Public Health, 2020). The CSHS is conducted biannually in randomly selected classrooms within randomly selected high schools throughout Connecticut.

Teen dating violence, controlling or abusive behavior by an intimate partner, occurs among school-age youth and young adults. CSHS results over a period of 7 years, 2013 through 2019, indicate that an average of 11.1% of students in grades 9 through 12 (range 10.0–11.8%) experience sexual dating violence which is described as being forced by someone they were dating or going out with to do sexual things that they did not want to, one or more times over a 12-month period. Additionally, an average of 7.9% of students (range 6.5–9.0%) experience physical dating violence by someone they are dating or going out with, one or more times during a 12-month period.

Finally, violence in school-age youth can be experienced as suicide ideation and suicide attempts in those youth who are currently depressed, who have other mental health issues, or who are having intimate partner problems, such as a sudden and unexpected break up of a girlfriend or boyfriend. CSHS results show that from 2009 through 2019, the percentage of high school students who seriously considered attempting suicide was 14.1% in 2009 and by 2019, the rate was 12.7%. Although this may be observed as a downward trend, the change was not statistically significant. On average, 7.5% of students attempted suicide, and there was no observed significant change in trend over a 10-year observation period between 2009 and 2019.

Firearm-Involved Violence Although firearms have many uses today, such as for protection of family and property, hunting and target shooting, and as collector's items, firearms are also a lethal weapon in both interpersonal and self-directed violence. Our schools, which are normally safe and secure places for children to learn and grow, are not exempt from lethal firearm-involved violence. An elementary school in Newtown, Connecticut was the scene of a horrific mass school shooting on December 14, 2012 when 20 first graders and six educators were murdered in a matter of a few minutes by one 20-year-old male shooter using an AR-15 semiautomatic assault rifle. Prior to the school shooting, he had shot his mother to death (Ray, 2019). Although school-based mass shootings are a "focus of media attention and raise awareness about the problem of firearm deaths among children and teens," they account for 1.2% of all homicides among children 5–18 years old (Zimmerman et al., 2019). Much can be written about mass school shootings in Connecticut and throughout the United States, but they are not the focus of this chapter.

Until recently, in Connecticut and the United States., the study of effective public health prevention initiatives to reduce and eliminate firearm-involved violence was basically curtailed due to lack of funding allocated by Congress. According to a recent article by Allen Rostron (Rostron, 2018), research on firearm violence has been limited in the United States due to restrictions that Congress placed on the federal level. In the early 1990s, the CDC started utilizing the public health approach to address violence and injury in the United States. The initial studies brought to light the issue of firearms in the home and the related association with homicide. The National Rifle Association (NRA) and other pro-gun lobby organizations were concerned that the media attention brought on by this new research was putting too much emphasis on firearm-involved violence, was anti-gun, and could lead to gun control. The Congressional restrictions were led by Representative Jay Dickey of Arkansas, and Congress added a provision to a 1996 spending bill allocated to the CDC that the CDC could not use the funds to advocate for gun control. This was known as the Dickey Amendment. For 22 years between 1996 and 2018, the CDC and other federal agencies, such as the National Institutes of Health, ceased funding research studies of firearm-involved violence and injury due to the concern that these studies would be perceived as advocating for gun control. However, in March 2018, a report added to the spending bill clarified that the funding from Congress earmarked to the CDC for injury and violence control and prevention could be used for firearm injury research, but the agencies were not to advocate for or promote gun control policy.

Despite the Dickey Amendment, since the early 2000s, the CDC has been providing state and local public health agencies funding for active public health surveillance of violent death. Connecticut was one of the first states in the United States to pilot this surveillance initiative (Lapidus et al., 2001; Borrup et al., 2008) which has now grown to include all 50 US states, Washington DC, and Puerto Rico. Although violent death surveillance is funded by the CDC, which include firearm-involved homicides and suicides, targeted evidence-based prevention and research efforts were not funded until 2020. Federal congressional representatives from

Connecticut have championed the research efforts of the CDC and the National Institutes of Health. In particular, Connecticut Congresswoman Rosa DeLauro who represents the 3rd District, and is Chair of the House Appropriations Subcommittee on Labor, Health and Human Services, and Education, led efforts to "secure $25 million for firearm violence prevention research…and to focus on firearm violence as a public health issue" (Project Longevity, 2020, January 18).

As stated previously, on average, about 15 individuals per 100,000 Connecticut residents die by violent death per year (IVSU, 2019). This rate includes the rate of firearm-involved violent deaths. In over half (62.5%) of the homicides in Connecticut, there was a firearm involved; and 28% of the suicides were carried out by a firearm (IVSU, 2019). According to an online article on the website www.TheTrace.org, "Firearms are the second leading cause of death among American children and adolescents, after car crashes. Firearm deaths occur at a rate more than three times higher than drownings" (Zimmerman et al., 2019).

Regarding nonfatal injuries in the United States, in the under 25-year-olds between 2014 and 2018, the average rate of violent firearm-involved injuries was 33.3 per 100,000 US population, and the average violent injury rate due to all causes was 745.03/100,000. Based on these rates, nonfatal firearm injuries are about 5% of injuries from all causes. Contrast this to fatal firearm injuries, where 62.5% of all homicides and 28% of all suicides in Connecticut are firearm involved. These data indicate that when firearms are involved in violence, the outcome is much more lethal than with other types of weapons or methods.

Recent nonfatal firearm-involved injury and death data reported by the Connecticut State Health Assessment 2025 (Connecticut Health Improvement Coalition, 2020a, pp. 278–280) indicated that between 2008 and 2016 firearm-involved deaths were on the downward trend, especially since 2011. The largest decrease was seen in the non-Hispanic Black population by about one-half the 2011 rate but were still the highest rates compared to other race and ethnicity groups featured in this chapter. Hispanic residents of any race also exhibited a downward trend by about one-half the firearm death rate from the year 2009. The trend in non-Hispanic Whites remained flat from 2008 through 2016.

The Connecticut State Health Assessment 2025 firearm-involved injury results showed that nonfatal firearm injuries treated and discharged from either the emergency department or after being admitted to the hospital were the highest in the 15- to 29-year-olds compared to the other age groups studied. Combined 2016 and 2017 data indicated that there were 396 nonfatal ED and hospitalization discharges in the 15- to 29-year-old age group, compared to 51 in the under 15-year-olds and 162 in the 30- to 44-year-olds. This translates to a 6.5 times higher rate of nonfatal firearm injury in the 15- to 29-year-olds compared to the younger age group and twice as high as the 30- to 44-year-olds. A 2017 study using trauma data from Yale-New Haven Hospital (YNHH) emergency department indicated that the age of people being treated for gunshot wounds at YNHH has increased in the last 13 years, from an average of 23.9 to 27.6 years old (Law et al., 2017).

Unintentional Firearm-Involved Injury and Death Although most fatal firearm injuries are due to violence against others or oneself, there are instances in which school-age children are unintentionally killed by firearms, either other-inflicted (i.e., killed by another) or self-inflicted (unintentionally). In a 2015 study, it was found that the principal danger comes from the availability of firearms to children, their siblings, and their child friends (Hemenway & Solnick, 2015). The authors stated that approximately two-thirds of the shootings [of children under 15 years of age] were other- inflicted, and in 97% of those cases, the shooter was a male. The typical shooter in other-inflicted shootings is a brother or friend and for children between 11 and 14 years of age, they are often shot in the home of friends.

Purpose

This chapter will focus on violence-related firearm-involved mortality, mainly in young people 10–24 years of age who make up the middle school, high school, and college-age grade levels. Twenty- to 24-year-olds are included in this report because recent research has shown that young adults are as likely or more likely than other age groups to engage in risk-seeking behavior due to poor impulse control, and faulty judgment and decision-making (Icenogle et al., 2019; Schiraldi et al., 2015). Although legally they are *adults*, it has been shown that their brains have not fully developed and matured. By about 16 years old, their cognitive ability is mature, but their psychosocial maturity, which helps to control and restrain impulsive behavior, is still developing until their mid-20s. This age group has some of the highest rates of violent behavior and violent injuries, and because of this, they are included in this chapter.

The main questions that are being considered here in this chapter are as follows:

1. Who are the victims who died from firearm-involved violence?
2. What are the suspected circumstances that surrounded these violent deaths?
3. Who are the offenders who used firearms and what are the relationships of the victims to their offenders, in the context of homicide?
4. What are effective ways to prevent violent deaths, especially death by firearm?
5. How can the public health approach be applied to reducing and eliminating firearm deaths?

Three different age groups or grade levels will be discussed: 10- to 14-year-olds (middle school age), 15- to 19-year-olds (high school age), and 20- to 24-year-olds (college age/post-secondary school). The types of deaths being reviewed are as follows: (a) firearm-involved homicides (including police-involved/legal intervention homicides), suicides, and deaths of undetermined intent (i.e., unable to discern if the death is intentional or unintentional) and (b) unintentional firearm-involved deaths.

A recent report released by the Connecticut Department of Public Health (DPH) Injury and Violence Surveillance Unit (IVSU) provides descriptive statistics of firearm-involved violent deaths in Connecticut between 2015 and 2017 (IVSU,

2019). The data from this violent death report come from the Connecticut Violent Death Reporting System (CTVDRS) database, which was established at DPH in 2015 through funding from the CDC, National Center for Injury Prevention and Control. The next section describes the CTVDRS database in more detail.

Connecticut Violence Death Reporting System

The CTVDRS is a public health surveillance database established in Connecticut in 2015 and comprises detailed information on decedents of violent death. The CTVDRS is part of the larger National Violent Death Reporting System (NVDRS) funded and coordinated by the CDC (CDC, National Violent Death Reporting System [NVDRS], 2019, November 27). The NVDRS links information about the "who, when, where, and how" from data on violent deaths and provides insights about "why" they occurred. Each CDC-funded state is expected to follow the NVDRS Implementation Manual (CDC, NVDRS, 2014) which guides a state or municipal government entity in how to establish a surveillance and reporting system on violent deaths, what data elements need to be collected and how to link them, and advice for building relationships with primary data providers. Three types of data sources need to be utilized for a comprehensive violent death data surveillance system. They are medical examiner or coroner case records, death certificates, and police investigation records.

Violent death information is collected according to data collection standards specified in the NVDRS Coding Manual (CDC, NVDRS, 2018). Data include demographics (e.g., age, sex, race, and ethnicity), date and location of fatal injury, intent of injury, types of weapons used, and circumstances of the incident. If the violent death is due to homicide, information on the offenders (i.e., perpetrators of the crime) is collected. Toxicology testing results are also collected for almost all the cases, unless they had been hospitalized for days to weeks before dying. In those cases, the Connecticut Office of the Chief Medical Examiner (OCME) may not be able to obtain the toxicology results upon admission to the hospital. NVDRS is the only state-based surveillance system that pools more than 600 unique data elements from multiple sources into a usable, anonymous database.

If a child under the age of 18 dies by homicide, suicide, or under suspicious circumstances, additional data specific to the child fatality are collected by the state Office of the Child Advocate (OCA). This office collects and analyzes data on caregiver(s), living situations, connection to the state Department of Social Services Child Protective Services, school attendance and disciplinary records, and other issues which may have contributed to their untimely deaths. Selected child death cases are reviewed by a statewide Child Fatality Review Panel (CFRP) coordinated by the OCA. The panel is made up of state agency representatives, state and local law enforcement, behavioral health professionals, and social workers.

Sources of CTVDRS Data. For inclusion in the CTVDRS database, new violent death cases are identified through monthly reports received from the OCME. Data abstractors review and extract information from death scene investigation narratives and record decedent demographics and characteristics. Next, state death certificate data are matched and linked to the existing records in the CTVDRS. Data variables from the death certificate that are entered into the CTVDRS include ICD10 cause-of-death codes, occupation and industry, level of education, birth state or country, and marital status.

The third type of CTVDRS data source is law enforcement reports which ranges from summary reports, such as the Supplemental Homicide Report (SHR) to police department investigation records. Local law enforcement records are reviewed in each of the 169 towns and cities in Connecticut where one or more violent deaths occurred. From these law enforcement data sources, key information is collected on weapons used, scene details, offender demographics, characteristics, and circumstances surrounding the violent death, such as in the case of a homicide, whether it could have been related to drugs, gang-violence, or a verbal argument that escalated to violence. In the case of a suicide, the police will usually state if a suicide note is found and the means of the suicide. SHRs from the Crime Analysis Unit at the Connecticut Department of Emergency Services and Public Protection (DESPP) provide additional information on offenders and the relationship between victim and offender.

These 600+ variables collected and linked together form one comprehensive look at many of the circumstances and factors that are associated with violent deaths, like homicide, legal intervention deaths, suicide, and unintentional firearm-involved deaths. These linked data provide an in-depth picture or profile of the person who died by violence which helps to better understand the circumstances surrounding their death. Much can be gleaned from these data, providing public health practitioners with valuable and useful information for focusing their prevention efforts with the goal of reducing violence-related injury and death.

Descriptive Statistics of Firearm-Related Violent Deaths

Violent Deaths In the CTVDRS, violent deaths comprise four main categories: homicides, suicides, deaths of undetermined intent, and unintentional firearm deaths. The CTVDRS also tracks deaths due to legal intervention and deaths due to terrorism. In Connecticut and elsewhere throughout the United States, there are more suicides than homicides, by a ratio of 3 or 4 to 1. In Connecticut, a resident is 3.5 times more likely to die by suicide than by homicide. Data collected on violent deaths between 2015 and 2017 indicated that overall, there were 1589 deaths over this 3-year period, which averages to about 530 deaths per year due to violence. Five hundred forty-four cases had information on firearm-related injuries, which is about 34.2% of the violent deaths overall (IVSU, 2019).

Violent deaths, by any weapon or means, when broken out by age group show that school-age youth are not at highest risk of violent death, but there is still a substantial number of violent deaths in individuals below the age of 25 which is of great concern. In the years 2015 through 2017, there were 233 violent deaths in Connecticut youth under 25 years old (IVSU, 2019). The highest percentage of deaths was in the 20- to 24-year-olds (51.1%), followed by 15- to 19-year-olds (33.9%) and 10- to 14-year-olds (5.6%). Of note is the percentage of violent deaths in children under 5 years of age (7.3%) which is higher compared to the 10- to 14-year-old age group. Deaths in children and young adults need to be analyzed and explored to understand how and why they happened, so that future tragic violent deaths among youth can be prevented.

Homicide Eighty Connecticut children and young adults between the ages of 10 and 24 years died by homicide in a 3-year period between 2015 and 2017. The homicide rate of 6.3 per 100,000 CT population in the 20- to 24-year-olds was 60% higher than in the 15- to 19-year-olds (at 4.0 per 100,000 CT population) (IVSU, 2019).

Firearm-Involved Homicide Recent CTVDRS data from 2015 through 2017 reveal that by far, the most common weapon used in homicide is the firearm (62.5%), whereas the next most common is a knife or other sharp instrument (11.8%), a ratio of 5.3 to 1. The remainder of homicides occur by poisoning of unknown type (6.3%), blunt instrument (3.3%), or motor vehicle (3.1%).

Youth as young as 8 years of age were victims of a firearm-involved homicide. Since 2015, there have been six Connecticut children ages 8–12 years of age who have been victims of lethal violence: three were males, three were firearm involved, and four were related to domestic violence or parental negligence of their children. In general, homicide in male victims is about four times higher than in females. When looking at homicide by race and ethnicity (Hispanic or non-Hispanic), the greatest rate of homicide is in the non-Hispanic Black population (13.9 per 100,000 CT population), followed by Hispanic, all races (4.0 per 100,000), non-Hispanic White (1.3 per 100,000), and finally non-Hispanic populations of other races (0.8 per 100,000). Other races include Asian, Pacific Islander, American Indian, Native Hawaiian, and Native Alaskan.

Of all the states in the Northeast US, Connecticut's average 3-year (2015–2017) age-adjusted rate of firearm-involved homicides of 2.10 per 100,000 CT population is closest to New York state's rate of 1.91 (CDC, WISQARS, Fatal Injury Reports, n.d.). The firearm-involved homicide rate in youth between 10 and 24 years old in Connecticut (2.56) is higher than the age-adjusted rate for all ages, almost 22% higher (see Table 19.1). In the Northeast, Connecticut's youth firearm-involved homicide rate differs by up to 3.8 times higher than the rates in Maine (0.98), New Hampshire (0.68), and Vermont (0.73).

Corresponding to these recent rates by state, in a study presented at the Council of State and Territorial Epidemiologists (CSTE) Annual Conference in June 2015 by representatives of the eight northeast state public health departments, University of Southern Maine, Brown University, and the Harvard School of Public Health, it was found that between the years 2007 and 2011, the average 5-year rate of

Table 19.1 Age-adjusted firearm-involved homicide rate by northeast region state, 2015–2017

State/Region	Age-adjusted Rate All ages	Age-adjusted Rate 10–24 years old
Connecticut	*2.10*	*2.56*
Maine	0.81	0.98[a]
Massachusetts	1.37	2.48
New Hampshire	0.71	0.68[b]
New Jersey	3.34	5.40
New York	1.91	3.13
Rhode Island	1.03	2.77[a]
Vermont	1.35	0.73[b]
Northeast	2.60	4.24
United States	4.45	6.64

Data Source: CDC, WISQARS, Fatal Injury Reports (n.d.)
[a]Based on 10-year time period 2009–2018
[b]Based on 20-year time period 1999–2018

firearm-involved homicides was greatest in Connecticut, New Jersey, and New York (NCIPN, 2015).

In a recent 2017 analysis of NVDRS data collected from sixteen US states between 2005 and 2012, an 8-year period (Hemenway & Solnick, 2017), the authors identified 154 child suspects under the age of 15 years old who perpetrated a homicide. They estimated that for all US states, there were 74 child suspects per year of homicide. Of the 154 child suspects studied in the NVDRS analysis, it was found that nearly 90% were boys, 79% were age 13–14 years old, 13% were age 11–12 years old, and they typically used firearms.

Suicide Although the northern-most states in the Northeast region of the United States, specifically Maine, New Hampshire, and Vermont, have fewer firearm-involved homicides than Connecticut, Table 19.2 demonstrates that each of these three states has higher rates of firearm-involved suicides (CDC, WISQARS, Fatal Injury Reports, n.d.).

Based on the 2015 study presented at the 2015 CSTE Annual Conference, the states with the highest rates of suicide by firearm were Maine, New Hampshire, and Vermont (NCIPN, 2015). At the time, the authors attributed these differences in suicide rates to the percentage of firearm ownership in each northeast state, with the highest percentage of firearms in the household in Maine (40%), New Hampshire (31%), and Vermont (44%). These percentages are two to three times higher than the other northeast states studied. In a more recent BRFSS survey in Vermont in 2018, results indicated that 45% of Vermont households contained at least one firearm and 65% of the loaded firearms were not properly secured (Vermont BRFSS, 2020). Thus, firearm ownership and presence of unsecured firearms in the household correlates with suicide by firearm.

In Connecticut, health disparities are seen with suicides, as they are with homicide, but these observed differences vary extensively from the disparities seen in

Table 19.2 Age-adjusted firearm-involved suicide Rate by northeast region state, 2015–2017

State/Region	Age-adjusted Rate All ages	Age-adjusted Rate 10–24 years old[a]
Connecticut	2.74	*1.14*
Maine	8.72	5.31
Massachusetts	1.82	0.78
New Hampshire	8.51	5.03
New Jersey	1.97	0.89
New York	2.10	1.19
Rhode Island	3.10	0.77
Vermont	9.28	5.11
Northeast	3.60	1.90
United States	6.72	3.77

Data Source: CDC, WISQARS, Fatal Injury Reports (n.d.)
[a]Based on 10-year time period 2009–2018

homicide. Whereas in homicide, the decedents are mainly young non-Hispanic Black males between the ages of 20 and 39 years old, the highest suicide rates are in middle age 50- to 59-year-olds (14.4 per 100,000), males (16.3 per 100,000 vs. 5.8 in females), and non-Hispanic Whites (14.0 per 100,000). These rates are higher relative to the overall suicide rate which was 10.9 per 100,000 Connecticut population during this time (IVSU, 2019).

For everyone involved, suicide is an incomprehensible reality that parents and loved ones struggle to come to terms with and can tear the surviving members of the family apart. Since DPH has started collecting these data in 2015, data have revealed that children as young as 11 years old have died by suicide. The current rate in youth between 10 and 19 years of age is 5.4 per 100,000 and in 20- to 24-year-olds, it is 11.7 per 100,000 (CDC WISQARS, 2020, July 1), so within a few years of age, the risk of suicide more than doubles in young adults. Compare these rates to individuals 25 years old and older (13.2), and the older the individual, the higher the rate of suicide. This trend occurs until about age 70 years old where it starts to level off and then decreases among the oldest age groups (IVSU, 2019).

According to Curtin and Heron, in many states throughout the United States, youth suicide is trending upward (Curtin & Heron, 2019). This reported increase has not been observed in Connecticut's youth, however. Although the trend among all age groups has been increasing in Connecticut over the last several years, the trend in youth under 25 years of age has remained stable between 2009 and 2018 (CDC WISQARS, Fatal Injury Reports, n.d.). One exception was the unexpected spike in suicides in males in 2017, but the rate returned to expected levels in 2018.

Nationwide YRBS statistics indicate that suicide ideation and suicide attempts are increasing year over year among high school students (Underwood et al., 2020, August 21). But in Connecticut between 2005 and 2017, the CSHS statistics indicate no increasing trend in suicide ideation or attempt among high school students surveyed. There are stark differences by sex: 2017 CSHS results show that suicide ideation is significantly higher among females (16.8%) than among males (10.3%).

Students in the 9th grade and those who are Hispanic are more likely to consider attempting suicide; however, the differences are not significant (Connecticut Health Improvement Coalition, Suicide Ideation, 2020b).

Firearm-Involved Suicide As with firearm-involved homicides, persons who die by suicide utilize firearms to a high degree, compared to other means or methods. Between 2015 and 2017, 28% of suicides in persons of all ages involved self-inflicted gunshot wounds. Asphyxia or suffocation by hanging was the most common method, causing 36% of suicides. Drug overdose was also a frequent mechanism of suicide (18%). Finally, non-drug poisoning and fall from a height were each involved in less than 5% of suicides during that time (IVSU, 2019).

In youth age 10–24 years old, 116 individuals died by suicide within a 3-year period (years 2015–2017). Seventeen (14.7%) utilized a firearm, being the second most common method among this age group. Other common methods included asphyxia by hanging ($n = 69$; 59.5%) and fall from a height ($n = 13$; 11.2%) (CDC WISQARS NVDRS, 2020, July 1).

Violent Deaths of Undetermined Intent In some cases, the Connecticut state Medical Examiner's Office rules the manner of death as a death of undetermined intent. "Undetermined death is a death resulting from the use of force or power against oneself or another person for which the evidence indicating one manner of death is no more compelling than the evidence indicating another manner of death" (CDC, NVDRS Coding Manual, 2018). In other words, the medical examiner may rule the death was of undetermined intent because there is no way to determine if the death was intentional (e.g., homicide or suicide), unintentional (i.e., an accident), or from natural causes. Currently only 4.4% of decedents examined are classified as undetermined manner of death, and this percentage has dropped substantially since 2015. The proportion of firearm deaths due to undetermined intent, is minimal, about 3% of the undetermined intent deaths, and 0.13% of all violent deaths.

Unintentional Firearm-Involved Deaths CTVDRS data analyzed for the years 2015–2019 indicated that five individuals died unintentionally from firearms, and all these deaths were self-inflicted, rather than other-inflicted. The victims were non-Hispanic White males with a median age of 24 years old whose ages ranged from 15 to 33 years old. The weapons used were three semiautomatic handguns, one handgun, and one rifle. A combination of alcohol and drugs was associated with the deaths of the four older males, ages 23 through 33. The different drugs being used were alcohol ($n = 4$), opiates ($n = 1$), marijuana ($n = 2$), PCP and LSD ($n = 1$), and amphetamines ($n = 1$). Using the firearms while under the influence of drugs and alcohol was associated with their reckless and dangerous use of the firearms which contributed to their deaths. The 15-year-old boy who died in 2018 did not use drugs or alcohol, but was handling his friend's firearm without adult supervision, prior firearm safety training, or any knowledge of how to safely handle a firearm.

These data points, rates, and health disparities reflect the scope of this public health issue, which is the first step of the public health approach, *defining the problem.* The next steps are to understand why, where, and to whom these violent events occur and how can we use public health prevention strategies and policy to reduce and prevent firearm-involved morbidity and mortality. In the next two sections, the questions which were presented at the beginning of the chapter will be addressed. Firstly, who are the victims of lethal firearm-involved violence and what are the suspected circumstances that surround these violent deaths? Secondly, in the situation of a homicide, who are the offenders or perpetrators of the homicide and what is the relationship between the offender and the victim? These descriptions and possible explanations can help the public health practitioner start to root out the causes of violence and begin to put interventions in place which can help to prevent future violent situations.

Victims of Lethal Firearm-Involved Violence and Circumstances Surrounding Their Deaths

Information from Table 19.1 which described the homicide rates by state in the northeast region of the United States indicated that Connecticut was one of three northeast states with a higher homicide rate compared to the other states in the region. The higher rate of homicides in these three states could be due to larger cities, lower socioeconomic status in the inner-city population, higher prevalence of violent injury and trauma, gang related, or illicit drug related. According to a recent 2019 study by Daniel Kim (Kim, 2019), it was concluded that firearm homicide rates in the United States were related to the gap between the poor and the wealthy, the community members' trust in government institutions at all levels (e.g., the police), the opportunity to achieve a better socioeconomic status, and the amount of public welfare spending in the community.

The WHO compendium of youth violence studies, which included studies on bullying, physical fights, sexual violence, domestic violence, and homicide, addressed major risk factors for these types of interpersonal violence. Based on the studies analyzed, the victims of violence were almost four times more likely to have a history of perpetrating violence, three times more likely to identify as LGBTQ+ (lesbian, gay, bisexual, transgender, queer (or sometimes questioning), and others), and almost three times more likely to be frequent internet users (WHO Youth Violence, n.d.). For persons who perpetrate violence, i.e., the "offenders," besides being 5.5 times more likely to have a history of perpetrating violence, they were 4.4 times more likely to exhibit delinquent behavior or have delinquent peers, and three times more likely to have substance use disorder or misuse drugs. Other youth violence risk factors described were a poor parent-child relationship and low parental supervision.

Connecticut youth who are victims of firearm-involved homicide are on average black males, 20–29 years old. These homicides mainly occur in the larger cities in Connecticut, such as Hartford, Waterbury, New Haven, and Bridgeport. An analysis of 2015 through 2017 CTVDRS data found that the primary circumstances surrounding their deaths (in order of frequency) were as follows: (1) the homicide was precipitated by another crime, (2) it started as a verbal argument which escalated to violence and death, (3) it was a physical fight between two people, (4) it was due to intimate partner violence, and (5) drugs were involved (IVSU, 2019).

In the aforementioned study of child homicide perpetrators by Hemenway and Solnick (2017), homicides by children under 15 years of age can occur by impulsive shooting during play, where the child typically shoots a sibling or friend. These shootings sometimes involve feelings of momentary anger toward the other person, but for the most part, these homicide cases are likely unintentional. The authors also found that homicides occur when a group of youth are trying to steal money, usually from an adult, or when youth are fighting other youth in a group assault.

For youth who die by firearm-involved suicide, they are primarily between 17 and 24 years old, and the highest rate in this age range are in the 20- to 24-year-olds. Circumstances associated with their suicides are a history of previous suicide attempts, mental illness, and current depressed mood. In a recent analysis of 2015–2019 Connecticut violent death data, among youth age 10–17 years old, the most common circumstances were as follows: (1) mental health condition, (2) current depressed mood, and (3) a family relationship problem. For youth between the ages of 18 and 24 years old, additional circumstances were an intimate partner problem, substance use disorder or drug misuse, and alcohol use disorder or alcohol misuse. These data indicate that as youth age into their late teens and early 20s, suicide decedents are more likely than their younger counterparts to have misused drugs and alcohol. In addition, the sudden breakup or problem in an intimate partner relationship can play a role in raising the risk of suicide among this older age group (Makowski, 2020).

Geographically, suicides are not focused on any particular city or region in Connecticut, and are usually more widespread throughout the state than homicides. An interesting phenomenon is that there are pockets of higher rates of suicide throughout Connecticut, which could be due to what sociologists refer to as *suicide contagion*. According to the federal Health and Human Services agency, suicide contagion is "*the exposure to suicide or suicidal behaviors within one's family, one's peer group, or through media reports of suicide and can result in an increase in suicide and suicidal behaviors. Direct and indirect exposure to suicidal behavior has been shown to precede an increase in suicidal behavior in persons at risk for suicide, especially in adolescents and young adults*" (Health and Human Services [HHS], n.d.).

Many researchers have studied the link between suicide ideation and behaviors and the reporting of suicides in the traditional news media, on social media, on the internet, and in online discussion forums. Dunlop et al. in 2011 found that although youth aged 14–24 years were exposed to all of these types of media and information sources for news about suicide, it was their involvement with online discussion forums with suicide-related content which were associated with an increase in suicide ideation (Dunlop et al., 2011). In Connecticut, geo-mapping of town-specific rates of suicides demonstrates clusters of higher than average suicide rates in two or three adjacent towns or cities within most regions of Connecticut. More research needs to be done to explore the cause of these clusters, and potential public health interventions to reduce and minimize these clusters.

The sites or locations of violent deaths depend on the manner of the death, whether it is homicide or suicide. Most suicides occur at home (70.7%) and much less frequently in a natural area (e.g., field, river, beach, and woods) (6.9%) or a motor vehicle (4.3%). Although most homicides also occur at home 37.8% of the time, the other sites where homicides occur are very different than for suicides. Specifically, homicides occur on the street, sidewalk, or in an alley (24%), in a motor vehicle (7.7%), or in a commercial establishment, like a grocery store or other retail outlet (4.4%) (IVSU, 2019).

Among the 81 violent deaths (homicides and deaths of undetermined intent) in children and young adults between the ages of 10 and 24 in Connecticut from 2015 through 2017, 66 (81.5%) died by firearm, 8 (9.9%) by blunt force injury, and 6 (7.4%) by stabbing. Of those who died when two people were arguing ($n = 7$), three of them died by sharp force injury (i.e., stabbing). The eight gang-related deaths were by firearm.

Access to weapons for school-age youth and young adults is a preventable circumstance which is all too commonplace. Weapons are even found on school property in Connecticut high schools, according to CSHS data. This school health survey includes questions on the presence of weapons, such as a firearm, knife, or club, on school property. The 2019 CSHS results showed that 3.5% of students carried a weapon on school property on at least 1 day during a 30-day period. This percentage has fortunately decreased in the last several years from the highest rate which was 6.6% in 2013. In 2019, 6.8% of students reported that they were threatened or injured with a weapon on school property one or more times over a 12-month period. This percentage has remained around 7% over the last 10 years since 2009.

As stated previously, access to firearms in the home is a risky circumstance. The 2004 Behavioral Risk Factor Surveillance System (BRFSS) survey results found that, depending on the state, 11–44% of households in the northeast region of the United States contained at least one firearm. Eighteen percent of Connecticut households in 2004 had at least one firearm and the 2018 CT BRFSS also indicated that 18% of households had at least one firearm (Zheng, 2019, October). The highest percentage of firearm ownership was in Vermont (44%) and the lowest percentage was in Massachusetts and New Jersey, both with 11% of households having a firearm (Northeast and Caribbean Injury Prevention Network [NCIPN], 2015).

Offenders Who Used Firearms and Their Relationships to the Victims

In a firearm-involved homicide in Connecticut, the offenders are usually acquaintances of the victim, but in many situations this information is not known at the time of the violent death report to the OCME and to DPH. A police investigation of the homicide provides scene details and possible circumstances of the homicide, but the offender, or perpetrator, is not always identified. In a CDC National Violent Death Reporting System (NVDRS) study of 32 U.S states conducted in 2019, it was found that the suspect in a homicide was most frequently an acquaintance or friend of a male victim, or a current or former intimate partner of a female victim (Ertl et al., 2019). In data collected by Connecticut law enforcement and medical examiner investigators on homicides in children and young adults 10–24 years of age, the results indicated that in many cases, the offender in a homicide is an acquaintance or friend of the victim (IVSU, 2019). In contrast to the Ertl, et al. study of NVDRS surveillance data which looked across the lifespan, the second most frequent relationship between a suspect and victim 10–24 years old was that they were rival gang members. Specifically, when the relationship between offender and victim was known, 50% were friends or acquaintances (who died by blunt force injury, stabbing, or gunshot wounds), 32.4% were rival gang members (all of whom died by gunshot wounds), and 8.8% were intimate partners (all victims were female and all died by gunshot wounds). In addition, two of the firearm deaths were due to legal intervention where police officers were in dangerous situations with the victims. Of the homicides in 10- to 24-year-olds in Connecticut, the relationship was unknown in 29.2% of cases.

Hemenway and Solnick, in their 2017 paper on child homicide perpetrators under the age of 15 years old, categorized the victims and their relationships to the offenders in several groups, which included the following: (1) an older child, usually a teenage boy, taking care of their infant sibling. A homicide of this type usually occurs in the home and the infant dies by blunt force trauma. (2) An adult family member, like a parent or grandparent is killed by the child, usually with a firearm or knife (Hemenway & Solnick, 2017). Other identified characteristics of offenders were as follows: they were mostly male (96%) and non-Hispanic Black (60%); twelve (25%) were non-Hispanic White; and nine (19%) were Hispanic, all races. One person was recently released from jail, otherwise none of the suspects had known previous contact with police.

In the next section, prevention strategies and new and current public health policy will be discussed as ways to curb the incidence of violent injuries and deaths and to reduce the number of unintentional firearm-involved injuries and deaths. The section is divided into three major injury and violence areas previously discussed: homicide, suicide, and unintentional firearm injuries. In each of the areas or subsections, current prevention initiatives in Connecticut will be highlighted. In addition, related public health policy and general statutes will be described and the potential impact of the policies. For instance, these selected policies and statutes were put in place with the intent of protecting the public from fatal violent injuries and unintentional hazards, such as accidentally shooting others or themselves. The public health approach plays a role in developing, implementing, and evaluating prevention strategies for each of these major areas. Practitioners who use this approach seek to expand successful and evidence-based strategies to a wider high-risk population and develop effective policies to ensure the public's safety.

Prevention Strategies and Public Health Policy

Preventing Violent Deaths

Prevention, intervention, and treatment are three methods that work together in a tiered and overlapping approach to address the key issue of firearm-involved violence in school-age youth and young adults. Prevention can be thought of as taking steps to impede the incident before it has a chance to occur. There is an opportunity to reach out to youth and families to address the risk factors that could lead a child to either become a perpetrator of violence or a victim of violence. Not only do risk factors need to be identified and dealt with, protective factors, such as encouraging connectedness, building resilience, teaching coping mechanisms, and providing educational and economic opportunities need to be instilled and taught to youth. Intervention is defined as interfering with an outcome or a process before a tragic event occurs. Examples of this are removing access to weapons, implementing risk warrants to seize firearms from people in serious risk of harming themselves or others, and installing high fencing on bridges and highway overpasses to obstruct suicide attempts by jumping off a high place. Finally, the treatment approach is providing clinical and social services and assistance needed to persons who have been victims of violence or who have been identified as having suicide thoughts and behaviors. Effective treatment practices can prevent the person from repeatedly being a victim and improving their quality of life. Perpetrators of violence can also be "treated" by encouraging them to go into appropriate treatment for their substance use disorders, providing them with viable alternatives to staying in a group or gang, and working with the families to improve their relationships with the youth and provide proper supervision.

Planning and implementing evidence-based prevention strategies and instituting public health policies are the final two steps of the public health approach. As the reader may recall, Step 3 of the public health approach is developing prevention strategies for use in a target population and evaluating the effectiveness of the strategy or strategies. The final Step 4 of this approach is to adopt the effective strategy/ies and implement them on a larger scale. Prevention strategies can also be incorporated into public health policy and legislation.

Preventing Homicide

Recent (2018) cause-of-death data from the CDC listed homicide as the third most common cause of death in teens and young adults 15–24 years of age. Homicide was the 5th most common cause in 10- to 14-year-olds. In 2016, experts from the CDC Division of Violence Prevention developed a technical package on preventing youth violence called "A Comprehensive Technical Package for the Prevention of Youth Violence and Associated Risk Behaviors" (David-Ferdon et al., 2016). Two of the approaches recommended in this expansive document are *Creating Protective Environments* (ibid., pp. 29–31) and *Intervene to Lessen Harms and Prevent Future Risk* (ibid., pp. 33–35). The authors explain that creating protective community environments in which young people can grow and thrive is a necessary step toward achieving population-level reductions in youth violence. One of the strategies listed in this approach is implementing community programs that utilize trained outreach staff to connect with neighborhood youth who have a history of violence, group membership, and criminal behavior. The outreach staff also provide education, link them to resources, and work to change the norms about using violence to solve arguments and help youth realize that any violence in a community is unacceptable.

The second prevention strategy recommended in the youth violence technical package is in the section on intervening to lessen harms and prevent future risk. The authors describe evidence-based approaches that prevent the continuation and escalation of violence and its associated risk factors, including hospital-community partnerships that provide community prevention services. Hospital trauma centers are most often the facilities treating acute interpersonal violence-related injuries from shootings, stabbings, or blunt force. If a hospital is affiliated with a community violence reduction program, hospital staff connect the acutely injured patient with staff from the community program, who provide follow-up services to the individual. This includes assessing their needs, providing assistance, such as social services, making referrals to mental health and substance abuse treatment, as needed, and discussing ways the individual can better cope with life stressors and manage themselves in high-risk situations.

These two youth violence prevention and intervention approaches have been in place in Connecticut in varying degrees since about 2004, when Saint Francis Medical Center in Hartford partnered with Hartford Communities that Care (HCTC), a nonprofit community services organization, to establish the Hartford Crisis Response Team/hospital-based violence intervention program. This model fits well with the second approach described in the CDC youth violence prevention technical package, with the objective of intervening with at-risk youth to lessen harms and prevent future risk of violence. Currently in 2020, Connecticut has several active hospital trauma center-, law enforcement-, and community-based organizations working toward reducing the rate of firearm violence among school-age children and young adults who are at most risk of being victims or perpetrators of violence. One evidence-based initiative that has taken hold in Connecticut cities is the "Cure Violence" model. This model takes the public health approach to reducing and preventing violent injuries and deaths within urban communities most affected by violence (Butts et al., 2015). The Cure Violence model is one of the violence prevention models recommended in the CDC technical package under *Creating a Protective Environment*. This model was developed in Chicago by Dr. Gary Slutkin, a physician and epidemiologist, formerly with the WHO, who founded the Cure Violence model in 2000. Based on the epidemiology of violence in Chicago and other areas in the United States, Dr. Slutkin saw patterns and trends that were very similar to a public health problem and was one of the first to view violence as a health epidemic (Cure Violence Global, Cure Violence Global Staff, 2020a). Information obtained from the Cure Violence Global webpage explains that violence is an epidemic, is contagious, and should be treated as a public health issue. Using the public health approach, this model seeks to (1) detect and interrupt the transmission of violence, (2) identify those at highest risk for violence and work to change their behavior, and (3) change community norms to discourage the use of violence (Cure Violence Global, The Big Idea, 2020b). This approach utilizes trained outreach workers and violence interrupters who try to stop the chain of violence before it happens.

The first metro-area in Connecticut to utilize the Cure Violence model was New Haven, called the Connecticut Violence Intervention Program (CTVIP), established in October 2018. CTVIP is "based on a mix of different evidence-based models from across the country; specifically, the Cure Violence program in Chicago and the Cease Fire program in Boston" and their mission is to "change group and community norms to interrupt violence among youth and the re-entry population in the community" (Connecticut Violence Intervention Program [CTVIP], 2020). Currently there are three hospital trauma center-based violence intervention programs (HVIPs) utilizing the Cure Violence model and functioning in two of the major urban, underserved areas in Connecticut, namely, Hartford and New Haven. The HVIPs work closely with nongovernmental organizations (NGO), such as HCTC, and train hospital program staff to intervene with the victim and provide them appropriate care and follow-up to try to change their violent behavior. HCTC has community outreach workers called "Interrupters," who are integral and trusted members of the community and who have lived experience with violence perpetration. HCTC's mission, which is based on the Prevention Institute's, 2018 Recommendations for Preventing and Reducing Gun Violence, is to provide "a nonviolent and drug free environment through the coordination and collaboration of services, promotion of education, healthy lifestyles, and practices and by the formation of effective partnerships with key members of the community" (HCTC, 2020a, b; Prevention Institute, 2018). The Prevention Institute advocates for a public health approach to reducing firearm violence and promotes a multi-faceted, multi-strategic policy and prevention approach to firearm violence.

Another NGO that functions in three Connecticut cities, Bridgeport, Hartford, and New Haven is Project Longevity, a statewide anti-violence initiative that was implemented in Connecticut through a joint effort of numerous partners spearheaded by the U.S. Department of Justice, the U.S. Attorney's Office, and Governor Dannel Malloy in 2012 (Department of Justice, 2012). Project Longevity's (PL) philosophy and approach is slightly different from the Cure Violence model because it relies on law enforcement closely connecting with community residents and social workers on focused deterrence of firearm violence among street groups. Groups, otherwise known as gangs, are the most likely to be victims and offenders of firearm violence. As stated previously, where the relationship between offender and victim was known, 32.4% of homicides were between rival gang members. The PL program is based on Boston's *Operation Cease Fire* initiative developed by criminologist David M. Kennedy in the mid-1990s. PL Connecticut's message is to encourage group members to stop the violence because community members want them to reach their potential rather than dying at a young age or becoming incarcerated. PL is there to offer group members the help they need to change their behavior and to support law enforcement in keeping their communities safe places to live (Project Longevity, 2020). Project Longevity has shown some initial success in New Haven, the first PL site, which started in November 2012. Over an 18-month study period which evaluated the effectiveness of PL in New Haven (Sierra-Arevalo et al., 2015; Sierra-Arevalo & Papachristos, 2015), the evaluators saw a sharp reduction in group member-involved shootings and homicides by an average of 4.6 incidents per month compared to the previous 22 months.

These approaches cannot be implemented and sustained without the commitment and involvement of multiple sectors, such as community programs, social services, all levels of government, including policy-makers and public health officials, healthcare, law enforcement, and justice systems, business, and the media.

Preventing Suicide

Suicide is the second most common cause of death (unintentional injury is the first) for US children and young adults 10–24 years of age. This cause-of-death ranking also rings true for Connecticut (Connecticut Department of Mental Health and Addiction Services, 2019). Connecticut has implemented a multi-faceted approach to suicide prevention, intervention, and response (SPIR). Much of this SPIR work is guided by the Connecticut Suicide Advisory Board (CTSAB) that was established in 2012 by merging the Youth Suicide Advisory Board with the Interagency Suicide Prevention Network. The members of the CTSAB were responsible for developing the statewide suicide prevention plans 2020 and 2025 (Heller & CTSAB, 2014; May & CTSAB, 2020) with goals, objectives, strategies, and recommendations for implementation and monitoring that follow the *continuum of care* model framed out by the Institute of Medicine in 1994 (Springer & Phillips, 2006). This model considers diverse populations with different needs, risk factors, and underlying circumstances related to behavioral health conditions and outcomes. The care continuum starts with health promotion and prevention, moves to intervention and treatment, and extends out to recovery and maintenance of wellness.

One component of the suicide prevention work currently being conducted in Connecticut is lethal means restriction planning and implementation. Lethal means restriction is reducing and preventing access to weapons and situations that could result in a suicide, such as firearms, prescription and over-the-counter medications, restricting public access to train tracks, and raising fencing on bridges, highway overpasses, and parking garages. In the years 2016–2018, suicide prevention and behavioral health organizations were involved in an evidence-based initiative to train and educate gun shop owners and staff at gun ranges on recognizing the signs of suicide. This initiative was modeled on a gun shop project implemented by the Harvard School of Public Health Injury Research Center, *Means Matter* campaign

(Harvard School of Public Health Injury Research Center, n.d.). It was a novel project that started in New Hampshire in 2009 to reach out to gun shop owners and staff and emphasize the role that they can play in suicide prevention. Like the project in New Hampshire, the Connecticut campaign offered gun shop owners and gun range staff QPR Gatekeeper training to help them identify the signs of someone in crisis. They were encouraged to provide their customers with written materials on firearm safety and suicide prevention. The awareness and training materials were co-developed by the CTSAB, the Connecticut Chapter of the American Foundation for Suicide Prevention (CT-AFSP), and the National Shooting Sports Foundation (NSSF).

In Connecticut, mental health promotion and social-emotional learning (SEL) strategies are embedded across the lifespan and in targeted communities and populations groups, including school-age youth and young adults. One such strategy is a mental health promotion toolkit and associated curriculum developed by the CTSAB and geared toward elementary school students called *Gizmo's Pawesome Guide to Mental Health* (CTSAB, 2017). The Gizmo curriculum features a therapy dog and K-9 first responder (Gizmo) that presents important mental health wellness messages and coping skills in a friendly and understandable way to young children. There is an opportunity for each child who participates in the program to develop their own mental health plan.

Middle school and high school-based initiatives include *4 What's Next* (Jordan Porco Foundation, 4 What's Next, n.d.-a), a primary prevention program for middle and high school students who may be experiencing stress and anxiety about upcoming life changes, such as transition from middle school to high school or what to expect after high school graduation. The program was developed and is supported by the Connecticut-based Jordan Porco Foundation. The program teaches resiliency and coping methods to students to help them handle their stress and distress now and in the future. In 2019, 60 Connecticut schools and 25 school-based health centers participated in the *4 What's Next* suicide prevention program.

A suicide prevention program for college students that started in Connecticut and has spread to almost every state in the United States is called *Fresh Check Day* (Jordan Porco Foundation, Fresh Check Day, n.d.-b), which was also developed by the Jordan Porco Foundation. It is a mental health promotion and suicide prevention event held by the university or college near the start of the college semester. It includes information booths, games and prizes, and free food, and peer advisors are available to help students learn about the mental health resources on campus to which they can connect and seek help if needed.

A suicide intervention strategy that is frequently utilized by residents in Connecticut is the National Suicide Prevention Lifeline, which is a call center for persons in crisis who may be seriously considering suicide. In 2020, the federal National Suicide Hotline Designation Act of 2020 (S.2661) was passed by Congress and signed into law by President Trump that will replace the toll-free 1-800 number with a universal three-digit 9-8-8 number, effective July 1, 2022. The bill, which became law on 10/17/2020 (Public Law No: 116-172), aims to reduce the stigma of suicidality, make it easier to remember a 3-digit number similar to 9-1-1, and provide a needed service to persons in crisis, especially high-risk populations, such as minorities, LGBTQ+ youth, and those living in rural areas.

Another suicide intervention and treatment strategy available to all residents is the *Zero Suicide* framework which is a mental health promotion and suicide prevention program (Zero Suicide, n.d.) embedded in many healthcare and behavioral health organizations across the state. Zero Suicide holds the belief that providers have an opportunity to prevent suicides among people in their care. Zero Suicide Academy-trained providers screen patients for suicide thoughts and behaviors, encourage care-seeking behavior, and build awareness of crisis resources in the community, such as the National Suicide Prevention Lifeline and United Way 2-1-1. Many healthcare staff in organizations embracing the Zero Suicide approach participated in Zero Suicide Academy training sessions and became members of the Zero Suicide Learning Community (ZSLC), coordinated by the CTSAB. As of June 2020, 120 staff representing 35 healthcare systems were members of the Connecticut ZSLC. For youth and young adults of all ages, Zero Suicide can make a big impact on identifying, treating, and reducing the rate of suicides.

New healthcare policy from the Joint Commission, which accredits US healthcare organizations and programs, released a Sentinel Event Alert (Sentinel Event Alert 56) in 2019 on detecting and treating suicide ideation in all healthcare settings (Joint Commission, 2019a). This Sentinel Alert was subsequently written into National Patient Safety Goal 15.01.01, effective July 2020, which is "Reduce the Risk of Suicide" (Joint Commission, 2019b). As a result of this Alert and the new healthcare organization recommendations by the Joint Commission, Connecticut Children's Medical Center initiated screening of children 10 and older who are seen in the emergency department. According to a presentation given by Dr. Steven C. Rogers, an emergency medicine physician and assistant professor at the University of Connecticut School of Medicine, the keys to preventing suicide in children are to (1) identify a child at risk, (2) connect them to the appropriate level of care required, and (3) counsel the child and their family on reducing the child's access to lethal means of suicide (Rogers, 2019; Brahmbhatt et al., 2019).

At Connecticut Children's Medical Center (CCMC), when children come to the emergency department, they are given a suicide risk screen called the ASQ (Ask Suicide Screening Questions) to identify their risk for suicide (National Institute of Mental Health, n.d.). The ASQ is a series of four questions related to one's wish to die, suicide ideation/thoughts, and suicide attempts. If a child screens positive based on the ASQ, they are assessed for degree of risk using the Columbia-Suicide Severity Rating Scale (C-SSRS) (Columbia-Suicide Severity Rating Scale, n.d.). The children at highest risk based on the C-SSRS are connected to immediate care at CCMC through a hospital social worker. Another way to connect all Connecticut children under 19 years of age who are in crisis is through the Emergency Mobile Psychiatric Services (EMPS). Within the hour of a call to EMPS, a clinician will come to wherever the child in crisis is located, such as their home, school, or hospital, and try to stabilize the crisis and provide immediate care and/or referral to services. Once the child is stabilized and starts behavioral health treatment, they and their family are provided lethal means counseling to reduce their access to firearms and medications around the household. The family is educated on safe and secure storage of firearms and medications in the home that could cause the child injury and death.

In 1999, landmark policy was passed in Connecticut that authorized law enforcement to remove firearms and ammunition from individuals who are at imminent risk of injuring themselves or others (C.G.S. § 29-38c, 1999). To seize the firearm(s) and ammunition, the police need to obtain a risk warrant from a judge. For this to be issued, the complainant(s) is required to provide clear and convincing evidence to a judge hearing the case of "(1) recent threats or acts of violence by such person directed toward other persons; (2) recent threats or acts of violence by such person directed toward himself or herself; or (3) recent acts of cruelty to animals ... by such person" (C.G.S. § 29-38c, 1999). The complainant's evidence, among other factors, are evaluated by the judge and if the judge believes that probable cause exists and there is an imminent risk of injury, he/she will issue a risk warrant.

A study was conducted by researchers in 2017 (Swanson et al., 2017) evaluating Connecticut's gun seizure law and its implications on the prevention of suicide. The researchers analyzed 762 gun-removal events occurring from October 1999 through June 2013 where a risk warrant was issued, and firearm(s) were removed. Of the 762 individuals studied, 702 had information on the reason for the risk warrant: 61% of the removals were due to risk of injury to self and 32% were for reasons of potential injury to others. An additional 9% was a combination of both types of imminent risk, harm to self and harm to others. Based on the study results and calculated likelihood of risk, the researchers estimated that for every 10–20 gun seizures, a suicide was averted.

When a suicide occurs, social services and other "postvention" services are provided to family and friends (aka loss survivors) of the person who died by suicide. Postvention refers to *"activities which reduce risk and promote healing after a suicide death.* Although postvention is implemented after a suicide it is essential that we prepare for postvention *before* a suicide" (Norton, 2015). After a loved one dies by suicide, loss survivors, such as family members, friends, classmates, teachers, co-workers, and others in the community, are affected in different ways. They experience emotions, such as sadness, blame, guilt, shame, and anger, as ways to deal with their loss. During the postvention period, trained mental health providers and social workers dispense information about community resources and services, make referrals to counselors and grief support groups, and connect loss survivors to others with lived experience. The CTSAB has several board members who are involved in promoting the postvention response by developing community postvention plans, each geared to a different type of situation. These include postvention plans for how a college or a high school community respond to a suicide death of a student or teacher, or how community leaders, social services, and local public health respond to a community member's suicide death. There may also be occupation-specific community postvention plans for organizations, like the Connecticut National Guard, the Coast Guard Academy, or law enforcement officer fraternal organizations impacted by suicide.

Postvention services help loss survivors heal from this painful experience and reduce the rare occurrence of associated suicides via suicide contagion. As discussed earlier in the chapter, suicide contagion occurs when an at-risk person who has a close relationship with a suicide decedent develops increased suicide thoughts and behaviors. This is especially true for at-risk teens and young adults (HHS, n.d.). Appropriate media coverage, sensitivity-trained first responders and medical providers, and culturally competent intervention services are ways to help prevent clusters of suicide behaviors and suicides.

Preventing Unintentional Firearm-Involved Deaths

Most firearm-involved deaths are due to interpersonal violence and self-directed violence. Rarely, someone is unintentionally killed by a firearm. Although those cases are few (three deaths in 2015–2017 in males ages 15–24 years old), implementing prevention practices, mandating firearms safety training before applying for a pistol permit, and enacting child-protective policies are tools that can be utilized to reduce these preventable deaths. Currently in 2020, there are many options and locations available for people applying for a pistol or handgun permit to attend a state of Connecticut-approved firearms training course. One of the only state of Connecticut-approved courses is the NRA certified pistol permit and firearms safety training course. This course teaches the basic knowledge, skills, and attitude needed for owning and using a pistol safely.

Connecticut gun laws were strengthened in 2013 and again in 2018 to protect children and victims of domestic and intimate partner violence. A summary of firearms laws was compiled in a document by the Connecticut State Police, Department of Emergency Services and Public Protection, entitled "Your Guide to Firearms and Permits in Connecticut" (Connecticut Department of Emergency Services and Public Protection, 2017).

A review of Connecticut firearm-related statutes (C.G.S. § 29-27 to 29-38p) indicated that current laws exist with the objective of keeping firearms away from people who may harm others or themselves. First, no application of a firearm permit will be approved for anyone: (a) under 21 years of age, (b) who does not pass a background check, (c) who has a history of being hospitalized for mental illness, (d) who has a restraining or protective order filed against them for assaulting, attempting, or threatening physical force against another person, (e) who is subject to firearm seizure (via a risk warrant), or (f) who is an undocumented immigrant. Second, the purchase of ammunition is limited to persons 18 years of age and older and only if they hold a current firearm permit. Third, when purchasing a firearm, the seller must equip the firearm with a gunlock or gun-locking device of sufficient material so as not to be able to easily break or disable the lock. Finally, a printed warning in block letters at least three inches high must be posted on the gun retail shop service counter which states, "*unlawful storage of a loaded firearm may result in imprisonment or fine.*" Each violation carries a fine of up to $500.

The 2018 case of the 15-year-old child killed at a friend's house received much publicity and led to new legislation in Connecticut in 2019, substitution bill C.G.S. § 29-37i, also known as "Ethan's Law" (Connecticut General Assembly, 2019). The existing statute was repealed and substituted with new language that defined a minor as a person under 18 years of age (changed from under 16 years of age) and made the firearm owner liable for damages even if the firearm was stored unloaded, but not secure. Prior to this change, the statute specified unsecure storage of "loaded" guns; this statute was changed to specify the unsecure storage of both loaded and unloaded firearms. Baseline survey data from the Connecticut Behavioral Risk Factor Surveillance System 2018 questionnaire, given randomly via phone call to adults 18 years and older, found that 17.9% of respondents said that they have at least one firearm in the household. When asked if their unloaded and loaded firearm(s) were securely stored away, 90.7% indicated that yes, they were. Finally, when asked if their ammunition was safely stored away in a separate location from their firearm(s), 81.7% responded in the affirmative. This questionnaire was given prior to the enactment of "Ethan's Law," and future surveillance studies on this topic will assess if this policy has had an impact on gun owners' secure storage behavior.

Section 4 of the same Public Act 19-5, which was enacted and written into statute C.G.S. § 10-18b, requires the State Board of Education to develop and provide firearm safety curriculum and extend this curriculum to grades 9 through 12, rather than ending it at grade 8 (formerly Kindergarten through 8). The proposed legislation stated that effective July 1, 2019, "the State Board of Education is required to develop guidelines to help local and regional boards establish firearm safety programs for public school students from kindergarten to high school." The public school system may incorporate these firearm safety guides into their existing curriculum. If a public school system offers firearm safety, students are not required to participate. C.G.S. § 10-18c states that parents and legal guardians can specify that they do not want their child to participate in this safety training.

Conclusions and Future Directions

In this chapter, several issues pertaining to violence-related morbidity and mortality and unintentional firearm deaths in Connecticut youth and young adults were reviewed and discussed. According to many health experts, violence is a health epidemic and needs to be treated as such, thus the development of the CURE Violence model in Chicago which used a public health approach to address gun violence in this city (Cure Violence Global, The Big Idea, 2020b). By applying this approach, public health practitioners, behavioral scientists, and others are able to determine the extent and scope of the problem by using data to identify vulnerable populations, and to learn about their risk factors and potential protective factors. When utilizing this approach, the practitioner develops, implements, and evaluates data-informed strategies that work to prevent or mitigate the risk factors and increase the protective factors within the vulnerable populations' environment. Another way to build prevention efforts into the community and the society at large is to write and enact effective state and federal policy that aims to address the public health issue of gun violence. Finally, successful evidence-based prevention approaches, shown to work through evaluation of effectiveness, are adopted and disseminated to a wider population so that other at-risk populations are positively impacted.

Since 2015, Connecticut has been closely tracking violent deaths, namely, suicides and homicides, by firearms which are being used to define the problem of firearm violence-related mortality in the state's vulnerable populations, including youth 10–24 years of age. Using multiple sources of demographic and circumstance data from police reports, medical examiners and investigators, and death certificates, DPH is starting to piece together and pinpoint the contributing risk factors and circumstances associated with these deaths.

One of the limitations of implementing a surveillance only data system, like the Connecticut Violent Death Reporting System, is that a major portion of the public health approach is not being utilized as it relates to identifying protective factors, implementing and evaluating prevention initiatives, and disseminating prevention efforts to a larger population. The surveillance data *are* being used by partnering state agencies and community organizations that have allocated homicide and suicide prevention and treatment resources and funding, but DPH has had limited funding and resources for prevention efforts. Typically, state and local funding for firearm violence is sourced from the U.S. Department of Justice, though grant programs such as the Victims of Crime Act (VOCA) and the Youth Violence Initiative (YVI). It was not until 2020 that the CDC was able to allocate public health funding and assistance for suicide prevention efforts and Connecticut was one of eight US states that received a 5-year grant award for this new funding opportunity, entitled "A Public Health Approach to Comprehensive Suicide Prevention in Connecticut." One of the key vulnerable populations that are a focus of this project is youth ages 10–24 years old.

Since early to mid-2020, Connecticut has seen an escalation of interpersonal violence and shootings in persons of all ages, in large part as a reaction to the worldwide pandemic of the SARS-CoV-2 virus (also known as Coronavirus 19 or COVID-19). Connecticut and the rest of the world are facing a major health threat which has been associated with widespread and excess infectious disease morbidity and mortality. The virus has caused hundreds of thousands of deaths in the United States and throughout the world in 2020 and this pandemic has brought to light many of the health and economic disparities experienced by minority populations in the United States. Specifically, there are higher rates of COVID-19 cases and deaths in non-Hispanic Black and Hispanic US residents, and the same is true for Connecticut. Fear of the spread of the virus, which is transmitted through the air and through direct contact with contaminated surfaces, has resulted in state government-mandated shutdowns of places where large groups congregate, such as work places, religious institutions, schools, colleges and universities, and entertainment facilities (restaurants, bars, theaters, etc.) to name a few. The shutdowns have impacted every aspect of a Connecticut resident's life and have led to increased interpersonal violence among community members and among family members in the home. In addition, increased feelings of anxiety, depression, isolation, and loneliness are a consequence of the pandemic which can have a negative effect on the incidence and prevalence of suicide ideation and self-directed violence.

During the pandemic, protests throughout the country have sprung up as a reaction to several deaths of Black people by law enforcement officers over several years in various parts of the United States. The pandemic seems to have been the match that lit a fire and exposed systemic racism in not only healthcare and access to healthcare for minority populations but also systemic racism that limits employment and educational opportunities, and impedes minority populations from receiving fairness and equity in the US justice system. Movements such as "Black Lives Matter" and other grassroots advocacy organizations are calling for societal change and to defund law enforcement agencies so that more funding, resources, and direct services are dedicated to preventing violence and intervening before it occurs. Unfortunately, several of the protests have escalated to vandalism and looting, violence against others on the opposing side, and against police officers.

Future Recommendations. In order to reduce firearm violence in youth and young adults ages 10–24 years, a more focused, multi-faceted approach to learning and understanding: (a) the root causes of firearm violence in this age group; (b) how best to reduce risk factors, such as employing lethal means restriction and other methods; and (c) how best to increase protective factors, such as improve quality of home life and nurture healthy relationships, promote family and community connectedness, teach coping skills, and identify trusted adults in school and elsewhere to talk to when feeling overwhelmed and depressed.

A second recommendation for addressing firearm violence in youth is actively promoting universal suicide screening and universal screening for interpersonal violence for children and adults 10 years of age and older, by assessing risks for suicidality, bullying, domestic violence, intimate partner violence, and gang violence. And for people who screen positive, having the resources and capacity at the ready so that at-risk persons are directly connected to services and provided continuity of care.

A third recommendation is to increase opportunities and access to treatment for persons with substance use disorder and mental illness, and access to social and protective services for victims of domestic and intimate partner violence. Practitioners must work toward reducing the stigma of substance misuse, mental illness, or being victims of violence, like domestic violence and intimate partner violence, including dating violence and partner intimidation, so that people are not ashamed or afraid to come forward and seek the help they need.

A fourth recommendation is to expand hospital- and community-based violence intervention programs (HVIPs and VIPs), which are proven to be effective, throughout Connecticut's urban areas to locations outside of just the Hartford and New Haven areas. Firearm violence and other types of violence occur in all areas throughout the state, although interpersonal gun- and other weapon-involved violence is concentrated in Connecticut's major cities: Bridgeport, Hartford, New Haven, and Waterbury.

A final recommendation is to further evaluate gun-related policy and determine its effectiveness in reducing gun-involved violence. As discussed, a recent study of Connecticut risk warrant laws reported a reduction in gun-involved suicides. To do this, effective evaluation methodology and models need to be applied not only to suicide by firearm but also firearm assaults and homicides. A comprehensive state-wide evaluation of gun-related policy has not been fully put in place to address all the new Connecticut gun laws enacted since 2013.

Other future considerations in evaluation of prevention initiatives and public health policy are including firearm secure storage questions in the BRFSS and CSHS surveys and questioning high school youth who have firearms in the home if they have received firearm safety training. It is also important to know who trained them – was it a parent, NRA training course, high school curriculum, other type of training, or a combination of these? Finally, high schools should be surveyed and curriculum assessed to see if they have initiated effective firearm safety training as mandated. The surveys and assessments would help understand the stages for planning and implementation of the curricula, the frequency of the training, and to which grade levels it is being taught.

By improving and expanding public health, social, clinical, and behavioral health services; providing community outreach, education, and training; and by actively addressing and negating systemic racism, Connecticut will reduce firearm-involved violence in youth and young adults, as well as in persons of all ages. Evidence has shown that addressing the root causes of firearm violence by using the public health approach and instilling protective factors early on in a child's life at the pre-school and elementary school level have a positive impact on how that child thrives throughout the rest of their life. Evidence has also shown that many of the current initiatives taking place on a smaller scale in Connecticut are effective, and by spreading out the good work throughout the state, lives will be saved and overall quality of life will be improved.

References

American Public Health Association. (2018, November 13). *Policy statement #20185: Violence is a public health issue: Public health is essential to treating and understanding violence in the U.S.* Retrieved from https://apha.org/policies-and-advocacy/public-health-policy-statements/policy-database/2019/01/28/violence-is-a-public-health-issue

Borrup, K., Banco, L., Gelven, E., Carver, W., & Lapidus, G. (2008). Violent death in Connecticut, 2001–2004. *Connecticut Medicine, 72*(4), 83–87.

Brahmbhatt, K., Kurtz, B. P., Afzal, K. I., Giles, L. L., Kowal, E. D., Johnson, K. P., et al. (2019). Suicide risk screening in pediatric hospitals: Clinical pathways to address a global health crisis. *Psychosomatics, 60*(1), 1–9. https://doi.org/10.1016/j.psym.2018.09.003

Burrows, S., Butchart, A., Butler, N., Quigg, Z., Bellis, M. A., & Mikton, C. (2018). New WHO violence prevention information system, an interactive knowledge platform of scientific findings on violence. *Injury Prevention, 24*(2), 155–156. https://doi.org/10.1136/injuryprev-2017-042694

Butts, J. A., Roman, C. G., Bostwick, L., & Porter, J. R. (2015). Cure violence: A public health model to reduce gun violence. *Annual Review of Public Health, 36*(1), 39–35.

CDC. (2014). *National violent death reporting system (NVDRS) implementation manual: A state's guide to starting and operating a violent death reporting system*. National Center for Injury Prevention and Control, Centers for Disease Control and Prevention. Retrieved from https://www.cdc.gov/violenceprevention/pdf/2014-NVDRS-Implementation-Manual-and-Appendix_Combined.pdf

CDC. (2018). *National violent death reporting system (NVDRS) coding manual revised [Online] 2018*. National Center for Injury Prevention and Control, Centers for Disease Control and Prevention. Retrieved from www.cdc.gov/injury

CDC. (2019). *National violent death reporting system (NVDRS)*. National Center for Injury Prevention and Control, Division of Violence Prevention. Retrieved 5 Oct 2020, from https://www.cdc.gov/violenceprevention/datasources/nvdrs/

CDC Web-based Injury Statistics Querying and Reporting System (WISQARS). (n.d.). *Fatal injury reports, national, regional and state, 1981–2018*. National Center for Injury Prevention and Control, Division of Violence Prevention. Retrieved 207 Aug 2020, from https://webappa.CDC.GOV/SASWEB/NCIPC/MORTRATE.HTML

CDC WISQARS. (2020, July 1). *National violent death reporting system: Violent deaths 2003–2017*. National Center for Injury Prevention and Control, Division of Violence Prevention. Retrieved from https://www.cdc.gov/injury/wisqars/nvdrs.html

CDC WISQARS. (n.d.). *Nonfatal injury reports, 2000–2018*. National Center for Injury Prevention and Control, Division of Violence Prevention. Retrieved 27 Aug 2020, from https://webappa.cdc.gov/sasweb/ncipc/nfirates.html

Centers for Disease Control and Prevention (CDC). (n.d.). *The public health approach to violence prevention*. Retrieved 14 Aug 2020, from https://www.cdc.gov/violenceprevention/publichealthissue/publichealthapproach.html

Columbia Suicide Severity Rating Scale. (n.d.). Retrieved from https://cssrs.columbia.edu/

Connecticut Department of Emergency Services and Public Protection (DESPP). (2017, November 28). *Your guide to firearms and permits in Connecticut*. Retrieved from https://portal.ct.gov/-/media/DESPP/CSP/files/StatePistolPermit/firearms_brochure_06-7-16.pdf?la=en

Connecticut Department of Mental Health and Addiction Services. (2019). *Suicide in youth*. Retrieved from https://www.ctclearinghouse.org/Customer-Content/www/topics/FINAL_Suicide_In_Youth.pdf

Connecticut Department of Public Health. (2020). *2019 youth risk behavior survey results: Connecticut high school survey 10-year trend analysis report*. Retrieved from https://portal.ct.gov/DPH/Health-Information-Systems%2D%2DReporting/Hisrhome/Connecticut-School-Health-Survey

Connecticut General Assembly (C.G.S.). (2019). *Public Act 19-5 (Section 1). Repealed C.G.S. 29-37i and substituted with new language. AKA "Ethan's Law"*. Effective October 1, 2019. Retrieved 29 Aug 2020, from https://www.cga.ct.gov/2019/act/Pa/pdf/2019PA-00005-R00HB-07218-PA.PDF

Connecticut Health Improvement Coalition. (2020a). *Firearm injuries and deaths. Behavioral health, trauma and injury. Healthy Connecticut 2025: State health assessment* (pp. 278–280). Connecticut Department of Public Health.

Connecticut Health Improvement Coalition. (2020b). *Suicide ideation. Behavioral health, trauma and injury. Healthy Connecticut 2025: State health assessment* (pp. 296–298). Connecticut Department of Public Health.

Connecticut Suicide Advisory Board. (2017). *Gizmo 4 mental health*. Retrieved from https://www.gizmo4mentalhealth.org/

Connecticut Violence Intervention Program. (2020). *Connecticut violence intervention program: About*. Retrieved 19 Sept 2020, from http://www.ctintervention.org/about/

CT Suicide Advisory Board (CTSAB). (2017). https://www.gizmo4mentalhealth.org/wp-content/uploads/2017/09/GizmoPawesome.pdf

Cure Violence Global. (2020a). *Cure violence global staff: Gary Slutkin, MD—founder and CEO*. Retrieved 13 Sept 2020, from https://cvg.org/who-we-are/

Cure Violence Global. (2020b). *The big idea: Violence is like an epidemic disease...and it can be effectively prevented using health methods.* Retrieved 13 Sept 2020, from https://cvg.org/the-big-idea/

Curtin, S. C., & Heron, M. (2019). *Death rates due to suicide and homicide among persons aged 10–24: United States, 2000–2017.* NCHS Data Brief, no 352. National Center for Health Statistics.

David-Ferdon, C., Vivolo-Kantor, A. M., Dahlberg, L. L., Marshall, K. J., Rainford, N., & Hall, J. E. (2016). *A comprehensive technical package for the prevention of youth violence and associated risk behaviors.* National Center for Injury Prevention and Control, Centers for Disease Control and Prevention.

Department of Justice. (2012). *Project longevity launched to reduce gun violence in Connecticut's cities.* DOJ Office of Public Affairs News Release. Retrieved from https://www.justice.gov/opa/pr/project-longevity-launched-reduce-gang-and-gun-violence-connecticut-s-cities

Dunlop, S. M., More, E., & Romer, D. (2011). Where do youth learn about suicides on the internet, and what influence does this have on suicidal ideation? *Journal of Child Psychology and Psychiatry, and Allied Disciplines, 52*(10), 1073–1080. https://doi.org/10.1111/j.1469-7610.2011.02416.x

Ertl, A., Sheats, K. J., Petrosky, E., Betz, C. J., Yuan, K., & Fowler, K. A. (2019). Surveillance for violent deaths – National Violent Death Reporting System, 32 states, 2016. *MMWR Surveillance Summaries, 68*(9), 1–36. https://doi.org/10.15585/mmwr.ss.6809a1

Hartford Communities That Care. (2020a). *HCTC: Hartford communities that care.* Retrieved 13 Sept 2020, from https://hartfordctc.org/

Hartford Communities That Care. (2020b). *About HCTC.* Retrieved 13 Sept 2020, from https://hartfordctc.org/new2020/index.php/about-us

Harvard School of Public Health Injury Research Center. (n.d.). *Means matter gun shop project: Suicide prevention: A role for firearm dealers and range owners.* Retrieved from https://www.hsph.harvard.edu/means-matter/gun-shop-project/

Health and Human Services. (n.d.). *What does "suicide contagion" mean, and what can be done to prevent it?* Retrieved 15 Aug 2020, from https://www.hhs.gov/answers/mental-health-and-substance-abuse/what-does-suicide-contagion-mean/index.html#:~:text=Suicide%20contagion%20is%20the%20exposure%20to%20suicide%20or,indirect%20exposure%20to%20suicidal%20behavior%20has%20been%20shown

Heller, N. R., & Connecticut Suicide Advisory Board. (2014). *State of Connecticut suicide prevention plan 2020.* Retrieved from, https://www.preventsuicidect.org/wp-content/uploads/2015/04/Suicide-Prevention-Plan.pdf

Hemenway, D., & Solnick, S. J. (2015). Children and unintentional firearm death. *Injury Epidemiology, 2*(1), 26. https://doi.org/10.1186/s40621-015-0057-0

Hemenway, D., & Solnick, S. J. (2017). The epidemiology of homicide perpetration by children. *Injury Epidemiology, 4*(5), 1–6. https://doi.org/10.1186/s40621-017-0102-2

Icenogle, G., Steinberg, L., Duell, N., Chein, J., Chang, L., Chaudhary, N., et al. (2019). Adolescents' cognitive capacity reaches adult levels prior to their psychosocial maturity: Evidence for a "maturity gap" in a multinational, cross-sectional sample. *Law and Human Behavior, 43*(1), 69–85. https://doi.org/10.1037/lhb0000315

Injury and Violence Surveillance Unit. (2019). *2015–2017 Connecticut violent death reporting system annual report.* Connecticut Department of Public Health.

Joint Commission. (2019a). *Sentinel event alert #56: Detecting and treating suicide ideation in all settings.* [Sentinel event alert retired February 2019.]

Joint Commission. (2019b, November 20 Updated). National Patient Safety Goal for suicide prevention, NPSG 15.01.01. Reduce the risk of suicide. *R3 Report,* Issue 18, 2018.

Jordan Porco Foundation. (n.d.-a). *4 what's next.* Retrieved from https://4whatsnext.org/

Jordan Porco Foundation. (n.d.-b). *Fresh check day.* Retrieved from https://freshcheckday.com/

Kim, D. (2019). Social determinants of health in relation to firearm-related homicides in the United States: A nationwide multilevel cross-sectional study. *PLoS Medicine, 16*(12), e1002978. https://doi.org/10.1371/journal.pmed.1002978

Lapidus, G., Merwin, D., Carver, H. W., & Banco, L. (2001). Firearm-related fatality surveillance in Hartford County, Connecticut. *Connecticut Medicine, 65*(2), 91–95.

Law, T., Seiver, S., Papachristos, A. V., & Violano, P. (2017). *Age of gunshot wound victims in New Haven, 2003–2015.* ISPS working paper ISPS17-03. Yale University Institution for Social and Policy Studies. https://isps.yale.edu/research/publications/isps17-03

Makowski, M. (2020). *Suicides: The Connecticut landscape 2015 to 2019.* Connecticut Department of Public Health. Presented at the Connecticut Suicide Advisory Board Meeting, September 10, 2020.

May, A., & Connecticut Suicide Advisory Board. (2020). *State of Connecticut suicide prevention plan 2020–2025.* Retrieved from https://www.preventsuicidect.org/wp-content/uploads/2020/09/Suicide-Prevention-Plan-2020-2025.pdf

National Institute of Mental Health. (n.d.). *Youth ASQ toolkit.* Retrieved 5 Oct 2020, from https://www.nimh.nih.gov/research/research-conducted-at-nimh/asq-toolkit-materials/youth-asq-toolkit.shtml#emergency

Northeast and Caribbean Injury Prevention Network (NCIPN). (2015). *Firearms by intent: A comparison of data in the Northeast U.S.* Presented at the Council of State and Territorial Epidemiologists (CSTE) Annual Conference in New York, July 17, 2015.

Norton, K. (2015). *Director's corner: Postvention as prevention.* Retrieved 5 Oct 2020, from https://www.sprc.org/news/postvention-prevention

Prevention Institute. (2018, March). *Prevention Institute's recommendations for preventing gun violence.* Retrieved from https://www.preventioninstitute.org/publications/prevention-institute-full-recommendations-preventing-gun-violence

Project Longevity. (2020, January 18). *Statewide Dir. Brent Peterkin joins Congresswoman Rosa DeLauro for gun violence research roundtable.* Retrieved 13 Sept 2020, from https://www.project-longevity.org/post/statewide-dir-brent-peterkin-joins-congresswoman-rosa-deluaro-for-gun-violence-research-roundtable).

Ray, M. (2019, December 7) *Sandy hook elementary school shooting.* Retrieved from https://www.britannica.com/event/Newtown-shootings-of-2012

Rogers, S. (2019). *Youth suicide: Improving identification, prevention, and care.* Retrieved 12 Sept 2020, from https://www.connecticutchildrens.org/wp-content/uploads/2019/10/rogers_suicide_presentation.pdf

Rostron, A. (2018). The Dickey Amendment on federal funding for research on gun violence: A legal dissection. *American Journal of Public Health, 108*(7), 865–867. https://doi.org/10.2105/AJPH.2018.304450

Schiraldi, V., Western, B., & Bradner, K. (2015). *Community-based responses to justice-involved young adults. New thinking in community corrections bulletin.* U.S. Department of Justice, National Institute of Justice, NCJ 248900.

Sierra-Arevalo, M., & Papachristos, A. V. (2015). *Focused deterrence strategy reduces group member involved shootings in New Haven, CT.* Institution of Social and Policy Studies (ISPS) Policy Brief ISPS15-025. Yale University Institution of Social and Policy Studies and Yale Law School Justice Collaboratory.

Sierra-Arevalo, M., Charette, Y., & Papachristos, A. V. (2015). *Evaluating the effect of project longevity on group-involved shootings and homicides in New Haven, CT.* Institution of Social and Policy Studies (ISPS) Working Paper ISPS15-024. Yale University Institution of Social and Policy Studies.

Springer, F., & Phillips, J. L. (2006). The IOM model: A tool for prevention planning and implementation. *Prevention Tactics, 8*(13). Retrieved from http://www.cars-rp.org/publications/Prevention%20Tactics/PT8.13.06.pdf#:~:text=The%20Institute%20of%20Medicine%20%28IOM%29%20continuum%20of%20care,and%20individuals%20with%20differing%20prevention%20needs%2C%20and%20aligning

Swanson, J. W., Norko, M. A., Lin, H., Alanis-Hirsch, K., Frisman, L. K., Baranoski, M. V., et al. (2017). Implementation and effectiveness of Connecticut's risk-based gun removal law: Does it prevent suicides? *Law and Contemporary Problems, 80*, 179–208. http://scholarship.law.duke.edu/lcp/vol80/iss2/8

Underwood, J. M., Brener, N., Thornton, J., Harris, W. A., Bryan, L. N., Shanklin, S. L., et al. (2020, August 21). Overview and methods for the youth risk behavior surveillance system — United States, 2019. *MMWR Supplement 2020, 69*(Suppl-1), 1–10. https://doi.org/10.15585/mmwr.su6901a1

Vermont Department of Health. (2020, January). Firearm storage. In *2018 vermont behavioral risk factor surveillance system report* (p. 67). Vermont Department of Health.

World Health Organization. (2017). *Prevalence studies of youth violence: Bullying.* Retrieved 30 Aug 2020, from https://apps.who.int/violence-info/studies?area=youth-violence&country=US

World Health Organization. (n.d.). *Youth violence: 635 studies.* Retrieved from https://apps.who.int/violence-info/youth-violence/

Zero Suicide. (n.d.). Retrieved from https://zerosuicide.edc.org/

Zheng, X. (2019, October). *Prevalence estimates for risk factors and health indicators: Selected summary tables, 2018. Connecticut behavioral risk factor survey report.* Connecticut Department of Public Health.

Zimmerman, M. A., Carter, P., & Cunningham, R. (2019). The facts on children and teens killed by guns: Firearm injuries are a leading cause of death for American kids. *Black youth face the worst violence.* https://www.thetrace.org/2019/08/children-teens-gun-deaths-data/

Chapter 20
Trauma-Informed Care as a Framework to Reduce Trauma and Violence in Schools

Ginny Sprang

The Centers for Disease Control and Prevention (2016a) defines school violence as youth perpetrated bullying, assaults, physical aggression, shootings, or gang violence that occur on school grounds, while traveling to or from school, and during school sponsored activities. The literature on school violence documents the trajectory of the problem over the past few decades and shows mixed results (Zhang et al., 2016; Musu et al., 2019). The majority of research on U.S. school violence documents declines in overall violence since the early 1990s; though some indicators show stable patterns of violence-related behaviors over time (Musu et al., 2019). Discrepancies in prevalence estimates are generally due to varying reporting sources, and varied foci related to age, and type of victimization. Anonymous student surveys are the most reliable and valid method of data collection due to concerns about privacy and reporting. For example, although comprehensive, the School Crime Supplement of the National Crime Victimization Survey (NCVS) focused only on youth between the ages of 12 and 17 years. Similarly, the Youth Risk Behavior Survey (YRBS) and the National Adolescent Health Survey focus on older youth and have a more limited scope. In general, those surveys with broader age inclusion include a more restricted set of victimization experiences (Schreck et al., 2003; Agnich & Miyazaki, 2013; Molcho et al., 2009; Wang et al., 2009).

Overall, studies identify significant declines in violent victimization at and away from school from 1992 to 2004, minor declines over the next 6 years, and variability in rates from 2010 to 2014 (Zhang et al., 2016). There is evidence of higher rates of violence in schools than in the communities where they are located. Notably, the 2017 National Crime Victimization Survey (NCVS), documented that adolescents

G. Sprang (✉)
Department of Psychiatry, College of Medicine, University of Kentucky, Lexington, KY, USA

Center on Trauma and Children, Department of Psychiatry, College of Medicine, University of Kentucky, Lexington, KY, USA
e-mail: sprang@uky.edu

T. W. Miller (ed.), *School Violence and Primary Prevention*,
https://doi.org/10.1007/978-3-031-13134-9_20

465

between the ages of 12 and 18 experienced 827,000 total victimizations (i.e., theft and nonfatal violent victimization) at school, compared to 503,800 total victimizations away from school. However, Finkelhor et al. (2016) note that evidence from the National Survey of Children's Exposure to Violence Study II reveals some of the most serious victimizations, such as sexual assaults and weapons assaults, occurred less frequently at school than in other contexts. Over the first two decades of this century, there were 296 casualties (137 killed and 159 wounded) in active shooter incidents at elementary, secondary, and postsecondary schools. During this same period, reports of gang activity at schools declined overall from 20% to 9%, decreases that were evident across rural, suburban, and rural areas. In the reporting period for 2015–2016, 47% of schools reported one or more crime incidents to police, lower than all prior survey years. However, the National Center for Education statistics reports that the percentages of high school students who have been involved in physical altercations at school has remained more stable (Musu et al., 2019).

Bullying, physical aggression, and harassment can be the precursor to eruptions in school violence (Espelage & Hong, 2019; Mongan et al., 2009; Wike & Fraser, 2009). The National Threat Assessment Center reports that in over two-thirds of the school shooting cases analyzed by that department, the attackers reported feeling persecuted, bullied, threatened, attacked, or injured by others prior to the incident (Bowman-Perrott et al., 2013; Vossekuil et al., 2000). Child on child violence, romantic rejection, or perceived teacher-perpetrated harassment or conflict can lead to feelings of helplessness, isolation, anger, and desperation in children and youth (Rapp & Wodarski, 2019). If the victimized child has a prior trauma history, these situations may be painful reminders of unresolved issues and longstanding feelings of otherness, humiliation, and shame (Cook et al., 2017; Mc Guckin et al., 2017). For adolescents, these responses are occurring in a context where peer pressure, puberty, sexual identity, separation from caregivers and other stage development tasks are occurring (Harter, 2003). In extremity, school shooters reported feeling that the adults in their life were no longer able to protect them, and that violence was their only recourse (Vossekuil et al., 2000). In their analysis of school shootings these researchers note, "A number of attackers had experienced bullying and harassment that was longstanding and severe. In those cases, the experience of bullying appeared to play a major role in motivating the attack at school" (p. 11).

How Trauma Impacts Children and Their Behavior and Can Lead to Violence

The *Diagnostic and Statistical Manual of Mental Disorders, Fifth Edition* (DSM-5) describes a traumatic event as exposure to actual or threatened death, serious injury, or sexual violence through direct experience, witnessing such an event, learning it has happened to a loved one or repeated and extreme exposure during the course of professional duties (American Psychological Association, 2013). Based on 2018 data from the National Data Archive on Child Abuse and Neglect Study (NCANDS) children and youth were classified as victims of child maltreatment at a rate of 6.8 per 1000, with the highest rates of maltreatment found in American Indian/Alaska Native and African American children (U.S. Department of Health and Human Services, 2020). Caregiver alcohol and drug abuse were identified as factors that increase the likelihood of risk of maltreatment in the families. Other large sample studies such as the National Survey of Children's Exposure to Violence note high rates of trauma exposure in children, over and above child maltreatment, including other forms of family and community violence, physical and sexual assaults, shootings, and stabbings (Finkelhor et al., 2015; Finkelhor et al., 2016). Studies that examine polyvictimization in children and youth demonstrate that a majority of children who have experienced trauma and/or maltreatment also experience multiple other forms of violence or victimizations that overlap with each other (Adams et al., 2016; Vachon et al., 2015). McLaughlin and Lambert (2017) identify mechanisms of action that link these exposures to subsequent disruptions in mental health, internalizing and externalizing behavior, and functioning: (1) heightened threat processing; (2) social information processing biases that produce over identification of environmental threats; (3) disturbances in learning central to the acquisition of fear; (4) increased emotional reactivity to real or imagined threats; and (5) diminished capacity to disengage from negative emotional states.

Multiple studies note that trauma exposure during childhood and adolescents can lead to post-traumatic stress symptoms (re-experiencing and avoidance symptoms, alterations in cognitions and mood and reactivity and arousal) and disturbances of the biochemical stress response system (Rosen et al., 2018; Cicchetti & Toth, 2005; McEwen & Wingfield, 2010). The Adverse Childhood Experiences Study is landmark research that clearly documents the negative short- and long-term impacts of adversity on the development of health risk behaviors, and poor health and mental health outcomes over the life course (Anda et al., 2006). A positive relationship has been documented between the number of adverse childhood events a person experienced, and the development of health risk behaviors (i.e., substance misuse, smoking, suicidality, and having more than 50 sex partners), which are also positively associated with psychiatric morbidity, disease states, and mortality (Centers for Disease Control and Prevention, 2016b). Cecil et al. (2014) conducted an analysis of the interactive relationships among maltreatment categories and community violence experiences using Latent Profile Analysis and uncovered additive effects of polyvictimization on the domains of externalizing behaviors, dissociation, and post-traumatic stress symptoms. These researchers also noted a significant interaction between child maltreatment experiences and community violence on child anger over time, suggesting that increased exposure may lead to heightened interpersonal sensitivity and unresolved negative emotional states (Cecil et al., 2014).

These responses to trauma can interfere with and alter brain development, perceptions of safety, and learning, which in turn can affect behavior, engagement, and performance at school (De Bellis & Zisk, 2014). A meta-analysis conducted by Fry et al. (2018) noted that victimization due to bullying is highly correlated with poor school attendance and school engagement. While some students may withdraw, others may react in more disruptive ways. Several decades of neurobiological research documents that individuals suffering from traumatic stress conditions may experience an altered psychological and physiologic response to stimuli that is interpreted as threatening (Sege, Amaya-Jackson, & the American Academy of Pediatrics Committee on Child Abuse and Neglect, 2017).

Consider the case of Johnny[1] who has been identified as a problem student based on his frequent, angry outbursts. Johnny's can be quiet and calm, but he will respond quickly and unexpectedly with violence if he perceives an interaction with another student to be threatening, even if the stimuli is benign. Last week a student bumped into him while walking down the aisle in the classroom. Johnny was concentrating on his work at the time, and startled by the encounter, he jumped up and physically attacked the student. It took almost an hour for Johnny to calm down. Later, in the counselor's office he described feeling the student was trying to "start something." Johnny described you have to stay "on guard" because people will "come at you for no reason." He recounted an experience at home the week before where a conflict over a dirty coffee cup ended in severe family violence and police intervention. Over time, Johnny revealed that these encounters were commonplace in his family, and had become "a way of life."

In Johnny's case, he had become hypervigilant due to the frequency and chronicity of his trauma exposures. As a result, he had an extreme physiological response in anticipation of danger, and did not have the insight needed to appropriately appraise the situation and/or the regulation skills to manage his extreme stress response. In this scenario, Johnny used externalizing behavior as a way to self-protect and fend off a perceived attack, a biologically based response that is conditioned and reinforced based on development, life experience, and situational context. Of course, Johnny's teachers, counselors, peers, and other school personnel have their own fight, flight, or freeze response, and instinctively respond to Johnny's outbursts in self-protective ways. This may include punitive attempts to control or manage Johnny, which may further reinforce for him that the world is indeed not safe. Actions toward him that he perceives as aggressive may also trigger a trauma response. Another common response strategy used by school personnel is to isolate Johnny from other student's in an attempt to minimize the impact of his externalizing behavior on others. While it temporarily solves the classroom management problem, this action removes Johnny from the potentially healthy benefits of relationships, and the corrective emotional experiences that may facilitate self-regulation and recovery. Ironically, both of these response patterns violate what we know to be fundamental to trauma recovery, the creation of safety, and the protective qualities of healthy emotional relationships. Ignoring opportunities to interact with Johnny in a manner that provides biopsychosocial stabilization may jeopardize his well-being and ultimately the safety of those around them.

---

[1] All names and other personal identifiers of this case have been changed to protect privacy and confidentiality.

Trauma Impacts Professionals and the Systems as Well and May Make Them Less Able to Respond

Imagine a classroom full of students like Johnny. School professionals are exposed to the trauma experiences of their students when they observe this type of dysregulation, fear, and suffering, witness bullying, and violence against vulnerable children and youth, when graphic details of the trauma are shared, and in their interactions with other professionals. Due to the amount of time school personnel spend with students, they can form important attachment relationships that could promote healing (Brend et al., 2013). However, this relational proximity may increase the risk of negative outcomes in teachers as the dose of indirect exposure to the student's trauma experience may increase. These indirect exposures can lead to secondary traumatic stress (STS), a condition that parallels Post-Traumatic Stress Disorder, but that can be experienced in mild to severe forms (Sprang et al., 2019). Recent research conducted by this author reveals that of 459 school personnel surveyed, 49.9% reported daily and 30.4% endorsed weekly exposure to the trauma experiences of their students. Rates of distress as measured by the Secondary Traumatic Stress Scale (Bride et al., 2004) revealed 10.5% reported they had trouble sleeping, and 12.9% has intrusive thoughts related to the trauma experiences of their students (Sprang, 2019). Risk factors for experiencing secondary traumatic stress include younger age or inexperience on the job (Van Hook & Rothenberg, 2009), prior trauma history (Hensel et al., 2015; Jenkins & Baird, 2002), type of work (Sprang et al., 2011), and female gender (Hensel et al., 2015; Sprang et al., 2007). STS, if left untreated, can interfere with the professional's capacity to assist the student in coping with their trauma-induced dysregulation because these interactions may serve as trauma reminders of the professional's own trauma experiences, and/or may activate traumatic stress symptoms that impede trauma-sensitive responding (e.g., avoidance and irritability).

Trauma-Informed Care

If children are to learn and function at their best in the school environment, they must feel safe and secure. This requires schools to be sensitive to the life experiences of their students and aware of how adversity and trauma can shape a child or youth's understanding of the world. How school personnel respond to trauma-exposed students can decrease the compounding effects of trauma, and can create a safer school experience for everyone (Espelage & Hong, 2019; Rivard et al., 2005). Trauma-informed care creates a culture where trauma is understood as an experience that shapes a child's understanding of and reaction to the world. School personnel, following the tenets of trauma-informed care, interact with students to promote and support coping in extreme situations, and to create a culture that reflects the trauma-informed principles of safety, trustworthiness, peer support, collaboration, empowerment and choice, and cultural competency (SAMHSA, 2014). These principles are adhered to in an ongoing process that requires awareness, constant monitoring, ongoing action, and data-driven organizational change. The activities of a trauma-informed school are guided by and reflect these principles.

The Trauma-Informed Systems Framework proposed here defines the essential elements of an approach that schools can use to focus organizational change, and integrates well with approaches already used in the educational systems, such as Multi-tiered Systems of Support. The framework proposed here draws heavily from best practice, and empirical evidence regarding how trauma impact the biopsychosocial functioning of a child, and recommended strategies to address these affects (NCTSN, 2016; SAMHSA, 2014). The National Child Traumatic Stress Network (NCTSN) defines a trauma-informed child and family service system in the following way:

> one in which all parties involved recognize and respond to the impact of traumatic stress on those who have contact with the system including children, caregivers, staff, and service providers. Programs and agencies within such a system infuse and sustain trauma awareness, knowledge, and skills into their organizational cultures, practices, and policies. They act in collaboration with all those who are involved with the child, using the best available science, to maximize physical and psychological safety, facilitate the recovery or adjustment of the child and family, and support their ability to thrive (2016, p. 1)

To be trauma-informed, schools/districts can follow a model that the Substance Abuse and Mental Health Services Administration (SAMHSA) calls the Four "Rs." This approach "*realizes* the widespread impact of trauma and understands potential paths for recovery; *recognizes* the signs and symptoms of trauma in clients, families, staff, and others involved with the system; *responds* by fully integrating knowledge about trauma into policies, procedures, and practices, and seeks to actively *resist* re-traumatization" (SAMHSA's Trauma and Justice Strategic Initiative, 2014, p. 9). This model guides the creation of an school culture that recognizes trauma's role in the development of altered neurodevelopment and compromised immune responses, the psychological and behavioral manifestations of distress, and impairments in social, emotional, relational, and academic functioning (Felitti et al., 1998; Shonkoff, Garner, Committee on Psychosocial Aspects of Child and Family Health, Committee on Early Childhood, & Section on Developmental and Behavioral Pediatrics, 2012).

Emerging research on the use of trauma-informed systems and methods across child serving systems of care yield some promising findings. Schmid et al. (2020) found that employees who did not receive trauma-informed care (TIC) training experienced significantly more physical aggression from clients and had significantly higher hair cortisol concentrations over time. Following implementation of trauma-informed practices and treatments, significant reductions in the use of physical restraint as a safety intervention were noted by Department of Juvenile Justice staff (Marrow et al., 2012). Similarly, a 67% reduction in the number of times children were placed in seclusion and/or in restraints were noted by residential treatment center staff following the implementation of a trauma-informed approach (Azeem et al., 2011). If fewer restraints are used, the risks of retraumatization in the school environment are minimized. In the education system, trauma-sensitive interventions were associated with improvements in trauma-related symptoms, positive classroom behavior, and improved physical and psychological safety for students (Kataoka et al., 2003; Bartlett et al., 2016; Stevens, 2012), and decreases in physical aggression incidents and out of school suspensions 5 years post-implementation (Dorado et al., 2016). More recently, Atallah et al. (2019) found that following implementation of trauma-informed principles and practices, senior leadership and school personnel reported significant changes in their policies and practices. Notably, these researchers recorded that faculty and staff reported increased efforts at assisting students develop social-emotional skills, and improved peer relationships with one another. Similarly, students reported an improved sense of belonging at school and more healthy connections to teachers and other staff. Atallah and colleagues state, "Within educator reports we observed the emergence of a rehumanizing relationality, which could be akin to building new social capital in school communities" (2019, p. 4). Efforts to attenuate violence in schools are certainly enhanced within this type of context.

A Data-Driven Approach to Implementing Trauma-Informed Care to Reduce Trauma and Violence in Schools

A data-based decision-making process can create the pathway between identified need and the mechanisms of action needed to address trauma and violence in schools. This data-driven approach allows for tailoring of activities to support school-based change based on unique socio-environmental characteristics, the perceptions of school personnel, students, family members, and other key stakeholders, and issues that emerge and change over time. Studies examining the planting of new programs in the educational system consistently find that even evidence-based, effective interventions will deteriorate over time if continuous feedback loops regarding performance are not put in place (Detrich, 2013). For example, School X conducted a baseline assessment to determine the degree to which their school was trauma informed using a set of organizational metrics. This data provided them with a blueprint for launching a trauma-informed care change initiative. Based on the results of this assessment, School X realized that students rated the safety of the school low, despite numerous efforts that had been initiated by leaders to increase building security and access. The school decided to focus their initial efforts at addressing the concerns of the students related to safety. A series of student-led focus groups revealed some serious concerns related to bullying and intimidating behavior that was occurring within the confines of school grounds, and outside of the awareness of school leaders. Based on this information, the school was able to modify its monitoring metrics to ask specifically about these behaviors at each data collection interval, and provide anonymity to students to ensure their privacy was protected and information was provided freely and without fear of reprisal. Because the school was particularly concerned about the prevention of violence, specific questions were added to the metrics regarding student perceptions of the risk of violence in the school. A series of interventions were developed based on data that was provided, including a trauma-informed psychoeducation campaign, increased surveillance, restructuring of cafeteria time, and additional trauma-focused intervention services for those who expressed need. Over the subsequent 6 months, student concerns began to diminish and student and faculty perceptions regarding the risk of violence subsided. While monitoring these trends and programming to address security continued, the school began to add other initiatives toward their goals of increasing safety. After 9 months, the schools scores related to the psychological and physical safety of the school had improved considerably, and the perceived risk of violence was decreased from baseline.

This case scenario illustrates some of the key elements of a data-driven, trauma-informed care approach to addressing trauma and violence in schools. Following these guidelines allows for full integration of a TIC approach that is flexible and nimble enough to respond to changes in the environment (see Box 20.1) and include the following:

Box 20.1 Essential Elements of a Data-Driven, Trauma-Informed Care Approach to Addressing Trauma and Violence in Schools

1. Full Integration of Trauma-Informed Care with Multi-tiered Systems of Support
2. A Data-Informed Implementation Plan
3. Repeated Assessment and Monitoring Using Trauma and Violence Specific Tools
4. Consideration of the Impact of Trauma and School Violence on Students and School Personnel
5. Sensitivity and Responsiveness to Culture and Experience, Past and Present, Broadly Defined

---

Trauma-Informed Care and Multi-Tiered Systems of Support

School professional can use a trauma-informed approach to managing externalizing behaviors, and in rare cases, violence that includes minimizing trauma reminders, preventing additional physical or psychological harms, and promotes recovery through the use of evidence-based, trauma-informed interventions (Foa et al., 2008). To accomplish this, a tiered, trauma-informed approach, grounded in the Multi-tiered Systems of Support (MTSS) is suggested (Fig. 20.1) (Sulkowski & Michael, 2014).

These tiers define the scope of work by specifying the potential intervention targets and data strategies to guide and monitor progress toward becoming trauma

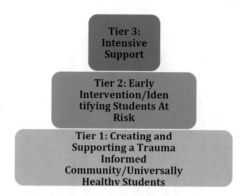

Fig. 20.1 Integrated MTSS and trauma-informed activity grid

informed within a MTSS approach (Blodgett & Dorodao, 2016; Chafouleas et al., 2016; Perfect et al., 2016).

Tier 1 activities include universal messaging and efforts toward creating and supporting a trauma-informed community of healthy students, prevention programs that develop and maintain safe environments for all students and staff. This foundational work is necessary to support the MTSS activities at Tiers 2 and 3. Tier 2 activities includes more focused efforts at identifying students at risk for negative outcomes due to trauma exposure at home or school, or traumatic stress responses that interfere with their functioning; as well as the provision of early intervention services for students and staff who are at risk for traumatic stress conditions. Tier 3 activities include targeted and intensive responses for highly affected students and staff via trauma-informed, evidence-based practices. At each level, a trauma-informed care approach can be applied to guide response strategies. These activities emphasize the principles and foci of trauma-informed care; provide metrics to guide and assess outcome, and build upon education's best practice approach to responding to need. Included in the approach are evaluation and practice routines, relationship building strategies, school- and district-wide policies and procedures, the inclusion of youth and families in decision-making, and community capacity-building strategies. Staff who are interacting with those with traumatic stress may have exposure to traumatic material (hearing stories of extreme abuse; seeing physical and emotional signs of trauma; hearing reports from others about these experiences). A trauma-informed educational system applies the same principles identified above to the care and protection of its workforce.

Even though the educational and mental health needs of trauma-exposed populations differ, the trauma-informed framework integrates these important concerns, and focuses attention on the best ways to address both perspectives. Table 20.1 identifies strategies to achieve the goals at every tier, and the key partners needed in collaboration.

Table 20.1 Strategies by tier

MTSS designation	Sample intervention strategies	Sample data strategies
Tier 1	Promoting a safe and positive school climate through mission, vision, and professional development of staff Safe crisis management strategies Psychological First Aid for students Post–crisis processing for school staff Bullying prevention and response Secondary Traumatic Stress education and response Resiliency building Psychoeducation about trauma Consideration of trauma during student interactions and decision-making Confidential self-referral options Organizational assessments of trauma-informed practices (including secondary traumatic stress) Partnerships with family and youth Promoting a sense of community at school Professional development to promote cultural competence Comprehensive, trauma-informed emergency response, bullying prevention plans Prevention and awareness of secondary traumatic stress Trauma-informed disciplinary actions Resource Mapping and Service Access that includes trauma-focused resources Low impact processing of stressful student interactions by staff	Knowledge, attitudes, and beliefs about TIC surveys e.g., attitudes related to trauma-informed care (Baker et al., 2016); Trauma-informed Beliefs measure (Traumatic Stress Institute, 1994) Organizational level assessment regarding activities, protocols, and policies consistent with trauma-informed care delivery TICOMETER (Bassuk et al., 2017) Trauma-informed Organizational Self-Assessment (http://www.traumainformedcareproject.org/) Trauma Responsive Systems Implementation Advisor (2011 www.epowerandassociates.com) Trauma Sensitive Schools Checklist (Guarino & Chagnon, 2018) Secondary Traumatic Stress Informed Organizational Assessment (pandemic version available) (Sprang et al., 2017)

MTSS designation	Sample intervention strategies	Sample data strategies
Tier 2	Screening those with behavioral, psychological, or academic difficulties for traumatic exposures, and subsequent trauma-informed management of positive cases Evidence-based early interventions/prevention practices (e.g., mindfulness groups; social skills, Child and Family Traumatic Stress Intervention, self-efficacy promotion) Trauma-Informed Behavior/Special Ed Support Plans/Trauma-informed Safety Plans Developmentally appropriate trauma-informed responses (e.g., classroom structure, supports) Peer support networks for students and staff Realign practices and protocols that may adversely impact students Peer or supervisory supports for educators to counteract secondary traumatic stress Multidisciplinary team approaches Threat assessments	Trauma screening tools UCLA PTSD Reaction Index for DSM-5 screening tool (Kaplow et al., 2020); Child Trauma Screen (Lang & Connell, 2017). Individual measures of staff wellness and trauma ProQol 5 measures STS, burnout and compassion satisfaction (Stamm, 2010) Student Subjective Wellbeing Questionnaire (Renshaw et al., 2015) Virginia Student Threat Assessment Guidelines manual (Cornell & Sheras, 2006; Cornell, 2020) Secondary Traumatic Stress Core Competencies for Trauma-Informed Supervision Self-rating tool (Sprang, 2018 available at www.nctsn.org)
Tier 3	Comprehensive trauma assessment Intensive individual, group, and family treatments (e.g., evidence-based trauma treatments, such as Trauma Trauma-focused Cognitive Behavioral Therapy, Cognitive Behavioral Therapy in Schools) Engaging families in treatment Creating safe spaces for students Trauma-informed crisis recovery services Secondary traumatic stress responses (e.g., through referrals to outside mental health resources such as Employee Assistance Programs) Adapting interventions to be culturally sensitive Restorative practices integrated with disciplinary protocols Consultation with community experts	Full trauma assessment using the UCLA PTSD Reaction Index (child/youth or caregiver report); Child PTSD Symptom Scale (child/youth and caregiver report) (Foa et al., 2001); Trauma Symptom Checklist for Children or Trauma Symptom Checklist for Young Children (caregiver report) (Briere, 1996) Fidelity metrics for intervention selected Outcome rating scale and session rating scale (Campbell & Hemsley, 2009) Secondary Traumatic Stress Scale (Bride et al., 2004)

A Data-Driven Implementation Plan

When launching a trauma-informed care initiative, a data-driven approach toward implementation of trauma-informed care is key. A good implementation plan guided by trauma and violence outcome data provides the structure needed for effective implementation of a trauma-informed care initiative that can be sustained long enough to impact student outcomes. There are many anecdotal accounts of new initiatives or programs that produce little change because they were not implemented at all; rather, they were simply presented to the school or district without any a defined implementation plan. A key strategy to ensure effective implementation is alignment of the internal and external supports that will sustain the implementation effort. This requires what the National Implementation Research Network (NIRN) calls facilitative administration, "the proactive, vigorous and enthusiastic attention by the administration to reduce implementation barriers and create an administratively hospitable environment for practitioners" (Blasé et al., 2015, p. 6). A data-driven approach of conducting an organizational assessment, using the results for goal setting, defining an action plan tailored to the unique needs of the school, and self-correcting based on repeated testing is a good example of facilitative administration.

An effective plan must be nimble enough to allow modifications to address individual, school, and community needs, while leaving the core elements intact, less the promise of the initiative is undermined (Kearney et al., 2019). Using the principle of trauma-informed care outlined earlier provides the essential context to guide all modifications. If senior leaders (administrators, superintendents, principals, etc.) are to understand the essential parameters of the approach, they must be well trained and have access to coaching and consultation with experts to identify possible strategies to address barriers that may arise.

Research suggests that innovations, such as trauma-informed care, have increased success at being adopted if they are introduced on a pilot basis, with good data collection processes in place to capture barriers to implementation (Rogers, 2003; Elliott & Mihalic, 2004). Those involved in the small-scale applications of trauma-informed care can become change champions, and early adopters who can assist with scale up and spread (Miech et al., 2018). By using repeated measurement of key indicators, emerging research demonstrates that these change champions can be effective in sustaining improvements in organizational as well as individual outcomes even after the implementation action period (Sprang et al., 2021).

The use of a data-driven approach requires that all school personnel interact with the data on an ongoing basis. This may feel intimidating to those who prefer other ways of knowing, so feedback accommodations should be made based on local preferences (Hojnoski et al., 2009). For example, Easton and Erchul (2011) in their study noted that educators had wide-ranging preferences for how often and in what format information would be provided, and the types of variables that were important when considering effectiveness. Ultimately, data about the impact of trauma-informed care on the school or districts unique set of outcomes must be displayed in a manner that has utility for those interacting with the information.

Repeated Assessment and Monitoring Using Trauma- and Violence-Specific Tools

A good assessment will query the presence and utilization of macro-level policies to micro-level strategies that can be used by schools wanting to become trauma responsive. These tools must also explicate the competencies that organizations should possess in order to become trauma informed. These organizational assessments are Tier 1 activities meant to prepare the environment for the delivery of the integrated MTSS/TIC process, and can and should be repeated over time to determine progress toward becoming trauma informed. These assessments should consider both the what and the how of trauma-informed care implementation. Detrich (2013) in his synthesis of research on school-based implementation notes that "any systematic effort at change will require ongoing measurement of both the important outcomes and the processes required to produce the outcomes" (p. 43). If done correctly, implementation will be iterative in nature, and will require ongoing data input so that decision-making is guided by pre-selected, reliable measures related to a specific outcome (trauma and violence), and not unknown and/or irrelevant factors.

Table 20.1 provides examples of measures and metrics that can be used to guide this data-driven, trauma-informed care approach to reducing trauma and violence in schools. As an anchor for all other measurement activities, the following tools can be useful at establishing a baseline (a Tier 1 Activity) to guide a school or districts efforts, as well as monitor its overall progress over time. These tools are free, and part of the public domain, so they require no financial investment to use.

The *Trauma-Sensitive Schools Checklist* (Guarino & Chagnon, 2018) is a 25-item inventory of trauma-informed care activities organized into five components involved in creating a trauma-sensitive school, including school-wide policies and practices, classroom strategies and techniques, collaborations and linkages with mental health services, family partnerships, and community linkages. Trauma-informed care teams rate the schools progress toward implementing the strategy on a scale of 1 (element is not at all in place) to 4 (element is fully in place). The items reflect the application of trauma-informed principles to the management of behavior by teachers, safety planning, the inclusion of family members as partners, and the way that collaborations occur with external providers.

The *Secondary Traumatic Stress Informed Organizational Assessment* (STSI-OA) (Sprang et al., 2017) is a 40-item measure of an organization's capacity regarding to STS prevention and intervention. The tool can be used to facilitate a school's self-assessment, create a blueprint for change consistent with their current capacity and need, and build off existing strengths. The tool allows school personnel to monitor change overtime, and create a collaboration with all faculty and staff in a process that shifts the focus from the individual's self-care responsibilities to shared accountability for sustained personnel wellness. Items on the STSI-OA are organized into domains of activity related to the school's promotion of resilience building activities in staff (7 items); the degree to which an organization promotes physical and psychological safety in the workplace (7 items); the degree to which the organization has STS relevant policies (6 items); how STS has informed leadership practices are (9 items); and routine school-based practices (11 items). Employees rate the degree to which the school (or district) addresses the item using the categories 1 = "Not at All," 2 = "Rarely," 3 = "Somewhat," 4 = "Mostly," and 5 = "Completely."

Consideration of the Impact of Trauma and School Violence on School Personnel as well as Students

The literature is replete with examples of how work with children and youth with traumatic stress responses can impact professional well-being (Lawson et al., 2019; Benuto et al., 2018; Sprang et al., 2011). Studies document high rates of secondary traumatic stress in educators and school personnel (Borntrager et al., 2012; Smith Hatcher et al., 2011), with student characteristics, class load size, and a personal history of trauma emerging as contributing and mitigating factors (Caringi et al., 2015). It is reasonable to assume that educators and school personnel cannot effectively enact trauma-informed care strategies with their students in an effective manner, if they are operating in an environment where their own trauma needs are ignored. Teachers and other school personnel are on the front lines in addressing the trauma responses of students, who may come to school with high rates of hyperarousal, may be triggered by bullying or perceived humiliation, or who feel desperate and out of control. If school professionals are to recognize and respond effectively, they must not be burdened by the avoidance, distress, or vulnerabilities associated with their own trauma response. Furthermore, there are examples in the literature that the collective experience of secondary traumatic stress in a school can negatively impact organizational climate (Tyler, 2012; Hormann & Vivian, 2005). Schools or districts that do not recognize or under-respond to employees with secondary traumatic stress may unwittingly cultivate an organizational climate that is not psychologically safe for workers (Bloom, 2006). Physical and psychological safety are key to a healthy student body and a high functioning, trauma-informed workforce, and can be considered an upstream organizational resource that is highly influenced by leadership (Dollard & Bakker, 2010). Based on findings from the organizational health literature, schools and districts who fail to prioritize safety in the student body and workforce may be less effective in their attempts to address trauma and minimize violence in the student body (Bakker & Demerouti, 2008).

Sensitivity and Responsiveness to Culture and Experience, Past and Present, Broadly Defined

Peter Drucker is often attributed to the quote, "culture eats strategy for breakfast." Trauma-exposed children and youth may have unique needs that are influenced by community, culture, and socio-environmental factors that may undermine the implementation of a trauma-informed violence prevention program if not addressed. To be successful, those charged with the task of implementation must consider the cultural variations within and among schools and districts. Any innovation introduced to create change will require tailoring to meet these differences. Following this principle, the school and/or district would take efforts to avoid the reenactment of stereotypes, biases, and discriminatory behavior fueled by racism, sexism, ageism, and negative actions based on sexual orientation, religious preferences, immigration status, ethnicity, etc. Furthermore, a trauma-informed approach recognizes the impact of historical trauma, the multigenerational trauma of certain groups due to their membership in a specific racial, cultural, or ethnic group. Events, such as slavery, the Holocaust, the compulsory sterilization of people with disabilities, and/ or the colonization of Native Americans that included extreme acts of violence and oppression, become part of the cultural narrative of these groups. Although not everyone is affected, these historical trauma experiences can influence expectations, assumptions, and well-being, and responses to new trauma exposures in families and communities (Brave Heart, 2003; De Gruy, 2005; Miller & Levine, 2013). The effects of historical trauma have been documented as including damaged cultural identity, decreased physical and psychiatric well-being, somatization, decreased sense of self-efficacy, depression, substance use disorders, increased risk of suicidality, and notably, a marked propensity for violent or aggressive behavior (Sotero, 2006; Danieli, 1980; Brave Heart, 2003; Miller & Levine, 2013).

It is important to recognize that these historical events have sometimes occurred within those systems that mean to promote and protect children, and have played out in professional relationships with others (US Department of Health and Human Services, 2014). Examples include denial and dismissal by others when attempting to share their stories (Danieli, 1980), being forbidden to speak a person's native language (Walters et al., 2002), reinforced otherness, and/or messages that one is not welcome or does not belong (Gordon & Johnson, 2003). This phenomenon is noteworthy, as the lingering effects of historical trauma can influence perceptions of current and ongoing racial and interpersonal trauma (the psychological effects of racism, discrimination, and bias). Racial violence precipitated by perceived social injustice, and a lack of fair and transparent response can fuel desperation and despair in students who already have a limited number of adaptive skills based on development and life experience.

Overcoming these effects requires leaning into the other trauma-informed principles of safety, trustworthiness and transparency, peer support collaboration and mutuality, empowerment, voice and choice, as well as being respectful of history, culture, and gender issues that may be evident in the student body and community

(US Department of Health and Human Services, 2014). In a trauma-informed environment, schools will acknowledge and respond to current racial trauma and the lingering effects of historical trauma through intentional discussion of these events and processing. The process begins by asking school personnel to self-assess their own prejudices, biases, and misperceptions, recognizing that every person has a set of heuristics that guides thinking and behavior that may elude their awareness. Schools can engage in implicit or unconscious bias training to cultivate a culture of tolerance and acceptance, and school-wide discussions about policies, practices, and protocols that may unwittingly reinforce negative perceptions, or otherness. Ultimately, self-exploration and awareness are key to a culturally sensitive response that can influence outcomes related to trauma and violence. Recognizing and acknowledge that trauma enters the school environment through an invisible backpack of thoughts, assumptions, and expectations about one's self, others, and the world provides the context for responding and connecting current and historical events to class material and discussions allows for an exploration of these ideas. Basic psychoeducation about the role that trauma plays in society, including the lingering effects of historical trauma, can raise awareness and provide validation of these experiences. Finally, school personnel must model courage by sharing feelings and questions about cultural identity and humbly acknowledging areas of targeted personal growth.

Culture sensitivity is not just a phenomenon relevant to the population of students and their families. Schools and school districts also create and maintain an internal culture that can greatly influence how trauma and violence may manifest, and the best ways to respond. Rogers (2003) counters the "better mousetrap fallacy" by suggestion that how an innovation is accepted and implemented is a function of social processes influence by culture as much as its features. Consideration of the values, beliefs, and norms of the organization is key to aligning the what with the how. Teachers, for example, may accept the premise of trauma-informed care but will ultimately have to reconcile the practice with issues, such as their perceptions of what constitutes effective pedagogy or behavior management, issues of time and logistics, the ease of implementation, and what they feel they have the skill and resources to implement (McIntosh et al., 2014). Additionally, the desired outcomes must address problems important to the school community. Therefore, connecting the implementation of trauma-informed care as a strategy to increase safety, decrease externalizing behavior, and prevent school violence is important in the orientation stages of rollout. Providing training and education to school personnel on the science of the stress response, the neurobiological effects of trauma exposure, the effects of this response on learning and impulse control, and the effectiveness of trauma interventions in the reduction of externalizing behavior provides an evidence-based rationale for implementation. If a trauma-informed approach is selected by administration, but does not have the buy-in and support from those responsible for its implementation, the likelihood of full implementation and sustainability is decreased (Fixsen et al., 2005). Indeed, there is evidence in the educational literature that innovations are more likely to be adopted if they match and respect the culture of the school (Kealey et al., 2000; Detrich et al., 2007).

Conclusion

Trauma-informed care is a viable approach for addressing student trauma and decreasing school violence because it creates a learning environment where the physical and psychological safety of students are foundational to the academic enterprise. If schools can respond to problem behaviors without re-traumatizing the student, efforts at de-escalation, remediation, and redirection are more likely to be effective. A data-driven approach to reducing trauma and school violence requires a nimble approach to implementing trauma-informed care that considers the culture of the school, the trauma responses of school personnel who may be exposed to indirect trauma, a continuous feedback loop using trauma- and violence-specific tools to guide implementation, and integration with existing Multi-Tiered Systems of Support services. For the child who has experienced child maltreatment, bullying, and community violence, trauma-informed care provides a window of opportunity to move away from the negative self-images of being broken, desperate, and misunderstood, to recovery, stabilization, and reconnection with adults who can positively change the course of their life. For those of us responsible for allowing the light in, trauma-informed care shows us the way.

References

Adams, Z. W., Moreland, A., Cohen, J. R., Lee, R. C., Hanson, R. F., Danielson, C. K., et al. (2016). Polyvictimization: Latent profiles and mental health outcomes in a clinical sample of adolescents. *Psychology of Violence, 6*(1), 145.

Agnich, L. E., & Miyazaki, Y. (2013). A multilevel cross-national analysis of direct and indirect forms of school violence. *Journal of School Violence, 12*(4), 319–339.

American Psychiatric Association (Ed.). (2013). *Diagnostic and statistical manual of mental disorders* (5th ed.). American Psychiatric Association.

Anda, R. F., Felitti, V. J., Bremner, J. D., Walker, J. D., Whitfield, C. H., Perry, B. D., et al. (2006). The enduring effects of abuse and related adverse experiences in childhood. *European Archives of Psychiatry and Clinical Neuroscience, 256*(3), 174–186.

Atallah, D. G., Koslouski, J. B., Perkins, K. N., Marsico, C., & Porche, M. V. (2019). *An evaluation of trauma and learning policy Initiative's (TLPI) inquiry-based process: Year three.* Boston University, Wheelock College of Education and Human Development.

Azeem, M. W., Aujla, A., Rammerth, M., Binsfeld, G., & Jones, R. B. (2011). Effectiveness of six core strategies based on trauma-informed care in reducing seclusions and restraints at a child and adolescent psychiatric hospital. *Journal of Child and Adolescent Psychiatric Nursing, 24*(1), 11–15.

Baker, C. N., Brown, S. M., Wilcox, P. D., Overstreet, S., & Arora, P. (2016). Development and psychometric evaluation of the attitudes related to trauma-informed care (ARTIC) scale. *School Mental Health, 8*(1), 61–76.

Bakker, A. B., & Demerouti, E. (2008). Towards a model of work engagement. *Career Development International, 13*(3), 209–223.

Bartlett, J. D., Barto, B., Griffin, J., Fraser, J. G., Hodgdon, H., & Bodian, R. (2016). Trauma-informed care in the Massachusetts child trauma project. *Child Maltreatment, 21*(2), 101–112.

Bassuk, E. L., Unick, G. J., Paquette, K., & Richard, M. K. (2017). Developing an instrument to measure organizational trauma-informed care in human services: The TICOMETER. *Psychology of Violence, 7*(1), 150–157.

Benuto, L. T., Newlands, R., Ruork, A., Hooft, S., & Ahrendt, A. (2018). Secondary traumatic stress among victim advocates: Prevalence and correlates. *Journal of evidence-informed social work, 15*(5), 494–509.

Blasé, K., van Dyke, M., & Fixsen, D. (2015). *Implementation drivers: Assessing best practices.* Adapted with permission by The State Implementation & Scaling-up of Evidence-based Practices Center (SISEP). Based on the work of The National Implementation Research Network (NIRN). University of North Carolina Chapel Hill.

Blodgett, C., & Dorado, J. (2016). A selected review of trauma-informed school practice and alignment with educational practice. CLEAR Trauma Center. San Francisco, CA: University of California, *1*, 1–88.

Bloom, S. L. (2006). Human service systems and organizational stress: Thinking and feeling our way out of existing organizational dilemmas. *Report for the trauma task force,* Philadelphia, PA.

Borntrager, C., Caringi, J. C., van den Pol, R., Crosby, L., O'Connell, K., Trautman, A., & McDonald, M. (2012). Secondary traumatic stress in school personnel. *Advances in School Mental Health Promotion, 5*(1), 38–50.

Bowman-Perrott, L., Benz, M. R., Hsu, H., Kwok, O., Eisterhold, L. A., & Zhang, D. (2013). Patterns and predictors of disciplinary exclusion over time: An analysis of the SEELS national data set. *Journal of Emotional and Behavioral Disorders, 21*, 83–96.

Brave Heart, M. Y. H. (2003). The historical trauma response among natives and its relationship to substance abuse: A Lakota illustration. *Journal of Psychoactive Drugs, 35*(1), 7–13.

Bride, B. E., Robinson, M. M., Yegidis, B., & Figley, C. R. (2004). Development and validation of the secondary traumatic stress scale. *Research on Social Work Practice, 14*, 27–35.

Briere, J. (1996). *Trauma symptom checklist for children* (pp. 00253–00258). Psychological Assessment Resources.

Brend, D., Fletcher, K., & Nutton, J. (2013). With Laura: Attachment and the healing potential of substitute caregivers within cross-cultural child welfare practice. First peoples child & family review: an interdisciplinary journal honouring the voices, perspectives, and knowledges of first peoples through research, critical analyses, stories, standpoints and media reviews, 7(2), 43–59.

Campbell, A., & Hemsley, S. (2009). Outcome rating scale and session rating scale in psychological practice: Clinical utility of ultrabrief measures. *Clinical Psychologist, 13*(1), 1–9.

Caringi, J. C., Stanick, C., Trautman, A., Crosby, L., Devlin, M., & Adams, S. (2015). Secondary traumatic stress in public school teachers: Contributing and mitigating factors. *Advances in School Mental Health Promotion, 8*(4), 244–256.

Cecil, C. A., Viding, E., Barker, E. D., Guiney, J., & McCrory, E. J. (2014). Double disadvantage: The influence of childhood maltreatment and community violence exposure on adolescent mental health. *Journal of Child Psychology and Psychiatry, 55*(7), 839–848.

Centers for Disease Control and Prevention. (2016a). *Understanding school violence*, downloaded on 6/9/2020 from https://www.cdc.gov/violenceprevention/pdf/school_violence_fact_sheet-a.pdf

Centers for Disease Control and Prevention. (2016b). *About the CDC-Kaiser ACE study: Major findings.* Retrieved from https://www.cdc.gov/violenceprevention/acestudy/about.html

Cicchetti, D., & Toth, S. L. (2005). Child maltreatment. *Annual Review of Clinical Psychology., 1*, 409–438.

Chafouleas, S. M., Johnson, A. H., Overstreet, S., & Santos, N. M. (2016). Toward a blueprint for trauma-informed service delivery in schools. *School Mental Health, 8*(1), 144–162.

Cornell, D. G. (2020). Threat assessment as a school violence prevention strategy. *Criminology & Public Policy, 19*(1), 235–252.

Cook, S. H., Valera, P., Calebs, B. J., & Wilson, P. A. (2017). Adult attachment as a moderator of the association between childhood traumatic experiences and depression symptoms among young Black gay and bisexual men. *Cultural Diversity and Ethnic Minority Psychology, 23*(3), 388.

Cornell, D., & Sheras, P. (2006). *Guidelines for responding to student threats of violence.* Sopris West.

Danieli, Y. (1980). Families of survivors of the Nazi Holocaust: Some long- and some shortterm effects. In N. Milgram (Ed.), *Psychological stress and adjustment in time of war and peace.* Hemisphere Publishing Corps.

De Gruy, J. (2005). *Post traumatic slave syndrome.* Uptone Press.

De Bellis, M. D., & Zisk, A. (2014). The biological effects of childhood trauma. *Child and Adolescent Psychiatric Clinics, 23*(2), 185–222.

Detrich, R. (2013). Innovation, implementation science, and data-based decision making: Components of successful reform. In M. Murphy, S. Redding, & J. Twyman (Eds.), *Handbook on innovations in learning* (pp. 31–48). Center on Innovations in Learning.

Detrich, R., Keyworth, R., & States, J. (2007). A roadmap to evidence-based education: Building an evidencebased culture. *Journal of Evidence-Based Practices for Schools, 8*(1), 26.

Dollard, M. F., & Bakker, A. B. (2010). Psychosocial safety climate as a precursor to conducive work environments, psychological health problems, and employee engagement. *Journal of Occupational and Organizational Psychology, 83*(3), 579–599.

Dorado, J., Martinez, M., McArthur, L., & Leibovitz, T. (2016). Healthy Environments and Response to Trauma in Schools (HEARTS): A whole-school, multi-level, prevention and intervention program for creating trauma-informed, safe and supportive schools. *School Mental Health, 8,* 163–176.

Easton, J. E., & Erchul, W. P. (2011). An exploration of teacher acceptability of treatment plan implementation: Monitoring and feedback methods. *Journal of Educational and Psychological Consultation, 21*(1), 56–77.

Elliott, D. S., & Mihalic, S. (2004). Issues in disseminating and replicating effective prevention programs. *Prevention Science, 5*(1), 47–53.

Espelage, D. L., & Hong, J. S. (2019). School climate, bullying, and school violence. In M. J. Mayer & S. R. Jimerson (Eds.), *School safety and violence prevention: Science, practice, policy* (pp. 45–69). American Psychological Association.

Finkelhor, D., Turner, H. A., Shattuck, A., & Hamby, S. L. (2015). Prevalence of childhood exposure to violence, crime, and abuse: Results from the national survey of children's exposure to violence. *JAMA Pediatrics, 169*(8), 746–754.

Finkelhor, D., Vanderminden, J., Turner, H., Shattuck, A., & Hamby, S. (2016). At-school victimization and violence exposure assessed in a national household survey of children and youth. *Journal of School Violence, 15*(1), 67–90.

Fixsen, D. L., Naoom, S. F., Blase, K. A., Friedman, R. M., & Wallace, F. (2005). Implementation research: A synthesis of the literature. Tampa, FL: University of South Florida, National Implementation Research Network.

Felitti, V. J., Anda, R. F., Nordenberg, D., Williamson, D. F., Spitz, A. M., Edwards, V., & Marks, J. S. (1998). Relationship of childhood abuse and household dysfunction to many of the leading causes of death in adults: The Adverse Childhood Experiences (ACE) Study. *American journal of preventive medicine, 14*(4), 245–258.

Foa, E. B., Johnson, K. M., Feeny, N. C., & Treadwell, K. R. (2001). The child PTSD symptom scale: A preliminary examination of its psychometric properties. *Journal of Clinical Child Psychology, 30*(3), 376–384.

Foa, E. B., Chrestman, K. R., & Gilboa-Schechtman, E. (2008). Prolonged exposure therapy for adolescents with PTSD emotional processing of traumatic experiences, therapist guide. Oxford University Press.

Fry, D., Fang, X., Elliott, S., Casey, T., Zheng, X., Li, J., et al. (2018). The relationships between violence in childhood and educational outcomes: A global systematic review and meta-analysis. *Child Abuse & Neglect, 75,* 6–28.

Gordon, J., & Johnson, M. (2003). Race, speech, and a hostile educational environment: What color is free speech? *Journal of Social Psychology, 34*(3), 414–436.

Guarino, K., & Chagnon, E. (2018). *Leading trauma-sensitive schools action guide. Traumasensitive schools training package.* National Center on Safe Supportive Learning Environments.

Harter, S. (2003). Development of self-representations during childhood and adolescence. In M. R. Leary & J. P. Tangney (Eds.), *The handbook of self and identity* (pp. 610–642). Guilford.

Hensel, J. M., Ruiz, C., Finney, C., & Dewa, C. S. (2015). Meta-analysis of risk factors for secondary traumatic stress in therapeutic work with trauma victims. *Journal of Traumatic Stress, 28*(2), 83–91.

Hojnoski, R. L., Caskie, G. I., Gischlar, K. L., Key, J. M., Barry, A., & Hughes, C. L. (2009). Data displaypreference, acceptability, and accuracy among urban Head Start teachers. *Journal of Early Intervention, 32*(1), 38–53.

Hormann, S., & Vivian, P. (2005). Toward an understanding of traumatized organizations and how to intervene in them. *Traumatology, 11*(3), 159–169.

Jenkins, S. R., & Baird, S. (2002). Secondary traumatic stress and vicarious trauma: A validational study. *Journal of Traumatic Stress, 15*, 423–432.

Kaplow, J. B., Rolon-Arroyo, B., Layne, C. M., Rooney, E., Oosterhoff, B., Hill, R., et al. (2020). Validation of the UCLA PTSD Reaction Index for DSM-5: A developmentally informed assessment tool for youth. *Journal of the American Academy of Child & Adolescent Psychiatry, 59*(1), 186–194.

Kataoka, S. H., Stein, B. D., Jaycox, L. H., Wong, M., Escudero, P., Tu, W., et al. (2003). A school-based mental health program for traumatized Latino immigrant children. *Journal of the American Academy of Child and Adolescent Psychiatry, 42*(3), 311–318.

Kealey, K. A., Peterson, A. V., Jr., Gaul, M. A., & Dinh, K. T. (2000). Teacher training as a behavior change process: Principles and results from a longitudinal study. *Health Education & Behavior, 27*(1), 64–81.

Kearney, C., Gonzálvez, C., Graczyk, P. A., & Fornander, M. (2019). Reconciling contemporary approaches to school attendance and school absenteeism: Toward promotion and nimble response, global policy review and implementation, and future adaptability (part 1). *Frontiers in Psychology, 10*, 2222.

Lang, J. M., & Connell, C. M. (2017). Development and validation of a brief trauma screening measure for children: The Child Trauma Screen. *Psychological trauma: theory, research, practice, and policy, 9*(3), 390.

Lawson, H. A., Caringi, J. C., Gottfried, R., Bride, B. E., & Hydon, S. P. (2019). Educators' secondary traumatic stress, children's trauma, and the need for trauma literacy. *Harvard Educational Review, 89*(3), 421–447.

Marrow, M. T., Knudsen, K. J., Olafson, E., & Bucher, S. E. (2012). The value of implementing TARGET within a trauma-informed juvenile justice setting. *Journal of Child & Adolescent Trauma, 5*(3), 257–270.

Mc Guckin, C., Lewis, C. A., Cummins, P. K., & Cruise, S. M. (2017). The stress and trauma of school victimization in Ireland: A retrospective account. *Psychology, Society, & Education, 3*(1), 55–67.

McEwen, B. S., & Wingfield, J. C. (2010). What's in a name? Integrating homeostasis, allostasis and stress. *Hormones and Behavior, 57*(2), 105.

McIntosh, K., & Turri, M. G. (2014). Positive Behavior Support: Sustainability and Continuous Regeneration. Grantee Submission. downloaded on Jan 10, 2022 from https://files.eric.ed.gov/fulltext/ED562561.pdf

McLaughlin, K. A., & Lambert, H. K. (2017). Child trauma exposure and psychopathology: Mechanisms of risk and resilience. *Current Opinion in Psychology, 14*, 29–34.

Miech, E. J., Rattray, N. A., Flanagan, M. E., Damschroder, L., Schmid, A. A., & Damush, T. M. (2018). Inside help: An integrative review of champions in healthcare-related implementation. *SAGE Open Medicine, 6*, 2050312118773261.

Miller, P. S., & Levine, R. L. (2013). *Avoiding genetic genocide: Understanding good intentions and eugenics in the complex dialogue between the medical and disabilities communities.* http://www.ncbi.nlm.nih.gov/pmc/articles/PMC3566260/

Molcho, M., Craig, W., Due, P., Pickett, W., Harel-Fisch, Y., Overpeck, M. D., & HBSC Bullying Writing Group. (2009). Cross-national time trends in bullying behavior: Findings from Europe and North America. *International Journal of Public Health, 54*, S225–S234.

Mongan, P., Hatcher, S. S., & Maschi, T. (2009). Etiology of school shootings: Utilizing a purposive, non-impulsive model for social work practice. *Journal of Human Behavior in the Social Environment, 19*(5), 635–645.

Musu, L., Zhang, A., Wang, K., Zhang, J., & Oudekerk, B. (2019). *Indicators of school crime and safety: 2018*. From https://ncvc.dspacedirect.org/handle/20.500.11990/1242

National Child Traumatic Stress Network. (2016). *What is a trauma-informed child and family service system?* Downloaded from https://www.nctsn.org/resources/what-trauma-informed-child-and-family-service-system

Perfect, M. M., Turley, M. R., Carlson, J. S., Yohanna, J., & Saint Gilles, M. P. (2016). School-related outcomes of traumatic event exposure and traumatic stress symptoms in students: A systematic review of research from 1990 to 2015. *School Mental Health, 8*(1), 7–43

Rapp, L. A., & Wodarski, J. S. (2019). Violence in schools. In *Empirically based interventions targeting social problems* (pp. 65–86). Springer.

Renshaw, T. L., Long, A. C., & Cook, C. R. (2015). Assessing adolescents' positive psychological functioning at school: Development and validation of the Student Subjective Wellbeing Questionnaire. *School Psychology Quarterly, 30*(4), 534.

Rivard, J. C., Bloom, S. L., McCorkle, D., & Abramaovitz, R. (2005). Preliminary results of a study examining the implementation and effects of a trauma recovery framework for youths in residential treatment. *Therapeutic Community: The International Journal for Therapeutic and Supportive Organizations, 26*(1), 83–96.

Rogers, E. M. (2003). *Diffusion of innovations* (5th ed.). Free Press.

Rosen, A. L., Handley, E. D., Cicchetti, D., & Rogosch, F. A. (2018). The impact of patterns of trauma exposure among low income children with and without histories of child maltreatment. *Child Abuse & Neglect, 80*, 301–311.

Schmid, M., Lüdtke, J., Dolitzsch, C., Fischer, S., Eckert, A., & Fegert, J. M. (2020). Effect of trauma-informed care on hair cortisol concentration in youth welfare staff and client physical aggression towards staff: Results of a longitudinal study. *BMC Public Health, 20*(1), 21.

Schreck, C. J., Miller, J. M., & Gibson, C. L. (2003). Trouble in the school yard: A study of the risk factors of victimization at school. *Crime & Delinquency, 49*(3), 460–484.

Sege, R. D., Amaya-Jackson, L., & American Academy of Pediatrics Committee on Child Abuse and Neglect. (2017). Clinical considerations related to the behavioral manifestations of child maltreatment. *Pediatrics, 139*(4), e20170100.

Shonkoff, J. P., Garner, A. S., Committee on Psychosocial Aspects of Child and Family Health, Committee on Early Childhood, Adoption, and Dependent Care, and Section on Developmental and Behavioral Pediatrics, Siegel, B. S., Dobbins, M. I., Earls, M. F., ... & Wood, D. L. (2012). The lifelong effects of early childhood adversity and toxic stress. *Pediatrics, 129*(1), e232–e246.

Smith Hatcher, S., Bride, B. E., Oh, H., Moultrie King, D., & Franklin Catrett, J. (2011). An assessment of secondary traumatic stress in juvenile justice education workers. *Journal of Correctional Health Care, 17*(3), 208–217.

Sotero, M. M. (2006). A conceptual model of historical trauma: Implications for public health, practice and research. *Journal of Health Disparities Research and Practice, 1*(1), 93–108.

Sprang, G. (2019). *Secondary traumatic stress in school personnel*. Presentation at the translational research forum on secondary traumatic stress, September 5, 2019. University of Kentucky Center on Trauma and Children.

Sprang, G., Clark, J. J., & Whitt-Woosley, A. (2007). Compassion fatigue, compassion satisfaction, and burnout: Factors impacting a professional's quality of life. *Journal of Loss and Trauma, 12*, 259–280.

Sprang, G., Craig, C., & Clark, J. (2011). Secondary traumatic stress and burnout in child welfare workers: A comparative analysis of occupational distress across professional groups. *Child Welfare, 90*(6), 149–168.

Sprang, G., Ross, L., Miller, B. C., Blackshear, K., & Ascienzo, S. (2017). Psychometric properties of the secondary traumatic stress–informed organizational assessment. *Traumatology, 23*(2), 165–171.

Sprang, G., Ford, J., Kerig, P., & Bride, B. (2019). Defining secondary traumatic stress and developing targeted assessments and interventions: Lessons learned from research and leading experts. *Traumatology, 25*(2), 72.

Sprang, G., Lei, F., & Bush, H. (2021). Can organizational efforts Lead to less secondary traumatic stress? A longitudinal investigation of change. *American Journal of Orthopsychiatry, 91*(4), 443–453. https://doi.org/10.1037/ort0000546

Stamm, B. H. (2010). *The ProQOL (Professional quality of life scale: Compassion satisfaction and compassion fatigue).* ProQOL.org.

Stevens, J. E. (2012). Lincoln high school in walla walla, WA tries new approach to school discipline— Suspensions drop 85%. *ACEs too high.* Retrieved from http://acestoohigh.com/2012/04/23/lincolnhigh-school-in-walla-walla-wa-tries-new-approachto-school-discipline-expulsions-drop-85/

Substance Abuse and Mental Health Services Administration. (2014). *SAMHSA's concept of trauma and guidance for a trauma-informed approach. HHS publication no. (SMA) 14–4884.* Substance Abuse and Mental Health Services Administration.

Sulkowski, M. L., & Michael, K. (2014). Meeting the mental health needs of homeless students in schools: A multitiered system of support framework. *Children and Youth Services Review, 44*, 145–151.

Traumatic Stress Institute. (1994). *The TSI belief scale.* Author.

Tyler, T. A. (2012). The limbic model of systemic trauma. *Journal of Social Work Practice, 26*(1), 125–138.

U.S. Department of Health & Human Services, Administration for Children and Families, Administration on Children, Youth and Families, Children's Bureau. (2020). *Child maltreatment 2018.* Available from https://www.acf.hhs.gov/cb/research-data-technology/statistics-research/child-maltreatment

US Department of Health and Human Services, Substance Abuse and Mental Health Administration. (2014). *Tips for disaster responders: Understanding historical trauma when responding to an event in Indian country.* Retrieved from https://www.acf.hhs.gov/trauma-toolkit/trauma-concept

Vachon, D. D., Krueger, R. F., Rogosch, F. A., & Cicchetti, D. (2015). Different forms of child maltreatment have comparable consequences among children from low-income families. *JAMA Psychiatry, 72*(11), 1135.

Van Hook, M. P., & Rothenberg, M. (2009). Quality of life and compassion satisfaction/fatigue and burnout in child welfare workers in community based care organizations in central Florida. *Social Work & Christianity, 36*(1), 36–54.

Vossekuil, B., Reddy, M., Fein, R., Borum, R., & Modzeleski, W. (2000). *U.S.S.S. Safe school initiative: An interim report on the prevention of targeted violence in schools.* U.S. Secret Service, National Threat Assessment Center.

Walters, K., Simoni, J. M., & Evans-Campbell, T. (2002). Substance use among American Indians and Alaska Natives: Incorporating culture in an "indigenist" stress-coping paradigm. *Public Health Reports, 117*(1), S104–S117.

Wang, J., Iannotti, R. J., & Nansel, T. R. (2009). School bullying among adolescents in the United States: Physical, verbal, relational, and cyber. *Journal of Adolescent Health, 45*, 368–375.

Wike, T. L., & Fraser, M. W. (2009). School shootings: Making sense of the senseless. *Aggression and Violent Behavior, 14*(3), 162–169.

Zhang, A., Musu-Gillette, L., & Oudekerk, B. A. (2016). *Indicators of school crime and safety: 2015.* (NCES 2016–079/NCJ 249758). National Center for Education Statistics, U.S. Department of Education, and Bureau of Justice Statistics, Office of Justice Programs, U.S. Department of Justice.

Chapter 21
Bullying as a Form of Abuse: Conceptualization and Prevention

Amanda B. Nickerson, Amanda Breese, and Jean M. Alberti

Historical Context

Bullying is not a new concept but rather a phenomenon that has been happening since recorded history (Allanson et al., 2015; Koo, 2007). The word "bully" was first recorded in the 1530s (Donegan, 2012), originally with positive connotations with definitions ranging from "sweetheart" to "fine fellow" (Allanson et al., 2015). It was not until the 1680s that "bully" was given the negative definition of "harasser of the weak" (Allanson et al., 2015). Since the change in definition, bullying has become ingrained in American society as a rite of passage, or just a part of growing up (Alberti, 2001; Allanson et al., 2015; Donegan, 2012). In order to address bullying, it is important to understand its historical context and its conceptualization.

School bullying has been well studied in many European and Asian countries since the early seventeenth century (Koo, 2007). In Asian countries like Korea and Japan, bullying has been well documented since the early seventeenth century. Bullying in Korea, or "myunsinrae," was first documented in writings from the Chosun Dynasty in the 1300s (Williams, 2014). Mostly seen in the military between new and superior officers, "myunsinrae" is an overt form of bullying to make a victim feel shame through physical and psychological insults (Koo, 2007). Common forms of "myunsinrae" or "playing invisible coat" include: hitting a victim with sticks, painting their faces with dirt, and riding the victim as if they were a horse (Koo, 2007). "Myunsinrae" lacked information or punishment until the sixth king of

A. B. Nickerson (✉) · A. Breese
Alberti Center for Bullying Abuse Prevention, University at Buffalo, The State University of New York, Buffalo, NY, USA
e-mail: nickersa@buffalo.edu

J. M. Alberti
Alberti Psychological Services, Glen Ellyn, NY, USA

the Chosun Dynasty died by suicide after having endured "myunsinrae" for over a year (Williams, 2014).

Bullying in Japan, "ijime," has been documented as early as 1603 (Koo, 2007). Japan is the only nation in Asia where bullying is well studied (Koo, 2007). "Ijime" takes the form of psychological isolation rather than physical harm or injury, the most common form being ostracism (Sakai, 1985; Koo, 2007). Often "ijime" was seen as a form of parenting or punishment. Common forms of punishment include: child isolation, familial separation, and threats to abandon the child (Sakai, 1985). The belief behind these punishments is that the child would learn how to survive through the punishment. The tradition of "ijime" quickly moved into school class-rooms where teachers and staff would encourage the children to ostracize others who were acting strange in an effort to teach assimilation (Williams, 2014). In the mid-1980s, "ijime" became the biggest social problem featured in the media (Koo, 2007). In 1986, newspapers and television shows presented the public with nine incidents of students' suicide notes which detailed their need for help with "ijime" (Naito & Gielen, 2005). Between 1985 and 1998, more than 1200 academic papers and over 400 books were written on "ijime" (Takatoku, 1999).

In the early nineteenth century, the United Kingdom considered the violence of bullying to be private, or a matter between individuals rather than the focus of national attention (Koo, 2007). However, toward the end of the nineteenth century, bullying began to gain national attention with *Tom Brown's Schooldays* by Thomas Hughes (Koo, 2007). Hughes' novel contains one of the first examples of bullying within UK schools and enlightened the general public about the violence that can occur in schools. The novel was widely read, which led to heated public debates and conjured repugnance toward and disapproval of bullying behaviors (Horton, 2014; Rigby et al., 2004; Sercombe & Donnelly, 2013).

In the United States before the early twentieth century, bullying was only consid-ered to be physical harassment in school children, commonly seen as strong boys being cruel to weak ones (Koo, 2007). The first known academic article to address bullying was written in 1897 by Frederic Burk at Clark University (Koo, 2007). Burk's article surveyed 156 school-aged children from a New Jersey school about their experiences with teasing and bullying, revealing around 1120 instances of bul-lying (Burk, 1897). Attention toward bullying and violence began to shift during World War II when the press coverage of the war increased the American people's awareness of crimes against the dignity of life when (Koo, 2007). The war helped to change the American people's perception of the treatment and acceptable behavior of others, including the human right to be free from violence and aggression (Koo, 2007; Williams, 2014).

While some school bullying research in the United States was conducted as early as 1885, it did not gain traction until the early 1970s in the United Kingdom and Scandinavia (Burk, 1897; Horton & Forsberg, 2015). Early Scandinavian research centered on the subset of bullying termed mobbing, or the collective behavior of harassing a victim (Koo, 2007; Monks & Coyne, 2011). The term mobbing, used originally to describe a group of birds that attack an individual, was adopted to describe the violence seen among school-aged youth (Monks & Coyne, 2011). Dan

Olweus, a leading figure in bullying research, used the term mobbing as his early research focused on children attacking individuals (Allanson et al., 2015; Monks & Coyne, 2011), including a systematic study he conducted in 1973 (Allanson et al., 2015). However, Olweus later realized that bullying between individuals was more common than mobbing behavior (Monks & Coyne, 2011). Olweus' research shifted and the term "bullying" became more prevalent in research and publications (Monks & Coyne, 2011). His work is considered to be the pioneering research on bullying. In 1993, Olweus provided the first widely used definition of bullying (Allanson et al., 2015; Koo, 2007). A person is bullied when he or she is exposed, repeatedly and over time, to negative actions on the part of one or more other persons, and he or she has difficulty defending himself or herself (Olweus, 1993). Currently, the term "mobbing" is more closely related to the mistreatment by colleagues in the workplace (Seo et al., 2012). Olweus also developed the first comprehensive school-wide bullying prevention program in Norway called the Olweus Bullying Prevention Program (OBPP; Olweus, 1993), discussed in more detail later in the chapter.

In the late 1990s, after a string of massacres in schools, bullying became a more urgent issue in the United States (Allanson et al., 2015). In 1999 at Columbine High School, Eric Harris and Dylan Klebold murdered twelve students and one teacher, which became the second most-covered news event of the decade (Larkin, 2009). The massacre evoked national outrage, sparking debates and awareness on bullying, school violence, and mental health issues because the perpetrators were reportedly bullied and rejected by their peers (Koo, 2007; Larkin, 2009). Due to the national attention that Columbine drew, school bullying came to be viewed as a public health epidemic and a threat to all students which spurred zero-tolerance and the criminalization of bullying (Cohen & Brooks, 2014).

By the beginning of the twenty-first century, bullying in schools had drawn national attention and awareness in the United States and around the world (Allanson et al., 2015). For example, similar to the United States, South Korea began studying bullying in the early 2000s after a number of suicides that were linked to bullying (Slee & Skrzypiec, 2016).

After the Columbine massacre, many schools across the country began instituting zero-tolerance policies toward bullying and school violence (Larkin, 2009). Prior to this time, teachers advised victims to tell an adult, walk away or tell the bully to stop (Elledge et al., 2010a), but by 2004, many schools adopted anti-bullying programs and sixteen states had passed anti-bullying laws (Allanson et al., 2015). Since the Columbine massacre, peer victimization and mental health moved to the forefront of attention in the United States, with corresponding legislation and prevention approaches discussed later in this chapter. In recent years, bullying has come to be considered the most prevalent form of violence in American schools (Allanson et al., 2015).

Cyberbullying is the newest form of bullying to be recognized. Due to the increase in popularity of the Internet and social media platforms, cyberbullying is at the forefront of national focus and research (Donegan, 2012; Langos, 2012). Cyberbullying was brought into mainstream focus after the online harassment resulted in multiple teen suicides (Donegan, 2012). In October 2006, Megan Meier, a thirteen-year-old from Missouri, died by suicide that was later attributed to cyberbullying. Meier's former friend created a fake account on MySpace, a popular social media platform of the time, to gather information about Meier which was going to be used to later humiliate her (Pokin, 2007). The former friend created the fake account under the name "Josh Evans" and was originally meant as a "joke" (Donegan, 2012). However, in October, the tone of the messages from "Josh" turned sinister with one reading, "[t]he world would be a better place without you" (Pokin, 2007). Megan's story caught national attention and sparked outrage after county prosecutors decided not to file any criminal charges in relation to cyberbullying. In 2008, the Missouri State Legislature voted to criminalize using the Internet to harass someone, and is now known as "Megan's Law." This was one of the first comprehensive cyberbullying and cyberstalking state laws passed to protect youth and adults from online harassment on social media platforms.

The Centers for Disease Control and Prevention (CDC), recognizing bullying as a major public health issue, convened a working group to develop a uniform definition as "any unwanted aggressive behavior that involves an observed or perceived power imbalance that inflicts physical, psychological, social or emotional harm or distress on a targeted youth" (Gladden et al., 2014). The CDC currently recognizes two modes of bullying and four types of bullying (Gladden et al., 2014). A mode of bullying (direct or indirect) is how the aggressive behavior is experienced by the victim. Direct bullying is aggressive behavior that occurs in the presence of the victim (Allanson et al., 2015; Gladden et al., 2014). Indirect bullying is aggressive behavior that is not directly communicated to the victim (Gladden et al., 2014). The types of bullying include: physical, verbal, relational, and damage to property. Physical bullying is defined as the use of physical force by the perpetrator against the target which includes hitting, kicking, and punching (Gladden et al., 2014). Verbal bullying is oral or written communication that causes harm like taunting and inappropriate sexual comments (Gladden et al., 2014). Relational bullying includes behaviors constructed to harm the relationships or reputations of another like spreading rumors and making derogatory comments (Gladden et al., 2014).

Cyberbullying is formally defined as "the willful and repeated harm inflicted through the use of computers, cell phones, and other electronic devices" (Hinduja & Patchin, 2014). Colette Langos (2012) suggests the two following definitions: (a) "cyberbullying is bullying transposed on a technological platform, and (b) "cyberbullying involves the use of information and communication technologies to carry out a series of acts as in the case of direct cyberbullying, or as an act as in the case of indirect cyberbullying, intending to harm another who cannot easily defend his/ herself." Although cyberbullying is difficult to define, it shares several commonalities with traditional bullying like existing as direct and/or indirect, and repetition as a key criterion (Langos, 2012).

Theories of Bullying

In order to better understand the phenomenon of bullying, many theories have been developed. Several theories focus on bullying as a learned behavior that is reinforced within their larger social contexts. Children often learn to use violence as a way to handle interpersonal problems (Alberti, 2001; Donegan, 2012), which may be modeled after and reinforced in the home, school, and larger society (e.g., media). In a school setting, students learn corrupt tactics (e.g., spreading social rumors, pressuring others for assignments) to get ahead in the highly competitive educational environment; if they are reinforced (e.g., becoming more popular, getting better grades), then they may become a habit (Donegan, 2012). Media influence and exposure to violence can reinforce children's learned behaviors (Piotrowski & Hoot, 2008) by providing a model for youth to follow (Anderson & Bushman, 2002) and enabling a perpetrator to justify their behaviors as a legitimate mode of problem-solving (Piotrowski & Hoot, 2008). There is ample evidence that other forms of abuse and violence are also learned behaviors (Bauman & Yoon, 2014; Bergman & Brismar, 1994; Fitch & Papantonio, 1983; Kruger & Valltos, 2002). We next review several theories on the motivation for bullying behaviors, which can be considered as falling broadly as focusing on learning and social cognitions; social capital, power, and dominance; and social-ecological theory.

Learning and Social Cognitive Theories

The social cognitive theory of bullying is based on Albert Bandura's work indicating that individuals learn behaviors through direct observations and the consequences that follow (Bandura, 1977; Swearer et al., 2014). Social cognitive theory suggests that individuals tend to avoid behaviors that are believed they will be punished for, and instead, engage in behaviors that will be rewarded (Bandura, 1977; Swearer et al., 2014). Youth learn social behavior like violence and aggression through observational learning (Bandura, 1977; Bandura et al., 1961), including watching violent media. In Bandura's classic Bobo doll experiment, some children were exposed to an adult model who acted aggressively (e.g., hitting, punching) toward a Bobo doll. After a period of time, the children were left alone with the doll, and those who were exposed to the aggressive model were more likely to also show aggressive behaviors toward the doll (Bandura, 1977). The results suggest that children can learn and then display aggressive or violent behaviors, like bullying, through mere observation, which can occur at home, in school, and in their neighborhoods.

Therefore, according to the social cognitive theory of bullying, those who engage in bullying behaviors have the belief that they will be rewarded (Swearer et al., 2014). An offshoot of social cognitive theory is moral disengagement (MD) theory. MD posits that bullying perpetrators' behavior is linked to their moral understanding of the consequences of the behavior (Hymel & Bonanno, 2014). Indeed, researchers have shown that MD was significantly related to bullying and aggressive behaviors (Gini et al., 2014).

Social Capital, Power, and Dominance Theories

These theories are closely related to Charles Darwin's theory of natural selection; the "strong" pick on the "weak" (Alberti, 2011; Allanson et al., 2015). The "weak" must learn to fight back in order to survive; or in a school setting, bullying victims must learn to defend themselves (Allanson et al., 2015). The social capital theory of bullying theorizes that people invest in social relationships in order to access and benefit from the resources embedded within the relationships (Evans & Smokowski, 2016). In the school setting, social capital is represented by one's social status and the number of friends one has. Bullies may turn to bully perpetration as a way to gain social capital and/or improve their own social status (Evans & Smokowski, 2016). According to the social capital theory, bully perpetrators will seek out those with minimal social capital as they may have few friends and a lower social status (Bagwell & Schmidt, 2011; Evans & Smokowski, 2016). Bullying perpetrators have an easier time gaining social capital by exerting power over their victims. Although disliked (Rodkin & Berger, 2008), bullying perpetrators are perceived as popular; this perception is a form of social capital that implies power and social status (Evans & Smokowski, 2016).

Dominance theory suggests that an individual's desire for dominance and power is the key motivating factor that drives bullying behavior (Evans & Smokowski, 2016). The theory claims that youth will engage in bullying behaviors in attempts to gain group favor while maintaining their perceived social status through repetition of the behaviors. Dominance theory is related to social norms theory, which suggests bullying behaviors are used to reinforce social norms (Blumenfeld, 2005; Hymel et al., 2014). Youth that challenges the social norms will likely experience group member resistance and bullying in order to maintain dominance (Hymel et al., 2014). Another theory that focuses on the social power dynamic is the theory of humiliation. The theory of humiliation centers on the concept that embarrassment requires action from an outside individual who creates feelings of powerlessness in the victimized individual (Evans & Smokowski, 2016). Humiliation not only impacts the victim but also the surrounding community/society. In an attempt to establish power, bullies will either physically, verbally, or relationally humiliate their victims and lower the victim's social status (Evans & Smokowski, 2016).

All the aforementioned theories are consistent with power being at the center of bullying (Hawley & Williford, 2015; Koo, 2007; Olweus, 1978; Vaillancourt & Hymel, 2006), which aligns closely with the roots and theories of traditional violence/abuse. Other forms of abuse, such as domestic violence, are also patterns of behaviors used to keep control and power over another (National Domestic Violence Hotline, n.d.). Like domestic violence and child abuse, bullying is also an urgent public health matter (Cohen & Brooks, 2014), and can be conceptualized as child abuse perpetrated by children (Alberti, 2011).

Social-Ecological Theory

One of the most comprehensive and current theories of bullying is the social-ecological theory that views bullying as embedded in larger social contexts including peers, school, family, neighborhood, and the larger society (Alberti, 2001; Bauman & Yoon, 2014). Based on the Bronfenbrenner model, the social-ecological model posits bullying behavior is not only the result of an individual's characteristics but is also influenced by relationships with peers, families, teachers, neighbors, and societal influences (Swearer & Hymel, 2015). According to this theory, bullying perpetrators and targets are part of a complex system and flow from the center to the various systems that shape the person (Hong & Espelage, 2012). Studies have found that bullying perpetrators experience problems within several areas like the family, the school, and their neighborhood/community (Swearer & Espelage, 2004).

Indeed, many of the aforementioned theories can be subsumed under the social-ecological theory and help further explain the processes that occur in adult-child, peer, and other relationships. As shown in Fig. 21.1, Dr. Jean Alberti (2020), benefactor of the University at Buffalo's Alberti Center for Bullying Abuse Prevention, has represented many aspects of these complex theories in a bullying tree. The tree shows the many roots, or contributors to bullying (e.g., Darwin's theory, social learning, community, and cultural influences), conceptualizes bullying as a form of abuse and demonstrates the long-lasting consequences that parallel those of other forms of physical and emotional abuse. Also aligned with this framework, organizational culture theory also posits that a positive school climate (e.g., the quality and character of a school in relation to learning, social relationships, emotional and physical safety) is associated with less bullying behaviors than a school with a negative climate (Lee & Song, 2012; Evans & Smokowski, 2016). Indeed, many of the practices discussed next focus on what schools can and should do to prevent and intervene with bullying.

Bullying Prevention Approaches and Best Practices

Although public attention to the problem has spurred various approaches to addressing bullying, there is the most promise for using the public health framework with a multi-tiered (i.e., universal, targeted, and indicated) approach to preventing and intervening with bullying (Bradshaw, 2015; Nickerson et al., 2013; Ttofi & Farrington, 2011). There is no federal legislation about bullying specifically, but schools are guided by state law and policy for bullying and related issues of harassment, intimidation, and bias. First, we provide a critical review of policy and

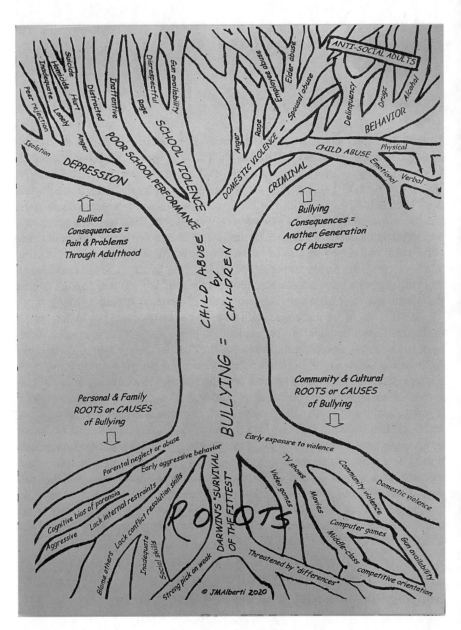

Fig. 21.1 Roots and consequences of bullying abuse. (Copyright © JM Alberti, 2020. Used with permission)

legislation regarding bullying. Then, multi-tiered bullying prevention approaches, with a focus on universal approaches implemented with all students to prevent bullying, as well as targeted and indicated prevention that work specifically with youth who are at-risk for or already involved in bullying as a perpetrator, target, or both.

Policies and Legislation

Since the late 1990s, every state in the United States has enacted legislation to address bullying, which guides school policies, actions, and systems-level interventions (Hall, 2017). Stopbullying.gov provides information on these state laws and policies, and how many of the U.S. Department of Education common components (e.g., prohibiting statement, definition, scope, protected groups, requirements for district policy, reporting and investigations, consequences, communication of policy, safeguards and supports, review and updates of policy, prevention education, and parent engagement) they include (https://www.stopbullying.gov/sites/default/files/StopBullying-Law-Policies-Regulations.pdf).

Most states require schools to implement a bullying policy, including procedures for investigating and responding (i.e., with sanctions) to bullying incidents. Some states also mandate education for students (e.g., bullying prevention programs, integrating bullying prevention in health education or social-emotional learning standards) and/or professional development for teachers and other school staff members (see https://www.stopbullying.gov/resources/laws; Sabia & Bass, 2017).

Despite the prevalence of legislation, there have been very few studies on the effectiveness of these policies. Hall (2017) conducted a systematic review of 21 studies of educator perceptions of effectiveness and the impact of anti-bullying legislation which revealed mixed results of policies. However, consistent results were found for anti-bullying policies that explicitly protected students based on sexual orientation and gender identity which related to lower rates of victimization for lesbian, gay, bisexual, transgender, and questioning/queer (LGBTQ) students and higher rates of intervention by educators (Hall, 2017).

Three relatively recent empirical studies revealed modest correlational support between compliance with legislative mandates and reduced bullying (Cosgrove & Nickerson, 2017; Hatzenbuehler et al., 2015; Sabia & Bass, 2017). Two studies (Hatzenbuehler et al., 2015; Sabia & Bass, 2017) conducted cross-sectional analyses of bullying and other forms of violence from the Youth Risk Behavior Surveys (YRBS) and compared with the comprehensiveness of state anti-bullying policies. Hatzenbuehler et al. (2015) found that students attending school in states with bullying policies that had at least one of the U.S. Department of Education's legislative components experienced reductions in bullying and cyberbullying (by 24% and 20%, respectively), compared to states without these legislative components. Sabia and Bass (2017) found that states with strong and comprehensive school district mandates compared to those that were less expansive and inclusive were associated with an 8–12% reduction in bullying, a 7–13% reduction in school violence, and a 9–11% reduction in students arrested for violent crimes. Cosgrove and Nickerson (2017) conducted a cross-sectional analysis of educators in New York State before and after the state's anti-bullying and harassment legislation was implemented, and they found that educators who reported their schools complied with more aspects of the state mandates also had less severe bullying and harassment and more positive school climate.

The way districts and schools develop, implement (including communication and training), and evaluate the policy is likely to contribute greatly to its effectiveness (Nickerson et al., 2013). For example, a district may adopt a policy developed by the state yet pay it only the bare minimum attention if it is perceived as an unfunded mandate that is not a high priority. Another district may prioritize this and go above the minimum requirements to: (a) develop a policy with the input of stakeholders (e.g., parents, teachers, school staff, and students) to increase support, personal investment, and commitment; (b) disseminate it widely to all stakeholders through newsletters, meetings, assemblies, handbooks, and websites; and (c) monitor progress, evaluate its effects, and revise continuously (Nickerson et al., 2013). The district that engages in meaningful practices around not only the letter but the spirit and intent of the law and policy, may be more likely to see a more positive school climate and reduced bullying. Indeed, according to the previously mentioned organizational culture theory of bullying, a positive school climate, where the entire school organization (e.g., teachers, staff, administrators, and parents) is committed to the mission is not only likely to decrease bullying behaviors, but also provide students with a sense of safety and support, and encourage bystander intervention (Evans & Smokowski, 2016). A school should be a learning organization that acquires and uses information from its employees and stakeholders to successfully plan, implement and evaluate its performance goals (Bowen et al., 2006; Evans & Smokowski, 2016).

Universal Prevention

These broad and systemic approaches are universal in that they are designed to reach the entire population of students in schools (as opposed to those who have already been identified as at-risk for bullying perpetration or victimization). We first provide information about bullying prevention programs and evidence of their effectiveness. Then, we describe approaches that are focused more broadly on teaching and reinforcing positive and prosocial behavior and teaching social-emotional skills, along with the evidence about their impact on bullying.

Bullying Prevention Programs A plethora of commercially available and school-created bullying prevention programs have emerged in the past two decades. Researchers have conducted several meta-analyses and systematic reviews to assess the effectiveness of anti-bullying programs, as detailed in Nickerson and Parks (2021). The first of these meta-analyses showed rather disappointing results, suggesting that bullying prevention programs, on the whole, had some effects on teacher perceptions and behaviors, but mixed or negligible effects on rates of bullying and victimization (e.g., Baldry & Farrington, 2007; Ferguson et al., 2007; Merrell et al., 2008; Smith et al., 2004). For example, Smith et al. (2004), Ferguson et al. (2007), and Baldry and Farrington (2007) found small and even negative effects of bullying prevention programs on students' bullying and victimization.

Merrell et al.' (2008) meta-analysis similarly indicated no significant reductions in bullying and victimization rates following bullying prevention programs, although there were significant increases in teacher knowledge, awareness, and perception of the ability to intervene.

More recent and comprehensive meta-analyses conducted by David Farrington, Maria Ttofi, and colleagues (Farrington & Ttofi, 2009; Gaffney et al., 2019; Ttofi & Farrington, 2011) have included more studies and revealed more encouraging results, with a 19–23% reduction in bullying perpetration and a 15–20% reduction in victimization. Farrington and Ttofi's (2009) study also revealed that approaches characterized by management (e.g., providing more and better playground supervision and structure, using consistent disciplinary methods, and using behavior management strategies in classrooms), anti-bullying rules for the school and classroom, training teachers, and including parents (e.g., sharing information, holding meetings, training) resulted in strongest effects. Comprehensive programs with multiple components, as well as longer programs, more intense training, greater dosage, and monitoring of intervention integrity were also associated with better outcomes (Farrington & Ttofi, 2009). A recent meta-analysis examining the effectiveness of bullying prevention programs with a parental component also found small but significant effects in reducing bullying victimization and perpetration (Huang et al., 2019).

As described in Nickerson and Parks (2021), the first comprehensive, whole-school bullying prevention program created in Norway, following several highly publicized suicides tied to bullying, was the Olweus Bullying Prevention Program (OBPP; Olweus, 1993). Implemented across the country of Norway, the OBPP includes comprehensive schoolwide components, such as establishing a committee, implementing anti-bullying rules, holding events, information sharing with parents, and improving playground supervision. It also includes classroom meetings and activities, and targeted interventions for perpetrators (e.g., non-hostile consequences, firm talking) and victims (e.g., providing support) of bullying. The Olweus Program has resulted in decreased student reports of bullying and other problem behaviors (e.g., fighting; Bauer et al., 2007; Limber et al., 2004; Olweus et al., 1999), increased intervention in bullying (Bauer et al., 2007; Limber et al., 2004), and improved school climate (Olweus et al., 1999) in elementary and middle schools. Results are more positive in Scandinavian countries as compared to the United States, likely of the homogeneity in these cultures and because the structure, priorities, and demands of the educational curriculum in the United States are incompatible with sustained, comprehensive efforts (e.g., frequent classroom meetings) required by the OBPP (Farrington & Ttofi, 2009; Smith et al., 2004).

Given these concerns about its effectiveness in the United States, two recent studies have been published of quasi-experimental extended age-cohort design of students grades 3–11 across schools in Pennsylvania that had implemented the OBPP, finding significant reductions in bullying perpetration and victimization (Limber et al., 2018; Olweus et al., 2019), including all forms of verbal, physical, indirect, sexual, and electronic/cyberbullying (Olweus et al., 2019). In addition, longitudinal analyses over the course of the program implementation revealed increases in students' expressions of empathy for targets of bullying and decreases in their willingness to join in bullying; students also perceived that their teachers were actively addressing bullying in their classrooms (Limber et al., 2018). Effects were stronger the longer the program was in place, and the program was also more effective for elementary and middle school as opposed to high school (Limber et al., 2018; Olweus et al., 2019), suggesting that starting early with prevention is important. Program effects were typically larger for White students, although in the Olweus et al. (2019) study comparable results were found for Black students on most program outcomes, whereas effects were somewhat weaker for Hispanic students.

KiVA is a more recent and increasingly well-researched and widely implemented anti-bullying program developed in Finland (see Nickerson & Parks, 2021). KiVA includes classroom materials, skill practice with computer games, information for parents, disciplinary strategies, and a large focus on increasing the self-efficacy of bystanders to serve as allies for victims (Williford et al., 2012). Studies in Finland have found decreased victimization of students (Garandeau et al., 2014; Kärnä et al., 2011; Williford et al., 2012), particularly for students in grades 1–6 compared to grades 7–9 (Kärnä et al., 2011). Results are also improved for students whose teachers report preparing and adhering more closely to lessons (Haataja et al., 2014). Implementation and evaluation are ongoing in other countries, including but not limited to Chile, Italy, South Africa, the Netherlands, the United Kingdom, and the United States (https://www.kivaprogram.net/kiva-around-the-world/). Some of the studies have been uncontrolled pre-post-test designs with convenience samples of schools that delivered the program after 1 year in both the United Kingdom (Clarkson et al., 2019) and New Zealand (Green et al., 2019). In the Clarkson et al. (2019) study, student reports of victimization were reduced from 18.1% at pre-test to 15.7% at post-test. Green et al. (2019) conducted anonymous online surveys prior to and one year after implementing KiVa with 1175 students aged 6–10 who attended 7 schools in New Zealand, finding decreases in self-reported rates of bullying, victimization, and cyberbullying victimization, although effects were stronger for girls.

In Italy, a randomized controlled trial (RCT) with more than 2000 students in grades 4 and 6 found reductions in bullying victimization and perpetration, as well as increases in pro-bullying attitudes, and the odds of students in the control schools being victimized by bullying were 1.93 greater than for students in the intervention schools (Nocentini & Menesini, 2016). Effects were greater in grade 4 compared to grade 6, and in grade 4 empathy toward victims increased where it did not in grade 6 (Nocentini & Menesini, 2016). In contrast, a recent randomized controlled trial involving over 3000 children from 21 primary schools in the United Kingdom did not find statistically significant effects on bullying victimization and perpetration or on related outcomes of child emotional and behavioral difficulties or absenteeism (Axford et al., 2020).

A three-level meta-analysis of bullying prevention programs found different developmental effects of bullying prevention programs that were implemented broadly across K-12 schools (Yeager et al., 2015). This meta-analysis found some effectiveness for students in 7th grade or lower, no effects for students in 8th grade, and harmful effects for students in 9th–12th grades, as described in Nickerson and Parks (2021). Using the same approach (particularly teacher-delivered content) across development levels may not be appropriate for adolescents given their need for autonomy (Nickerson & Parks, 2021; Yeager et al., 2015). With adolescents, training peer leaders to shift peer norms and behaviors regarding bullying, harassment, and prejudice holds promise (Paluck, 2011; Polanin et al., 2012). For example, Paluck and colleagues (Paluck, 2011; Paluck & Shepherd, 2012) found that training peer leaders to model anti-harassment/anti-prejudice behavior (e.g., verbal condemnation, confrontation) using activities such as skits, announcements, posters, and wristbands of messaging resulted in more prosocial norms and increases in student leaders' and their peers' behaviors to confront teasing, insults, and prejudice. In addition, a meta-analysis revealed that school-based bystander intervention programs have the strongest effects in high school (Polanin et al., 2012), again suggesting the importance of attending to developmental considerations in bullying prevention (Nickerson & Parks, 2021).

Together, results from systematic reviews and meta-analyses of bullying prevention programs reveal some positive impacts on teacher attitudes and behavior and student bystander intervention, although effects on actual rates of bullying and victimization are mixed. There are some promising results for comprehensive and systematically implemented programs developed in Scandinavia, although results are more variable when implemented and evaluated outside of the contexts in which they were developed. It is clear that the comprehensiveness and fidelity of the programs make a difference, as well as their developmental appropriateness.

Given the findings about specific anti-bullying prevention programs, the success of public health models of prevention, and the need for schools to be efficient with their time, resources, and focus (e.g., it is not practical to have separate programs on bullying prevention, substance use prevention, pregnancy prevention, social-emotional and behavioral skills, etc.), most experts recommend a public health approach to the prevention of bullying (Bradshaw, 2015; Nickerson, 2017; Nickerson et al., 2013; Ttofi & Farrington, 2011). This includes universal and targeted prevention approaches to teach and reinforce positive behavior and social-emotional skills (as opposed to programs that focus more specifically on bullying), which are discussed in the following sections.

School-Wide Positive Behavior Support (SWPBS) SWPBS is aimed at creating psychologically healthy educational environments (McIntosh & Lane, 2019) that facilitate healthy prosocial development and academic achievement of children (Sprague & Horner, 2012). This multi-tiered approach focuses on both staff and student behavior and is implemented to increase positive, prosocial behavior, thereby reducing problem behaviors (e.g., noncompliance, bullying; Sugai & Horner, 2006). SWPBS involves directly and proactively teaching expectations, monitoring students' behaviors and skills, and providing specific and immediate feedback across multiple settings in the school (e.g., classrooms, hallways, cafeterias, buses; Kern et al., 2016; Sugai & Horner, 2006). SWPBS focuses on student outcomes using research-validated behavioral practices within a systems approach that includes the active collection and utilization of data to make decisions. There is a large body of research indicating that SWPBS decreases problem behaviors and discipline referrals (Bradshaw et al., 2010; Nese et al., 2014; Noltemeyer et al., 2019) and results in a more positive school climate (Bradshaw et al., 2009; Horner et al., 2009). In terms of the impact of SWPBS on bullying, Waasdorp et al. (2012) conducted a 4-year RCT and found that although both bullying and peer rejection increased as children progressed through elementary school grades, schools in the SWPBS condition had lower rates of bullying and peer rejection (according to teacher reports) than the control schools.

SWPBS has also been adapted to address bullying in elementary and middle schools through the Bullying Prevention in Positive Behavioral Interventions and Supports (BP-PBIS) which uses the PBIS approach more specifically for bullying in elementary and middle schools. This approach takes the SWPBS principles and makes them specific to bullying and cyberbullying, such as implementing school-wide rules and teaching students how to respond (Good et al., 2011). Studies have found BP-PBIS to lead to reduced bullying and victimization, decreased office discipline referrals and suspensions for bullying, and improved perceptions of safety and school climate (Good et al., 2011; Ross & Horner, 2009).

Social Emotional Learning (SEL) Another approach that can be applied universally to all students in schools is teaching social and emotional skills such as self-awareness, self-management, relationship awareness, and decision-making (Collaborative for Academic, Social, and Emotional Learning [CASEL], 2018). SEL is a school-based preventative approach to promote student resiliency and reduce the risk factors that may contribute to problem behaviors, including bullying perpetration and victimization (Fredrick et al., 2022). Meta-analyses of hundreds of studies of SEL programs have found that they improve academic performance and social competence, as well as decrease disruptive behavior, emotional distress, and suspension rates (Durlak et al., 2011; Taylor et al., 2017). Although SEL is not designed to reduce bullying specifically, there is increasing support that teaching SEL skills can be important contributor to bullying and violence prevention efforts (Fredrick et al., 2022; Nickerson, 2018; Nickerson et al., 2019; Smith & Low, 2013).

SEL skills can be taught even to young children, and early childhood programs often emphasize teaching the whole child, including skills related to recognizing and managing emotions and getting along with others. The Early Childhood Friendship Project (ECFP) is an example of an SEL approach that includes social and emotional skills training, the use of puppets and stories to model problem-solving and resolving conflicts, and using reinforcement in preschool classrooms (Ostrov et al., 2009, 2015). RCTs have revealed that the ECFP leads to reduced relational aggression (Ostrov et al., 2009, 2015) and increased prosocial behavior (Ostrov et al., 2009).

The most well-researched SEL program examining bullying outcomes is Second Step (Committee for Children, 2001, 2008). This classroom SEL curriculum has been shown to reduce bullying by 19.3% after 6 months and 31.4% 1 year later in elementary schools (Frey et al., 2005, 2009). Students in schools who received the intervention compared to those in the control schools were also less likely to accept bullying and were more likely to have positive interactions and assume responsibility as bystanders (Frey et al., 2005). Adults in the intervention schools were also more responsive to bullying incidents than those in the control schools (Frey et al., 2005). In another RCT, Second Step has been found to result in 42% reduced physical aggression after 1 year (Espelage et al., 2013), and lower homophobic name-calling and sexual harassment after 2 years (Espelage et al., 2014). Importantly, the program has also resulted in reduced bullying perpetration for students with disabilities (Espelage et al., 2015). In addition, delinquency decreased in the first 2 years of program implementation, which then drove significant reductions from the first year to the third year in homophobic name-calling, bullying, and cyberbullying.

Targeted and Indicated Prevention for Bullying Perpetrators and Targets

Although universal or primary prevention is the ultimate goal so that youth are taught the crucial skills from a young age that will prevent bullying from occurring, given its prevalence, there is a need for targeted and indicated approaches to intervene with perpetrators and targets of bullying. Most research on bullying prevention and intervention has been conducted at the universal level, but the following section describes approaches used to intervene with bullying perpetration and victimization at an individual level, including the problems associated with these experiences.

Perpetrators Intervening with perpetrators of bullying involves applying appropriate and proportionate consequences for behavior (Thompson & Smith, 2011; Ttofi & Farrington, 2011), as well as teaching and supporting prosocial skills incompatible with bullying (Chin et al., 2012). Garandeau et al. (2014) found that adult intervention through either direct sanctions (e.g., sending a strong message about bullying being wrong and needing to stop) or approaches that engaged perpetrators and bystanders in concern for the target and suggested improvements in the situation stopped bullying in 78% of cases according to reports from victims. The direct sanction approach was more effective for short-term victimization in middle and high school. The latter approach is based on the No-Blame Approach (Support Group Method; Robinson & Maines, 2008) and the Method of Shared Concern (Pikas, 2002) which involves adults meeting with bullying perpetrators and bystanders to communicate concerns, gather additional information about the situation and elicit suggestions for and commitment to making the problem better for the victim. Garandeau et al. found this to be more effective for longer-term victimization and in elementary schools (Garandeau et al., 2014). Allen (2010a, b) implemented and evaluated a very similar method to engaging in shared concern for the victim in a high school, which led to decreased bullying and fear of being bullied, as well as increased disclosures of victimization, more empathy for victims, and improvements in staff knowledge of how to respond to bullying.

Restorative justice approaches are also being used increasingly in schools to address discipline issues (e.g., aggression, bullying) by formulating consequences to repair the harm caused to others (Smith, 2008; Song & Swearer, 2016). Although there is variability in restorative justice approaches, they all include a facilitator who uses a circle that includes the initiator of the process (typically the one who has been targeted by the bullying), others from the school or community (peers, allies, teacher), and the perpetrator(s) in order to explore the harm that occurred, the resulting needs, and the obligations to repair the damage and relationships. Unfortunately, research falls far behind the practice with regard to implementing restorative justice in schools, and its implementation, conceptualization, and effects are quite varied and in need of further study (Song & Swearer, 2016).

Another approach that offers an alternative to more problematic exclusionary school discipline is the Target Bullying Intervention Program (T-BIP; Swearer et al., 2009). In T-BIP, the bullying perpetrator engages in a 3-h session with a mental health professional that includes an assessment and a psychoeducational lesson (e.g., video and teaching about more effective ways of behaving; Strawhun et al., 2013). The professional prepare a follow-up report, meets with parents, and makes recommendations for further intervention. These recommendations are based on the specific areas of concern for the perpetrator (e.g., anger and other aggressive behaviors, hostile attribution bias), as T-BIP is built on the assumption that treating underlying conditions such as internalizing problems, aggression, cognitive distortions, and skill deficits can help reduce bullying behaviors (Swearer et al., 2009).

Targets Youth victimized by bullying are also likely to have other social difficulties with peers, such as rejection and lack of acceptance (Salmivalli et al., 1996). In addition, peers are less likely to assist bullied children who lack friendships or who have social connections with other victims (Boulton et al., 1999; Salmivalli et al., 1997). Indeed, targets of bullying are at higher risk for other forms of victimization (e.g., sexual abuse, sexual harassment, physical and emotional maltreatment), by parents and others (Duncan, 1999; Holt & Espelage, 2003).

Because targets of bullying experience other difficulties with peers, interventions often focus on social skill development or increasing support from peers. Social skills instruction for social withdrawal behavior focuses on teaching children to make friends, increasing positive prosocial strategies, regulating anxiety, and being assertive (Bienert & Schneider, 1995). Group social skills training has been implemented with targets of bullying to increase prosocial beliefs and behaviors, assertiveness, and coping skills (DeRosier, 2010; Hall, 2006). There is some evidence that social skills training can improve self-worth, decrease social anxiety, and increase peer liking of targets of bullying (DeRosier, 2010; Fox & Boulton, 2003), although it may not impact future victimization or social skills (Fox & Boulton, 2003).

Other interventions have focused on increasing peer support for targets of bullying. Cowie and colleagues (Cowie, 1998; Cowie & Wallace, 2000; Naylor & Cowie, 1999; Sharp & Cowie, 1998) evaluated the impact of training peer helpers to offer listening and companionship to children who are targeted by bullying. This training has led to increases in the peer helpers' confidence, sense of responsibility, and communication and improvements in the overall school climate (Cowie, 1998; Naylor & Cowie, 1999). However, training peer helpers has not led to reductions in bullying rates (Menesini et al., 2003; Naylor & Cowie, 1999). In fact, in Ttofi and Farrington's (2011) meta-analysis, many programs using peer-facilitated approaches (e.g., peer-mediation, peer mentoring) resulted in *increased* victimization, possibly because without adult intervention the power dynamics between peers may allow the abuse to continue to become worse.

More success has been found in providing mentorship or support guided by adults. In a study with fourth- and fifth-grade targets of bullying, those paired with college students who visited twice weekly during lunch reported fewer instances of victimization than peers who had not participated (Elledge et al., 2010b). Non-confrontational approaches, adult-led interventions like the support group method, where adults in the school meet with the perpetrators and bystanders (i.e., potential allies to encourage support of the target), have been found to reduce victimization, decrease internalizing symptoms, and increase peers' positive perceptions of targets (Williford et al., 2012). In an exploratory qualitative study of a brief solution-focused support group for early adolescent targets of bullying, Kvarme et al. (2013) found decreased bullying and safety concerns and more peer support as reported by targets after the intervention and at a follow-up.

Interventions for Problems Associated with Bullying

Although beyond the scope of this chapter, perpetrators, and targets of bullying often have mental health or relational difficulties that contribute to or result from the bullying experiences, such as internalizing problems (e.g., anxiety, depression) or externalizing problems (e.g., anger, reactive aggression; see Nickerson & Orrange-Torchia, 2015). Therefore, evidence-based treatment approaches for these problems based on individual needs are very appropriate. For example, cognitive–behavioral interventions have been shown to reduce depression and anxiety symptoms (Albano & Kendall, 2002; Van Starrenburg et al., 2013), and have also resulted in decreased reports of distress and peer relation problems for targets of bullying (McElearney et al., 2013). Perpetrators of bullying and other aggressive behavior may also benefit from cognitive–behavioral therapy programs and techniques (e.g., teaching emotion awareness and recognition, social problem-solving, anger management), which have been shown to reduce anger, aggression, and externalizing behaviors and improve social competence (Lochman et al., 2011; McCart et al., 2006; Sukhodolsky et al., 2004).

For perpetrators of bullying, behavior management strategies may also be helpful. Within a PBIS framework, behavior education programs including daily check-ins, checkouts, and behavioral progress monitoring have been found to be effective (McCurdy et al., 2007). Functional behavioral assessments can also be used to gather systematic information about behavior setting events, antecedents, and consequences to facilitate the development of an individualized behavior intervention plan (BIP) to identify appropriate replacement behaviors, teach alternative skills, change antecedents, and alter consequences in order to reduce problem behaviors (Goh & Bambara, 2012; Steege & Watson, 2003). In addition, one of the most well-established interventions for children with aggressive problems is parent training (Ttofi & Farrington, 2009). For example, The Incredible Years Parent Program has shown to not only improve parenting skills, but also increase children's prosocial behaviors and socioemotional competence, as well as reduce conduct problems (Menting et al., 2013; Posthumus et al., 2012). Although further research is needed to evaluate the effectiveness of these interventions for bullying, in particular, their success with aggression and related problems associated with bullying hold promise in helping to ameliorate this important problem.

References

Albano, A. M., & Kendall, P. C. (2002). Cognitive behavioural therapy for children and adolescents with anxiety disorders: Clinical research advances. *International Review of Psychiatry, 14*, 129–134. https://doi.org/10.1080/09540260220132644

Alberti, J. M. (2001). *Three steps to ending school violence*. Presented at the Pi Lambda Theta Biennial Conference.

Alberti, J. M. (2011). *Guiding philosophy for the Dr. Jean M Alberti center for the prevention of bullying abuse and school violence* [Paper] University at Buffalo, Buffalo.

Alberti, J. M. (2020). *Bullying tree*. Author.

Allanson, P. B., Lester, R. R., & Notar, C. E. (2015). A history of bullying. *International Journal of Education and Social Science, 2*, 31–36. http://www.ijessnet.com/uploades/volumes/1576145463.pdf

Allen, K. P. (2010a). A bullying intervention system: Reducing risk and creating support for aggressive students. *Preventing School Failure, 54*, 199–209. https://doi.org/10.1080/10459880903496289

Allen, K. P. (2010b). A bullying intervention system in high school: A two-year schoolwide follow-up. *Studies in Educational Evaluation, 36*, 83–92. https://doi.org/10.1016/j.stueduc.2011.01.002

Anderson, C. A., & Bushman, B. J. (2002). Human aggression. *Annual Review of Psychology, 53*, 27–51. https://doi.org/10.1146/annurev.psych.53.100901.135231

Axford, N., Bjornstad, G., Clarkson, S., Ukoumunne, O. C., Wrigley, Z., Matthews, J., Berry, V., & Hutchings, J. (2020). The effectiveness of the KiVa Bullying Prevention Program in Wales, UK: Results from a pragmatic cluster randomized controlled trial. *Prevention Science, 21*, 615–626. https://doi.org/10.1007/s11121-020-01103-9

Bagwell, C. L., & Schmidt, M. E. (2011). *Friendships in childhood and adolescence*. Guilford Press.

Baldry, A. C., & Farrington, D. P. (2007). Effectiveness of programs to prevent school bullying. *Victims and Offenders, 2*, 183–204. https://doi.org/10.1080/15564880701263155

Bandura, A. (1977). *Social learning theory*. Prentice Hall.

Bandura, A., Ross, D., & Ross, S. A. (1961). Transmission of aggression through imitation of aggressive models. *Journal of Abnormal and Social Psychology, 63*, 575–582. https://doi.org/10.1037/h0045925

Bauer, N., Lozano, P., & Rivara, F. P. (2007). The effectiveness of the Olweus bullying prevention program in public middle schools: A controlled trial. *Journal of Adolescent Health, 40*, 266–274. https://doi.org/10.1016/j.jadohealth.2006.10.005

Bauman, S., & Yoon, J. (2014). This issue: Theories of bullying and cyberbullying. *Theory Into Practice, 53*, 253–256. https://doi.org/10.1080/00405841.2014.947215

Bergman, B., & Brismar, B. (1994). Hormone levels and personality traits in abusive suicidal male alcoholics. *Alcoholism: Clinical and Experimental Research, 18*, 311–316. https://doi.org/10.1111/j.1530-0277.1994.tb00019.x

Bienert, H., & Schneider, B. H. (1995). Deficit-specific social skills training with peer-nominated aggressive-disruptive and sensitive-isolated preadolescents. *Journal of Clinical Child Psychology, 24*, 287–299. https://doi.org/10.1207/s15374424jccp2403_6

Blumenfeld, W. J. (2005). *Cyberbullying: A variation on an old theme*. Paper, CHI 2005 Abuse Workshop from Portland, OR.

Boulton, M. J., Trueman, M., Chau, C., Whitehead, C., & Amatya, K. (1999). Concurrent and longitudinal links between friendship and peer victimization: Implications for befriending interventions. *Journal of Adolescence, 22*, 461–466. https://doi.org/10.1006/jado.1999.0240

Bowen, G. L., Rose, R. A., & Ware, W. B. (2006). The reliability and validity of the school success profile learning organization measures. *Evaluation and Program Planning, 29*, 97–104. https://doi.org/10.1016/j.evalprogplan.2005.08.005

Bradshaw, C. P. (2015). Translating research to practice in bullying prevention. *American Psychologist, 70*, 322–332. https://doi.org/10.1037/a0039114

Bradshaw, C. P., Koth, C. W., Thornton, L. A., & Leaf, P. J. (2009). Altering school climate through school-wide Positive Behavioral Interventions and Supports: Findings from a group-randomized effectiveness trial. *Prevention Science, 10*, 100–115. https://doi.org/10.1007/s11121-008-0114-9

Bradshaw, C. P., Mitchell, M. M., & Leaf, P. J. (2010). Examining the effects of school-wide positive behavioral interventions and supports on student outcomes: Results from a randomized controlled effectiveness trial in elementary schools. *Journal of Positive Behavior Interventions, 12*, 133–148. https://doi.org/10.1177/1098300709334798

Burk, F. L. (1897). Teasing and bullying. *The Pedagogical Seminary, 4*, 336–371. https://doi.org/10.1080/08919402.1897.10534145

Chin, J. K., Dowdy, E., Jimerson, S. R., & Jeremy Rime, W. (2012). Alternatives to suspensions: Rationale and recommendations. *Journal of School Violence, 11*, 156–173. https://doi.org/10.1080/15388220.2012.652912

Clarkson, S., Charles, J. M., Saville, C. W., Bjornstad, G. J., & Hutchings, J. (2019). Introducing KiVA school-based antibullying programme to the UK: A preliminary evaluation of effectiveness and programme cost. *School Psychology International, 40*(4), 347–365. https://doi.org/10.1177/0143034319841099

Cohen, J., & Brooks, R. (2014). *Confronting school bullying: Kids, culture, and the making of a social problem*. Lynne Rienner.

Collaborative for Academic, Social, and Emotional Learning. (2018). *What is SEL?* https://casel.org/what-is-sel/

Committee for Children. (2001). *Steps to respect: A bullying prevention program*. Author.

Committee for Children. (2008). *Second step: Student success through prevention program*. Author.

Cosgrove, H., & Nickerson, A. B. (2017). Anti-bullying/harassment legislation and educator perceptions of severity, effectiveness, and school climate: A cross-sectional analysis. *Educational Policy, 31*, 518–545. https://doi.org/10.1177/0895904815604217

Cowie, H. (1998). Perspectives of teachers and pupils on the experience of peer support against bullying. *Educational Research and Evaluation, 4*, 108–125. https://doi.org/10.1076/edre.4.2.108.6958

Cowie, H., & Wallace, P. (2000). *Peer support in action: From bystanding to standing by.* Sage Publications.

DeRosier, M. S. (2010). Building relationships and combating bullying: Effectiveness of a school-based social skills group intervention. *Journal of Clinical Child and Adolescent Psychology, 33*, 196–201. https://doi.org/10.1207/S15374424JCCP3301_18

Donegan, R. (2012). Bullying and cyberbullying: History, statistics, law, prevention and analysis. *Elon Journal, 3*, 33–42. https://www.elon.edu/docs/e-web/academics/communications/research/vol3no1/04doneganejspring12.pdf

Duncan, R. D. (1999). Maltreatment by parents and peers: The relationship between child abuse, bully victimization, and psychological distress. *Child Maltreatment, 4*, 45–55. https://doi.org/10.1177/1077559599004001005

Durlak, J. A., Weissberg, R. P., Dymnicki, A. B., Taylor, R. D., & Schellinger, K. B. (2011). The impact of enhancing students' social and emotional learning: A meta-analysis of school-based universal interventions. *Child Development, 82*, 405–432. https://doi.org/10.1111/j.14678624.2010.01564.x

Elledge, L. C., Cavell, T. A., Ogle, N. T., Malcolm, K. T., Newgent, R. A., & Faith, M. A. (2010a). History of peer victimization and children's response to school bullying. *School Psychology Quarterly, 5*, 129–141. https://doi.org/10.1037/a0020313

Elledge, L. C., Cavell, T. A., Ogle, N. T., & Newgent, R. A. (2010b). School-based mentoring as selective prevention for bullied children: A preliminary test. *The Journal of Primary Prevention, 31*, 171–187. https://doi.org/10.1007/s10935-010-0215-7

Espelage, D. L., Low, S., Polanin, J. R., & Brown, E. (2013). The impact of a middle-school program to reduce aggression, victimization, and sexual violence. *Journal of Adolescent Health, 53*, 180–186. https://doi.org/10.1016/j.jadohealth.2013.02.021

Espelage, D. L., Low, S., & Jimerson, S. (2014). Understanding school climate, aggression, peer victimization, and bully perpetration: Contemporary science, practice, and policy. *School Psychology Quarterly, 29*, 233–237. https://doi.org/10.1037/spq0000090

Espelage, D. L., Rose, C. A., & Polanin, J. R. (2015). Social-emotional learning program to reduce bullying, fighting, and victimization among middle school students with disabilities. *Remedial and Special Education, 36*, 299–311. https://doi.org/10.1177/0741932514564564

Evans, C. B. R., & Smokowski, P. R. (2016). Theoretical explanations for bullying in school: How ecological processes propagate perpetration and victimization. *Child and Adolescent Social Work Journal, 33*, 365–375. https://doi.org/10.1007/s10560-015-0432-2

Farrington, D. P., & Ttofi, M. M. (2009). *School-based programs to reduce bullying and victimization.* (Campbell Systematic Reviews No. 6). Campbell Corporation. https://doi.org/10.4073/csr.2009.6

Ferguson, C. J., Miguel, C. S., Kilburn, J. C., & Sanchez, P. (2007). The effectiveness of school-based anti-bullying programs: A meta-analytic review. *Criminal Justice Review, 32*, 401–414. https://doi.org/10.1177/0734016807311712

Fitch, F. J., & Papantonio, A. (1983). Men who batter: Some pertinent characteristics. *Journal of Nervous and Mental Disease, 171*, 190–192. https://doi.org/10.1097/00005053-198303000-00011

Fox, C. L., & Boulton, M. J. (2003). Evaluating the effectiveness of a social skills training (SST) programme for victims of bullying. *Educational Research, 45*, 231–247. https://doi.org/10.1080/0013188032000137238c

Fredrick, S. S., Traudt, S., & Nickerson, A. B. (2022). Social emotional learning practices in schools and bullying prevention. In J. Liew, T. Spinrad, & D. Fisher (Eds.), Encyclopedia of Education. Routledge. https://doi.org/10.4324/9781138609877-REE171-1

Frey, K. S., Hirschstein, M. K., Snell, J. L., Edstrom, L. V., EP, M. K., & Broderick, C. J. (2005). Reducing playground bullying and supporting beliefs: An experimental trial of the Steps to Respect program. *Developmental Psychology, 41*, 479–491. https://doi. org/10.1037/0012-1649.41.3.479

Frey, K. S., Hirschstein, M. K., Edstrom, L. V., & Snell, J. L. (2009). Observed reductions in school bullying, nonbullying aggression and destructive bystander behavior: A longitudinal evaluation. *Journal of Educational Psychology, 101*, 466–481. https://doi.org/10.1037/a0013839

Gaffney, H., Ttofi, M. M., & Farrington, D. P. (2019). Evaluating the effectiveness of school-bullying prevention programs: An updated meta-analytical review. *Aggression and Violent Behavior, 45*, 111–133. https://doi.org/10.1016/j.avb.2018.07.001

Garandeau, C. F., Poskiparta, E., & Salmivalli, C. (2014). Tackling acute cases of school bullying in the KiVa anti-bullying program: A comparison of two approaches. *Journal of Abnormal Child Psychology, 42*, 981–991. https://doi.org/10.1007/s10802-014-9861-1

Gini, G., Pozzoli, T., & Hymel, S. (2014). Moral disengagement among children and youth: A meta-analytic review of links to aggressive behavior. *Aggressive Behavior, 40*, 56–68. https://doi.org/10.1002/ab.21502

Gladden, R. M., Vivolo-Kantor, A. M., Hamburger, M. E., & Lumpki, C. D. (2014). *Bullying surveillance among youth: Uniform definitions for public health and recommended data elements, version 1.0*. National Center for Injury Prevention and Control, Centers for Disease Control and Prevention and U.S. Department of Education.

Goh, A. E., & Bambara, L. M. (2012). Individualized positive behavior support in school settings: A meta-analysis. *Remedial and Special Education, 33*, 271–286. https://doi. org/10.1177/0741932510383990

Good, C. P., McIntosh, K., & Gietz, C. (2011). Integrating bullying prevention into schoolwide positive behavior support. *Teaching Exceptional Children, 44*, 48–56. https://njbullying.org/documents/BullyingPosBehSupports.pdf

Green, V. A., Woods, L., Wegerhoff, D., Harcourt, S., & Tannahill, S. (2019). An evaluation of the KiVa anti-bullying program in New Zealand. *International Journal of Bullying Prevention, 2*(3), 225–237. https://doi.org/10.1007/S42380-019-00034-6

Haataja, A., Voeten, M., Boulton, A. J., Ahtola, A., Poskiparta, E., & Salmivalli, C. (2014). The KiVa antibullying curriculum and outcome: Does fidelity matter? *Journal of School Psychology, 52*, 479–493. https://doi.org/10.1016/j.jsp.2014.07.001

Hall, K. R. (2006). Using problem-based learning with victims of bullying behavior. *Professional School Counseling, 9*, 231–237.

Hall, W. (2017). The effectiveness of policy interventions for school bullying: A systematic review. *Journal of the Society for Social Work and Research, 8*, 45–69. https://doi.org/10.1086/690565

Hatzenbuehler, M., Schwab-Reese, L., Ranapurwala, S. I., Hertz, M. F., & Ramirez, M. R. (2015). Associations between antibullying policies and bullying in 25 states. *JAMA Pediatrics, 169*(10), e152411. https://doi.org/10.1001/jamapediatrics.2015.2411

Hawley, P. H., & Williford, A. (2015). Articulating the theory of bullying intervention programs: Views from social psychology, social work, and organizational science. *Journal of Applied Developmental Psychology, 37*, 3–15. https://doi.org/10.1016/j.appdev.2014.11.006

Hinduja, S., & Patchin, J. W. (2014). *Bullying beyond the schoolyard: Preventing and responding to cyberbullying*. Corwin.

Holt, M. K., & Espelage, D. L. (2003). A cluster analytic investigation of victimization among high school students: Are profiles differentially associated with psychological symptoms and school belonging? *Journal of Applied School Psychology, 19*, 81–98. https://doi.org/10.1300/J008v19n02_06

Hong, J. S., & Espelage, D. L. (2012). A review of research on bullying and peer victimization in school: An ecological system analysis. *Aggression and Violent Behavior, 17*, 311–322. https://doi.org/10.1016/j.avb.2012.03.003

Horner, R. H., Sugai, G., Smolkowski, K., Eber, L., Nakasato, J., Todd, A. W., & Esperanza, J. (2009). A randomized, wait-list controlled effectiveness trial assessing school-wide positive behavior support in elementary schools. *Journal of Positive Behavior Interventions, 11*, 133–144. https://doi.org/10.1177/1098300709332067

Horton, P. (2014). Portraying monsters: Framing school bullying through a macro lens. *Discourse: Studies in the Cultural Politics of Education, 37*, 204–214. https://doi.org/10.1080/0159630 6.2014.951833

Horton, P., & Forsberg, C. (2015). Essays on school bullying: Theoretical perspectives on a contemporary problem. *Confero: Essays on Education, Philosophy and Politics, 3*, 6–16. https://doi.org/10.3384/confer.2001-4562.1501988

Huang, Y., Espelage, D. L., Polanin, J. R., & Hong, J. S. (2019). A meta-analytic review of school-based anti-bullying programs with a parent component. *International Journal of Bullying Prevention, 1*, 32–44. https://doi.org/10.1007/s42380-018-0002-1

Hymel, S., & Bonanno, R. A. (2014). Moral disengagement processes in bullying. *Theory Into Practice, 53*, 278–285. https://doi.org/10.1080/00405841.2014.947219

Hymel, S., McClure, R., Miller, M., Shumka, E., & Trach, J. (2014). Addressing school bullying: Insights from theories of group processes. *Journal of Applied Developmental Psychology, 37*, 16–24. https://doi.org/10.17105/15-0133.1

Kärnä, A., Voeten, M., Little, T. D., Poskiparta, E., Alanen, E., & Salmivalli, C. (2011). Going to scale: A nonrandomized nationwide trial of the KiVa antibullying program for grades 1–9. *Journal of Consulting and Clinical Psychology, 79*, 796–805. https://doi.org/10.1037/a0025740

Kern, L., George, M. P., & Weist, M. D. (2016). *Supporting students with emotional and behavioral problems: Prevention and intervention strategies*. Paul H. Brookes Publishing.

Koo, H. (2007). A time line of the evolution of school bullying in differing social contexts. *Asia Pacific Education Review, 8*, 107–116. https://files.eric.ed.gov/fulltext/EJ768971.pdf

Kruger, K. J., & Valltos, N. G. (2002). Dealing with domestic violence in law enforcement relationships. *FBI Law Enforcement Bulletin, 71*, 1–7. https://www.ncjrs.gov/App/Publications/abstract.aspx?ID=195903

Kvarme, L. G., Aabø, L. S., & Sæteren, B. (2013) "I feel I mean something to someone": solution-focused brief therapy support groups for bullied schoolchildren. Educational Psychology in Practice: Theory, *Research and Practice in Educational Psychology, 29*(4), 416–431. https://doi.org/10.1080/02667363.2013.859569

Langos, C. (2012). Cyberbullying: The challenge to define. *Cyberpsychology, Behavior and Social Networking, 15*, 285–289. https://doi.org/10.1089/cyber.2011.0588

Larkin, R. W. (2009). The columbine legacy: Rampage shootings as political acts. *American Behavioral Scientist, 52*, 1309–1326. https://doi.org/10.1177/0002764209332548

Lee, C. H., & Song, J. (2012). Functions of parental involvement and effects of school climate on bullying behaviors among South Korean middle school students. *Journal of Interpersonal Violence, 27*, 2437–2464. https://doi.org/10.1177/0886260511433508

Limber, S. P., Nation, M., Tracy, A. J., Melton, G. B., & Flerx, V. (2004). Implementation of the Olweus bullying prevention program in the southeastern United States. In P. K. Smith, D. Pepler, & K. Rigby (Eds.), *Bullying in schools: How successful can interventions be?* (pp. 55–79). Cambridge University Press.

Limber, S. P., Olweus, D., Wang, W., Masiello, M., & Breivik, K. (2018). Evaluation of the Olweus bullying prevention program: A large-scale study of U.S. students in grades 3-11. *Journal of School Psychology, 69*, 56–72. https://doi.org/10.1016/j.jsp.2018.04.004

Lochman, J. E., Powell, N. P., Boxmeyer, C. L., & Jimenez-Camargo, L. (2011). Cognitive-behavioral therapy for externalizing disorders in children and adolescents. *Child and Adolescent Psychiatric Clinics of North America, 20*, 305–318. https://doi.org/10.1016/j.chc.2011.01.005

McCart, M. R., Priester, P. E., Davies, W. H., & Azen, R. (2006). Differential effectiveness of behavioral parent training and cognitive-behavioral therapy for antisocial youth: A meta-analysis. *Journal of Abnormal Child Psychology, 34*, 527–543. https://doi.org/10.1007/s10802-006-9031-1

McCurdy, B. L., Kunsch, C., & Reibstein, S. (2007). Secondary prevention in the urban school: Implementing the behavior education program. *Preventing School Failure: Alternative Education for Children and Youth, 51*(3), 12–19. https://doi.org/10.3200/PSFL.51.3.12-19

McElearney, A., Adamson, G., Shevlin, M., & Bunting, B. (2013). Impact evaluation of a school-based counselling intervention in Northern Ireland: Is it effective for pupils who have been bullied? *Child Care in Practice, 19*(1), 4–22. https://doi.org/10.1080/13575279.2012.732557

McIntosh, K., & Lane, K. L. (2019). Advances in measurement in school-wide positive behavioral interventions and supports. *Remedial and Special Education, 40*, 3–5. https://doi.org/10.1177/0741932518800388

Menesini, E., Codecasa, E., Benelli, B., & Cowie, H. (2003). Enhancing children's responsibility to take action against bullying: Evaluation of a befriending intervention in Italian middle schools. *Aggressive Behavior, 29*, 1–14. https://doi.org/10.1002/ab.80012

Menting, A. T. A., de Castro, B. O., & Matthys, W. (2013). Effectiveness of the Incredible Years parent training to modify disruptive and prosocial child behavior: A meta-analytic review. *Clinical Psychology Review, 33*, 901–913. https://doi.org/10.1016/j.cpr.2013.07.006

Merrell, K. W., Gueldner, B. A., Ross, S. W., & Isava, D. M. (2008). How effective are school bullying intervention programs? A meta-analysis of intervention research. *School Psychology Quarterly, 23*, 26–42. https://doi.org/10.1037/1045-3830.23.1.26

Monks, C. P., & Coyne, I. (2011). *Bullying in different contexts*. Cambridge University Press.

Naito, T., & Gielen, U. P. (2005). Bullying and ijime in Japanese schools: A sociocultural perspective. In F. L. Denmark, H. H. Krauss, R. W. Wesner, E. Midlarsky, & U. P. Gielen (Eds.), *Violence in schools: Cross-national and cross-cultural perspectives* (pp. 169–190). Springer.

National Domestic Violence Hotline online. (n.d.). *What is domestic violence?* https://www.thehotline.org/is-this-abuse/abuse-defined/

Naylor, P., & Cowie, H. (1999). The effectiveness of peer support systems in challenging school bullying: The perspectives and experiences of teachers and pupils. *Journal of Adolescence, 22*, 467–479. https://doi.org/10.1006/jado.1999.0241

Nese, R. N., Horner, R. H., Dickey, C. R., Stiller, B., & Tomlanovich, A. (2014). Decreasing bullying behavior in middle school: Expect respect. *School Psychology Quarterly, 29*, 272–286. https://doi.org/10.1037/spq0000070

Nickerson, A. B. (2017). Preventing and intervening with bullying in schools: A framework for evidence-based practice. *School Mental Health, 11*, 15–28. https://doi.org/10.1007/s12310-017-9221-8

Nickerson, A. B. (2018). Can SEL reduce school violence? *Educational Leadership, 76*, 46–50. http://www.ascd.org/publications/educational-leadership/oct18/vol76/num02/Can-SEL-Reduce-School-Violence%C2%A2.aspx

Nickerson, A. B., & Orrange-Torchia, T. (2015). The mental health impact of bullying. In P. Goldblum, D. Espelage, J. Chu, & B. Bongar (Eds.), *The challenges of youth bullying and suicide* (pp. 39–49). Oxford University Press.

Nickerson, A. B., & Parks, T. (2021). Preventing bullying in schools. In P. J. Lazarus, S. Suldo, & B. Doll (Eds.), *Fostering the emotional well-being of our youth: A school-based approach* (pp. 338–354). Oxford University Press. https://doi.org/10.1093/med-psych/9780190918873.003.0017

Nickerson, A. B., Cornell, D. G., Smith, J. D., & Furlong, M. J. (2013). School antibullying efforts: Advice for policymakers. *Journal of School Violence, 12*, 68–282. https://doi.org/10.1080/15388220.2013.787366

Nickerson, A. B., Fredrick, S. S., Allen, K. P., & Jenkins, L. N. (2019). Social emotional learning (SEL) practices in schools: Effects on perceptions of bullying victimization. *Journal of School Psychology, 73*, 74–88. https://doi.org/10.1016/j.jsp.2019.03.002

Nocentini, A., & Menesini, E. (2016). KiVa anti-bullying program in Italy: Evidence of effectiveness in a randomized controlled trial. *Prevention Science, 17*, 1012–1023. https://doi.org/10.1007/s11121-016-0690-z

Noltemeyer, A., Palmer, K., James, A. G., & Wiechman, S. (2019). School-wide positive behavioral interventions and supports (SW-PBIS): A synthesis of existing research. *International Journal of School and Educational Psychology, 7*, 253–262. https://doi.org/10.1080/21683603.2018.1425169

Olweus, D. (1978). *Aggression in the schools: Bullies and whipping boys*. Hemisphere.

Olweus, D. (1993). *Bullying at school: What we know and what we can do*. Blackwell.

Olweus, D., Limber, S., & Mihalic, S. (1999). *The bullying prevention program: Blueprints for violence prevention*. Center for the Study and Prevention of Violence.

Olweus, D., Limber, S. P., & Breivik, K. (2019). Addressing specific forms of bullying: A large scale evaluation of the Olweus bullying prevention program. *International Journal of Bullying Prevention, 1*, 70–84. https://doi.org/10.1007/s42380-019-00009-7

Ostrov, J. M., Massetti, G. M., Stauffacher, K., Godleski, S. A., Hart, K. C., Karch, K. M., Mullins, A. D., & Ries, E. E. (2009). An intervention for relational and physical aggression in early childhood: A preliminary study. *Early Childhood Research Quarterly, 24*, 15–28. https://doi.org/10.1016/j.ecresq.2008.08.002

Ostrov, J. M., Godleski, S. A., Kamper-DeMarco, K. E., Blakely-McClure, S. J., & Celenza, L. (2015). Replication and extension of the early childhood friendship project: Effects of physical and relational bullying. *School Psychology Review, 44*, 445–463. https://doi.org/10.17105/spr-15-0048.1

Paluck, E. L. (2011). Peer pressure against prejudice: A high school field experiment examining social network change. *Journal of Experimental Social Psychology, 47*, 350–358. https://doi.org/10.1016/j.jesp.2010.11.017

Paluck, E. L., & Shepherd, H. (2012). The salience of social referents: A field experiment on collective norms and harassment behavior in a school social network. *Journal of Personality and Social Psychology, 103*, 899–915. https://doi.org/10.1037/a0030015

Pikas, A. (2002). New developments of the shared concern model. *School Psychology International, 23*, 307–326. https://doi.org/10.1177/0143034302023003234

Piotrowski, D., & Hoot, J. (2008). Bullying and violence in schools: What teachers should know and do. *Childhood Education, 84*, 357–363. https://doi.org/10.1080/000904056.2008.10523043

Pokin, S. (2007). Megan's story. *Megan meier foundation.* https://www.meganmeierfoundation.org/megans-story

Polanin, J. R., Espelage, D. L., & Pigott, T. D. (2012). A meta-analysis of school-based bullying prevention programs' effects on bystander intervention behavior. *School Psychology Review, 41*, 1–19. https://doi.org/10.3102/0034654316632061

Posthumus, J. A., Raaijmakers, M. A., Maassen, G. H., Van Engeland, H., & Matthys, W. (2012). Sustained effects of incredible years as a preventive intervention in preschool children with conduct problems. *Abnormal Child Psychology, 40*, 487–500. https://doi.org/10.1007/s10802-011-9580-9

Rigby, Ken, Peter K. Smith, and Debra Pepler. 2004. "Working to prevent school bullying: Key issues." In Peter K. Smith, Debra Pepler, and Ken Rigby Bullying in schools: How successful can interventions be?, 1–12. : Cambridge University Press.

Robinson, G., & Maines, B. (2008). *Bullying: A complete guide to the support group method*. Sage.

Rodkin, P. C., & Berger, C. (2008). Who bullies whom? Social status asymmetries by victim gender. *International Journal of Behavioral Development, 32*, 473–486. https://doi.org/10.1177/0165025408093667

Ross, S. W., & Horner, R. H. (2009). Bully prevention in positive behavior support. *Journal of Applied Behavior Analysis, 42*, 747–759. https://doi.org/10.1901/jaba.2009.42-747

Sabia, J. J., & Bass, B. (2017). Do anti-bullying laws work? New evidence on school safety and youth violence. *Journal of Population Economics, 30*, 473–502. https://doi.org/10.1007/s00148-016-0622-z

Sakai, T. (1985). Child welfare in Japan today. *Japan Quarterly, 32*, 18–22. http://www.worldcat.org/title/japan-quarterly/oclc/1754204

Salmivalli, C., Lagerspetz, K., Björkqvist, K., Österman, K., & Kaukiainen, A. (1996). Bullying as a group process: Participant roles and their relations to social status within the group. *Aggressive Behavior, 22*, 1–15. https://doi.org/10.1002/(SICI)1098-2337

Salmivalli, C., Huttunen, A., & Lagerspetz, K. M. J. (1997). Peer networks and bullying in schools. *Scandinavian Journal of Psychology, 38*, 305–312. https://doi.org/10.1111/1467-9450.00040

Seo, Y. N., Leather, P., & Coyne, I. (2012). South Korean culture and history: The implications for workplace bullying. *Aggression and Violent Behavior, 17*, 419–422. https://doi.org/10.1016/j. avb.2012.05.003

Sercombe, H., & Donnelly, B. (2013). Bullying and agency: Definition, intervention and ethics. *Journal of Youth Studies, 16*, 491–502. https://doi.org/10.1080/13676261.2012.725834

Sharp, S., & Cowie, H. (1998). *Counselling and supporting children in distress.* Sage Publications.

Slee, P. T., & Skrzypiec, G. (2016). Bullying and victimization: A global perspective. In *Well-being, positive peer relations and bullying in school settings.* Springer.

Smith, J. D. (2008). Promoting a positive school climate: Restorative practices for the classroom. In D. Pepler & W. Craig (Eds.), *An international perspective on understanding and addressing bullying, PREVNet series* (Vol. 1, pp. 132–143). PREVNet.

Smith, B. H., & Low, S. (2013). The role of social-emotional learning in bullying prevention efforts. *Theory Into Practice, 52*, 280–287. https://doi.org/10.1080/00405841.2013.829731

Smith, J. D., Schneider, B., Smith, P. K., & Ananiadou, K. (2004). The effectiveness of whole-school anti-bullying programs: A synthesis of evaluation research. *School Psychology Review, 33*, 548–561. https://eric.ed.gov/?id=EJ683748

Song, S. Y., & Swearer, S. M. (2016). The cart before the horse: The challenge and promise of restorative justice consultation in schools. *Journal of Educational and Psychological Consultation, 26*, 313–324. https://doi.org/10.1080/10474412.2016.1246972

Sprague, J. R., & Horner, R. H. (2012). School-wide positive behavioral interventions and supports: Proven practices and future directions. In S. R. Jimerson, A. B. Nickerson, M. J. Mayer, & M. J. Furlong (Eds.), *Handbook of school violence and school safety: International research and practice* (pp. 447–462). Taylor and Francis.

Steege, M. W., & Watson, T. S. (2003). *Conducting school-based functional behavior assessments: A practitioner's guide.* Guilford Press.

Strawhun, J., Fluke, S., & Peterson, R. (2013). *The target bullying intervention program [Program brief].* Student Engagement Project, University of Nebraska–Lincoln and the Nebraska Department of Education.

Sugai, G., & Horner, R. (2006). A promising approach for expanding and sustaining school-wide positive behavior support. *School Psychology Review, 35*, 245–259. https://www.icareby.org/sites/www.icareby.org/files/spr352sugai.pdf

Sukhodolsky, D. G., Kassinove, H., & Gorman, B. S. (2004). Cognitive-behavioral therapy for anger in children and adolescents: A meta-analysis. *Aggression and Violent Behavior, 9*, 247–269. https://doi.org/10.1016/j.avb.2003.08.005

Swearer, S. M., & Espelage, D. L. (2004). Introduction: A social-ecological framework of bullying among youth. In D. L. Espelage & S. M. Swearer (Eds.), *Bullying in American schools: A social-ecological perspective on prevention and intervention.* Lawrence Erlbaum Associates.

Swearer, S. M., & Hymel, S. (2015). Understanding the psychology of bullying: Moving toward a social-ecological diathesis-stress model. *American Psychologist, 70*, 344–353. https://doi.org/10.1037/a0038929

Swearer, S. M., Espelage, D. L., & Napolitano, S. A. (2009). *Bullying prevention and intervention: Realistic strategies for schools.* Guilford.

Swearer, S. M., Wang, C., Berry, B., & Myers, Z. R. (2014). Reducing bullying: Application of social cognitive theory. *Theory Into Practice, 53*, 271–277. https://doi.org/10.1080/00405841.2014.947221

Takatoku, S. (1999). *Ijime mondai handobukku.* [Handbook of bullying problems]. Translated by Takashi Naito and Uwe P. Gielen. Tsugeshyoboushinshya.

Taylor, R. D., Oberle, E., Durlak, J. A., & Weissberg, R. P. (2017). Promoting positive youth development through school-based social and emotional learning interventions: A meta-analysis of follow-up effects. *Child Development, 88*, 1156–1171. https://doi.org/10.1111/cdev.12864

Thompson, F., & Smith, P. K. (2011). *The use and effectiveness of anti-bullying strategies in schools. DFE-RR098.* Department for Education.

Ttofi, M. M., & Farrington, D. P. (2009). What works in preventing bullying: Effective elements of anti-bullying programmes. *Journal of Aggression, Conflict, and Peace Research, 1*, 13–24. https://doi.org/10.1108/17596599200900003

Ttofi, M. M., & Farrington, D. P. (2011). Effectiveness of school-based programs to reduce bullying: A systematic and meta-analytic review. *Journal of Experimental Criminology, 7*, 27–56. https://doi.org/10.1007/s11292-101-9109-1

Vaillancourt, T., & Hymel, S. (2006). Aggression and social status: The moderating roles of sex and peer-valued characteristics. *Aggressive Behavior, 32*, 396–408. https://doi.org/10.1002/ab.20138

Van Starrenburg, M. L., Kuijpers, R. C., Hutschemaekers, G. J., & Engels, R. C. (2013). Effectiveness and underlying mechanisms of a group-based cognitive behavioural therapy-based indicative prevention program for children with elevated anxiety levels. *BMC Psychiatry, 13*, 183. https://doi.org/10.1186/1471-244X-13-183

Waasdorp, T. E., Bradshaw, C. P., & Leaf, P. J. (2012). The impact of schoolwide positive behavioral interventions and supports on bullying and peer rejection: A randomized controlled effectiveness trial. *Archives of Pediatrics & Adolescent Medicine, 166*, 149–156. https://doi.org/10.1001/archpediatrics.2011.755

Williams, B. D. (2014). *Federal efforts on bullying in schools* (Master's thesis). John Hopkins University, Baltimore, Maryland.

Williford, A., Boulton, A., Noland, B., Little, T. D., Antti, K., & Salmivalli, C. (2012). Effects of the KiVa anti-bullying program on adolescents' depression, anxiety, and perception of peers. *Journal of Abnormal Child Psychology, 40*, 289–300. https://doi.org/10.1007/s10802-011-9562-y

Yeager, D. S., Fong, C., Lee, H. Y., & Espelage, D. (2015). Declines in efficacy or anti-bullying programs among older adolescents: Theory and a three-level meta-analysis. *Journal of Applied Developmental Psychology, 37*, 36–51. https://doi.org/10.1016/j.appdev.2014.11.005

Chapter 22
Mindfulness Strategies for Primary Prevention

Brian Simmons

Introduction

No textbook on school violence would be complete without a serious consideration of the role of mindfulness. Yet, there is an inescapable irony to my authoring a chapter on the topic. On the one hand, I am a seasoned educator who pioneered the use of mindfulness as a classroom teacher for many years, and later implemented it to significantly lower school violence as the head of discipline at a public High School for inner-city kids in Manhattan, and then as Assistant Principal of School Culture and Climate in a suburban High School suffering the painful aftermath of a violent student tragedy just a few months before my arrival. But long before all that, I was a kid with a penchant for fistfighting. Much to the chagrin of my teachers and parents, many of these early incidents occurred in classrooms, lunchrooms, and playgrounds, depending on who or what was pushing my buttons on any given day. What I would have loved to have known back in the 1980s is that there was a way to harness impulsive reactions to unpleasant feelings and situations and that there were more options available to me than the narrow ones that I could see in the moment. Mindfulness is one way. After developing an intensive personal meditation practice since the 1990s, under the careful training of some of the most credible mindfulness teachers on earth, I can say with certainty that it is a potent one.

B. Simmons (✉)
New York Insight Meditation Center, New York, NY, USA

Mount Vernon High School, Mount Vernon City School District, Mount Vernon, NY, USA
e-mail: brian@brian-simmons.org

© The Author(s), under exclusive license to Springer Nature   513
Switzerland AG 2023
T. W. Miller (ed.), *School Violence and Primary Prevention*,
https://doi.org/10.1007/978-3-031-13134-9_22

The March of Mindfulness

The emergence of mindfulness, with roots in Ancient India, has been exploding through the West for the past four decades, gaining speed, traction, and scientific validity with each passing year. Once considered the folly of the hippie generation seeking new modes of ecstasy and spiritual transcendence, mindfulness is now considered a legitimate endeavor by everyday people, one worthy of serious investment by scientists, CEOs, physicians, and entrepreneurs alike. It is blazing a fast trail through the hard sectors of science, technology, health care, and business. Yet, nowhere is the promise and hope of mindfulness more evident than in classrooms across America.

From the hardscrabble inner-city schools of New York City and Los Angeles to quaint suburbs and sprawling cities across America, mindfulness is increasingly becoming a buzzword in education. With its promise of promoting well-being, calm, and even higher academic outcomes, educators are betting on mindfulness to tackle an increasing number of challenges. Among them are student attention, the negative effects of heightened technology consumption, emotional regulation, and lowering school violence. This is all without mentioning the massive potential to benefit in myriad ways the teachers, administrators, and support staff charged with serving students and their families while also navigating sweeping educational reforms and the pressures of high-stakes testing and increasingly stringent measures of teacher evaluation. In short, educators are hoping that mindfulness can help everybody.

Periods of scheduled inner reflection time, meditation classes, wellness assemblies, after-school stress reduction programs, and school-wide mindfulness breaks are becoming the norm in many schools. The hope amongst school leaders is that these low-cost interventions can help to level the achievement gap, differentiate instruction for learners with different needs and abilities, build community and provide social and emotional learning for young people facing unparalleled stress in an age of unprecedented distractions. Yet, what is mindfulness?

What Is Mindfulness?

According to Dr. Jon Kabat-Zinn, mindfulness is "the awareness that arises from paying attention, on purpose, in the present moment and non-judgmentally" (Kabat-Zinn, 2003). This ability to harness one's attention "on purpose" is a skill that can be developed and deepened over time. You might say that mindfulness is a training of the mind, where presence is achieved by bringing the mind's attention back to the present moment repeatedly over the course of time. In order to pay attention to the present moment, one must focus one's attention on the things that are occurring in the present moment at any given point in time. These "objects" of attention can be sights, sounds, physical sensations, breathing patterns, moods, feelings, and even thoughts. One simply brings one's attention back to the mindfulness object each time it slips into mental distractions and preoccupations. Over the course of time, the mind can become still and settled. Yet calmness is only one benefit.

The ability to see clearly is one of the hallmarks of mindfulness. It reflects things without distortions, much like a pristine mirror. This clarity allows for a person to make better assessments and decisions, and not act upon destructive impulses that are often triggered in educational settings. The "non-judgmental" awareness allows for feelings and situations to be known and felt without automatically being pulled into cycles of reactivity. It is clear how this ability to see clearly and not act out of impulse would be a valuable skill for students to learn in school. Most acts of violence in schools are born out of emotional reactivity in the heat of the moment. Mindfulness is a powerful antidote as it provides clarity and context to complex feelings which ultimately allows for better decisions and healthier relationships. Amazing, that a practice as simple as meditation can offer such promise. Yet, mindfulness is far more than meditation.

Mindfulness Versus Meditation

One of the most common misconceptions about mindfulness is that it is a mind state that is limited to periods of formal meditation practice. Yet mindfulness has more profound potential than an isolated mind state experienced during scheduled periods of the day when we take a few minutes to sit or lie down with our eyes closed. Rather, Mindfulness is a portable awareness that can be honed and developed during formal meditation practice and utilized informally throughout the rest of the day in any situation we find ourselves in. You might say meditation is the training ground where we intentionally develop mindfulness on purpose. Yet, the practical value of mindfulness is that it can be employed during the most challenging and stressful times of our day. Rather than making unpleasant feelings vanish, mindfulness allows us to engage with difficult emotions in ways that are honest and provide clarity, equanimity, and appropriate options for action or non-action. This measured restraint is central to the lowering of violence in schools.

Another common misconception is that the purpose of mindfulness is to conquer unpleasant experiences by creating pleasant feelings of bliss or happiness. While it is possible that under certain conditions mindfulness practice may incline the mind to pleasurable experiences, this will frequently not happen and is certainly not the point. In fact, meditation practice can often be difficult or painful! The promise of mindfulness is far more humble and profound than feeling good. Rather than making bad feelings disappear, or contrive happier ones in their place, the goal of mindfulness is to ground ourselves in the truth of the moment, which is often painful. This intentional grounding is a precursor to the development of resilience and inner fortitude. Mindfulness provides us the clarity and balance to engage with the full range of human emotions we could ever experience without needing them to be different from how they are. It changes how we relate to our experience, which provides us with greater power, resilience, and self-determination. The intention of mindfulness is to understand what is happening as it is happening without getting pulled into the current of strong feelings. This is what is meant by *non-judgmental awareness*.

Mindfulness makes no preference of experience. Its only goal is to see clearly into the nature of what is happening in each moment: a thought, an emotion, a bodily sensation, or an impulse. Through seeing clearly, we are able to navigate a straight path through discomfort, and even injustice, by remaining clearheaded and aware of the consequences of our actions on others, regardless of their actions on us. In this way, we remain more effective under trying circumstances. Rather than turning us into passing victims of circumstance on the one hand, or lost in destructive reactivity patterns on the other, mindfulness refines our view of the situation we find ourselves in and empowers us to adjust, adapt and respond intelligently to injustice through reasoned actions informed by dignity and a strong commitment to justice. The ability to tune in to what is happening inside of themselves and outside of themselves in real-time provides students with a sense of agency over their habitual reactions and lowers the likelihood of blind reactivity and violence. Not surprising, since the foundation of mindfulness comes from a history of non-harm.

The Origins of Mindfulness and Non-Violence

Many spiritual traditions have some form of contemplative practice at the center of their faith to promote harmony for the group and relief from stress and suffering for the individual. The roots of Mindfulness stem back 2600 years to Southeast Asia. From its earliest inception, mindfulness was considered a powerful technology amongst ancient Buddhists for the cultivation of peace, non-harm, and personal liberation. The Sanskrit term *Ahimsa* refers to non-violence and respect for all living things and was a central aim of mindfulness practice. It was thought that Mindfulness was a highly refined method to tame the destructive impulses of the human mind and cultivate a sense of goodwill and compassion toward others in the community. This orientation created social order and cohesion. Rather than a solitary practice to exclusively benefit the self, as is sometimes emphasized in modern applications, the original teachings of mindfulness were contained in a much larger canon and doctrine of practices that promoted peace and harmony for the entire community. More than a standalone practice, mindfulness was viewed as a path to live one's entire life and a roadmap for how to show up in the world. Even though the modern secular view of mindfulness often leaves out a great deal of the original context, the potential for mindfulness to develop habits of social harmony remain.

Mindfulness and Ethics

The original training on mindfulness were paired with teachers on moral conditioning. This meant that mindfulness was never excluded from the development of wholesome behavior, speech, and action in the pursuit of other benefits. In fact, they could not be understood apart from one another. When an ancient Buddhist student was learning mindfulness, it was generally preceded by teachings on generosity and living one's life in a way that was primarily kind, compassionate, and beneficial to others as much to oneself. From a technical point of view, this makes perfect sense. Mindfulness allows us to observe our intentions and motivations in the present moment before speaking or acting. This clarity allows us the chance to redirect our words or actions in ways that de-escalate conflict and promote well-being. If we act in ways that cause tension, we will inevitably sow the seeds of regret, and it will therefore be harder to concentrate the mind in meditation. This will work against the development of mindfulness, and short-circuit our progress and benefits. Therefore, harm to others works against our own self-interest. Yet, from a common-sense view, it is clear that acting out of harm works contrary to the spirit of mindfulness. I raise this point early on because mindfulness should not be considered an isolated technique to troubleshoot academic and behavioral problems. Rather, it is meant as a holistic approach to the moral development of a person and community. This ancient awareness practice provides a powerful example and history to positively shape the culture of a school building toward collaboration and away from violence. Yet, how can this happen?

Equity

A major focus of education in America is leveling the Achievement Gap between students of different income levels, disabilities, geographies, races, sexual orientations, and gender identities. In this way, schools are the front lines of the social inequities, evils, and injustices plaguing the nation at large. These injustices frequently unfold in schools and reflect inequitable funding and allocation of resources, not to mention the negative views different members of groups may harbor toward other groups. Yet, the primary role of any educator is to provide the resources for all students to be successful based on their individual needs in order to level the playing field. This is the essence of equity.

This conundrum is compounded by social unrest in response to perceived law enforcement inequities erupting in cities, streets, and screens across the nation. The result is a country divided along lines of race and resources with our most precious national commodity, our students, caught in the cross-hairs. These conflicts frequently unfold within school buildings and can cause mistrust between students and teachers, and at times, violence amongst students.

Cultural Awareness and Responsiveness

Cultural awareness and inclusion are commonly the go-to strategies to bridge this divide within school buildings and districts. These efforts promote tolerance and understanding through targeted efforts such as diversity initiatives, heritage celebrations, and other well-meaning efforts to unite school communities. In classrooms, teachers provide culturally relevant resources and assessments to differentiate learning for all students. Student-centered approaches to instruction transfer learning to the hands of students and allow them to authentically relate to materials from their own diverse cultural experiences in ways that are rich and empowering. Open and candid conversations around race, equity, and intolerance in classrooms can often be uncomfortable for both teachers and students, yet are highly effective opportunities to set norms and share values of respect and inclusion.

All of these strategies serve as precursors to promote civic responsibility and social activism where students are empowered to learn about injustice and to take action in order to promote equitable conditions for a better school and society. These efforts strike at the heart of lowering violence. Yet, doing so takes considerable courage and resilience.

This is where mindfulness has a significant role to play, in concert with an *equity consciousness*, for an even greater impact. While cultural awareness has traditionally limited focus to diversity and inclusion, mindfulness purposefully embedded into a school community provides even greater potential for positive outcomes. Perhaps what is needed most to lower violence is a more fundamental change of thinking in education – a paradigm shift from "cultural awareness" to a *Culture of Awareness*.

A Culture *of* Awareness

Years ago I created the concept a *Culture of Awareness* is to define a school climate that develops, nurtures, and weaves the clinical benefits of mindfulness into the fabric of School Culture, alongside an *equity consciousness*, that allows for all students to succeed. It celebrates the values of inclusion as outlined above, and combines it with purposeful awareness of one's inner experience and the outer world. In this expanded vision of cultural awareness, all stakeholders in a school community aspire to be active stewards of how they show up each moment with each other based on mindfulness and meditation training, with its deep roots in presence, wisdom, compassion, and non-harm.

This combination has the power to shift how all members of a school community relate to their own unfolding experience in each moment (thoughts, feelings, moods, etc.), as well as to the diverse experiences of others they are sharing space with. Over the course of time, it redefines how students and teachers navigate the sticky waters of cultural differences through curiosity, respect, restraint, and mindful speech. And it offers the promise to lower the rate of conflict and violence in school. For an entire school community to shift in this direction, mindfulness training must be authentically provided, practiced together, reinforced on a regular basis, and bought in by all stakeholders involved. But how?

Building a Culture of Awareness

Mindfulness Training for Students

In order for students to develop the skills of mindful awareness, quality instruction and guidance must be authentically provided by qualified teachers or other professionals trained in mindfulness from within the school, or visiting partners from outside the school community. Such instruction can be offered in a variety of structures and settings, each with its own benefits and drawbacks.

Afterschool mindfulness programs allow the opportunity for students to connect with others in a social atmosphere and develop relationships with likeminded peers willing to stay after school hours and commit to learning and practicing the skills of meditation and stress reduction. A major benefit of this approach is that students who show up for this kind of voluntary program tend to be very committed and take the initiative more seriously. This combination can make for a richer and more rewarding learning opportunity, which tends to produce better and more lasting results. Students in these programs also tend to serve as strong support partners for each other based on the shared values of growth, self-reflection, and non-harm. These relationships often extend to the school day, deepen over time, and silently serve against the forces of conflict and violence. Yet, the downside of this approach is that the numbers of interested students tend to be somewhat limited, and are generally reserved for older students in middle or high school.

Another approach to providing mindfulness in a school is the offering of *curriculum-based mindfulness courses* scheduled within the school day. In these classes, sometimes accredited, there is more time and space provided for students to take a deeper dive into mindful practices, on a daily or semi-weekly basis, over the course of a semester or year. I have personally found semi-weekly courses to be much better received by students. The day off in between classes gives students more time to digest what they are learning, and to practice mindfulness on their own, and it lessens the likelihood that they will take the class for granted as they might if it was offered every day. For many students, a longer-term structured mindfulness course can significantly deepen their understandings of self-awareness through consistent guided meditation practice, reinforcement of key concepts, and rich discourse on a variety of related topics with the teacher and other students. Many of these topics, such as kindness and compassion, directly teach the values of non-violence. The combination of learning about these ideas, while also practicing mindfulness on a regular basis, can be quite powerful for students, and impactful for the school community. One such course that I created from scratch many years ago brought High School students through an intensive and engaging curriculum through daily mindfulness practice periods and scaffolded units and lessons designed to develop a strong sense of self-awareness and social-awareness with a deep understanding of how the mind, body and nervous system interact. I called the curriculum **Mindful Fitness** and saw it change too many lives to count over the course of many years.

For some students, the experience of a longer course can be positively life-changing. I have seen the lives of students change right before my eyes, and in some cases, they have even reported that their family dynamics had shifted because they were now setting a new example at home, and it was having a ripple effect on their parents and siblings. This can be one of the most rewarding aspects of teaching mindfulness to students.

A curriculum-based class also provides many opportunities for a deeper exploration of the neuroscientific underpinnings of mindfulness with rich opportunities for interdisciplinary connections to other subject areas, including science and literature. As an English teacher, I taught *The Catcher in the Rye* by J.D. Salinger for many years through the lens of mindfulness and social-emotional learning. This matched perfectly with the content I was teaching some of the same students in **Mindful-Fitness** class. It was a powerful learning experience because students could make direct connections between what they were observing in their own minds during meditation and what the character, Holden Caulfield, was experiencing in the book. This led to deep insights and rich conversations in both classes. One potential drawback of a mindfulness class is that some students may not possess the same interest or maturity level to handle the experience of meditation on a frequent basis, which can present significant challenges for teachers to address, especially during periods of quiet time.

Push-in mindfulness breaks can also be practiced in the midst of traditional academic subjects. For example, providing students the ability to settle and breathe together for 5 min before an exam can be an effective way to lower anxieties in the room. For younger students, practicing a few mindful minutes after recess can help reset the energy in the room at a time when restlessness typically spills over and makes instruction all but impossible. Finally, *school-wide moments of silence* can be facilitated through morning announcements for the entire school community to practice mindfulness together. This can set the morning on a positive note, build community and calm the tone of the building as students arrive from different circumstances and home environments which encompass a full spectrum of mindsets and emotions.

Mindfulness Training for Teachers

Central to creating a *Culture of Awareness* is the training of teachers in mindfulness. A common mistake when attempting to introduce mindfulness into a school is providing in-depth training for students, and either neglecting the teachers or limiting the offering to one-time training opportunities that do not develop over time. Teachers hold much sway in schools, and their involvement is crucial. If teachers are buying in to an initiative, students are likely to follow suit. Sadly, the reverse is often also true.

Practicing mindfulness together in *Professional Learning Communities* provides rich opportunities for teachers to deepen relationships with colleagues around their shared humanity. Too often teachers rally around grievances, shared stress, and overwhelm from professional responsibilities and difficulties with colleagues. This is to be expected in a job as emotionally demanding and draining as teaching. Yet, mindfulness is a powerful agent for colleagues to connect around strategies for resilience, restoration, and relief. When people are fully present with one another they tend to be more honest, authentic, and vulnerable. Practicing mindfulness with colleagues provides the space for these moments to organically happen within a container of learning and support.

Teachers set the tone of the classroom and school building based on how they carry themselves and what they are carrying inside of them. When teachers operate out of the values of mindfulness and non-violence it is inevitable that the overall tone of the building will improve. And when teachers are more focused, relaxed, and authentic they are far more likely to meet the needs of the students in front of them. Why? Because they are seeing things more clearly. Most negative interactions between teachers and students occur when the teacher is not fully grounded in his/her feelings, or attentive to the subtle dynamics of interaction, and therefore misdiagnoses a situation, or blows it out of proportion. It can be easy to lose patience with a student when the teacher is not fully present. Sadly, the power of a teacher's mood to impact a student is more powerful than we sometimes realize in the moment. And we often are not fully aware of the consequences.

When students feel "dehumanized" or humiliated they are far more likely to take these feelings out on others. Conversely, when they feel inspired and joyous, they are far more likely to engage in positive interactions with teachers and peers. Teachers have a tremendous amount of influence over which of these seeds are nourished in their students and themselves.

The old saying applies, "hurt people *hurt* people." And hurt people are far more likely to engage in violence in school. When teachers practice mindfulness, they are better poised to see the battle brewing inside themselves and to make the wiser choice. This level of self-awareness helps to manage the stress of the job and to de-escalate their own conflicts with the students they teach, as well as their interactions with colleagues which can often be the source of much invisible tension in a school building. And they are far more likely to notice the seeds of conflict brewing between students in classrooms, hallways, gymnasiums, and cafeterias, and intervene, long before they bloom into violence. This is the power of awareness. It takes note of what is happening inside and outside and responds in ways that are healthy and healing.

Mindfulness training for teachers can occur in a variety of different settings. One effective and convenient platform is during *Professional Development sessions* (PDs). Teachers typically regard PD as a chore, oftentimes related to tedious compliance issues, or other content deemed as non-essential to instruction. Using these shared times for mindfulness training can provide a pleasant alternative for teachers to learn something truly empowering for both their professional and personal lives. It can be a welcome relief for a teacher to settle into a "professional" learning opportunity that provides them with training and time to decompress and reset their attention.

Another opportunity for teachers to practice mindfulness together on an ongoing basis is in the opening minutes of *staff meetings*. These are powerful opportunities to reframe the intention behind professional meetings and recommit to the values of non-violence. This small investment of time to regularly practice mindfulness together can shift the outcomes of meetings in subtle but profound ways, much like a large ship can change its entire destination by altering its rudder by one or two degrees. Just a few minutes of mindfulness can settle the room down and center the attention of the group in ways that promote active listening and authentic interactions, especially after a long day of teaching. My own experiences have revealed that meetings that begin with a few mindful minutes tend to be far more enjoyable, warm, and productive for all involved. Doing this on a regular basis normalizes the practice of mindfulness for the entire staff, deepens the skills of purposeful attention, builds community and collectively reinforces the values of non-violence.

Still, another opportunity for teachers to practice mindfulness together is during afterschool *stress reduction groups*. I created one of these groups many years ago at *Food and Finance High School* in Manhattan and found it to be a welcome offering for teachers to connect 1 day a week and rejuvenate on a drop-in basis. The voluntary nature of the group made it low pressure, and the teachers who chose to attend seemed to appreciate it more. I frequently observed teachers engaging in the meaningful discourse during and after the sessions, teachers who otherwise may not have had much connection with each other. Out of these moments of stillness often arose spontaneous conversations about shared interests, which sometimes resulted in creative planning opportunities for the kids. It was a pleasant reminder that when professionals drop the veil for a minute and become authentic with one another, everybody benefits. The teachers were being productive even though they did not feel like they were "working." And their mindful interactions together contributed to a larger cohesion in the building.

Administrators

In order for any initiative to succeed in a school, the administration must be fully committed. It is obvious that administrators hold the purse strings, schedule the classes and approve or deny initiatives in a school. But more importantly, administrators set the values of a school. This is not always an overt process. On paper, a principal, assistant principal, or superintendent may greenlight a program in a school or district, or pay lip service to it, but then distance themselves from it in ways that are clear and demotivating. This unconscious (and in some cases conscious) signaling can be felt by teachers, students, and families. In the case of mindfulness, when administrators are not visibly participating or modeling mindfulness in ways that are apparent to others in the community, there is a disconnect. This can be a major impediment to shifting to a culture of awareness. I have had the experience of administrators allowing me free reign to create robust mindfulness initiatives in a school, but then not personally engaging with them, at least not publicly. Yet, once I raised this concern with a fair amount of clarity and persistence, they chose to become more directly involved over time. Soon others began to notice and became much more receptive, and also began to participate. Oftentimes people are afraid of new initiatives in a workplace, especially something as vulnerable and personal as mindfulness. Seeing a school leader lower the guard and become vulnerable has a powerful effect on the staff. It allows professionals to be human beings. And it creates a sense of safety and trust, which can pay huge dividends for staff morale.

Another benefit of administrators practicing mindfulness in a school is the effect it has on their leadership. School principals are under exceeding pressure these days with expanded roles and sweeping educational reforms. Unlike years ago, when administrators focused primarily on building management, modern administrators are expected to be instructional leaders in addition to building managers who are tasked to solve seemingly endless daily crises. They are the public faces of district policies, family outreach efforts as well as human resource professionals. All of these hats must be competently worn while navigating through shifting local, state, and national political winds. This can take a huge toll on anyone.

From high-stakes testing and onerous teacher evaluations to a host of other high-pressure daily demands, the job of a building leader requires clear vision and a cool head in the midst of turmoil, change, and unpredictability. By practicing mindfulness, school leaders shore up their own inner resources and are better poised to meet the needs of the teachers, students, and families they serve. When leaders embody mindfulness, their example sets a tone in the building that ripples out to everyone. They become the calm in the storm. And this signals a commitment to, and respect for, de-escalation and non-violence.

Families

It was previously mentioned how families can positively benefit when students practice mindfulness. I have observed students sharing techniques and ideas learned in **Mindful Fitness** class that made visible improvements in the lives of their parents and siblings. In one example a few years ago, a student and her Mom both shared with me that the mother began employing breathing techniques when she was driving that she had learned from her daughter. The daughter had learned them in class to deal with anxiety she was experiencing around schoolwork stress and perfectionism. Mindfulness was helping her to accept herself, and apparently, it was helping her Mom too. Both happily reported that the Mom was now experiencing a clear reduction in road rage, a dangerous chronic habit. For the first time in her life, my student felt safe driving with her Mom! To me, this alone was clear evidence for the power of a Culture of Awareness, the ripple effect that organically unfolds when people begin sharing strategies that they learned in class. Family members often become naturally curious after observing a child or sibling growing more patient or caring in the house. This can open the door to healthy conversations and better relationships. They can be powerful moments when one family member inspires another to learn and grow.

In some cases, entire family dynamics can change. I will never forget when a 10th grade student of mine explained, "My relationship with my mother has gotten better. I do not argue with her as much. I learned how to listen to her and I actually see where she is coming from, and not stress her out as much. She has a lot on her plate." This was an important insight that changed their relationship forever. It did not take years of therapy to open to this insight; it was a moment of clear seeing that changed her entire perspective. And yet, teaching mindfulness directly to parents is another powerful option to promote peace and non-violence.

When schools create opportunities for parents to learn mindfulness skills everybody can benefit. On many occasions, I have facilitated mindfulness training at P.T.A. (parent-teacher association) meetings and they have been very well received. Most parents expressed appreciation and enthusiasm, especially after anticipating a tense and politically charged atmosphere, which can be common in these settings. Participants can have dramatically different goals and agendas which can create a great deal of underlying tension, uncertainty, and even dread. Many parents find the school to be a stressful place to visit for a variety of reasons. This is often true for parents in inner-city schools, especially ones that struggle with English, as they often feel intimidated by teachers they fear may not understand their concerns. Yet, somehow, practicing mindfulness together with teachers can lower the barriers, and reframe the entire experience and relationship. Parents can feel more settled, welcomed, and grateful for the opportunity to learn a valuable skill to help with their own stresses and enable them to relate more authentically to the struggles of their child. Mindfulness helps to parent from a position of strength and balance versus stress and overwhelm. It opens the door to trust between parents and teachers, and between parents and their children.

Above all else, trust is the cornerstone of a *Culture of Awareness*. Stakeholders organically develop empathy by practicing mindfulness. They become curious about the experience of others by paying attention on purpose and becoming more intimate with their own direct experience. That is what can be built when all stakeholders commit to being more fully aware, compassionate, and kind to one another. It takes vulnerability, practice, and strong leadership, but the rewards can ripple through an entire building, district, and community. This can shift an entire culture away from the seeds of violence, and provide greater opportunities for de-escalation, restoration, and perhaps most fundamental to the goal of education, *learning*, when conflict inevitably arises.

Mindfulness: The Essence of Learning

When you think about mindfulness, what is the first word that comes to mind? *Calm*? *Relaxation*? *Peace*? Mine would be *learning*. But mindfulness is no ordinary kind of learning. It deeply discerns the truth of the moment by seeing things exactly as they are both inside and out. This is a primal and powerful learning. You might even say it is the essence of critical thinking. Without some degree of present moment awareness would it even be possible to solve a complex math problem or analyze a text? Socrates famously warned to "know thyself." But he did not say how. Mindfulness is a technology to do just that.

Just think for a moment about the power of awareness. When another person really sees you, really hears you, and is really curious about you, what effect does their awareness have on how you feel? Does it make you feel more connected or less? More open or more shut down? More peaceful or more agitated? More curious or more contracted? Now imagine the power of an entire community really seeing one another? Really listening. How can this not lessen conflict and violence? In physics, they call this *the observer effect*: the mere observation of a phenomenon inevitably changes that phenomenon. This is the power of mindfulness. It influences events simply by seeing them more clearly. You might even call it a primary form of intelligence.

This understanding of intelligence is an important distinction from traditional views of education where intellect is prized above all else. Of course, information acquisition is important. Yet, mindfulness is something that already exists inside of every human being. It is our birthright. Nobody is born without awareness of themselves and the world around them. Everybody has had the experience of being fully present for a sunset, a meal or the smile from a loved one. Yet, mindfulness teaches us that we can systematically develop this potential for clarity, compassion, and non-violence. A school culture that actively trains these skills redefines the whole purpose of learning and reinforces it in daily action. Awareness is the building block of everything we could ever know about ourselves and the world. In this way, mindfulness educates students in a way that is fundamental to both critical thinking and non-violence.

Discipline Redefined

No school escapes conflict and violence. Humans, especially younger ones, misbehave from time to time. It is the "cost of doing business" in education. No program, philosophy, or technique will ever fully eradicate bad behavior. Yet, traditional methods of discipline have often over-relied on the "sticks" of detention, suspension, and other punitive measures to remediate bad behavior. This is not to say that traditional progressive discipline should be disregarded or demonized. It is very necessary to maintain order in a community; accountability must be maintained. However, if the purpose of education is clearly to learn, one must question how much learning is occurring when the first lines of defense are removal and punishment. Rather, what can mindfulness and social-emotional learning strategies teach us about the potential to utilize moments of negative behavior to restore the community and develop lasting learning lessons that will serve all involved?

Relationship-Building

When I first became the head of Discipline at Food and Finance High School in Manhattan, I sought fresh ways to reimagine how behavior was managed. Prior to that, there was a chronic level of discipline infractions in the school, some of them high profile, and there was a collective sense among students and teachers that the building was spiraling out of control. One of the first things I did was to change my title to "Dean of Mindfulness and Restorative Interventions." This unusual title received some eye rolls from colleagues at first, yet seemed a little closer to my aspirations. The intention was to utilize a whole range of options in handling discipline matters. The first of those options was relationship building. Simply getting to know kids, and showing them that you care about their lives and experiences, is half the battle. Everybody wants to be understood and appreciated. When kids begin to see that they are valued, they begin to trust the adults who serve them. Trust is primary to lowering violence, and it is a process that takes time to unfold.

Over the next 3 years, a very talented and supportive Assistant Principal named Michael Bollati and I made it our business to build authentic relationships with kids, and things slowly began to shift in the school culture. Students would routinely pop in my office to inform me that something was about to happen in the building because they bought in to our approach and wanted to preserve the community. These "heads-ups" gave us invaluable time to intercede, and in some cases, to prevent a physical altercation between students. Over time I learned the value of prevention, and how eager kids are to help when they know that you really care, and you are not faking it. And when students did violate a rule and were in trouble, they were significantly more cooperative with us because they trusted we would be fair. This was a dramatic reversal from the school's historical climate, where kids would frequently roam the hallways with impunity, ignore, and in many cases, curse at adults asking them to return to class. Over the course of time, the hallways progressively grew quiet, orderly, and largely empty, as the kids were too busy learning in classrooms to find trouble elsewhere. Most violent incidents typically occur in the hallways, and they started to drop. The shift was palpable to building visitors and the sense of safety dramatically improved. The security agents in the campus building began requesting stations in our school as they came to rely on us for a calm break.

We also gained insights into the planning of fights outside the school. Kids are smart. Often, they know enough to contain their aggression inside the school building only to have it erupt outside. In the case of Food and Finance High School, that often meant fighting in midtown Manhattan, something that is unthinkably dangerous for both students and pedestrians on the street. Soon, we were gaining knowledge of what was going to happen and where it was going to happen because kids were telling us ahead of time. This gave us time to intervene, contact parents and prevent incidents before students were released. And it all came down to the trust that students were now placing in us, and the value they had for the community. They knew that an altercation outside the building was just as much a violation, and they had faith in us to share what they knew. They wanted to be part of the solution.

Mindful Listening

One major factor that played a pivotal role in this transformation, was that we began really listening to students and hearing what they had to say. We became very curious about the forces that were causing kids to break the rules in the first place, or resort to violence as a solution. I do not think it is an exaggeration to say that in nearly all incidents there was some kind of emotional pain underlying misbehavior. This was especially true in acts of violence. Sometimes kids would fight, threaten other students, or even punch a wall or window. In each one of these incidents, there was a story of pain from home, a relationship gone sour, or some form of teasing, that finally built to a boiling point. In those moments, the student simply could not see any options and reacted out of momentary blindness. We have mentioned several times throughout this chapter that mindfulness enables a person to identify their feelings and surroundings more clearly. In most cases of violence, a little clarity would have stopped things in their tracks. But the student was too caught in cycles of reactivity, based on unresolved pain, with a chronic lack of awareness or empathy. The window of vision was too narrow to see a way out.

When the potential for conflict in the building was high, we would frequently hold mediations with the students involved, including, in many cases, the outer players, who would often stoke the conflict in subtle and direct ways. The purpose of these meetings was to create a space where all involved could share their perceptions and be heard. When it seemed appropriate, and the timing seemed right, we would often lead the students in mindful breathing techniques before we even considered having a conversation, which dramatically brought down the temperature in a relatively quick amount of time. But we only did this when the students indicated a sincere willingness, or else it would have been hollow and therefore, ineffective. Similarly, we never forced a solution or a fake truce amongst students caught in a conflict, which would have been counterproductive and for appearance only. We emphasized the right for students to authentically feel their feelings, and choose whom they liked or disliked, without any coercion from the adults. Yet, we insisted on their agreement to abide by the rules and values of the school no matter how they were feeling. This was non-negotiable. I can remember as a kid being ordered by an adult to shake another kid's hand after a fight or a conflict, which only heightened my rage, and delayed its inevitable reigniting. Suppressing feelings is not a pathway to peace. Instead, our intent was to create the space for students to authentically see and hear each other's perspectives, with no expectations for an ongoing relationship. Often, we decided to table the conversation for the following day when tensions were just too high. What we found, much to my surprise when we began this practice, was that kids almost always rose to the challenge when given the space, time, and respect to make their own decisions. They intuitively wanted to take the higher path, and respected the faith we placed in them to choose for themselves. Had we forced a solution, I am highly doubtful peace would have prevailed, at least not for the long term. But in most situations, it did. And it made our jobs much easier.

Another approach that the Assistant Principal and I began to use, was an open-door, "venting" policy. If any student needed to blow off steam, they could stop by either one of our offices and scream their heads off *at us* until they were ready to calm down. And many of them did! After the steam would pass, oftentimes tears would follow. Sometimes the kids wanted to speak about the issue, other times they wanted us to hear about the real pain they were experiencing at home. Sometimes they just wanted to sit in silence. During these moments of engaged stillness, we frequently offered the option to practice conscious breathing together for a few moments, which would help us to calm down and see things more clearly, as much as it did for the students. But we never forced the idea. Similarly, we never forced conversations. Rather, we listened, breathed, held the space, and respected what the student needed to share or not share. On occasions when we sensed that a student did not relate to either of us, perhaps because we are both white and male, or for any other reason, we would recruit a teacher or guidance counselor, or in some cases a security guard, that the student felt comfortable with. The important thing was they were heard, and they knew that we cared. This was mindfulness in action, and the students felt it. Like *the observer effect*, something seemed to shift inside of them in these moments, simply because they were seen and heard without judgment. Who does not need that?

In the third year, I developed a plan to lower suspensions by giving students an opportunity to learn about and practice mindfulness. Students who faced suspensions were given the choice to lower the number of suspension days they had to serve by agreeing to attend an afterschool stress reduction class led by me. The element of choice was the key to success because it was decided by the student and not imposed on them by adults. It put them in the driver's seat and gave them ownership of their path to restoration and learning. Since the class was open to anyone on a drop-in basis, nobody knew why others were attending, unless they chose to share. This made the environment much less stigmatizing and embarrassing for the student who was in trouble. It allowed them to blend in, feel the care of the group, and learn powerful strategies to calm down and see things more clearly in the heat of the moment. It also gave me the opportunity to build stronger relationships with these kids, which invariably resulted in more trust and leverage with them, and ultimately, better behavior. Most surprising of all, parents began calling to thank me when they learned that their child had been given a choice, and was serving less suspension days because of the agreement. It was a revelation the first time a parent called to thank me for suspending their child! I realized we were onto something.

What the whole experiment showed me was that mindfulness is the real "discipline." It teaches without punishment and provides clarity for students seeking to find a better way. It develops character, resilience, and valuable life lessons that will endure well beyond school-age years. In short, mindfulness *is* education.

At the end of year three, discipline incidents at Food and Finance High School dropped by more than 40%. Sadly, two years later, the safety issues and discipline incidents skyrocketed in just a few short months when a new administrator came on and failed to support the players, policies and measures that had worked like magic. I learned the hard way that school culture can dramatically improve or suddenly nosedive depending on trust, leadership and support.

Reacting Versus Responding

At the heart of behavioral change is understanding a simple but critical distinction between *reacting* versus *responding*. This is a key factor in determining whether a student will act violently or choose healthier options when faced with conflict and aggression in school. *Reacting* is impulsively speaking or acting without taking into consideration the long-term welfare of the self, others, and the greater good. Whereas *responding* is taking a simple pause to reflect on the possible consequences of speech or action. As I like to tell my students, this moment can be the difference between making a decision that will secure or sabotage your future. Your clarity and calm are the decisive elements.

Fight or Flight

Reacting is a survival mechanism rooted in our primal brain. When faced with impending danger the brain scans for threats and reacts quickly on impulse. In the wild, this tendency kept our ancient ancestors alive when facing the numerous natural dangers facing them. When a lion or bear is about to attack you, swift action is what is needed most, without the benefit of time to deliberate. The nervous system quickly activates the fight/flight reaction in order to mobilize the body's resources and prepare to fight the predator or flee the scene. This capacity is invaluable for safety and protection and is largely responsible for the survival of the human species. Yet, in modern life, we often mistake social and emotional threats for physical ones. On an evolutionary level, our nervous systems often cannot tell the difference and instinctively reacts the exact same way. Without the benefit of momentary grounded awareness, this is a recipe for disaster. And it is compounded for young people whose brains are still developing. They often do not have the context or clarity in the moment to understand that an insult or feeling of embarrassment in front of peers is not actually a physical threat, even though it may very much feel like one. And that lack of context can sometimes trigger a violent reaction. Therefore, acting on aggressive impulses that seem to make sense in the heat of conflict, without taking a moment to consider the consequences, can be responsible for a lot of unnecessary tension, and even violence, in a school building.

Reactions are largely based on beliefs, biases and prejudices in the unconscious, which are hardly reliable indicators of skillful or beneficial action. Generally, these forces are unexamined and often filled with corrupted and conflicted motives, hardly a recipe for de-escalation and sane decision making. When students react to a situation out of anger it invariably boils down to a closing of perceived options that they were able to see. The thoughts, emotions, mood, mental state, home-life situation, relationship history, academic pressures, identity issues, physical health, insecurities, appearance, perception of social status and sense of self, all sit beneath the surface and can get triggered quickly and violently when confronted by an obnoxious classmate or a challenging situation. When these intense feelings are not examined, held, and understood clearly, they can serve as a powder keg.

The job of mindfulness is to see clearly what is happening internally and externally. Knowing that you are having a bad day, or feeling particularly volatile or vulnerable, may inform the situations you choose to avoid and provide more clarity and wisdom when something unexpectedly happens in the moment. My own experience has shown me time and again that when I am not fully aware of my inner state, or feelings in the moment, I am far more likely to misdiagnose a situation and over-react. There have been occasions when I have spoken more aggressively to someone than they deserved, and was shocked afterward, simply because I did not realize or acknowledge how much emotional weight I was carrying. I suspect this is probably true for most people. Mindfulness provides us with an accurate forecast of our feelings, and this information can help steer us away from situations we are not capable of handling on a given day.

I have often asked my students if they have ever said something to a loved one in the heat of the moment that they wish they could take back. Invariably, every single hand in the room gets raised. This is what happens when we react blindly. Others get hurt, and so do we. The effects can last for a long time, and sometimes relationships can be ruined. And yet it all comes down to a single decisive moment.

Responding, on the other hand, is the ability to pause in the heat of conflict as you feel the tendency to say or do something harmful. It is sometimes referred to as a *sacred pause*, where you take one simple in-breath and out-breath at a decisive moment, and reflect on the consequences of your next word or action. This pause is the space between *stimulus and response*. It is incredibly valuable because it gives us the power to choose, and interrupts the momentum of emotion, impulse, and rage that impels us forward. It is a moment of awareness, of clear seeing. And the more students practice mindfulness on a regular basis, and become familiar with the terrain of their own thoughts and feelings, and become grounded in their bodies, the more frequently sacred pauses organically arise when they are needed most. Mindfulness trains the brain to override destructive tendencies that often feel good and right in the moment, yet create much suffering later on. When an entire school is practicing in this way, violence can dramatically drop because students are more attuned to their own anger before it comes out as aggression toward others.

The historical Buddha is reported to have described anger like this: "honey-tipped with a poisoned root." I think that sums it up accurately. Responding allows us to pass on the "honey" of aggression so we can forgo the poisons of harm and regret.

Bias

Earlier we mentioned the brain's evolutionary tendency to make snap decisions in the moment. These judgments allow us to simplify complex information into usable data, which often motivates our behavior. This capacity can be used for harm or good. Yet, biases in our perceptions of other people color our interactions in ways that are often very harmful. This can take root in a variety of ways. Educators can hold false perceptions about the race, gender, sexual orientation, and ability levels of their students. These judgments can impact the quality and fairness of the instruction they provide. This can create resentments and manifest as negative self-beliefs. Students also carry these biases, which affect their interactions with other students in a building. Often, biases result in behaviors that can be discriminatory and the cause of conflict and violence, in a school. There are two types of biases, *conscious* and *unconscious bias*. Both can be destructive to a school community.

Conscious Bias

In the case of explicit or *conscious bias*, the person is aware of his/her negative attitudes and feelings regarding the members of another group. This bias is clearly identifiable due to its overt nature. Explicit bias can lead to hostile speech or actions specifically targeting members of a different group. Other times, the behavior can be less obvious, especially in cases of social exclusion. Yet, the participant is aware of his/her intentions and bias. As destructive as these behaviors can be, the more pernicious bias is often unconscious, because the behaviors are more difficult to identify, even to the person carrying the bias. Therefore, they tend to persist unchallenged.

Unconscious Bias

Unconscious bias is an attitude, judgment, or prejudice we carry without even knowing it. It can result in a host of behaviors that inflict harm on others in ways that are invisible, and continue without realizing it. Unconscious bias is perpetuated through *stereotypes, prejudice,* and *discrimination. Stereotypes* are exaggerated images or distorted truths of members of a different social group. They are often rooted in distorted portrayals of groups of people in the media, and the inability to understand the individual nature and natural variation of all humans, regardless of group identity. *Prejudice* is an attitude, belief, or orientation toward people based on their membership in a group, and is generally negative. An example of prejudice would be for a teacher to falsely assume the lower academic ability of a black or brown student from the inner city, or underestimate the potential of a female student in science class. *Discrimination* is behavior that acts in ways that are unfair and harmful to others based on stereotypes or prejudice. In the example above, a teacher might call less on the inner-city kids in class, or provide fewer enrichment opportunities in a science class for the female student, without even realizing it.

As harmful as these behaviors appear when viewed through an academic lens, they can also ignite tension and conflict in a school. Left unchecked, they can threaten the fabric of the school's culture, especially when students discriminate against each other. Social and collaborative work interactions are often colored by the attitudes and beliefs students unknowingly carry. This can pit classmates against each other, and groups of students against other groups in small and large ways. In extreme cases, this can cause direct violence. Yet, the underlying stress and tension can persist without a clear and obvious cause. Therefore, biases need to be clearly examined and understood if peace is to be expected. Yet, how can schools work with something that is unconscious?

You guessed it. Mindfulness is a powerful strategy to address the unconscious biases that we all carry around. Non-judgmental awareness is a potent agent in seeing clearly our own biased thoughts, beliefs, and opinions of other people. It also enables us to see the harmful effects of our actions. When we are more conscious, we are less likely to cause unintentional harm. We are more likely to question our own assumptions about other people, and become curious about them as individuals, rather than relying on fixed stereotypes or preconceptions that often prove to be false under closer examination.

Blind Spots and Beginner's Mind

Mindfulness wakes us up to how we think, feel and treat others. This is not easy but a necessary first step to change. All humans carry around *blind spots*, hidden emotions and beliefs that drive our unconscious impulses. Seeing them can be painful but illuminating. When we pay attention to how many subtle preferences and judgments our mind is carrying, we can get a glimpse into how often our behavior is slanted toward one thing or against another. This puts us in touch with a humility that understands that we usually do not know as much as we think we know. And we are not often as fair-minded as we would like to believe. And that our lack of objectivity affects those around us in potentially harmful ways. Yet, rather than beating ourselves up over it, or becoming defensive, mindfulness opens us up to the wisdom of not knowing. In classical traditions of mindfulness, this has been described as *beginner's mind*, an open orientation to life that is inherently curious and seeks to understand what is happening, rather than reflexively imposing meaning on everything that is perceived. Mindfulness develops this ability naturally, and it strikes closely at the heart of education. It is a powerful attitude from which to approach academic knowledge, and a prerequisite for critical thinking. It is also a healthy and cohesive way to approach other people. It has the power to promote peace, build strong ties between students from different groups, and ultimately, to lower school violence. When we know our own heart and minds, and see into the harmful views and assumptions we are carrying, we are in a much better position to understand and care about each other. Ultimately mindfulness reveals our own conditioning, and seeing it clearly enough over the course of time helps us to transform it.

Developing Empathy and Compassion

Empathy is the key to becoming curious about another person, and crucial to building strong bonds. When we do not see our biases clearly, and the unconscious beliefs that support them, we can lose a sense of empathy. Without empathy, it becomes much easier to marginalize another person or group. Once this happens, violence is significantly more likely to occur.

Mindfulness of Breathing

Most mindfulness practices rely on the observation of passing phenomena and seeing clearly into their changing natures. One of the most common techniques is mindfulness of breathing. In this form of meditation, we observe the raw physical sensations of respiration from one moment to the next. It might be the rising and falling of the abdomen during the in-breath and out-breath, or the sensations of air entering and exiting our nostrils. This simple practice can settle our minds, relax our bodies and clarify our perception of what is happening in each moment by narrowing our focus. The point is simply to observe what is happening without interfering or manipulating anything. There are similar practices that rely on awareness of sights, sounds, feelings, and a host of other meditation objects.

What they all share in common is the simple observation of the present moment. Yet, there are also mindfulness practices that involve actively generating thoughts or intentions for the purpose of creating harmonious states of mind. Building empathy is at the heart of all of them. Cultivating these specific practices can actively work against the harmful effects of bias and promote peace and non-violence in a school. Below are three that I have found to be particularly effective at creating connection and harmony.

Lovingkindness

Loving Kindness is a mindfulness practice that actively develops feelings of empathy. The practice requires generating intentions of warmth and goodwill to ourselves and other beings in a systematic way. These "beings" can be people, animals, and even insects. This practice is particularly useful when we are struggling with afflictive emotions like anger, fear, or anxiety. It is more active than breathing meditation and can sometimes be easier to do when the mind is having trouble focusing attention.

In *loving kindness meditation*, one sits or lies down and brings the mind's attention to the heart region in the chest. Once the attention has settled down, the meditator calls to mind an image of themselves. The image can be recent or from their childhood. With this image in mind, he/she begins repeating well-wishing phrases internally. Some common phrases might be "May I be happy and healthy" or "May I be relaxed with ease of mind." The specific wording is less important than the intentions behind them to promote peace, well-being and generosity. In some cases, the meditator might skip the phrases and visually imagine colors representing goodwill blanketing themselves. After a few minutes, the meditator then progressively replaces the image with one of a benefactor, followed by a neutral person, an individual they have had a conflict with, and finally, all beings in the world. The intention for all categories is to send positive feelings in an unbiased way, realizing that everybody has pain and hardship in life and that we all deserve some relief, even people we are in opposition with. It reminds us that we are fundamentally connected to all beings in the world, even though we might be at odds with some of them. Yet, the purpose is not for anything to happen outwardly as a result of this practice, but just to develop a sense of goodwill, which will ultimately benefit ourselves. Over time, this practice can be a powerful antidote for hostility and negativity toward others and even anger toward oneself. Self-aggression is an internal form of violence, increasingly far more common for students, and lovingkindness can help build a sense of self-worth and kindness. It actively promotes compassion and non-violence.

Forgiveness

Forgiveness meditation can also be a powerful antidote to resentment and anger. During this meditation, the meditator spends a few minutes calming the mind by focusing on the breath. Once the mind is calm and clear he/she spends time reflecting on his/her own positive qualities, and offers words of forgiveness for "all the ways I have knowingly and unknowingly harmed myself." This meditation may be challenging for some students, and adults too. The patterns of self-judgment are deep in many of us. Yet, the value in allowing ourselves to be human, in the face of all the ways we have come up short, is very valuable. In my many years of teaching meditation to both adults and kids, I have observed that people generally have a harder time forgiving themselves than other people. Carrying around this amount of self-hatred can be very difficult. This meditation allows people to move closer to healing by recognizing our good qualities as well as the mistakes we have made. After this, the meditator then imagines a person he/she has harmed in the past. During this round, the meditator asks forgiveness "for all the ways I have harmed you, knowingly and unknowingly." Lastly, the meditator calls to mind a person he/she has been harmed by in the past. Like the first two, in this round, the meditator offers forgiveness for all the ways the person has "knowingly or unknowingly harmed me." A word of caution is necessary here. This meditation can bring up intense feelings, especially if the student has experienced trauma or abandonment. A great degree of sensitivity and common sense must be exercised when offering this meditation to students. It is highly advised for the instructor to ask students if they are okay with this kind of meditation before leading them through it. It is also beneficial to advise students to not begin with the most challenging examples in their own lives. Rather, they can work their way up over time if they feel comfortable doing so. It is also beneficial for students to spend more time forgiving themselves if extending to others is too challenging. As with all meditations, please allow students the option to switch activities if these exercises bring up too much intensity or pain from the past. This flexibility is compassion in action, and students will feel it.

Gratitude

One of the evolutionary mechanisms that has allowed humans to survive is a *negativity bias*. Simply put, our brains react more strongly to bad news than good news. This makes sense when you understand the primary role of the nervous system to scan for and protect us from threats in the environment. So, while the negativity bias is very good news on an evolutionary level, it can keep us fixated on the negative events and people that occupy our world. This can predispose us to anxiety, conflict, and even violence.

Gratitude can be a powerful way to compensate for the negativity bias and routinely focus our attention on the things that are working in our lives to balance out this disparity. There is only a certain amount of mental bandwidth available to any one of us in each moment, and when we routinely remember the things that we are happy about, the more frequently our brains will notice the good and not the band. One of the ways we can do this is by taking some time each day to jot down the big and small things that we are happy about in our lives in a *gratitude journal*. It can be something as big as the love of another person, or simply how much we enjoyed our lunch. The key is to regularly jot these thoughts down every day on a consistent basis. My students have reported year after year that their outlook on life, as well as their relationships with others, have dramatically improved from this simple practice. A powerful adjunct to a gratitude journal is *gratitude meditation*. This practice can combat the brain's negativity bias by spending some time contemplating the people, things, and situations that are serving us. Doing this over time can convince our subconscious minds that the world is a safe place, despite its many problems and injustices, and that we belong. In this meditation, students focus their attention on breathing for a few minutes and settle down. Once the attention is relaxed, the instructor leads the students through a progressive guided gratitude reflection. The reflections can invoke the trivial pleasantries of day-to-day life, such as a good meal or a sunny day, all the way up to the profound gift of life itself. The purpose is to actively contemplate the aspects of life that are working in one's own favor.

Mindful Communication

When most people think of mindfulness they tend to conjure a serene image of a yogi with eyes closed in the lotus position, blissing out on a mountaintop. Much of this distorted view has been proliferated by the media's portrayal of a largely isolated practice that benefits only the individual. Yet, most of our lives are spent interacting with other people. This is clearly the case in schools. Therefore, any mindfulness practice we engage in must account for how we relate to others. This is where mindful communication comes in. When we speak and listen from a position of purposeful awareness we are far more likely to build positive bonds with others than when we blurt out the first impulse that comes to mind. As the head of the discipline in a High School, I have learned that nearly every act of violence in a school comes down to a word that was spoken out of turn or a comment that was delivered in a way that did not fully reflect what the student was intending to say. How we communicate matters. When we are mindful our words can create harmony. When we are mindless, they can sow division and cause conflict and violence in a school.

Group Circles and Talking Sticks

Mindful speaking is a skill that can be practiced and developed over time. One method to practice on a regular basis in class (and staff meetings) is to form a group circle with a *talking stick* or other props. Only the person holding the prop can speak. This forces the speaker to be more conscious of his/her words, and make the most of the opportunity. It also encourages others to consider the intentions behind their words before abruptly speaking out of impulse. The circle focuses group attention directly on the speaker, which can be a strong validation for what is being said. This configuration can feel very vulnerable for both the speakers and listeners and increase group empathy. I have used this technique for many years in **Mindful Fitness** class, and during conflict meditations, and have found it to be a powerful way to engage group presence around the skill of communication.

Mindful Communication Pairs

Another way to develop this skill is to create opportunities for students to mindfully speak together on purpose with a partner. This is a very rich learning opportunity for students. I have seen it used to great effect, where students gain insights into their own communication patterns in a safe environment. Once students are partnered up, the teacher leads the students through a brief minute or two mindful breathing exercises, with their eyes closed. During the silence, the teacher provides a talking prompt and assigns one student the role of speaker, and the other the role of listener. When the bell rings again, the communication begins.

The speaker's job is to speak authentically to the prompt and to notice any sensations in the body that arise while speaking. For example, the speaker might notice tension in the throat, or heat in the face when something personal is revealed. There is no right or wrong way to do this. Rather, the point is to practice mindful presence while speaking. When students are grounded in their own bodies during speech, and aware of their partner's body language, they are far more likely to speak in presence. In this way, the communication has a better chance of connecting both parties, even around difficult topics, and increases feelings of empathy. It can also reveal how often we are not present when we speak. *Purposeful pausing* is something that is encouraged by the instructor. Rather than rambling through thoughts and ideas, when the speaker feels momentarily confused, disconnected, or just out of words, the instruction is to momentarily pause and take a breath or two. This can be very challenging as it works against the deeply ingrained habit of mindless speaking. It allows for a moment to reconnect to one's own breath and body, as well as to the listener.

While the speaker is speaking, the listener's job is to remain silent and attentive to the speaker's body language. This may sound easy, but it can actually be quite challenging to not interrupt with comments such as "I know what you're saying" and "I've had that happen too". Rather, *mindful listening* is becoming aware of the impulse to interrupt, and grounding the attention in the body, while continuing to actively listen with curiosity. For the listener, sometimes this involves watching his/her breath while also paying attention to the speaker's body language and vocal intonations. For most people, this is complex at first, but can be learned over time so that mindful listening becomes a habit in daily life.

When the bell rings, both students close their eyes and bring awareness to the lingering thoughts in their minds and the sensations in their bodies. This too can be quite revealing. Feelings of regret for sharing too much, or agitation for something the partner said, can come up and grab hold of the mind. Just seeing how sensitive we are to communication can be a powerful exercise, and train us to be more attentive in daily life interactions. It can reveal the complexities of communication between people, and give students a clearer perspective on the power of their words, and the impact of empathic listening. Becoming intimately aware of both can promote peace and connection in a school.

Technology

Perhaps more than any other development in the past few decades, technology is responsible for a growing amount of conflict in schools. With all of its incomparable contribution to academics, technology poses a significant risk to cohesion, emotional safety, and student health. The mindful communication strategies outlined in the previous section all depend on the active engagement of two cooperating students in direct union with one another under the guidance of a qualified instructor. Social media platforms completely sidestep these parameters and provide endless opportunities for students to communicate online in ways that require little to no presence or forethought. The results can be highly destructive and can often lead to *cyberbullying*. Students can post inflammatory comments to, or about other students, or groups of students, in relative isolation and anonymity, without having to look anyone in the eye. This can make it significantly easier to act out of violent instincts and create a great deal of tension in a school. Worse yet, students can do it at all hours of the day or night. Situations can spiral out of control quickly, and in extreme cases contribute to self-harm and even suicide. This can create a nightmare situation and one that requires an incredible amount of school resources to prevent. Who can monitor all students long after they have left the school building? Yet, that is exactly what school administrators are expected to do.

Technology Addiction

To compound this problem, students are increasingly becoming more and more addicted to cell phones. Rather than engaging with one another directly, they often retreat into the surface safety of a cell phone. This instinct is driven by the immediate gratification to avoid unpleasant situations and difficult inner feelings. Yet, it comes at a great cost. It creates a great deal of disconnection and isolation among students, which can also be a source of conflict. And it is compounded by the addictive natures of many social media sites that build reward systems into their programs, intentionally targeting the developing brains of young people and creating dependencies. The cost of all of this technology overload is alienation from the real world of interacting with people. At risk on the one hand are conflict and potential violence between students after posting nasty things online. On the other hand, is the risk of inner harm to a student's self-worth when they are regularly comparing their lives to the false images that other people portray on social media. Most everyone knows the problem. Yet, how can mindfulness begin to address the crisis?

Technology Fasts

Awareness can be a powerful ally in this regard. When students become aware of the destructive nature of social media, and its potential for harm, they can make better choices by limiting the amount of content they consume. This can be a rich area of inquiry, learning, and discussion in school settings, where students can brainstorm their own strategies to combat the problem under the guidance of a teacher. One strategy I have seen students use successfully is periodic *technology fasts*. During these periods, students consciously choose blocks of windows to drop technology. A common window is 15 min after waking up in the morning and 15 min before going to bed. This can be a powerful way to begin the day fresh, and head to sleep with a clear head.

Over time, these windows can extend into a couple of hours or even a full day. The mindfulness instructor can incentivize technology fasts into learning projects where students consciously engage in an activity without a cell phone, such as taking a walk and later journaling about the experience. *What did the colors look like? How did you feel? Was there any anxiety? How many times did you think about your cell phone?" What thoughts were you thinking?* When students are encouraged to approach these periods from a place of curiosity and scientific inquiry, they are more likely to keep an open mind and give it a shot. It allows them to investigate their chronic distraction habits, and compare them to the experience of not being hooked on technology. Seeing the difference can reveal a lot. Comparing how both experiences physically feel *in the body* can show how much tension is being caused by technology addiction. Conversely, most students report a refreshing feeling of relief when they finally drop their devices for a few minutes and absorb their surroundings with full presence. This can be an opening. It can demonstrate very clearly the price of constantly looking at a screen, and dispel the false illusion of happiness that drives the addiction. This insight can create a degree of disenchantment with technology. It can lessen our passion to mindlessly consume stimuli at the cost of disconnecting from the world and from ourselves. And it can make clear the cost we are paying in terms of satisfaction and authenticity. In this way, mindfulness can begin to weaken technology addiction by seeing clearly how much pain it is causing us in the moment, and how much freedom is possible without it.

Pragmatically speaking, it is clear that students are not likely to drop technology usage for extensive periods of time simply based on the request of their teacher. Yet, even small windows can make a big difference. They are golden opportunities to experience life more fully and can yield powerful insights for students into their own levels of technology dependency. Seeing this clearly can motivate change.

Another helpful reminder I like to offer to students is to take three deep breaths before replying to a text message or email, and then pay attention to how this pause can relax their minds and improve their communication. The impulse to reply automatically to electronic communication without a pause can be the source of much stress and conflict. When we look closely, we see that it does not feel good. Like all mindfulness practices, the purpose is for students to bring awareness to their experience and understand that each moment contains many options. Some of those options are healthy. Others cause harm. When they begin to see for themselves the difference, with the benefit of some clarity and presence, students are more likely to make the wiser choice. In this way, students learn how to use technology mindfully and not be used by it. In addition, there are many apps that offer guided meditations and incredibly helpful resources to develop awareness and build healthier habits. Like anything else, technology is not inherently bad. If approached mindfully, it can be highly beneficial for students. A conscious inquiry around technology can reduce unnecessary conflict and violence that spills over into the school day, not to mention the inner violence of feeling isolated and alienated.

Calm and Connected

During the COVID-19 Pandemic of 2020, I learned the true value of technology in helping students become more mindful. Faced with the sudden closure of schools and overnight switch to remote learning, without any training beforehand, I was highly concerned how to meet the emotional needs of students over a computer. My strategy was to create an online Zoom interview show rooted in mindfulness and driven by online polls I would submit to my students each week that assessed their levels of anxiety and difficulties during the pandemic. Each week I interviewed a guest expert, which included some of the most famous meditation teachers in the world. They would generously lead us through a guided meditation and address the students' questions regarding the stresses they were living through in quarantine. It was an incredibly rich opportunity for the school community to participate each week. Through this show, and the mindful community we were building, we were able to engage in deep and relevant conversations about emotional difficulties and social injustice, especially when nationwide protests erupted around the Minneapolis police murder of George Floyd. Many students reported that they were using the weekly show as an invaluable resource to navigate through the biggest crisis of their lives. They were learning effective strategies to calm down and learn about themselves during a period of extremely high stress. Week after week we tackled the issues they were most struggling with. I walked away from this experience convinced that online technology can be used to authentically teach and practice mindfulness while engaging in difficult conversations in ways that offered profound benefits to students and the entire school community. The interviews are currently available at: https://www.youtube.com/c/BrianSimmonsMindfulness

Considerations for the Mindfulness Educator

Providing mindfulness to students can be extremely rewarding, daunting, and at times, exhilarating. There is something deeply affirming about practicing awareness with young people. Oftentimes, educational leaders ask for the magic recipe. Unfortunately, there are no guarantees in bringing mindfulness to a school community. It is a delicate endeavor that requires a lot of work, patience, and planning. However, there are certain elements that can greatly contribute to success.

As a person who has taught mindfulness for many years, and practiced intensely for decades, I can say with certainty that the number one priority for the mindfulness educator is *embodiment*. As an English teacher, I could easily read the chapter of a new book a day before the students, and competently deliver a lesson with perfect authenticity. Yet, this is *not* the case with teaching mindfulness. Presence is something that must be sincerely developed over time, practiced regularly, and committed to in one's own life. If it is not, there will inevitably be a disconnect, and others will feel it. Simply stated, mindfulness is a way of life. It is not just a lesson to be delivered, and there is not a shortcut. Anyone can buy a bell and ring it, yet credibility cannot be faked. Not too long ago, bringing mindfulness into a school building was a risky maneuver that required great courage. It was perceived by many to be something on the fringe and was looked at with a healthy dose of skepticism, and even ire. Yet, now it has become a buzzword. With this opportunity can come the temptation to jump right in and reap the career benefits of its newfound popularity. Yet, it is doubtful who this will ultimately benefit. It is highly advisable to take several months, or longer, to develop a personal mindfulness practice, to seek out proper guidance and resources, and commit to a daily practice, before ever bringing it to students or staff. This requires honesty and humility. Everyone will benefit from your embodiment of mindfulness, including you.

Student choice has been mentioned several times throughout the chapter, yet it bears repeating. Meditation is an intimate practice that can raise feelings of discomfort and self-consciousness. Not all students, or staff members, are ready for it, and that is okay. Providing options is crucial. Some students might choose to journal during the meditation period or put their heads down. Allowing them the space and autonomy to make these decisions for themselves will add to the buy-in of the program, and model compassion in action. Ultimately, this degree of flexibility strengthens the container of the class, staff, or group practicing mindfulness. Others pick up on these accommodations from the leader, and it increases trust for everybody. I have observed that students who sit in the room respectfully and choose not to participate in the formal meditation, can also benefit from just being in the environment. There is something mysterious and wonderful that happens when people practice mindfulness together, and the job of the leader is to create the conditions for mindfulness to do its work. Offering choice, and honoring the different needs of everybody, is a top priority.

Final Thoughts

With all its promise to reduce school violence, mindfulness is not a panacea. Educators tend to look for the one magic pill to solve the problems of the day, and sadly, mindfulness is not that. Nothing ever is. There is not one complete way to solve any problem, especially one as complex as violence in schools. Yet, mindfulness brings to the table a profoundly potent option at a time of great need. It has endured over two millennia and traversed continents, oceans, and vastly different cultures to land here in the west at this exact moment in time. I do not feel it an exaggeration to call this a miracle. It is a time of truly great possibility for educators looking to tap into ancient wisdom for solutions to modern problems. The window of youth is brief, and offering students the gift of seeing clearly and calmly into themselves, and learning how to de-escalate conflict at a young age, from a position of presence, is something that can change their lives forever.

The promise of mindfulness is not just to fix the problems of today in a school, but to infuse the larger society with citizens who can transcend their own base impulses, and contribute positively to those around them. I opened the chapter by recanting my own youthful history of violence. It is clear to me after decades of seeing deeply into my own mind, and watching the transformation of countless others around me, that the potential for change in humans is vast and deep. Providing this gift to students and stakeholders has the power to shift the culture of the school community, and profoundly change many, many lives. Most of all, *yours*. To quote one of my former students, a guarded but determined young woman, with a particularly traumatic personal history, "When I do this, I. AM. FREE."

Reference

Kabat-Zinn, J. (2003). Mindfulness-based interventions in context: Past, present, and future. *Clinical Psychology: Science and Practice, 10*(2), 144–156. https://doi.org/10.1093/clipsy.bpg016

Chapter 23
Equipping Students' Minds with a Cognitive Training Program for Preventing School Violence

Carol T. Brown

Introduction

It should not be surprising to learn that 80% of behavior incidents occur in the class-room where academic instruction and academic frustration coincide (Kentucky Department of Education, 2019). Students may have difficulty following multi-step directions, exhibit poor self-regulation, inattentiveness, disorganization, impulsive behavior, and difficulty planning. These cognitive deficits negatively impact a student's success in school (Alloway, Gathercole, & Elliott, 2010; Carretti et al., 2009; Cramer et al., 2014) leading to academic failure and frustration in the classroom which is a significant predictor of students who exhibit delinquent, disruptive, and aggressive behavior (Gray, 2000; Maguin & Loeber, 1996; Rodney et al., 1999; Kaufman et al., 2000). This chapter[1] describes the importance of addressing cognitive deficits by implementing the Equipping Minds Cognitive Development Curriculum (*EMCDC*), a research and evidenced-based cognitive training program (Brown, 2018a; Brown, 2018b) to reduce or prevent violence-based behaviors by children in schools. The author has published research using the *EMCDC* demonstrating far transfer effects on verbal abilities, nonverbal abilities, IQ composite, and academic skills. For this reason, the author suggests that the missing component to improve cognitive deficits and academic skills is the inclusion of a cognitive training program, *EMCDC*. By equipping schools to increase cognitive abilities and

---

[1] Parts of this chapter, including cases 1–6, have published previously in: Brown (2018c), licensed under the terms of the Creative Commons Attribution 4.0 International License (http://creativecommons.org/licenses/by/4.0/).

C. T. Brown (✉)
Equipping Minds™, Frankfort, KY, USA
e-mail: Cbrown@equippingminds.com

© The Author(s), under exclusive license to Springer Nature Switzerland AG 2023
T. W. Miller (ed.), *School Violence and Primary Prevention*,
https://doi.org/10.1007/978-3-031-13134-9_23

facilitate academic success, frustration in the classroom will be decreased resulting in a reduction of violent behaviors and promoting school safety.

EMCDC has been used with students diagnosed with neurodevelopmental learning disabilities: specific learning disorders (SLD), attention deficit hyperactivity disorder (ADHD), autism spectrum disorders (ASD), speech and language disorders, and intellectual abilities, which are served under the Individuals with Disabilities Act (IDEA) or Section 504 of the Rehabilitation Act (Brown, 2018a; Brown, 2018c; Brown,2018d). Learners with diagnosed neurodevelopmental disorders have deficits in cognitive functions, such as, working memory, attention, executive functions, processing, and fluid reasoning which impact reading, writing, mathematics, and behavior (de Vries et al., 2021; Alloway, 2006; American Psychiatric Association, 2013). This chapter includes an overview of the *EMCDC*, the author's quantitative research study using the *EMCDC* with SLD learners, seven case studies of learners with neurodevelopmental disorders, and the implementation of *EMCDC* in the classroom for all learners.

School Climate and Safety

In 2018–2019, 7.1 million or 14% of students received special education services under IDEA through an Individualized Education Plan (IEP) or 504 Plan (National Center for Education Statistics, 2020). The US Department of Education, Office for Civil Rights, collected data in 2015–2016 and 2017–2018 on *School Climate and Safety*. The purpose of the report was to evaluate the safety of students at school and the number of serious offenses, referrals to law enforcement, expulsion, out of school suspension, harassment or bullying, restraint, and seclusion incidents. For the purposes of this chapter, the students with disabilities under the Individuals with Disabilities Act (IDEA) and Section 504 of the Rehabilitation Act, who represented 14% in 2015–2016 and 16% in 2017–2018 of overall student enrollment will be examined as their incidents are disproportionately higher than their peers. Students with disabilities (IDEA) represented 28% of students referred to law enforcement or school-related arrest, 26% of students who had out-of-school suspension, 24% of students who were expelled, 25% of the students disciplined for bullying and harassment, and 51% of those students who were harassed or bullied. Alarmingly, students with disabilities (IDEA) represent 71% of the students who were restrained in 2015–2016 and 80% in 2017–2018 and represented 66% of the students who were placed in seclusion in 2015–2016 and 77% in 2017–2018 (US Department of Education, Office of Civil Rights, 2018; US Department of Education, Office of Civil Rights, 2020).

These behaviors and practices impact academic performance causing students to often drop out of school, display delinquent and abusive behavior, and violate the law putting them at a higher risk of entering the criminal justice system and being incarcerated (Cramer et al., 2014). Specifically, the dropout rate for students with disabilities is 18% which is 3 times greater than their peers (National Center for Education Statistics, 2020).

Treatment and Prevention of Violence in Schools

In the past decade, schools have implemented numerous school-wide preventive efforts to reduce violence. These have included positive discipline approaches, social skills training, creating emotionally and physically safe learning environments, community-based mentoring programs, peer tutoring, parent training, and training for school personnel on specialized instructional methods and techniques including additional school psychological services.

Academic Intervention

The visible co-occurrence between academic failure and behavior difficulties is undeniable. Researchers have suggested that evidence-based interventions targeting academic deficits should be implemented (Scott et al., 2001; Witt et al., 2004). Bowman-Perrott et al. (2014) meta-analyzed 24 studies that examined the benefits of peer tutoring on social skills, behavior, and academics. Improvements in social skills and the reduction of disruptive behaviors were greater than academic engagement. To further the analysis of research on the effects of academic intervention modifications on student behavior, Warmbold-Brann et al. (2017) reviewed over 32 studies. The interventions to impact academic skills included instruction in reading, math, and writing, modifying task difficulty, and performance-based feedback. When the interventions were delivered 1-on-1 the greatest impact on behavior was reported. Modification in task difficulty and changes in instruction were linked to a moderate decrease in disruptive behavior.

Maguin and Loeber (1996) meta-analyzed academic and behavior research and identified three compelling relationships. First, poor academic performance correlates with delinquency and high academic performance extinguishes delinquent behaviors. Second, there is a reduction in delinquency when interventions improve academic performance. Finally, cognitive deficits and inattentiveness are significantly associated with poor academic performance and delinquency.

Individualized Education Plan (IEP)

Students with disabilities have an Individualized Education Plan (IEP) which provides academic intervention, remediation of subject content, accommodations, strategies, modifications, and specialized therapies. However, these interventions rarely address the underlying cognitive deficits in processing, working memory, executive functioning, fluid reasoning, and attention. The author suggests that to prevent and decrease school violence in students with learning disabilities, schools should include a cognitive training curriculum. Improving cognitive skills will impact behavior and academic performance. Cognitive training can empower victims of school violence by developing the cognitive abilities that will equip them in navigating possible encounters with bullies and other perpetrators at the elementary, secondary, and college level. Cramer et al. (2014), suggested that academic success would also decrease the dropout rate which would, in turn, decrease the incarceration rate.

Disability Categories

The US Department of Education identified 13 disability categories for students receiving special education services through an Individualized Education Plan (IEP) or 504 Plan. Some 33% of students are diagnosed with a specific learning disorder (SLD), 19% with communication disorder/speech or language impairments, 15% with other health impairments which includes ADHD, 11% with autism, 7% with developmental delay, 6% with intellectual disability, and 5% with emotional disturbance. Students with multiple disabilities, hearing impairments, traumatic brain injuries, visual impairments, orthopedic impairments, and deaf/blindness each account for 2% or less of learners served under IDEA (NCES, 2020).

According to the *Diagnostic and Statistical Manual of Mental Disorders, fifth Edition* (*DSM*-5), many of these categories are neurodevelopmental learning disorders (NLD) which are characterized by developmental deficits that produce impairments of cognitive, personal, social, academic, or occupational functioning. The range of developmental deficits varies from those of average to above average intelligence with very specific limitations of learning or control of executive functions to global impairments of social skills or intelligence (American Psychiatric Association (APA), 2013). For the purposes of this chapter, the five most prevalent NLDs will be described by diagnostic criteria, common interventions, and cognitive deficits as shown in Table 23.1.

Cognitive Skills Impact on Academics and Behavior

Educators and psychologists agree that cognitive abilities control and regulate behavior, attention, and impact academic success. Cognitive skills equip students to learn complex tasks, to perform mental math problems, to ignore distractions, to follow multiple-step directions, and to plan and think strategically. Specifically, executive functions have received a great deal of interest and research over the last decade (Chein et al., 2010; Diamond & Ling, 2016; von Bastian & Oberauer, 2013). There are three components of executive functions: inhibitory control, working memory, and cognitive flexibility. *Inhibitory control* allows the learner to think before acting or speaking and give a thoughtful response. Deficient inhibitory control can lead to impulsivity and making poor decisions which may result in illegal or destructive acts (Moffitt et al., 2020; Diamond, 2013).

Table 23.1 Learning disabilities, interventions, and cognitive deficits

Learning disabilities & diagnostic criteria	Interventions	Cognitive deficits
Attention deficit hyperactivity disorder (ADHD) neurodevelopmental disorder defined by inappropriate levels of inattentive and/or hyperactive/impulsive behaviors that persist across more than one environment. ADHD is also associated with reduced school performance, social isolation, conduct disorder in adolescence, and increased risk for incarceration (APA, 2013).	Behavior therapy and classroom strategies, modifications, accommodations	The primary cognitive impairments associated with ADHD are deficits in executive functioning, in particular behavioral inhibition, which involves suppressing a prepotent (automatic) or irrelevant response (APA, 2013). Individuals with ADHD typically perform below the average range in measures of verbal working memory, visuospatial short-term memory, and working memory. (Alloway, Elliott, & Place, 2010; Holmes et al., 2014; Holmes & Gathercole, 2009).
Autism spectrum disorder (ASD) was revised in the *DSM*-5. There was a spectrum of clinical profiles associated with this diagnosis ranging from autism, Asperger syndrome, and pervasive developmental disorder not otherwise specified (PDD-NOS) which are now integrated into the broad category of ASD (Reichenbe, 2014).	Interventions are based on the severity of the disorder. Speech and occupational therapy, behavior therapy, academic remediation, visual checklist, rules, and schedule are recommended (Meltzer, 2007)	General ability (measured by IQ tests) plays an important role in determining where individuals fall in this spectrum. There is a lack of social and communication skills as well as planning and organization skills which negatively impact learning. Students with ASD perform within age-expected levels for visuospatial, short-term, and working memory. However, they fall below the average range in measures of verbal short-term memory and working memory. This profile is consistent with the idea that verbal memory may be linked to deficits in communication (Belleville et al., 2006).
Intellectual disability includes deficits in intellectual and adaptive functioning in conceptual, social, and practical domains. There are four levels of severity which include mild, moderate, severe, and profound. An IQ score of 65–75 (70+ or –5) is the criterion for the diagnosis and further assessments by a clinician are needed to determine the severity level (APA, 2013).	Depending on the severity, behavior therapy, speech therapy, occupational therapy, life skills, academic modifications	Cognitive challenges are present in visual and auditory processing, working memory, comprehension, fluid reasoning, abstract thinking, executive functioning, and visual-spatial reasoning skills. (APA, 2013).

(continued)

Table 23.1 (continued)

Learning disabilities & diagnostic criteria	Interventions	Cognitive deficits
Communication disorders include specific language impairment (SLI) also known as developmental language disorder, language delay, or developmental dysphasia. It is more prevalent in boys and has disproportionate difficulty in learning language despite having normal hearing, normal intelligence, and no known neurological or emotional impairment (APA, 2013).	Speech therapy	SLI children typically have below-average performance in tests of verbal short-term memory and working memory (Archibald & Gathercole, 2006). Their visuospatial memory skills are not impaired, and performance is at the same levels as their peers in tests of both visuospatial, short-term memory, and visuospatial working memory. This suggests that the difficulty that SLI children have in processing and storing information is specific to the verbal domain Alloway, 2011a).
Specific learning disorder (SLD) combines the diagnosis of dyslexia or reading disorder, dyscalculia or mathematics disorder, written expression disorder, and learning disorder not otherwise specified. These students have normal levels of academic functioning. (APA, 2013).	Remediation of academic skills.	There are also functional negative consequences for students with an SLD including higher rates of high school dropout, lower academic achievement, and poor overall mental health (APA, 2013).
Dyslexia is a specific learning disability characterized by unexpected difficulties in accurate and/or fluent word recognition, decoding, and spelling (APA, 2013).	Remediation of reading skills. Some schools may implement a specialized reading curriculum and teach in small group or individual setting.	Dyslexia: auditory processing, visual processing, and comprehension challenges may be present. (APA, 2013). There are verbal working-memory impairments, but relative strengths in visuospatial working memory. Verbal working memory deficits impact reading ability as reading requires considerable working memory "space" to keep all the relevant speech sounds and concepts in mind. This process can exceed the capacity of the dyslexic individual and ultimately result in frustration when they encounter new vocabulary words or challenging texts (Alloway, 2011a).

(continued)

Table 23.1 (continued)

Learning disabilities & diagnostic criteria	Interventions	Cognitive deficits
Dyscalculia, or mathematics disorder, is where students struggle to learn or understand mathematics. An estimated 5–8% of children are dyscalculia with an equal representation of boys and girls affected. Students with dyscalculia find it difficult to decipher math symbols (e.g., +, −), understand counting principles ("two" stands for 2, for instance), and solve arithmetic problems. (Gersten et al., 2005).	Remediation of math skills. Some schools may implement a specialized math curriculum and teach in small group or individual settings.	Struggle with telling time and recognizing patterns. Poor verbal working memory is usually only linked to dyscalculia in younger children (Gersten et al., 2005). Once they reach adolescence, verbal working memory is no longer significantly linked to mathematical skills (Reuhkala, 2001). Visuospatial, working-memory problems are linked to dyscalculia as it supports number representation, such as place value and alignment in columns in counting and arithmetic tasks (D'Amico & Guarnera, 2005). Poor working memory is thought to be one explanation for dyscalculia, because it limits the ability to remember mathematical rules, from basic concepts like counting in ascending and descending order to more complicated algebraic functions (Alloway & Passolunghi, 2011; Peng et al., 2016, Raghubar et al., 2010).
Dysgraphia is characterized by difficulties with written expression including spelling, grammar and punctuation accuracy, and clarity or organization of written expression.	Remediation of writing skills and occupational therapy may also be used.	Struggles in working memory and executive functioning.

Working memory has been defined as the ability to hold onto two or more pieces of information in your mind while performing a mental operation (Camos, 2008). Efficient working memory allows learners to listen and take notes, remember the teacher's question, steps to a math problem, and what they read, as well as follow the classroom discussion. Deficient working memory impacts reading and spelling as the learner is unable to hold on to letters or visualize the story they are reading (Alloway & Passolunghi, 2011; Carretti et al., 2009; Peng et al., 2016).

Cognitive flexibility refers to altering your views as situations change. It is also necessary to consider other creative options when problem solving (Diamond, 2013). Research has found reliable correlations between executive functioning abilities to fluid reasoning, intelligence, comprehension, language, reading, and mathematics (Carretti et al., 2009; Jaeggi et al., 2008; Alloway, 2011b). Executive functioning skills are a stronger indicator of a learner's academic and personal potential than an IQ test (Diamond, 2013; Alloway & Alloway, 2014). Despite the research demonstrating this correlation, cognitive training in executive functioning skills is not explicitly taught in schools (Meltzer, 2007). Academic intervention continues to be the focus for students with deficient cognitive functions and learning disabilities.

Cognitive Plasticity

According to Strobach and Karbach (2021) and Novick et al. (2020), the discoveries in neuroscience confirming the cognitive and neural plasticity of the brain to change throughout one's lifetime have ignited research in cognitive training. Specifically, there has been a focus on computerized brain training programs targeting working memory and executive functioning training. While the research has shown some near transfer effects such as being more proficient on the trained task, far transfer effects to nontrained tasks and generalization to academic abilities remains elusive with computer- based programs (Melby-Lervag & Hulme, 2013).

An alternative approach, absent in the current literature on cognitive training, involves the use of a human mediator. Over 50 years ago, Reuven Feuerstein (1921–2014), a clinical and cognitive psychologist, theorized that intelligence was changeable and modifiable regardless of age, genetics, neurodevelopmental conditions, and developmental disabilities with a human mediator even if the condition is generally considered irrevocable and irreparable (Feuerstein et al., 2010). Feuerstein's theory is known as Structural Cognitive Modifiability (SCM). The Feuerstein Institute has conducted research for the last five decades that confirm cognitive abilities can be modified with a cognitive training instrument, Feuerstein Instrumental Enrichment (FIE) using mediated learning (Tan & Seng, 2008).

Mediation Learning Experience and Cognitive Training Research

Feuerstein believed a human mediator is essential to take the learner beyond the natural limitations to reach his or her full cognitive potential and generate new cognitive structures. Higher order cognitive skills and executive functions are developed through this experience. The mediated learning experience (MLE) is an interaction between the learner and the mediator who possesses knowledge and intentionally conveys a particular skill or meaning. The learner is then encouraged to relate the meaning to another experience or thought. Meaningful human interaction with a mediator also impacts social and emotional development (Feuerstein et al., 2010; Feuerstein et al., 2015).

FIE can be implemented in a classroom, as a therapeutic intervention in a small group, or on an individualized basis. Studies have been conducted on learners with attention deficit disorders (Kaplan & Kreiger, 1990; Roth & Szamoskozi, 2001), autism (Martin, 2001; Gross & Stevens, 2005), and specific learning disabilities (Brainin, 1982; Sanches, 1994).

Another study by Kozulin et al. (2010) was conducted with 104 learners from Canada, Belgium, Italy, and Israel who had neurodevelopmental disabilities, cerebral palsy, genetically based intellectual impairments, autism, or ADHD. The FIE Basic program that is designed for young learners was used over 30–45 weeks. The intervention emphasizes systematic perception, self-regulation, conceptual vocabulary, planning, decoding emotions, and social relationships that are transferred to principles in daily life. The research subjects showed statistically significant improvements in the WISC-R subtests of similarities, picture completion, and picture arrangement, as well as on Raven's Colored Matrices. Bohács (2014) also studied learners from 2 to 14 years of age with mild to moderate intellectual developmental disorders, including genetic syndromes, cerebral paresis, ADHD, and autism. Significant changes in cognitive development and growth in domains necessary for school readiness were demonstrated as well as gains in general intelligence on the Raven's Colored Matrix.

Cognitive Functions

Feuerstein looked beyond academic and psychological testing as he saw these as static assessments. He did not focus on academic skills or even define cognitive skills in terms of executive functioning, visual-spatial reasoning, fluid reasoning, processing, working memory, or verbal comprehension. Rather, he examined the cognitive function underlying intelligence regarding what is going on in the learner's mind (Feuerstein et al., 2006).

Cognitive functions are defined by Feuerstein as "thinking abilities" that can be taught, learned, and developed. Hence, they are the prerequisites of thinking and learning. There are three phases of cognitive functions: input, elaboration, and output. This model can be used by trained teachers and parents to better understand and help the child who is experiencing learning difficulties. Teachers can differentiate errors due to a lack of knowledge or a deficient cognitive function (Feuerstein et al., 2006; Feuerstein et al., 2015). For example, if a child is struggling with a concept, it may be due to underdeveloped cognitive functions, such as imprecise data gathering at the input phase or poor communication skills at the output phase. The following list outlined in Table 23.2, as defined by Feuerstein, identifies, and describes the deficient cognitive functions (Feuerstein et al., 2006).

Feuerstein sought to identify and correct these deficits to enable students to reach their full cognitive potential, as well as to increase their internal motivation, personal confidence, academics, and behavior. By using mediated learning and a cognitive training program, these deficient functions can be corrected, formed, and modified in significant ways (Feuerstein et al., 2010; Feuerstein,R. & Lewin-Benham, A. 2012).

Equipping Minds Cognitive Development Curriculum

(*EMCDC*) was developed by the author and is based on Feuerstein's theory of Structural Cognitive Modifiability (SCM), Mediated Learning Experience (MLE), and affirms that cognitive skills can be developed in the classroom or therapeutic setting in person or online, through a human mediator. The cognitive training program is designed to help any individual wanting to strengthen their ability to learn; from learners 3 to 90 years of age and from gifted learners to those with neurodevelopmental disorders including specific learning disorders, attention deficit hyperactivity disorder, Down syndrome, post-concussion syndrome, traumatic brain injury, fetal alcohol syndrome, communication and language disorders, auditory processing disorder, visual processing disorder, intellectual and developmental disorder, and memory challenges. *EMCDC* also employs a holistic approach to cognitive development that includes primitive reflex exercises and sensory-motor developmental exercises in addition to the cognitive training exercises.

Reflex Integration Exercises

Primitive reflex exercises are done 5–7 days a week for 6–12 weeks and take 15 minutes a day using the *Maintaining Brains Everyday* (Johnson, 2015). Primitive reflexes act as a foundation for more complex muscle movements and later cognitive tasks. The reflexes are integrated in a sequential fashion in utero and during the first year of life. The lack of integration can interfere with processing and affect learning, movement, and attention impacting cognitive and academic skills. The visual motor system is intimately involved in the transition from primitive reflexes to control of movement patterns. By replicating the stages of development, the neural pathways can be strengthened, allowing for treatment to be successful (Goddard Blythe, 2005a, b).

Table 23.2 Deficient cognitive functions

Input – taking in information	Elaboration – working on the problem	Output – communicating a response
Deficient: Blurred and sweeping perception of essential information occurs. The learner struggles to gather the correct information.	Deficient: Lack of ability to recognize the existence and definition of an actual problem.	Deficient: Egocentric communication modalities are present. It is difficult for the learner to relate to others and to see things from another's perspective.
Deficient: Difficulty in temporal and spatial orientation occurs. The learner lacks the ability to organize information realistically and to describe events in terms of where and when they occur.	Deficient: Inability to select relevant vs. nonrelevant cues or data in defining a problem is present.	Deficient: Lack of ability to repeat an attempt after a failure or blocking is present.
Deficient: The learner is lacking skills in precision and accuracy.	Deficient: Difficulty in comparative behavior is present. This may be due to slow processing and inability to make comparisons between two or more things.	Deficient: Difficulty in projecting virtual relationships.
Deficient: Inability to identify an object when there is a change in size, shape, quantity, or orientation, though it is the same object.	Deficient: A narrow mental field is present. There is an inability to combine, group, and coordinate information.	Deficient: Use of trial-and-error responses, which leads to failure to learn from previous attempts, is present.
Deficient: Lack of capacity for considering two or more sources of information at once is present. This is reflected in dealing with data in a piecemeal fashion rather than as a unit of organized facts.	Deficient: The projection of virtual relationships is impaired. The ability to perceive the relationship between events is difficult.	Deficient: Lack of, or impaired tools for communicating adequately elaborated responses.
Deficient: Impulsive and unplanned exploratory behavior is present.	Deficient: The absence of or need for logical evidence, inferential-hypothetical thinking, and hypothesis development occurs.	Deficient: Lack of self-control, impulsive, or acting-out behavior is demonstrated.
	Deficient: Inability to visualize and create mental images is present.	Deficient: Lack of, or impaired, need for precision and accuracy in communicating one's responses.
	Deficient; Difficulty defining goals, planning behavior, and taking steps in problem solving occurs.	Deficient: Lack of self-control, impulsive, or acting-out behavior is demonstrated.

Sensory-Motor Development

Sensory-motor development includes visual processing and auditory processing. Visual processing includes visual tracking, visual localization and fixation, visual coordination, and visual cognitive problem-solving skills. Students with poor visual motor development have a hard time finding the words for objects they are viewing. Alternatively, if they are asked to get an object, they might look right at it and say they cannot find it. Although they are seeing the object, their brains are not efficiently processing the fact that they are seeing it (Ayers, 2005). *EMCDC* includes numerous visual processing exercises.

Effective auditory processing is foundational for speech, phonemic discrimination, working memory, language, and learning. Auditory processing exercises benefit learners with reading, language, and fluency disorders by providing auditory feedback to help the students detect their errors (articulation, phonological processing), help to regulate vocal intensity, self-monitor their reading fluency and increasing their auditory memory. A student may hear what is being said, but the brain does not process it fast enough or accurately enough. The result is that the student misunderstands what was said or it takes a long time to process what was said (Doidge, 2015; Joundry & Joundry, 2009; Joundry, 2004). Throughout the *EMCDC*, auditory processing exercises are implemented.

Some learners with auditory processing disorders, ADHD, and sensory disorders benefit from listening to sound therapy to rehabilitate the auditory system. Sound therapy was developed by Alfred Tomatis, MD, to strengthen the auditory system. He discovered that playing filtered classical music directly into the ear increased learning ability, brain function, coordination, and emotional health (Joundry, 2009). Students wear sound therapy while doing the *EMCDC* cognitive exercises.

Cognitive Training Exercises

The cognitive training and developmental exercises set aside academic content to correct and strengthen deficient cognitive functions. Learners participate in interactive games and paper-and-marker activities which are organized in a progressive and challenging manner to strengthen cognitive functions as outlined by Feuerstein. These activities also strengthen the cognitive skills of working memory, long-term memory, processing speed, visual processing, auditory processing, executive functioning, attention, language, fluid reasoning, visual-spatial reasoning, and comprehension.

Playing games is a powerful therapeutic tool for developing self-regulation, awareness of others, and cognitive functions (Porges & Dand, 2018; Purvis, 2007). A trained mediator encourages the learner to "think aloud" and verbalize what they are processing and thinking. Verbalization increases language processing. The mediator and learner also take turns when playing the numerous sorting, memory, and strategic card games and exercises which strengthen cognitive functions, social and emotional skills, hence impacting academic skills, behavior, and relationships.

The structure for mediating within the curriculum is specified in the *EMCDC* and summarized in Table 23.3. The mediator follows the *EMCDC* full program as the intervention is typically 60 hours over 24 weeks (Brown, 2018a). Brown combines the work of Feuerstein with Aristotle's *Ten Categories of Being* to guide the

Table 23.3 Equipping minds mediation questions based on Feuerstein's *Cognitive Functions* and Aristotle's *Ten Categories of Being*

Collecting	Processing	Expressing
What or who do you see, hear, feel, taste, touch, and smell? What can you visualize or imagine in your mind? What do you see yourself doing? What is the name of what you see or are thinking? Where are you starting? Do you have the correct materials? What parts do you need, and what order will you need to follow to make the finished product? What do you know to be true, or what is constant and does not change? What is to your right? What is to my right? If you are facing in this direction, what is to your right? Left? Front? Back? East? West? North? South? Northwest? Southeast? When do you see this happening – past, present, future? How long did the event occur? In what order did it happen?	What am I to do? Problem, what problem? What do you need to figure out? What is relevant to the problem? What is needed, and what can be ignored/omitted? What is similar? What characteristics are different? Consider: number, color, shape, size, direction, position, and feeling What different categories do you see? How are these related to each other? Ask: What is your plan? What are the steps you will follow and the reasons? Avoid trial and error! Have a plan. Does this make sense? If this is true, then what else must be true? Are there different possibilities? How can you see if this is true?	What does the other person believe and why? How does the other person feel? Can you imagine how you would feel in their position? How would the other person want to be viewed and treated? Have you thought through what you want to say or write? Are your words relevant to the situation? Is your language clear to the audience? Do you need to take a break and attempt later or tomorrow?

Source: Brown (2018b)

mediator through the *EMCDC* exercises and games (Brown, 2018a). While the implementation is the same for all learners, individualization will occur based on the learner's progression. By using mediation, these cognitive functions can be corrected, formed, and modified in significant ways enabling students to reach their full cognitive and academic potential (Mentis et al., 2009).

Aside from the academic benefits of the *Ten Categories of Being* and mediated learning questions, schools are reporting significant benefits in social and emotional skills. It is essential for students to maintain positive relationships and navigate the stress and anxiety of learning. A student may feel threatened or embarrassed when conflict arises between a peer or teacher or when they are experiencing academic frustration leading to poor decisions as seen in negative reactions and violent behaviors. Schools report that the *EMCDC* has been beneficial in laying the foundation for social and emotional learning skills as it fosters a safe place to practice the basic skills needed to analyze and respond to relationships. Through the daily practices, high level analysis is occurring as they start to develop reasoning skills that easily transfer to relationships. Hence, when schools are implementing a formal social and emotional learning program which seeks to teach students to manage emotions, have empathy, solve problems, make responsible decisions and maintain healthy relationships, the student's participation has been significantly improved since doing the *EMCDC*.

Stroop Effect and N-Back Training

In developing the *EMCDC*, Brown reviewed the research conducted to increase working memory and executive functions. One of the first cognitive training exercises was developed by psychologist John Ridley Stroop in the 1930s. The Stroop test asks learners to view a list of words that are printed in a different color than the actual word (Stroop, 1935). EMCDC integrates the original Stroop exercise with colored words and incorporates additional elements alternating the color, word, number, animal, and symbol associated with the color or word. Dr. Eric Chudler also created three variations of the Stroop Effect with animals, directions, and numbers which are included in the *EMCDC* seen in Table 23.5 (Chudler, 2012).

In 1958, a single *n*-back task emerged to train working memory and executive functions followed by a dual *n*-back task (Jaeggi et al., 2003). Some studies have reported near transfer effects but failed to demonstrate far transfer effects confirming that generalization remains elusive (Jaeggi et al., 2008; Jaeggi et al., 2014). Brown developed an adaptive *n*-back with nine tasks or the "Brown Six-Nine *N*-Back" in which learners were asked to associate animals, letters, vowels, numbers, presidents, and sounds with symbols and colors as well as identify directions of left, right, up, and down. To Brown's knowledge, there has not been a nine *n*-back task in which the learner hears auditory instructions, uses their hands to write or place a cube while holding a pattern for nine categories, processing the information visually, and verbalizing what they are doing. There are over 60 possible items the learner is retrieving from their long-term memory while using their working memory to hold onto multiple pieces of information from regions of the brain which contain letters (A-I), vowels (a, e, i, o, u), sounds, numbers, pictures or images of animals and presidents, symbols, directions, and colors. If the learners succeeded at a particular level of n, the task was made incrementally more difficult by increasing the size of n to nine as seen in Tables 23.4, 23.5, 23.6, 23.7, and 23.8, and Fig. 23.1 which are included in *EMCDC*.

Table 23.4 Brown Six-Nine *N*-Back Equipping Minds Cognitive Development Curriculum

Cognitive functions targeted	Exercise	Description
		Mediator states 1–2 directions, e.g.: "I see you putting a circle around the one…" What do you see yourself doing? Learner replies, "I see myself putting a circle around the one" and performs the action. Use a page protector and dry erase marker.
Visual processing, auditory processing, working memory, visual motor coordination, receptive and expressive language, visual-spatial reasoning, abstract thinking, refraining impulsivity	Stroop Animals	Circle around bear, box around snake, X on fish, triangle around cat, line under elephant, line above turtle and continue for 20 directions. *N*-Back- Read Set 2 and say the animal, word, symbol, letter of animal, classification Recreate the directions on a blank grid.
Projection of relationships, numerical awareness, comparisons, visualization, expressive language, long-term memory, and working memory	Presidents "Yo Millard Fillmore" book	Describe the pictures of the 46 US presidents stating what and who, quantities, qualities, time, where, clothing, feelings, action, positions, and relationships.
Working memory, visual and auditory processing, long-term memory, attention, expressive and receptive language, abstract thinking, visual motor coordination, refraining impulsivity, logical thinking	Numbers 1–5	Use a page protector and dry erase marker. First, place symbols and then cubes with corresponding numbers. Circle/green cube on 1, x / blue cube on 2, box /red cube on 3, yellow/underline 4, black/ line above 5. Remove page protector and read symbols alternating saying the number, color, animal, vowel, vowel sound, symbol, president, letter- an 8 *n* back.
Working memory, visual and auditory processing, long-term memory, attention, expressive and receptive language, abstract thinking, visual motor coordination, refraining impulsivity, logic thinking	Number 1–9	Use a page protector and dry erase marker. First, place symbols and then cubes with corresponding numbers. Circle/green cube on 1, x/ blue cube on 2, box /red cube on 3, yellow / underline 4, black/ line above 5. Orange/slash on 6, brown / (on 7, white / ( ) on 8, and purple / line in the middle of nine. Remove page protector and read symbols back by alternating saying the number, color, animal, letter, letter sound, president, symbol

(continued)

Table 23.4 (continued)

Cognitive functions targeted	Exercise	Description
Working memory, visual and auditory processing, long-term memory, attention, expressive and receptive language, abstract thinking, phonemic processing, refraining impulsivity, logical thinking, spontaneous comparison	Vowels a–e	First, place symbols and then cubes with corresponding letters. Circle/green cube on a, x/ blue cube on e, box /red cube on i, yellow / underline o, black / line above u. Remove page protector and read symbols back by alternating saying the vowel, sound, color, number, animal, president- a 7 n back. Also do the 7 n back with the cubes covering the letters.
Working memory, visual and auditory processing, long-term memory, attention, expressive and receptive language, abstract thinking, phonemic processing, refraining impulsivity, logical thinking, spontaneous comparison	Letters A–I	First, place symbols and then cubes with corresponding letters. Circle/green cube on A, x/ blue cube on B, box/red cube on C, yellow/ underline D, black/line above E. Orange/slash on F, brown/(on G, white/() on H, and purple/ line in the middle of I. Remove page protector and read symbols back by alternating saying the letter, sound, color, number, animal, president, symbol a 7 n back. Also do the 7 n back with the cubes covering the letters.
Spatial concepts of left, right, up, down, Inductive thinking, inductions of rules, seriation, working memory, long-term memory, auditory and visual processing, abstract thinking, Systematic approach to new information and object, refraining impulsivity, logical thinking, spontaneous comparison	Colored Arrows *5 colors & 9 colors	Say the direction of the arrow, then the color, then alternate color, direction. Add the corresponding number and say number, color, direction. Add the corresponding animal and say number, color, animal, direction. Add the corresponding vowel and say the number, color, animal, vowel, vowel sound, and direction. Add the president sequentially and say the number, color, animal, vowel, vowel sound, president, letter, symbol, and direction. 9 n-back

Source: Brown (2018b)

Table 23.5 Animals

Stroop Animals
Circle the Bear
Box the Snake
X the Fish
Underline the Elephant
Line above the Turtle

Table 23.6 US Presidents (Brown, 2018b)

Basic US Presidents
1. Washington green and circle
2. Adams blue and X
3. Jefferson red and box
4. Madison yellow and underline
5. Monroe black and line above
Advanced US Presidents are said sequentially for n–back
1. Washington
2. Adams
3. Jefferson
4. Madison
5. Monroe
6. John Quincy Adams
7. Jackson
8. Van Buren
9. Harrison
10. Tyler
11. Polk
12. Taylor
13. Fillmore
14. Pierce

Table 23.7 1–5 Numbers (Brown, 2018b)

2 1 5 4 3 circle the 1 and place a green cube
5 3 2 4 1 X the 2 and place a blue cube
3 1 4 2 5 box the 3 and place a red cube
5 4 3 1 2 line under the 4 and place a yellow cube
4 2 5 3 1 line above the 5 and place a black cube

Table 23.8 Vowels a, e, i, o, u (Brown, 2018b)

e a u o i circle the a and place a green cube and the sound is a short "a"
u i e o a X the e and place a blue cube and the sound is a short "e"
i a o e u box the i and place a red cube and the sound is a short "i"
u o i a e line under the o and place a yellow cube and the sound is a short "o"
o e u i a line above the u and place a black cube and the sound is a short "u"

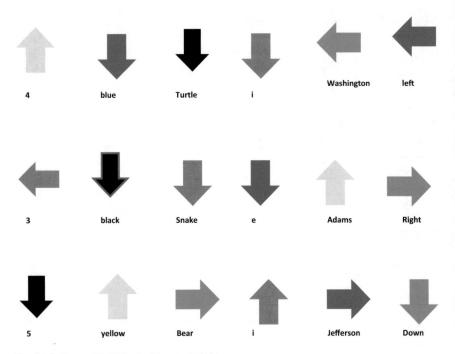

Fig. 23.1 Brown Six N Back. (Brown, 2018b)

Multi-Component, Multi-Domain, and Multi-Task Training

In using all nine variables of *n, EMCDC* is a multi-task, multi-component, and multi-domain cognitive training program with a mediator providing social engagement. Multi-task components include visually scanning the information, writing numbers, letters, and symbols with a dry erase marker, placing the corresponding- colored cubes, and verbalizing what they are doing when holding onto a sequence of 2–9 categories. *EMCDC* also uses various card games which train multiple cognitive skills. These multi-component elements include focused attention interfacing with long-term memory, visual and auditory processing, working memory, and reasoning. By working these cognitive functions in multi-domains through the reflex exercises, sound therapy, and the cognitive games which require eye-hand coordination with verbalization, there is an increase in functional connectivity among various regions of the brain (Kuo et al., 2018; Cao et al., 2016).

Say the number, color, animal, vowel, president(sequentially), direction. Using a page protector and dry erase marker, say and mark the six items. Place a point at the tip of the arrow for the direction. Remove the page protector and read the symbols: number, color, animal, letter, president (sequentially), and direction (Brown, 2018b).

Cognitive Neuroscience and Education

According to cognitive neuroscientist Stanislas Dehaene (2013), learning uses symbols to process letters, sounds, colors, numbers, and images which correlates with the Brown-*n* backs relationship of symbols to numbers, colors, sounds, letters, vowels, and images of animals and presidents. The four pillars of learning identified by cognitive psychologists include focused attention to relevant information, active engagement between the teacher and the learner, feedback to overcome errors successfully which instills internal motivation by providing positive verbal encouragement, and consolidation or transfer of acquired skills and information to knowledge (Dehaene, 2013). The four pillars overlap with Feuerstein's cognitive functions, mediated learning experience, and the *EMCDC* program. The combination of these components lays the foundation for academic success in the classroom.

Implementation and Benefits of Equipping Minds

Since 2010, professional development workshops have been conducted for educators, parents, interventionists, and therapists in person, online, and through prerecorded online courses. Participants receive the Equipping Minds Cognitive Development Curriculum and Equipping Minds Student Workbook. Schools are implementing 30 minutes a day in the classroom for all students. Students who are experiencing learning challenges also use Equipping Minds in tiered intervention for an additional 20–30 minutes a day. Small group and individual interventions are done with students with learning disabilities. Schools report the following benefits: increased reading fluency and comprehension, improved math and writing abilities, focused attention, increased participation in class and confidence, thinking before speaking and acting, improved relationships and self-regulation, and the ability to follow multi-step directions.

Specifically, students with disabilities (IDEA) have an IEP. *EMCDC* is being included in public and private school IEPs. Table 23.9 includes the cognitive abilities tested on psychological testing, the implications for academics, the goals for cognitive training, and the corresponding *EMCDC* exercises to implement. The author suggests using this template for all students under IDEA to target their cognitive skills which will impact academics reducing frustration in the classroom.

Table 23.9 Cognitive abilities and Equipping Minds Cognitive Training Intervention

Cognitive ability	Implications for academics	Goals	Equipping Minds Cognitive Training Intervention
Comprehension-knowledge (*Gc*) verbal/crystallized intelligence The ability to communicate one's knowledge of word meanings, factual information, comprehension, concepts, rules, and relationships. The ability to reason using previous learned experiences, procedures, and knowledge obtained through one's life experiences, school, and work.	Highly predictive of academic success. Strong and consistent relationship to reading, writing, and math throughout school: learning vocabulary, answering factual questions, comprehending oral/written language.	Increase comprehension, retain information, understand relationships, and reason. Visualize, retain, and express what they hear and read.	**Exercises to increase comprehension, retain information, understand relationships, and reason**: Follow Aristotle's *Ten Categories* of Being: what/who, quantities (numerical value), qualities (size, color, shape), action, time, where, relationships, feelings, position, clothing/accessories as your guide to discuss everything. Begin with a picture using the *STARE Jr.* cards, *Yo, Millard Filmore* president's book. ead short stories, Aesop's fables, and ask questions base on the *Ten Categories.* Recall the Stroop Animal directions from memory saying forward and backwards. Build comprehension through vocabulary exercise

(continued)

Table 23.9 (continued)

Cognitive processing speed (*Gs*) The ability to automatically and fluently perform cognitive tasks, particularly when measured under pressure to maintain focused attention. The ability to accurately identify and quickly scan and discriminate visual information to make and implement decisions.	There is a significant impact to reading, writing, and math: completing assignments on time, processing information quickly, copying from the board, and taking timed test.	Increase processing rate and fluency. Increase Rapid Automatic Naming pictures, letters, numbers, colors, shapes. Increase language processing by say what you're doing when sorting the cards and reading the charts/pages. Increase time when saying what you're doing when reading a page of numbers, vowels, letters, colors, directions, shapes, animals. Increase hand-eye coordination sorting	**Exercises to increase processing rate and fluency:** Sort Blink cards, SET, or a deck of cards naming numbers, colors, and shapes/suit. Sort Qwitch cards naming letters and numbers. Read Animal Set 1, Direction Set 1, and Number Set 1 of Stroop Effect. Read the colors of the arrows and then the directions. Read Number Hunt 1–5 and 1–9 numbers.
Auditory processing (*Ga*) The ability to perceive, analyze, manipulate, compare, discriminate, and synthesize patterns among auditory stimuli (speech sounds). The ability to employ auditory information in task performance. It includes phonological awareness, processing, sensitivity, and coding.	There is a significant relationship to reading, writing, and spelling: acquiring phonics, sequencing sounds, listening, learning a foreign language, musical skill. A weakness in phonological processing and awareness is a common factor among learners with reading challenges.	Increase phonemic awareness. Increase ability to retain and manipulate speech sounds.	**Exercises to increase phonemic awareness and auditory processing:** Read the vowels and say the sounds in Vowel Hunt. Use a phonics phone when learning the sounds. Teacher should speak directly into the learner's right ear. Read the letters and say the sounds Letter Fluency for A-H. Read Letters (b, d, p, q, m, w) exercises to say the direction, letter name, and sound. Sound therapy can be very beneficial for increasing auditory processing abilities.

(continued)

Table 23.9 (continued)

Cognitive ability	Implications for academics	Goals	Equipping Minds Cognitive Training Intervention
Short-term & working memory (*Gwm*) The ability to apprehend, hold, and manipulate visual and auditory information in immediate awareness while performing a mental operation on it. Requires attention, auditory and visual discrimination, and concentration. **Auditory working memory:** The ability to hold auditory information in immediate awareness while performing a mental operation on the information. **Visual memory:** The ability to hold visual information in immediate awareness while performing a mental operation on the information.	There is a significant impact to reading, writing, and math: following multi-step directions, recalling sequences, memorizing information, listening, and comprehending, taking notes, remembering math steps, holding letters and sounds in place for reading and spelling.	Recall and complete three and four step directions. Verbalize what he is doing when alternating a sequence of three and four qualities Recall the Stroop Animals forward and backwards Recall numbers from memory forwards and backwards? 6–3–8-1, then 9,4,2,7,6. Show 3 Blink cards. Turn them over and ask to recall. Then ask to recall 2 minutes later. Verbalize a sequence of 4–9 items on the Brown *n*-back	**Exercises to increase working memory and following multi-step directions:** When giving directions, begin with "I see you… What do you see yourself doing?" Blink/Cards: Alternate saying the number, color, and shape/suit. Qwitch: Alternate saying =, +, − ALL Stroop Exercises: Sets 1 and 2. Colored Arrows alternating number, color and direction. Vowel and Number Hunt exercises: Begin with one direction and build on from there. Use b, d, p, q, and other direction exercises Brown 4–9 *n*-back sequence on Arrows, Number Hunt 1–5 and 1–9, Vowels and Letter Fluency Auditory and Visual Working Memory Find it, Write it, & Say it: Use any list & build on it daily. Do not progress without mastery, and don't add too much too fast. Say 2-4-7, /2-4-7-3; and 5-1-6-9, / 5-1-6-9-2 Xtreme Memory with linking cubes, letters, numbers, and symbols Xtreme Tic Toe Visual and Auditory Recall Stare Cards: Ten Categories Presidents

(continued)

Table 23.9 (continued)

Long-term memory (Glr) The ability to store information (ideas, names, concepts) in one's mind and fluently retrieve it later in the process of thinking. Retrieval should be done easily, quickly, and using association.	There is a significant relationship to reading, writing, and math, especially during basic skill acquisition of learning numbers, letters, colors, shapes, sounds, and animals. Organization and classification of information is needed to make recall possible.	Increase the number of items the learner can recall. Name as many animals or any category as fast as you can in 1 minute. Learn the presidents and recall forwards and backwards Categorize animals and other categories	**Exercises to Increase long-term memory retrieval:** Play Make a List. Name as many animals as you can in 1 minute. Use any category in which you have information in your long-term memory and recall. Recall and categorize the items in Make a List, Spot It cards, Stroop Animals Finger exercises for the Palmer reflex daily. Recall stories you have heard and pictures you have seen over a 1-month period. Recall the President's full name, number, and picture from *Yo Millard Fillmore.*
Fluid reasoning (Gf) The type of thinking an individual may use when faced with a relatively new task that cannot be performed automatically. The ability to reason, form concepts, detect underlying relationships and rules among objects to solve problems.	Significant relationship to higher level skills in reading, writing, and math; problem solving, drawing inferences, cognitive flexibility, transferring and generalizing, thinking conceptually.	Apply problem-solving strategies and procedures. Verbalize the thought process when playing Set, Color Code, Blink, Tic Tac Toe, Perplexors, and Critical Thinking exercises.	**Exercises to increase fluid reasoning:** Color Code Blink Game SET Xtreme Tic Tac Toe Perplexor Puzzles Critical Thinking K-3 and 4–7 with verbalization
Visual processing (Gv) The ability to perceive, analyze, and synthesize visual patterns, including the ability to store and recall visual images. **Visual-spatial reasoning** The ability to evaluation visual details and to understand visual spatial relationships to construct geometric designs from a model.	There is a significant relationship to reading, writing, and math, especially during basic skill acquisition of learning numbers, letters, colors, shapes, sounds, and animals. Organization and classification of information is needed to make recall possible.	Read letters, numbers, and words without skipping lines Read letters, numbers, and words fluidly and calmly Verbalize his thought process when playing Color Code	**Exercises to increase visual processing and visual-spatial reasoning:** Color Code Xtreme Memory Xtreme Tic Tac Toe Tangrams

Case Studies with Equipping Minds

Since 2010, *EMCDC* has been implemented 1-on-1, demonstrating far transfer effects to cognitive and academic gains. Eight case studies[2] of learners with a neurodevelopmental disorder will be examined.[3] Brown utilized the following data collection techniques: clinical observations of the learners, examining and analyzing the psychological and educational documents, and interviewing the parents, the learners, and teachers. Academic and psychological testing ranged from 1 to 6 years providing significant insights into the impact cognitive training had on each learner. Seven of the eight cognitive developmental therapy sessions, i.e.., cognitive training, were conducted online. Three of the eight were international adoptions at 4 and 5 years of age. It should also be noted that English was their second language, and each had experienced trauma at a young age.

Case 1. Marie: Down Syndrome and Intellectual Disability

Marie[4] was born with a neurodevelopmental disorder: Down syndrome.

Assessment
Academic testing was conducted over a 4-year period using the Measures of Academic Progress (MAP), Kentucky Performance Rating for Educational (KPREP), Stanford Ten National Assessment Ranking, and Student Growth Profiles.

Intervention
Equipping Minds Cognitive Development Curriculum (*EMCDC*) was done from 2011 to 2015. In September 2010, the author worked with Marie an hour of every school day for 12 weeks.

Results After Intervention
At the end of 9 weeks, the principal reported that Marie had increased by 20 points in reading, 11 points in math, 16 points in science, and 17 points in language arts on the Measures of Academic Progress (MAP). The gains were unprecedented as students typically increase 3–5 points on the MAP.

Marie would continue the EMCDC cognitive developmental exercises and continue to progress academically for the next 4 years. Below are the results of the MAP tests after the first 9 weeks and over the next 4 years. Figures 23.2, 23.3, 23.4,

---

[2] Parts of this chapter, including cases 1–6, have published previously in: Brown (2018c) and Brown (2018d), licensed under the terms of the Creative Commons Attribution 4.0 International License (http://creativecommons.org/licenses/by/4.0/).

[3] These case studies are a revised version of an earlier publication by Brown (2018c) shared with Merrick's permission.

[4] All names and other personal identifiers in the case studies have been changed to protect privacy and confidentiality.

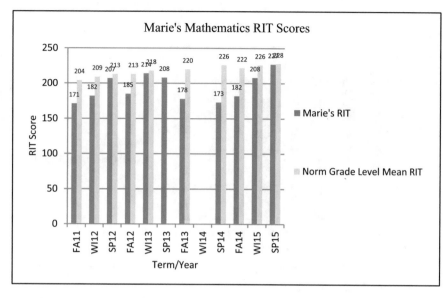

Fig. 23.2 Marie's mathematics RIT scores

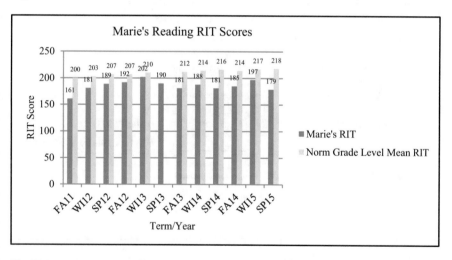

Fig. 23.3 Marie's reading RIT scores

and 23.5 illustrate re-creations of the MAP test results which demonstrate significant gains in academic abilities or far transfer effects. It should be noted that the only accommodation she received on MAP testing was extended time and having a reader for math, science, and language. She read the reading assessments herself.

Her Kentucky Performance Rating for Educational (KPREP) scores showed gains in math, reading, and writing on-demand. Marie's Kentucky Performance Rating for Educational Progress (KPREP) scores in sixth grade showed strong growth. The KPREP test is more comprehensive and has historically been difficult

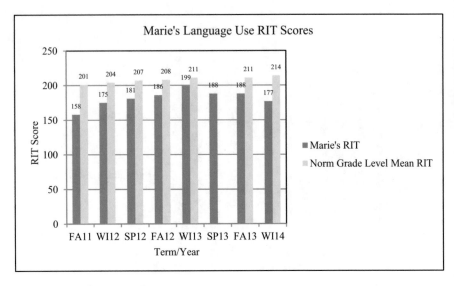

Fig. 23.4 Marie's language RIT scores

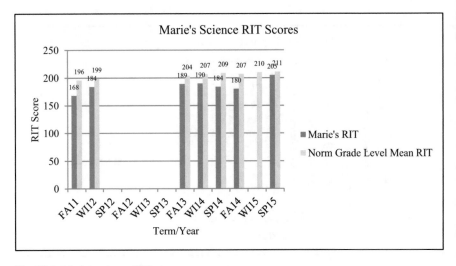

Fig. 23.5 Marie's science RIT scores

for Marie. In seventh grade, she scored two points above the state mean in mathematics and was one point from a proficient status. The apprentice level for the seventh grade states that a student can compute a percent of a number, use ratios to solve problems, evaluate mathematical problems using order of operations with integers, solve two-step equations, evaluate algebraic expressions with two or more variables using order of operations, select and apply basic geometric formulas, identify cross sections of a 3-D object taken parallel to a base, identify an appropriate sample for a population, and compute measures of central tendency. The recreation of her KPREP scores is illustrated in Figs. 23.6, 23.7, and 23.8.

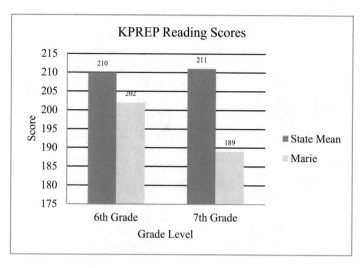

Fig. 23.6 KPREP reading scores

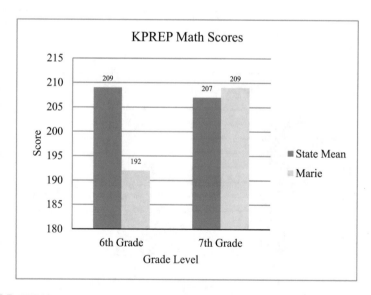

Fig. 23.7 KPREP math scores

Marie's student growth percentile (SGP) in reading was 93 percent in sixth grade and 7 percent in seventh grade. Her SCP was 63 percent in math as a sixth grader and 93 percent in seventh grade. Figure 23.9 illustrates a re-creation of the SCP for sixth and seventh grade. In 2015, as a seventh grader, she scored in the 39th percentile in mathematics, 36th percentile in science, and the seventh percentile in reading on the Stanford Ten National Assessment Ranking. Figure 23.10 illustrates a re-creation of the Stanford National Ranking.

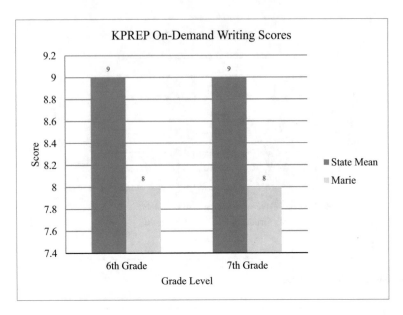

Fig. 23.8 KPREP on-demand writing scores

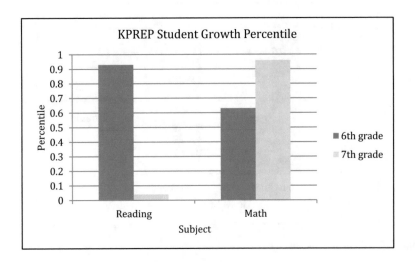

Fig. 23.9 K PREP student growth percentile

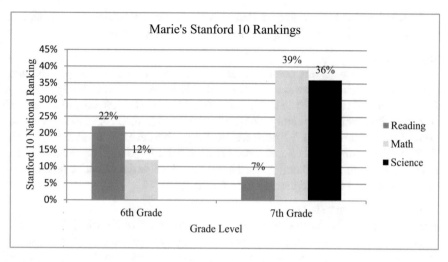

Fig. 23.10 Marie's Stanford 10 rankings

Case 2. Joseph: Fetal Alcohol Syndrome, Mixed Expressive/ Receptive Language Disorder, Developmental Coordination Disorder (Dysgraphia)

At the age of five, Joseph was adopted from Poland. He was removed from his biological mother due to alcohol abuse and neglect which was traumatic. He was diagnosed with fetal alcohol syndrome, a language processing disorder with impairments in both expressive and receptive channels, and developmental coordination disorder. English is his second language.

Assessment

Joseph received an extensive evaluation of his cognitive abilities in 2015 at 8 years of age and further evaluations in 2016 at 10 years of age. The examiner believes that Joseph's difficulties are consistent with a diagnosis of a Mixed Expressive/Receptive Language Disorder (ICD 10: F80.1). This profoundly impacts his ability to learn in a classroom environment (i.e., receptive language) as well as severely limits his capacity to participate in class or group-based activities (i.e., expressive language).

- Very weak visual-spatial processing skills as well as poor fine-motor control, which is likely to profoundly impact his ability to learn, unless accommodations are made to support this challenge. His difficulties are consistent with a diagnosis of developmental coordination disorder (i.e., dysgraphia, ICD 10 Code: F82).
- Some weakness for sustaining attention and executive functioning, that while likely to significantly impact his daily life at school, is likely to be related to the specific learning challenges described above. At this time, although these challenges would typically be indicative of an attention disorder, it is the examiner's

impression that his learning challenges are a better explanation for why he has weakness in tasks of working memory and processing speed.

Intervention

Joseph had been receiving occupational therapy, speech therapy, and educational support at his school. However, he was not able to work independently in class. Brown reviewed the academic and psychological testing showing cognitive deficits in processing, working memory, comprehension, and perceptual reasoning. From April 2015 to January 2017, Joseph received cognitive developmental therapy with *EMCDC* for 30-minute sessions, 5 days a week for 150 hours. The sessions were conducted via online teletherapy. During this time, he also did primitive reflex exercises and listened to sound therapy for a few months.

Results After Intervention

Previously, Joseph's working memory was an index score of 80, which is the ninth percentile. In contrast to the 2015 evaluation, the working memory index score increased to 103 and the 58th percentile in the average range conducted in December 2016. The processing speed is considerably higher on the 2016 evaluation, increasing from an index score of 83 to 98 and from the 13th to 45th percentile in the average range (see Table 23.10).

In March 2017, the Kaufman Test of Educational Achievement-third Edition-Form A (KTEA-3) was administered. The KTEA-3 is composed of subtests that measure a student's academic achievement in the areas of reading, written language, and math. Joseph is performing in the average range in all academic areas. When compared to grade norms, Joseph's scores are higher. While he demonstrated average comprehension abilities when reading expository passages and literal questions, he demonstrated weaknesses when reading fictional passages and answering inferential questions. Math concepts and applications are a relative strength for Joseph while math computations are a relative weakness. Joseph performed equally well with written expression and spelling. (see Table 23.11).

Table 23.10 Results of WISC IV and WISC V of Joseph

Scale WISC – IV 01–02/2015	Percentile	Composite score	Scale WISC –V 12/2016	Percentile	Composite score	Composite difference
Verbal Comprehension	32nd	93	Verbal Comprehension	18th	86	-7
Working Memory	9th	80	Working Memory	58th	103	23
Processing Speed	13th	83	Processing Speed	45th	98	15
Perceptual Reasoning	14th	84	Visual Spatial	30th	92	8
			Fluid Reasoning	8th	79	
			Full Scale IQ	21st	88	

Table 23.11 Results of KETA-3 of Joseph

Scale KETA-3 03/2017	Standard score	Percentile
Reading Composite	99	47
Math Composite	96	42
Written-Language Composite	98	45

The current scores are in some way like previous results and in some ways dissimilar. The WISC-V has a different format than the WISC-IV. With one exception, each of the index scores has at least one and sometimes two subtests within the average range, suggesting that Joseph's potential is at least in the average range in all the tested areas, except for one. Joseph's Vocabulary score was in the middle of the average range. However, as he did on the 2015 WISC-IV, he had extreme difficulty in understanding superordinate concepts. In other words, understanding the relationship to how things are similar. Another way of saying it would be that he had difficulty detecting the conceptual relationship among objects. In the 2015 report, Joseph had very poor visual-spatial ability. However, on this measure, there is an addition of another subtest not given on the WISC-IV. On the Block Design subtest, which is a visual-spatial task or a task of perceptual analytic reasoning, he scored in the average range and was in the low average range previously. The same is true for a task in which he had to analyze and synthesize visual objects. The index score of 92 falls in the average range. Thus, visual-spatial reasoning or perceptual analytic abilities are in the average range, albeit at the lower end of average (see Table 23.10).

Joseph had the most difficulty in Fluid Reasoning. These tasks require him to detect underlying conceptual relationships among visual objects and then use reasoning to identify and apply the rules. Similarly, as already mentioned, Joseph had difficulty understanding conceptual relationships on a verbal task (Similarities subtest). It should be noted that the examiner who administered the WISC V was not familiar to Joseph and noted significant impulsivity and anxiety during the testing.

However, at 10 years of age, Joseph was administered the Kaufman Brief Intelligence- 2 (KBIT-2) in September 2016 by Brown who had been working with him daily for 1.5 years. The test was given over 2 days. Joseph exhibited no impulsivity or anxiety and was extremely thoughtful in his responses. The KBIT-2 is a brief intelligence test that measures verbal and nonverbal intelligence for individuals from 4 to 90 years of age and yields three scores: verbal, nonverbal, and IQ composite. The Verbal scale is composed of two subtests that assess receptive vocabulary and general information (Verbal Knowledge) as well as comprehension, reasoning, and vocabulary knowledge (Riddles). Joseph had a standard score of 102 in the 55th percentile and average range. The Nonverbal scale uses a Matrices subtest to measure the ability to solve new problems by accessing an individual ability to complete visual analogies and understand relationships (Kaufman & Kaufman, 2004). Joseph had a standard score of 112 in the 79th percentile in the average range. The IQ composite had a standard score of 109 in the 73rd percentile also in the average range (see Table 23.12). This is the only assessment administered by

Table 23.12 Results of KBIT-2 of Joseph

Scale KBIT-2 02/2016	Standard score	Percentile
Verbal	102	55
Nonverbal	112	79
IQ	109	73

Brown. It is Brown's opinion that the difference in fluid reasoning scores on the WISC V and KBIT 2 is a result of the cognitive training and having a relationship with the examiner allowing Joseph to complete the test in optimum conditions.

These gains demonstrate the impact of EMCDC on working memory, fluid reasoning, and processing speed. Furthermore, the psychological examiner notes the Full-Scale IQ cannot be used as a fixed figure. There are several indicators on the measure that would suggest average intellect. This would agree with Brown's assessment on the KBIT-2 placing Joseph in the average range.

In conclusion, Joseph has shown strong cognitive modifiability throughout the program with *ECMDC*. He has an incredible work ethic and maintains a positive growth mindset. Joseph's visual and verbal memory, visual-spatial memory, working memory, processing, and reasoning skills have developed significantly. He is giving more attention to detail, following 3- to 4-step directions, and verbalizing his thought process.

Case 3. David: Autism, Apraxia, Anxiety, and Hashimoto's Disease

David is a 11-year-old boy with a diagnosis of Autism and verbal apraxia at 2 years, 8 months of age. He was also diagnosed with Hashimoto's disease in December of 2010. David's school performance is below average. He has received Applied Behavior Analysis (ABA) therapy, speech therapy, and occupational services for many years. He struggles with anxiety, atypical social behavior, and preservation of topics.

Assessment
At the age of 8, David received an extensive evaluation of his cognitive abilities in 2015 and further evaluations in 2016. In 2015 the processing speed index (PSI) of the WISC IV was given to David with a PSI of 73 as seen in Table 23.13. The Kaufman Brief Intelligence- 2 (KBIT-2) was also given in 2015. The verbal scale is composed of two subtests that assess receptive vocabulary and general information (Verbal Knowledge) as well as comprehension, reasoning, and vocabulary knowledge (Riddles). David had a standard score of 61 in the below-average range. The Nonverbal scale uses a Matrices subtest to measure the ability to solve new problems by accessing an individual ability to complete visual analogies and understand relationships (Kaufman & Kaufman, 2004). David had a Nonverbal standard score

Table 23.13 Results of WISC IV, WISC V and KBIT-2 of David

Scale WISC – IV 01/2015	Composite score	Scale WISC –V 09//2016	Composite score	Difference	
		Verbal Comprehension	62		Below average
		Working Memory	74		Below average
Processing Speed	73	Processing Speed	77	4	Below average
		Visual Spatial	97		Average
		Fluid Reasoning	85		Average
KBIT-2 IQ composite	58	Full Scale IQ	72	14	Below average

Table 23.14 Results of KBIT-2 of David

KBIT-2 01/2015	Standard score	KBIT-2 09/2016	Standard score	Difference	
Verbal	61	Verbal	69	8	Below average
Nonverbal	66	Nonverbal	122	56	Average
IQ composite	58	IQ composite	95	37	Average

Table 23.15 Results of WIAT-III of David

Scale WIAT-III 01/2015	Standard score	Scale KETA-3 09/2016	Standard score	Difference
Early Reading Skills	40	Reading Composite	73	33
Word Reading	70	Letter and Word Recognition	77	7
Listening Comprehension	53	Reading Comprehension	71	18
Receptive Vocabulary	66	Silent Reading Fluency	78	12
Expressive Vocabulary	55	Math Composite	73	18
Math Problem Solving	51	Math Concepts and Application	68	17
Numerical Operations	71	Math Computation	81	10
Spelling	83	Spelling	86	3

of 66 in the below-average range. The IQ composite had a standard score of 58 also in the below-average range for an intellectual disability as seen in Table 23.14.

The Wechsler Individual Achievement Test-III was given to David in 2015. The examiner noted severe difficulties academically with severely impaired scores in early reading, math problems, and listening comprehension. Spelling was in the low average range and alphabet writing in the average range. Word reading and numerical operations were in the moderately impaired range as seen in Table 23.15.

Intervention

David received cognitive developmental therapy with Equipping Minds Cognitive Development Curriculum from February 2015 to May 2017 for 20- to 30-minute sessions, 5 days a week for a total of 160 hours. The sessions were conducted via online teletherapy.

Results After Intervention

After receiving cognitive intervention with *EMCDC* for 1.5 years, David was referred for a psycho-educational re-evaluation in September 2016 to determine continued special education eligibility and placement. He was previously identified as a student with an autism spectrum disorder.

The WISC-V was the assessment given for the reevaluation to assess David's performance across five areas of cognitive ability. As measured by the WISC-V, his overall FSIQ score fell in the below-average range when compared to other children his age (FSIQ = 72) which was an increase of 14 points from the FSIQ of 58 in 2015. Furthermore, he showed average performance when working with primarily visual information and the VSI demonstrates an area of strength relative to his overall ability (VSI = 97). When compared to his fluid reasoning (FRI = 85), working memory (WMI = 74), and processing speed (PSI = 77) performance, visual spatial skills emerged as a particular strength (see Table 23.13).

Results of standardized achievement testing on the Kaufman Test of Educational Achievement-third Edition-Form A given in 2016 suggest that David is performing within the average range for the area of spelling. The areas of letter/word recognition, silent reading fluency, reading comprehension, math computation, and math concepts/applications were found to be within the below-average range. The assessment instruments used provide a comprehensive set of individually administered norm-referenced tests for measuring academic achievement. It should be noted that norm-referenced assessments do not test curriculums benchmark, or the amount of instruction needed to achieve benchmarks. These tests provide a measure of David's academic achievement as compared to peers of the same age using a standard score. His test performance can be generalized to similar, non-test, age-level tasks (see Table 23.15).

In analyzing the results on the Wechsler Individual Achievement Test-III given in 2015 and the Kaufman Test of Educational Achievement-third Edition-Form A given in 2016, David made significant gains in reading abilities, letter/word recognition, silent reading fluency, reading comprehension, math computation, and math concepts/applications moving from severely impaired in 2015 to below-average range 1.5 years later. Spelling moved from below-average to the average range (see Table 23.15). In conclusion, the academic and cognitive gains which David has shown indicate strong cognitive modifiability in many areas. His social skills also improved, impacting his relationships with peers.

Case 4. Kay: General Learning Disorder

Assessment

Kay's parents have been concerned about her cognitive abilities since the first evaluation when she was 7 years of age. At that time, her Full-Scale IQ on the WISC-IV was 72. Her Verbal Comprehension Index is 79, Perceptual Reasoning is 94, Processing Speed is 73, and Working Memory is 56 as seen in Table 23.16. Kay performs better on nonverbal than verbal reasoning tasks. At the age of 15 years, Kay had another educational evaluation. On the Slosson Full-Range Intelligence test, Kay received a Full-Range IQ score of 85. The verbal index score was 88, the memory index standard score was 80, and the performance index standard score is 84. All three of these index scores: 88, 84, and 80 are consistent with Kay's overall IQ score of 85 as seen in Table 23.17.

Academic testing had been done with the Woodcock Johnson Test of Achievement III (WJ-III) from 2010 to 2016. In April 2010, the WJ-III results indicated Kay was in the average range in broad math and math calculations. Oral language, brief and broad reading, written expression, and understanding directions were in the low average range (see Tables 23.19) . She has been home-schooled by her mother for her academic career. In 2013, the Peabody Individual Achievement Test was given. Kay had a standard score of 84 (14th percentile) in general information, a standard score of 71 (third percentile) in reading recognition, a standard score of 70 (second percentile) in reading comprehension, a standard score of 67 (first percentile) in total reading, a standard score of 74 (fourth percentile) in mathematics, a standard score of 76 (fifth percentile) in spelling, and a standard score of 71 (third percentile) in written language (see Table 23.18).

Table 23.16 Results of WISC IV for Kay

Scale WISC –IV 12/2005	Composite score	Percentile	
Verbal Comprehension	79	8	Low
Working Memory	56	0.2	Low
Processing Speed	73	4	Low
Perceptual Reasoning	94	34	Average
Full Scale IQ	72	3	Low

Table 23.17 Results of Slosson for Kay

Scale 03/2013	Composite score	Percentile	
Verbal Index	88	8	Low
Memory Index	80	0.2	Low
Performance Index	84	4	Low
Full Scale IQ	85	3	Below average

Table 23.18 Peabody Individual Achievement Test for Kay

2013	Standard score	Percentile
General Information	84	14
Reading Recognition	71	3
Reading Comprehension	70	2
Mathematics	74	4
Spelling	76	5
Written Expression	71	3

Intervention

Kay received cognitive developmental therapy with *EMCDC* from September 2015 to May 2016 for 30-minute sessions, 5 days a week for 60 hours. The sessions were conducted via online teletherapy. She was 17 years of age.

Results After Intervention

After completing 60 hours with EMCDC, Kay took the Woodcock Johnson Test of Achievement III as she does every year as seen in Table 23.19. In analyzing the results from 2010 to 2014, Kay typically made gains of 6 months to 1 year. At a 9.8 grade level in 2014, Kay's scores ranged from 4.2 to 7.0 in most subjects putting her 2 to 5 years below grade level. However, Kay made significant gains in Grade Equivalent (GE) and Age Equivalent (AE) on the 2016 assessment where she was 11.8 GE and 18.2 AE in the following areas:

- Oral language went from 4.4 GE to 17.6 GE for a gain of 13.2 years
- Written expression went from 7.6 GE to 12 GE for a gain of 4.4 years
- Understanding Directions which encompasses working memory went from 4.5 GE to 18 GE for a gain of 13.5 years
- Math Calculations went from 9.5 GE to 11.2 GE for a gain of 1.7 years
- Writing Fluency went from 7 GE to 13 GE for a gain of 6 years
- Story Recall went from 5.6 GE to 13 GE for a gain of 7.4 years

The same examiner has given the test for numerous years and indicated that gains of this magnitude had not been seen and are atypical of someone with Kay's long academic history of learning challenges. The gains correspond with the cognitive developmental therapy with EMCDC which Kay received from September 2015 to May 2016. She had previously been receiving academic tutoring alone. In conclusion, the academic gains which Kay has shown indicate strong cognitive modifiability in many areas. As her processing and working memory abilities increased, Kay was able to successfully complete her high school coursework and start her own photography business.

Table 23.19 Results Woodcock Johnson III Normative Tests of Achievement of Kay

	GE:5.8	GE:6.8	GE:7.8	GE:9.8	Score after intervention Grade: 11.8	Difference
	2010	2011	2012	2014	2016	
Oral Language	3.7	3.5	4.6	4.4	17.6	13.2
Brief Achievement	3.2	3.7	4.2	4.6	6.5	1.9
Broad Reading	2.8	3.1	3.9	4.7	6.6	1.9
Broad Math	5.2	5.7	6.3	7	7.2	0.2
Broad written language	3.3	4.3	4.8	6.3	8.9	2.6
Brief Reading	2.9	3.3	4.1	4.8	7	2.2
Brief Math	5.1	5.5	6.3	6.6	7.2	0.6
Math Calc Skills	6	6.4	8.1	9.2	9.2	0
Brief Writing	3	4.1	4.7	5.9	8.1	2.2
Written expression	3.9	5.1	5.5	7.6	12	4.4
Academic Skills	3.6	4	5.1	5.5	7.8	2.3
Academic Fluency	3.6	4.3	4.7	6.4	7.6	1.2
Academic Apps	3.6	4.5	4.7	5.9	6.7	0.8
Academic Knowledge	3.4	3.4	4.5	4.8	7.1	2.3
Letter Word ID	3	3.2	4.2	4.3	7.2	2.9
Reading Fluency	2.4	2.4	3.2	4.3	5.5	1.2
Understanding Directions	4.1	2.4	5.1	4.5	18	13.5
Calculations	6.4	6.4	9.5	9.5	11.2	1.7
Math Fluency	5.4	6.7	6.6	8.7	7.5	−1.2
Spelling	2.7	3.4	3.7	4.8	6.9	2.1
Writing Fluency	3.9	4.9	4.9	7	13	6
Passage Com	2.7	3.5	3.9	6	6.7	0.7
Applied Prob	4.2	4.7	4.5	4.8	5.2	0.4
Writing Sample	3.8	5.5	6.7	8.7	11.4	2.7
Story Recall	1.8	1.8	2.7	5.6	13	7.4
Academic Knowledge	3.4	3.4	4.5	4.8	7.1	2.3

Case 5. Steven: Fetal Alcohol Spectrum Disorder, Post-traumatic Stress Disorder, Autism, Mixed Receptive-Expressive Language Disorder, ADHD, Specific Learning Disorder, Anxiety

Steven was adopted from Russia at the age of 5 years. He has a history of mild alcohol-related neurodevelopmental disorder in addition to psychosocial growth failure and post-traumatic stress disorder. English is his second language.

Assessments
Steven has been evaluated by the pediatric endocrinologist for growth issues as he has been below the tenth percentile which was consistent with the initial neuropsychological evaluation. Steven is on medication for ADHD and has Lyme disease. He has a history of strabismus with residual exotropia which was addressed in

developmental optometry. The diagnostic conclusions indicated a mixed receptive-expressive language disorder; multi-sensory neuropsychologically-based processing deficits related to an alcohol-related neurodevelopmental disorder/static encephalopathy in addition to multiple learning disabilities in the category of developmental dyslexic disorder. Steven certainly had a great deal of anxiety which is very commonly seen in children who have multi-sensory neurocognitive deficits.

Steven's overall neuropsychological history indicates that he was evaluated at the age of 10 years with a pattern of global weaknesses in receptive and expressive language as well as processing and learning deficits. Many of these issues were related to mild alcohol-related neurodevelopmental disorder with some quasi-autistic characteristics in addition to multisensory information processing impairments. After the neuropsychological evaluation, Steven received special education services throughout his school years and was re-evaluated at the start of his tenth-grade year in January of 2012.

Steven's initial intellectual testing completed in 2005 yielded a verbal comprehension score of 75; perceptual reasoning score of 92; working memory score of 77; processing speed score of 97; and a Full-Scale IQ score of 81. Gaps and inconsistencies in nonverbal learning aptitudes and abilities, as well as receptive and expressive language, were evident.

In the updated evaluation in 2012, Steven was administered the Wechsler Intelligence Scale for Children – Fourth Edition and obtained a verbal comprehension score of 79; perceptual reasoning score of 88; working memory score of 83; processing speed score of 94; and a Full-Scale IQ of 81 which was the sale score in 2005 (See Table 23.20).

Steven also showed ongoing indications of a mild Autistic Disorder given his difficulties in relating to others as well as anxiety, stress, and struggles with adapting to change as well as expressive pragmatic language. He also had definite problems in comprehension and higher-level listening responses in addition to gaps and inconsistencies in attention, memory, learning, and overall information processing and problem solving. Academic-achievement abilities indicated weaknesses in reading style, rate, and written language with relative strengths in mechanical math but difficulties in mental calculations and word problems. Steven always struggled with expressive writing in addition to memory processing and consolidation in both auditory and visual spheres. He also had significant patterns of executive dysfunction. Over the years, Steven has been receiving special education services through his school district and has made gradual progress.

Intervention

Steven received cognitive developmental therapy with *EMCDC* from January 2015 to May 2015 for 60-minute sessions, 5 days a week for 60 hours. The sessions were conducted via online teletherapy. Steven also did 15–20 minutes of primitive reflex integration therapy and 60 minutes of sound therapy daily for a few months.

Results After Intervention

After completing cognitive developmental therapy with *EMCDC*, his parents stated that Steven showed reduced anxiety, increased eye contact, was more socially

Table 23.20 Results of WISC IV for Steven

Scale WISC – IV	Composite score 2005	Composite score 2012	Composite score 07/2015	Difference
Verbal Comprehension	75	79	76	−3
Working Memory	77	83	80	−3
Processing Speed	97	94	106	12
Perceptual Reasoning	92	88	97	9
Full Scale IQ	81	81	89	8

aware, and demonstrated a sense of humor and math sense. His overall language and language arts abilities have improved with cognitive therapy, and he has improved in his overall academic performance and cognitive abilities (See Table 23.20). Steven no longer needs to take ADHD medication.

In July 2015, Steven was administered the Wechsler Adult Intelligence Scale – Fourth Edition and showed a more stable pattern in his overall intellectual abilities which are now within the Average Range although he has a 21-point discrepancy between verbal comprehension and perceptual reasoning which indicates an ongoing language weakness pattern. As a general summary statement, there is no question that Steven has improved on a global perspective in terms of neurocognitive or neuropsychiatric functioning after completing 60 hours of *EMCDC*. His processing speed increased by 12 points, his perceptual reasoning increased by 9 points, and his IQ increased by 8 points as seen in Table 23.20. He is much more alert, oriented, and interactive as well as motivated to do well with a lessening of the neurocognitive effects of a fetal alcohol spectrum disorder in addition to his autistic spectrum disorder which has always been at the "higher-functioning spectrum." In terms of pure academic-achievement abilities, Steven is at the middle school level in overall reading, reading comprehension, spelling, written language, and mathematics. This certainly is a significant improvement as it shows that he has enough neurocognitive and academic skills in order to function at the technical-vocational training level. His strengths are in the areas of hands-on visual assimilative learning which is his area of interest and strength. Steven graduated from high school and is currently employed.

Case 6. Bryant: Post-traumatic Concussion Syndrome

At 18 years of age, Bryant experienced a head injury during a rugby game. The doctors recommended antidepressants and extended rest. As the symptoms increased, he tried various treatments over the next 4 years from acupuncture to chiropractic treatments. However, the symptoms were not alleviated. He then took 1 year off and had given up. He was 23 years of age when beginning cognitive training with *EMCDC*.

- Assessment   Interview with learner
- Equipping Minds Learning Screening Checklist
- Equipping Minds Primitive Reflex Checklist

Below is a list of the most prominent symptoms Bryant experienced after the concussion.

- Fogginess: One of my most prominent symptoms is what can only be described as a feeling of fogginess. When in this state, it is hard to complete most mental tasks. It felt as if my neurons were trying to fire and make connections but didn't have a clear pathway to do so.
- Difficulty with concentration and attention: Within this state, Bryant had a difficult time concentrating on tasks and paying attention for extended periods of time.
- Poor working memory: Difficulty following multiple-step directions
- Long-term memory retrieval: Difficulty remembering names of people
- Language retrieval and processing: Difficulty recalling vocabulary
- Extreme physical and mental fatigue: Mental fatigue is like fogginess but manifests itself in fatigue-like symptoms. For example, during reading Bryant would have to fight off an intense desire to sleep and could no longer concentrate on whatever was being read.
- Depression

Intervention

In October of 2016, Bryant contacted Brown to discuss using *EMCDC* to strengthen his cognitive deficits because of post-traumatic concussion syndrome. According to Bryant he has tired numerous interventions over the last 5 years with little relief. Brown agreed to have an EMCDC mediator begin working with Bryant using *EMCDC*. Bryant received cognitive developmental therapy with EMCDC from September 2016 to April 2017 for 30- to 60-minute sessions, 5 days a week for a total of 100 hours. The sessions were conducted via online teletherapy. Bryant also did 15–20 minutes of primitive reflex integration therapy and 60 minutes of sound therapy on a daily basis during this time.

Results After Intervention

After completing 100 hours of intervention with *EMCDC,* Bryant reported the following results.

- Decreased fogginess: After working with EMCDC, the periods and intensity of fogginess have significantly decreased. The exercises we focused on strengthened those connections and helped my brain work around its deficits.
- Increased concentration and attention: Bryant reports having a much easier time holding attention and concentrating on specific tasks.
- Increase in working memory: Able to follow multi-step directions
- Long-term memory: Able to store information and retrieve information much easier
- Increased stamina and energy: His stamina and energy have significantly improved while performing cognitive tasks.
- Enjoying reading and learning
- Spending extended time outside without being symptomatic

Bryant's improvements continue and he can work full-time and is asymptomatic.

Case 7. Scott: Anxiety, Autism, Developmental Coordination Disorder, Borderline Intellectual Functioning

At the age of 2.5 years, Scott was adopted from China. English is his second language.

Assessment
At 6 years of age, Scott received a cognitive evaluation in 2010 and further evaluations in 2015 at 10 years of age, 2017 at 12 years of age, and 2020 at 15 years of age. The examiner believes that Scott's difficulties are consistent with a mixed diagnosis of Anxiety, Autism, and Developmental Coordination Disorder. Scott had received physical therapy, speech therapy, occupational therapy, and Applied Behavior Analysis (ABA) therapy. He has been homeschooled and has attended a private school.

Intervention
Scott received cognitive developmental therapy with *EMCDC* from June 2019 to March 2020 for 60-minute sessions, 5 days a week for a total of 60 hours. The sessions were conducted via online teletherapy. Scott also did 15–20 minutes of primitive reflex integration therapy and 60 minutes of sound therapy daily for 10 months.

Results After Intervention
Scott made unprecedented gains on his cognitive testing. Table 23.21 includes cognitive testing over 10 years. His Full-Scale IQ increased 41 points from 80 in 2017 to 121 in 2020 moving him from a borderline intellectual disability to the superior range. His verbal comprehension increased 19 points, visual spatial increased 30 points, fluid reasoning increased 32 points, working memory increased 28 points, and processing speed increased 10 points. He was faithful in doing the primitive reflex exercises and listening to the sound therapy daily. Due to the pandemic of 2020, the school did not conduct year-end academic testing. However, he made all A's and a B+ in geometry. His social skills were also significantly impacted.

Table 23.21 Results of WISC IV and WISC V for Scott

	Oct. 2010	Feb. 2015	March 2017	May 2020	
Verbal Comprehension	VIQ 88	103	89	108 average	+19
Visual Spatial		78	92	122 superior	+30
Fluid Reasoning	PIQ 82	100	74	106 average	+32
Working Memory		76	97	125 superior	+28
Processing Speed		77	98	108 average	+10
Full Scale	83	89	80	121 superior	+41

Case 8. Jackson: Specific Learning Disorder with Impairment in Reading, Specific Learning Disorder with Impairment in Written Expression, ADHD, Other Specified Anxiety Disorder

Jackson is an 8-year-old boy. In 2019, an evaluation determined he met criteria for Specific Learning Disorder with impairment in reading (Dyslexia) and impairment in written expression and Other Specified Anxiety Disorder. In 2021, he was diagnosed with attention deficit/hyperactivity disorder. He received speech therapy in kindergarten to address articulation.

Assessment
Cognitive results from the WISC-V indicated an overall Full-Scale IQ (SS = 119; 98th percentile) at the top of the High Average range, Extremely High Comprehension (SS = 133; 99th percentile), Average Visual Spatial (SS = 97; 42nd percentile), High Average Fluid Reasoning (SS = 115; 84th percentile), Average Working Memory (SS = 91; 27th percentile) and Average Processing Speed (SS = 92; 30th percentile). The Wechsler Individual Achievement Test (WIAT)III indicated a Reading Composite (83; 13th percentile), Word Reading (90; 25th percentile), PseudoWord Reading (76; fifth percentile), and Spelling (89; 23rd percentile).

Intervention
Jackson received cognitive developmental therapy with Equipping Minds Cognitive Development Curriculum from August 2020 to March 2021 for 30-minute sessions, 5 days a week for a total of 70 hours. He also did a phonics-based reading intervention for an hour a day, 4 days a week. These sessions were conducted via online teletherapy. He also received occupational therapy twice a week for part of the school year.

Results After Intervention
In March 2021, Jackson completed a virtual administration of the core WISC-V subtests with the exception of Block Design with Dr. Brown. Results from this administration indicated a Very High overall Full Scale IQ (SS = 128; 97th percentile) which was a gain of 9 points, Extremely High Verbal Comprehension (SS = 142; 99th percentile) which was a gain of 9 points, High Average Fluid Reasoning (SS = 118; 88th percentile) which was a 3-point gain, High Average Working Memory (SS = 117; 87th percentile) which was a 26-point gain, and Average Processing Speed (SS = 108; 70th percentile) which is a 16-point gain. Additional testing was also done at the testing center which had conducted the assessments in 2019. The Kaufman Brief Intelligence Test, Second Edition (KBIT-2) placed Jackson in the High Average for his overall intellectual abilities (88th percentile) with his verbal skills in the High Average range (SS = 112; 79th percentile) and nonverbal skills in the High Average range (SS = 119; 90th percentile) which is consistent with the WISC-V. The WIAT-III showed improvements in several areas since his 2019 testing. Specifically, Jackson's Total Reading Composite increased from 83 and the 13th percentile to 92 and the 39th percentile. Word Reading increased from 90 and the 25th percentile to 101 and the 51st percentile. Pseudoword Reading increased from 76 and the fifth percentile to 92 and the 30th percentile.

Spelling scores improved from 89 and the 23rd percentile to 94 and the 34th percentile placing him in the Average range and High Average range in Reading Comprehension with a score of 113 and the 81st percentile.

The results from the cognitive testing indicate that overall abilities are at the utmost end of the High Average range with significant gains in processing speed and working memory. The severity of his reading disorder is considered mild at this time. The combination of cognitive training with the Orton-Gillingham phonics-based reading instruction proved beneficial for Jackson cognitively and academically demonstrating far transfer effects.

Discussion

Cognitive and academic gains are demonstrated in each of the learners. These results confirm that learners who have multiple neurodevelopmental disabilities benefit from a multi-component and multi-domain cognitive training program. Whereas six of the seven learners received the program through an online format, it expands the options for implementation by interventionists and educators. Finally, three of the learners were international adoptions, experienced trauma, and English was their second language which were additional challenges that impacted learning for each of them.

Research with Specific Learning Disorders Using Equipping Minds

The purpose of the author's doctoral research (Brown, 2016) was to examine the effect of the *Equipping Minds Cognitive Development Curriculum* (*EMCDC*) on working memory in students diagnosed with specific learning disorder (SLD), a neurodevelopmental learning disorder, and whether an increase in working memory resulted in transfer effects within an educational setting, measured by standardized tests of academic attainment and nonverbal and verbal abilities. Additionally, this study explored differences with gender and age (Brown, 2016).

Strengths of the Research Design Method

In response to the critiques of cognitive training research, the following concerns were addressed (Melby-Lervag & Hulme, 2013; Novick et al., 2020). First, the research design was a true quantitative experimental design with a random allocation of 32 participants into a training and active control group. The training group received 30 hours of cognitive training and the active control group participants received 30 hours of academic training with a teacher for 60 minutes, 5 days a week for 7 weeks in a small group strengthening the results. The statistical analysis was done by a statistician, and a regression output was used to determine if the difference in pre- to post-test scores could be statistically attributed to the training strengthening the validity of the intervention with *EMCDC*.

At the time of the pre-test, the participant's allocation into the groups had not been disclosed to the participants or testers, which was also a strength. Second, another strength of the design was the cooperative attitude, commitment, and fidelity to the intervention by the school administration, faculty, parents, mediators, and participants. No compensation was given to the participants. All 32 participants completed the entire study. The participants in the training and active control group had rapport with the testers, which brings out the participants' best performance. Third, multi-measures of testing examined verbal and visuospatial working memory, verbal and nonverbal abilities, IQ composite, and academic attainments in nine areas. Finally, utilizing the school's yearly academic test, *Terra Nova*, allowed a comparison of 2 years of testing strengthening the finding that *EMCDC* has statistically significant gains in academics.

Weaknesses of the Research Design

The major weakness of the research design was the time constraint. For optimum results from the *EMCDC*, Brown recommends a minimum of 60 hours of intervention over a 12- to 24-week period which was done in the case studies with *EMCDC*. The participants were limited to a 9-week period to complete the pre-testing with the *AWMA*-2 and *KBIT*-2, the 30 hours of intervention, and the post-testing with the *AWMA*-2 and *KBIT*-2. The participants had Spring break the first week of April and then the *TerraNova* testing. Finally, the time for the study did not allow follow-up assessments to determine if the gains were maintained.

Method

In phase one, a private school that serves learners with SLD initiated contact with Equipping Minds which allowed access to potential participants in the study. The initial information about the study was delivered to the school administration to confirm the willingness of the school, parents, and students to participate in the study. The school administration identified 32 potential participants in grades 4–8 who were between 9 and 14 years of age and had completed the *TerraNova* academic testing in 2015 at the school. The school administration provided the diagnostic assessments on each student which also included IQ scores with working memory subtest scores. It was confirmed that potential participants had a diagnosis of SLD and had completed the 2014–2015 *TerraNova* academic assessment prior to the beginning of the study. The parents of the 32 potential participants completed a Student Participation Consent Form prior to beginning the study. The eight training groups required 4 *EMCDC* mediators who were trained in *EMCDC* for the study.

In phase two, the school administration randomly allocated the 32 participants to either the active control or the training group upon receipt and examination of all the participation forms. The decision was made to place 16 participants in the training group with 7 males and 9 females: and 16 participants in the active control group with 7 males and 9 females. It should be noted that all 32 participants completed the entire research study. Qualified professionals administered a pretest with the *Kaufman Brief Intelligence Test,* 2nd ed. (*KBIT*-2), a brief intelligence test which measures verbal and nonverbal intelligence for individuals from 4 to 90 years of age. The test takes 15–30 minutes to administer and yields three scores: verbal, nonverbal, and IQ composite. The Verbal scale is composed of two subtests that assess receptive vocabulary and general information (Verbal Knowledge) as well as comprehension, reasoning, and vocabulary knowledge (Riddles). The Nonverbal scale uses a Matrices subtest to measure the ability to solve new problems by accessing an individual ability to complete visual analogies and understand relationships (Kaufman & Kaufman, 2004). At the time of the pre-test, the participant's allocation into the groups had not been disclosed to anyone testing the participants. The testing took place at the school and took approximately 30 minutes for each participant to complete.

Qualified professionals administered a pretest with a beta version of the *Automated Working Memory Assessment 2nd ed.* (*AWMA*-2) on a computer in the school's computer lab. At the time of the pre-test, the participant's allocation into the groups had not been disclosed to anyone testing the participants. The *AWMA*-2 was designed to provide classroom teachers and specialists with a tool to identify working memory difficulties quickly and easily. The tests used in the computerized *AWMA*-2 battery were selected based on research establishing that they provide reliable and valid assessments of verbal and visual-spatial short-term and working memory. The *AWMA*-2 was piloted with children and adults with autism spectrum disorders, ADHD, dyslexia, and motor disorders. The tests were also piloted on two groups of children: young children (4–5 years) and older children (9–10 years). The tests were adjusted to ensure that both the practice and test trials were age-appropriate and extensive practice trials with visuals were included. The *AWMA*-2 was field tested for 5 years and the feedback received from educators, psychologists, and other professionals helped to refine the current version. The *AWMA*-2 was standardized to include individuals aged 5–79 years (Alloway, 2011a).

As noted, all the participants had completed the *TerraNova* academic testing in 2015. *TerraNova* is a standardized academic assessment for second-12th grade students in reading, mathematics, language, science, social studies, and spelling. The *TerraNova* is a respected and valid national achievement test for reading, mathematics, language, science, social studies, and spelling. *TerraNova* features 2011 norms from a national study. These are the most current and accurate norms, which allow educators to compare achievement results between groups of students. With item alignments to state standards, educators can review student results in the context of common school and district criteria. The academic assessment the school already had in place was used, as it would have been a burden on the school and participants to add an additional academic assessment. This also strengthened the results of the academic assessments as all the students attended the same school for 2 years. The only difference between the students was either 7 weeks of intervention in the training group with cognitive developmental training or 7 weeks of intervention in the active control group with academic training.

In phase three, the participants in the training group received cognitive developmental training for 60 minutes, 5 days a week for 7 weeks in a small group of two participants with a trained mediator using *EMCDC*. The *"Maintaining Brains Everyday"* program for the primitive reflex exercises (Johnson, 2015) was done by the participants at home or at school for 15 minutes a day. The sensory-motor development exercises included the use of sound therapy (Joundry, 2004) which the participants wore during the one-hour intervention sessions while doing the cognitive developmental exercises. The mediators follow an abbreviated format of the *EMCDC* full program as the intervention was limited to 30 hours. Brown observed the training groups on a weekly basis to assure fidelity to the *EMCDC* research protocol. Brown was also available to answer questions from the mediators and observe the participants' progression. The participants in the active control group received academic training with a teacher for 60 minutes, 5 days a week for 7 weeks in a small group. All participating learners continued to receive standard special educational support services because of their learning difficulties.

In phase four, a qualified professional administered a post-test with the *KBIT*-2 which took approximately 30 minutes for the active control group as noted in the pretest. However, the training group took approximately 45 minutes to complete the post-test. Those administering the test noted more thoughtful responses by those in the training group. The *AWMA*-2 was administered on a computer by qualified professionals. The *TerraNova* academic testing was administered by the school administration and faculty over a 2-week period. The school principal confirmed the completion of *TerraNova* by the participants.

Data Analysis

In phase five, the results of all three tests were compiled on Excel spreadsheets. A statistician then conducted a statistical analysis of the data collected on the *AWMA-2*, the *KBIT*-2, and the *TerraNova*. To examine the gains as a function of cognitive developmental training, a statistician subtracted the pre-test scores from the post-test scores and compared the difference in scores (Time 2-Time 1) as a function of the group. Scores below 0 indicate a worse performance on the post-test. Scores above 0 indicate improvements the group made after training. A regression analysis was performed to determine the effect of training using *EMCDC*.

Findings

Research Question 1 asked, "What, if any, are the effects on working memory when applying the *Equipping Minds Cognitive Development Curriculum?*" The results demonstrate that there was a statistically significant improvement in Verbal Working Memory test scores for the students in the training group ($t_{(15)}$ = 2.459, p = 0.0265). Students in the training group also showed improvement in the Visuospatial Working Memory but the improvements were not statistically significant. The students in the active control group only showed improvement in Verbal Working Memory but the improvements were not statistically significant and showed a decrease in visuospatial working memory (see Table 23.22).

When applying a regression analysis, the results demonstrate that we are unable to conclude that the training provided by the *Equipping Minds Cognitive Development Curriculum* made a significant effect on the improvement in test scores for the students on the two Working Memory tests. While the average gain made by students in the training group was larger than the active control group on each Working Memory test, the difference that can be attributed to the training is not statistically significant (see Table 23.23).

In response to Research question 1, "What, if any, are the effects on working memory when applying the *Equipping Minds Cognitive Development Curriculum?*" one must conclude there is no statistically significant effect on working memory when applying the *Equipping Minds Cognitive Development Curriculum.*

Research question 2 asked, "What, if any, are the effects of changes in working memory to academic abilities in learners using the *Equipping Minds Cognitive Development Curriculum?*" The results demonstrate that there was a statistically significant improvement in the reading ($t_{(15)}$ = 2.249, p = 0.0399), science

Table 23.22 Working memory scores for SLD

Measures	Active control			Training group		
	M	$t_{(15)}$	Pre-to-post (p)	M	$t_{(15)}$	Pre-to-post (p)
Verbal WM	2.125	1.152	0.2671	3.875	2.459	0.0265 *
Visuo-Spatial WM	−1.063	−0.327	0.7480	4.313	1.519	0.1495

Note: M = Mean of the post- minus pre-test scores; p = p-value for the two-mean t-tests for the difference in pre- and post-test scores; * = significant at the 5% level

Table 23.23 Regression analysis: effect of training on working memory scores for SLD

Measures	Training B (S.E.)	p	r^2
Verbal WM	1.750 (2.425)	0.4761	0.0171
Visuospatial WM	5.375 (4.313)	0.2223	0.0492

Note: B = regression coefficient of the training effect on the difference in post- minus pre-test scores; SE = standard error of the regression coefficient; p = p-value for the significance of the training on the difference in test scores; * = significant at the 5% level

$(t_{(15)} = 4.050, p = 0.0010)$, and spelling $(t_{(15)} = 3.735, p = 0.0019)$ test scores for the students in the training group. Students in the training group showed improvement on each academic test aside from computation, but the other improvements were not statistically significant. The improvement shown by students on any of the academic tests in the active control group was not statistically significant. (see Table 23.24). When applying the regression analysis, the findings demonstrate that we are able to conclude that the training provided by the *Equipping Minds Cognitive Development Curriculum* made a significant effect on the improvement in test scores for the students on the science test $(r^2 = 0.1273, p = 0.0450)$. While the average gain made by students in the training group was larger than the active control group on every test other than math and computation, the difference that can be attributed to the training is not statistically significant for any of the other tests see Table 23.25).

Table 23.24 Grade equivalent academic scores for SLD

Measures	Active control			Training group		
	M	$t_{(15)}$	Pre-to-post (p)	M	$t_{(15)}$	Pre-to-post (p)
Reading	0.250	0.324	0.7508	1.069	2.249	0.0399 *
Vocabulary	0.150	0.204	0.8411	0.806	1.241	0.2336
Language	1.081	1.674	0.1148	1.169	1.722	0.1055
Mechanics	−0.594	−0.754	0.4624	1.131	1.498	0.1549
Math	0.819	1.622	0.1256	0.500	1.191	0.2521
Computation	0.775	1.449	0.1679	−0.113	−0.234	0.8181
Science	0.019	0.032	0.9745	1.438	4.050	0.00105 **
Social Studies	0.844	1.260	0.2268	0.950	1.239	0.2345
Spelling	0.656	1.361	0.1935	1.875	3.735	0.00199 **

Note: M = Mean of the difference in the grade equivalencies of the pre- and post-test scores; $p = p$-value for the two-mean t-tests for pre- and post-test scores; * = significant at the 5% level; ** = significant at the 1% level

Table 23.25 Regression analysis: effect of training on the grade equivalent academic scores for SLD

Measures	Training B (S.E.)	P	r^2
Reading	0.819 (0.907)	0.3740	0.0264
Vocabulary	0.656 (0.981)	0.5088	0.0147
Language	0.0875 (0.937)	0.9262	0.00029
Mechanics	1.725 (1.091)	0.1244	0.0769
Math	−0.319 (0.656)	0.6308	0.0078
Computation	−0.888 (0.719)	0.2267	0.0483
Science	1.419 (0.678)	0.0450*	0.1273
Social Studies	0.1063 (1.018)	0.9176	0.00036
Spelling	1.219 (0.6960)	0.0901	0.0927

Note: B = regression coefficient of the training effect on the difference in post- minus pre-test scores; SE = standard error of the regression coefficient; $p = p$-value for the significance of the training on the difference in test scores; * = significant at the 5% level

In response to Research question 2, "What, if any, are the effects of changes in working memory to academic abilities in learners using the *Equipping Minds Cognitive Development Curriculum?*" one must conclude that there were no statistically significant changes to working memory using the *Equipping Minds Cognitive Development Curriculum*, therefore there cannot be a correlation between working memory and the statistically significant changes found in the science scores.

Research question 3 asked, "What, if any, is the effect of working memory on nonverbal and verbal abilities?" The findings in Table 23.23 demonstrate that there was a statistically significant improvement in Verbal test scores for the students in the active control group ($t_{(15)} = 2.979, p = 0.0094$ and the training group ($t_{(15)} = 5.179$, $p = 0.0001$). The improvement shown by students in the training group on the nonverbal test ($t_{(15)} = 6.015, p < 0.0001$) and the IQ composite ($t_{(15)} = 7.239, p < 0.0001$) was statistically significant, while the improvement shown by students in the active control group was not statistically significant on either the nonverbal test or the IQ composite (see Table 23.26).

When applying the regression analysis, the findings in Table 23.24 conclude that the training provided by the *Equipping Minds Cognitive Development Curriculum* made a significant effect on the improvement in test scores for the students for the verbal ($r^2 = 0.1816, p = 0.0150$), nonverbal ($r^2 = 0.2624, p = 0.0027$), and IQ composite ($r^2 = 0.3927, p = 0.0001$) (see Table 23.24).

In response to Research question 3, "What, if any, is the effect of working memory on nonverbal and verbal abilities?" one must conclude there were no statistically significant changes to working memory, and there cannot be a correlation between working memory and the statistically significant changes found in the verbal, nonverbal and IQ composite scores.

Research question 4 asked, "What, if any, is the effect of the participant's gender on working memory using the *Equipping Minds Cognitive Development Curriculum?*" Research Question 5 asked, "What, if any, is the effect of the participant's age on working memory using the *Equipping Minds Cognitive Development Curriculum?*" An interaction regression model can determine the significance of the training interacting with gender and age on the differences between pre- and post-test scores.

Table 23.26 Verbal and nonverbal scores for SLD

| Measures | Active control | | | Training group | | |
	M	$t_{(15)}$	Pre-to-post (p)	M	$t_{(15)}$	Pre-to-post (p)
Verbal	5.313	2.979	0.00937 **	13.438	5.179	0.000112 ***
Nonverbal	1.125	0.308	0.7620	15.813	6.015	0.0000237 ***
IQ composite	1.500	0.580	0.5706	16.813	7.239	0.00000288 ***

Note: M = Mean of the post- minus pre-test scores; p = p-value for the two-mean t-tests for the difference in pre- and post-test scores; * = significant at the 5% level; ** = significant at the 1% level; *** = significant at the 0.1% level

Table 23.27 Regression analysis: effect of training on verbal and nonverbal scores for SLD

Measures	Training B (S.E.)	P	r^2
Verbal	8.125 (3.149)	0.0150 *	0.1816
Nonverbal	14.688 (4.495)	0.00272 **	0.2624
IQ composite	15.313 (3.476)	0.000124 ***	0.3927

Note: B = regression coefficient of the training effect on the difference in post- minus pre-test scores; SE = standard error of the regression coefficient; p = p-value for the significance of the training on the difference in test scores; * = significant at the 5% level; ** = significant at the 1% level; *** = significant at the 0.1% level

The findings in Table 23.28 signify that training interacting with gender was not a significant factor in affecting how the students responded to the training provided by the *Equipping Minds Cognitive Development Curriculum*, as evidenced by the improvement shown on the tests in verbal and visuospatial working memory, verbal and nonverbal abilities, and IQ composite. However, gender did play a significant role in two of the Academic tests: reading (r^2 = 0.1901, p = 0.0355) and science (r^2 = 0.3242, p = 0.0514). In each of these cases, the improvement in scores was more significant for males in the training group than for females. There were 7 males in the training and the active control group and 9 females in the training and in the active control group (Table 23.27).

Thus, in response to Research question 4, "What, if any, is the effect of the participant's gender on working memory using the *Equipping Minds Cognitive Development Curriculum?*" one must conclude there were no statistically significant changes to working memory, there cannot be a correlation between working memory and the participant's gender when using *the Equipping Minds Cognitive Development Curriculum*.

The findings in Table 23.28 signify that training interacting with age is a significant predictor in the difference in test scores only for the Verbal Working Memory test (r^2 = 0.1941, p = 0.0247). The students ranged from 9 to 14 years of age. More specifically, older students in the training group were more likely to exhibit significant improvement in test scores on the Verbal Working Memory test. Age was not a significant factor in affecting how the students responded to the training provided by the *Equipping Minds Cognitive Development Curriculum*, as exhibited by the improvement of test scores, for any of the other tests.

In response to Research question 5, "What, if any, is the effect of the participant's age on working memory using the *Equipping Minds Cognitive Development Curriculum?*" one must conclude there were no statistically significant changes to working memory, there cannot be a correlation between working memory and the participant's age.

Table 23.28 Regression output: significance of training interacting with gender and age on scores

Measures	Training: age B (S.E.)	P	Training: gender (M)B(S.E)	p	r^2
Verbal WM	5.714 (2.396)	0.0247 *	−0.0973 (5.200)	0.9852	0.1941
Visuospatial WM	−6.604 (4.311)	0.1377	8.748 (9.358)	0.3585	0.2020
Reading	−0.127 (0.903)	0.8893	4.345 (1.959)	0.0355 *	0.1901
Vocabulary	0.805 (1.049)	0.4496	−1.613 (2.276)	0.4849	0.0547
Language	0.206 (0.941)	0.8282	3.815 (2.043)	0.0731 #	0.1526
Mechanics	0.366 (1.117)	0.7456	−0.517 (2.424)	0.8326	0.1877
Math	−0.056 (0.653)	0.9318	2.319 (1.418)	0.1141	0.1744
Computation	−0.281 (0.770)	0.7186	0.161 (1.671)	0.9240	0.0835
Science	−0.552 (0.651)	0.4047	2.886 (1.413)	0.0514 #	0.3242
Social Studies	0.030 (1.056)	0.9777	0.787 (2.291)	0.7338	0.0974
Spelling	0.484 (0.715)	0.5046	−2.230 (1.552)	0.1626	0.1957
Verbal	−3.364 (3.110)	0.2893	8.560 (6.322)	0.1874	0.3660
Nonverbal	1.229 (4.199)	0.7721	−6.607 (8.536)	0.4459	0.4890
IQ composite	−4.006 (3.506)	0.2636	5.485 (7.128)	0.4486	0.5094

Note: B = regression coefficient for the interaction of term of Training with Age or with Gender; SE = Standard Error of regression coefficient; p = p-value for the significance of the interaction term; * = significant at the 5% level

Discussion

Guided by the five research questions, the following list is a summary of the implications derived from the researcher's evaluation of the analysis of the findings:

1. Students with SLD have low working memory scores which impact academic performance (see research question 1).
2. Working memory training does not seem to have a causative effect in relationship to verbal, nonverbal, and academic abilities when using *EMCDC* for 30 hours of intervention (see research question 1).
3. Thirty hours of intervention with *EMCDC* significantly improves science scores demonstrating far transfer effects in learners with a SLD (see research question 2 and Table 23.29).
4. *EMCDC* increases cognitive abilities of verbal (13 points), nonverbal (15 points), and IQ composite (16 points) despite insignificant measurable changes in working memory (see research question 3 and Table 23.29).

Table 23.29 Group profiles and means for pre- and post-training assessments

Measures	Active control group			Training group		
	Pre-test M (S.E.)	Post-test M (S.E.)	Pre-to-post p	Pre-test M (S.E.)	Post-test M (S.E.)	Pre-to-post p
Verbal WM	93.88 (8.55)	96.00 (10.30)	0.2671	88.31 (11.94)	92.19 (11.50)	0.0265
Visuospatial WM	101.31 (15.12)	100.25 (15.73)	0.7480	93.69 (15.81)	98.00 (15.99)	0.1495
Verbal Short-Term Memory	94.31 (11.25)	96.75 (11.43)	0.4342	89.31 (11.31)	92.50 (14.76)	0.1188
Visuospatial Short-Term Memory	104.50 (19.17)	101.25 (17.81)	0.3542	103.13 (14.60)	104.25 (13.14)	0.7224
Reading	6.156 (2.489)	6.406 (2.641)	0.7508	4.131 (0.980)	5.200 (1.904)	0.0399
Vocabulary	6.988 (2.496)	7.138 (2.253)	0.8411	5.044 (1.663)	5.850 (2.132)	0.2336
Language	6.494 (2.760)	7.575 (2.460)	0.1148	4.525 (1.055)	5.694 (2.575)	0.1055
Mechanics	6.038 (3.096)	5.444 (1.982)	0.4624	4.500 (2.260)	5.631 (3.091)	0.1549
Math	5.094 (1.912)	5.913 (2.198)	0.1256	4.275 (0.904)	4.775 (2.050)	0.2521
Computation	5.581 (1.843)	6.356 (2.716)	0.1679	4.556 (1.301)	4.444 (1.352)	0.8181
Science	6.444 (2.179)	6.463 (1.810)	0.9745	4.700 (1.726)	6.138 (1.810)	0.00105
Social Studies	6.081 (2.196)	6.925 (2.349)	0.2268	4.763 (2.852)	5.713 (2.378)	0.2345
Spelling	5.175 (2.037)	5.831 (2.178)	0.1935	4.038 (1.527)	5.913 (2.459)	0.00199
Verbal	101.25 (10.38)	104.19 (13.49)	0.00937	94.56 (10.51)	108.00 (15.99)	0.000112
Nonverbal	104.69 (10.62)	104.19 (13.76)	0.7620	100.81 (10.17)	116.00 (10.77)	0.0000237
IQ composite	103.69 (8.55)	105.06 (12.35)	0.5706	97.13 (9.84)	113.94 (14.08)	0.00000288

5. Human-mediated learning using a cognitive development curriculum, *EMCDC*, increases cognitive abilities of verbal, nonverbal, and IQ composite scores in learners with a SLD (see research question 3).
6. Gender is not a significant factor in a student's response to the training provided by *EMCDC* in verbal and visuospatial working memory, verbal and nonverbal abilities, and IQ composite (see research question 4).
7. *EMCDC* impacts males more significantly than females in reading and science (see research question 4).

8. Older students are more likely to exhibit significant improvement in test scores on the Verbal Working Memory test (see research question 5).

The first research question examined the effects on working memory when applying the *EMCDC*. The implication suggested by research over the last 20 years is that children with an SLD have low working memory (WM) which impacts academic performance. To determine the participants working memory scores, the *AWMA*-2 was the assessment used for both pre-test and post-test scores for working memory. The verbal working memory scores for the pre- and post-testing for participants in the training group were statistically significant ($t_{(15)} = 2.459, p = 0.0265$) and while the active control group made gains in verbal working memory, the change was not statistically significant. In regard to the visuospatial working memory pre- and post-testing, the training group continued to make gains, but the active control group decreased. However, the regression analysis demonstrated it is not possible to conclude that the training provided by *EMCDC* had a significant effect on the participants in verbal or visuospatial working memory in the 30 hours of intervention during a 7-week period. Therefore, the implication from the present research is that working memory training does not have a causative effect in relation to verbal, nonverbal, and academic abilities when using *EMCDC*.

In response to the second research question, having found that working memory did not significantly increase, significant gains were not expected in academic abilities. However, this assumption was incorrect. The results demonstrated that there was a statistically significant improvement in the reading ($t_{(15)} = 2.249, p = 0.0399$) science ($t_{(15)} = 4.050, p = 0.0010$) and spelling ($t_{(15)} = 3.735, p = 0.0019$) test scores for the students in the training group without significant gains in working memory. Students in the training group showed improvement on each academic test aside from computation, but the other improvements were not statistically significant. There was no statistically significant improvement on any of the academic tests in the active control group which received 30 hours of additional academic training.

The regression analysis reveals that the training provided by the *Equipping Minds Cognitive Development Curriculum* made a statistically significant improvement in test scores for the students on the science test ($r^2 = 0.1273, p = 0.0450$) and tend toward statistical significance on the spelling test ($r^2 = 0.0927, p = 0.0901$).

It is important to note that the annual academic assessment with *TerraNova* had been given in April of 2015 and April of 2016. The participants in the study had attended the same school for students with learning challenges for a minimum of 2 years. The teachers and interventionists at the participants' school are trained in numerous reading, mathematics, language, science, and spelling curricula designed for students with learning challenges. The participants in the training and active control group had received identical academic instruction for the entire school year. While the training group had participated in the study from February 2016–April 2016, *EMCDC* is void of academic content. While the findings were not statistically significant for language and reading, the training group did make stronger gains in these areas than the active control group. This implies that 30 hours of intervention with *EMCDC* significantly improve science scores demonstrating far transfer effects in learners with an SLD.

Having found that working memory did not significantly increase, significant gains in verbal and nonverbal abilities and IQ composite were not expected. The literature on working memory training with computerized cognitive training shows minimal transfer to verbal and nonverbal abilities even when gains in working memory are significant (Melby-Hulme, 2013). In response to the third research question, the findings have implications for a question that was not being asked: "Can IQ be increased in learners with an SLD using *EMCDC* independent of gains in working memory?" There was a statistically significant improvement in verbal test scores for the students in the active control group ($t_{(15)} = 2.979$, $p = 0.0094$) and the training group ($t_{(15)} = 5.179$, $p = 0.0001$). Applying the regression output, the improvement shown by students in the training group on the nonverbal test and the IQ composite was extremely statistically significant, with $p < 0.0001$ and <0.0001, respectively, while the improvement shown by students in the active control group was not statistically significant on the nonverbal test nor on the IQ composite. The research concludes, and the findings support, that the training provided by the *Equipping Minds Cognitive Development Curriculum* makes a significant effect on the improvement in test scores for the students in verbal ($r^2 = 0.1816$, $p = 0.0150$), nonverbal ($r^2 = 0.2624$, $p = 0.0027$), and IQ ($r^2 = 0.3927$, $p < 0.0001$). This implies that *EMCDC* increases verbal abilities, nonverbal abilities, and IQ composite despite insignificant measurable changes in working memory.

The results of the research support a holistic approach with *EMCDC* by training cognitive functions and the cognitive skills of working memory, processing, comprehension, and reasoning abilities to increase verbal abilities, nonverbal abilities, IQ composite, and academics. This implies that human-mediated learning using a cognitive development curriculum, such as *EMCDC*, increases cognitive abilities of verbal, nonverbal, and IQ composite scores in learners with a SLD.

The fourth research question examined whether a participants' gender impacted working memory, when using the *EMCDC*. The findings indicate that gender was not a significant factor in how the students responded to the training provided by the *Equipping Minds Cognitive Development Curriculum*, as evidenced by the improvement shown on the tests in verbal and visuospatial working memory, verbal and nonverbal abilities, and IQ composite. However, gender did play a significant role in two of the academic tests: reading ($r^2 = 0.1901$, $p = 0.0355$) and science ($r^2 = 0.3242$, $p = 0.0514$). In each of these cases, the improvement in scores was more significant for males in the training group than for females. There were seven males in the training and the active control group and nine females in the training and in the active control group. These findings imply *EMCDC* impacts males more significantly than females in reading, language, and science.

The fifth research question examined how a learner's age influenced working memory when using the *EMCDC*. The findings signify that training interacting with age is a significant predictor in the difference in test scores only for the verbal Working Memory test ($r^2 = 0.1941$, $p = 0.0247$). The students ranged from 9 to 14 years of age. More specifically, the findings imply older students are more likely to exhibit significant improvement in test scores on the verbal Working Memory test. Age was not a significant factor in affecting how the students responded to the training provided by the *Equipping Minds Cognitive Development Curriculum*, as exhibited by the improvement of test scores for any of the other tests.

Conclusion

Additionally, the study demonstrated that it is possible to use *EMCDC* to raise the cognitive abilities of learners to an extent that has previously not been linked to learners with these disorders in 30 hours over 7 weeks. The current research found that training in working memory, processing, comprehension, and fluid reasoning with a holistic approach does provide convincing evidence for the generalization of verbal abilities (13 points), nonverbal abilities (15 points), and IQ composite (16 points). Similarly, far transfer effects to academic abilities in science were substantiated.

Lessons Learned: Reasons for Implementing Cognitive Training

Finally, the existing research demonstrates the effectiveness of cognitive training to increase cognitive skills in the verbal and nonverbal reasoning realm. The implications for educators and psychologists are substantial since cognitive skills, intelligence, and academics can be developed when a mediator teaches and trains students of all ages and abilities. School administrators, teachers, and parents should be educated on the theory of structural cognitive modifiability and how to be an effective mediator of the environment without over-stimulating the child. Educators need to be trained in mediated learning and the Equipping Minds Cognitive Development Curriculum. A combination of cognitive training and curricular studies should result in significant advancement of both cognitive and domain-specific skills of all students.

Cognitive skills are the key to learning, social and emotional skills, attention, self-regulation, and decision-making. When students move from frustration in the classroom to success, in turn, negative behavior incidents decrease. As students' processing, memory, and problem-solving skills increase, their attention, self-regulation, and decision-making will improve as well. A cognitive training program can improve academic skills which should reduce the dropout rate and delinquent classroom behaviors hence, providing a safer and successful learning environment for all students.

References

Alloway, T. P. (2006). Introduction. In T. P. Alloway & S. E. Gathercole (Eds.), *Working memory and neurodevelopmental disorders*. Psychology Press.

Alloway, T. P. (2011a). *Alloway working memory assessment manual* (2nd ed.). Pearson Education.

Alloway, T. P. (2011b). *Improving working memory: Supporting students' learning*. Sage Publications.

Alloway, T. P., & Alloway, R. (2014). *The working memory advantage: Train your brain to function stronger, smarter, faster*. Simon & Schuster.

Alloway, T. P., Bibile, V., & Lau, G. (2013). Computerized working memory training: Can it lead to gains in cognitive skills in students? *Computers in Human Behavior, 29*(3), 632–638. https://doi.org/10.1016/J.chb.2012.10.023

Alloway, T., Elliott, J., & Place, M. (2010). Investigating the relationship between attention and working memory in clinical and community samples. *Child Neuropsychology, 16*, 242–254.

Alloway, T. P., Gathercole, S. E., & Elliott, J. (2010). Examining the link between working memory behaviour and academic attainment in children with ADHD. *Developmental Medicine & Child Neurology, 52*, 632–636.

Alloway, T. P., & Passolunghi, M. C. (2011). The relations between working memory and arithmetical abilities: A comparison between Italian and British children. *Learning and Individual Differences, 21*(1), 133–137.

American Psychiatric Association. (2013). *Diagnostic and statistical manual of mental disorders* (DSM-V:5th ed.). Arlington, VA: Author.

Archibald, L. M., & Gathercole, S. E. (2006). Short-term and working memory in children with specific language impairments. *International Journal of Language and Communication Disorders, 41*(6), 675–693.

Ayers, J. A. (2005). *Sensory integration and the child*. Western Psychological Services.

Belleville, S., Menard, E., Mottron, L., & Menard, M. C. (2006). Working memory in autism. In T. P. Alloway & S. E. Gathercole (Eds.), *Working memory and neurodevelopmental disorders* (pp. 213–238). Psychology Press.

Bohács, K. (2014). *Clinical applications of the modifiability model: Feuerstein's mediated learning experience and the instrumental enrichment program* (Doctoral dissertation). Graduate School of Educational Sciences, University of Szeged, Hungary.

Bowman-Perrott, L., Burke, M., Zhang, N., & Zaini, S. (2014). Social and behavioral outcomes: A meta-analysis of single-case research. *School Psychology Review, 43*(3), 260–285.

Brainin, S. (1982). *The effects of instrumental enrichment on the reasoning abilities, reading achievement, and task orientation of 6th grade underachievers* (Unpublished doctoral dissertation). Columbia University.

Brown, C. T. (2016) *Equipping minds: Applying a biblically base curriculum for improving working memory* (Doctoral dissertation). Southern Baptist Theological Seminary.

Brown, C. T. (2018a). Cognitive development curriculum increases verbal, nonverbal and academic abilities. In: Brown, C.T., & Merrick, J. (Eds.). (2018). Equipping minds cognitive development [Special issue]. *Journal of Alternative Medicine Research, 10*(2), 155–170.

Brown, C. T. (2018b). *Equipping minds cognitive development curriculum*. Author.

Brown, C. T. (2018c). Equipping minds cognitive development training in learners with neurodevelopmental disorders: Case studies. In: Brown, C.T., & Merrick, J. (Eds.). (2018). Equipping minds cognitive development [Special issue]. *Journal of Alternative Medicine Research, 10*(2), 171–193.

Brown, C. T. (2018d). Computer training or human mediator. In:Brown,C.T., & Merrick, J. (Eds). (2018) Equipping minds cognitive development [Special issue]. *Journal of Alternative Medicine Research, 10*(2),125–138.

Cao, W., Cao, X., Hou, C., Li, T., Cheng, Y., Jiang, L., et al. (2016). Effects of cognitive training on resting-state functional connectivity of default mode, salience, and central executive networks. *Frontier Aging Neuroscience, 8*, 70. https://doi.org/10.3389/fnagi.2016.00070

Carretti, B., Borella, E., Cornoldi, C., & DeBeni, R. (2009). The role of working memory in explaining the performance of individuals with specific reading comprehension difficulties: A meta-analysis. *Learning and Individual Differences, 19*(2), 246–251.

Camos, V. (2008). Low working memory capacity impedes both efficiency and learning of number transcoding in children. *Journal of Experimental Child Psychology, 99*, 37–57.

Chein, J. M., & Morrison, A. B. (2010). Expanding the mind's workspace: Training and transfer effects with a complex working memory span task. *Psychonomic Bulletin & Review, 17*(2), 193–199.

Chudler, E. (2012). *Neuroscience for kids*. Retrieved March 03, 2021, from https://faculty.washington.edu/chudler/words.html#seffect

Cramer, E., Gonzalez, L., & Pellegrini-Lafont, C. (2014). From classmates to inmates: An integrated approach to break the school-to-prison pipeline. *Equity & Excellence in ducation, 47*(4), 461–475. https://doi.org/10.1080/10665684.2014.958962

D'Amico, & Guarnera, M. (2005). Exploring working memory in children with low arithmetical achievement. *Learning and Individual Differences, 15*, 189–202.

Dehaene, S. (2013). Did neuroscience find the secret of learning? *Paris Innovation Review.* http://parisinnovationreview.com/articles-en/did-neuroscience-find-the-secrets-of-learning

de Vries, M., Kenworthy, L., Dovis, S., & Geurts, H. (2021). Cognitive training in children with neurodevelopmental conditions." In T. Strobach & J. Karbach,. Cognitive training: An overview of features and applications. : Springer. 351–364.

Diamond, A. (2013). Executive functions. *Annual Review of Psychology, 64*, 135–168.

Diamond, A., & Ling, D. (2016). Conclusions about interventions, programs, and approaches for improving executive functions that appear justified and those that don't despite much hype, do not. *Developmental Cognitive Neuroscience, 18*, 34–48.

Doidge, N. (2015). *The Brain's way of healing*. Viking Press.

Feuerstein, R., Falik, L. H., & Feuerstein, R. S. (2015). *Changing minds & brains*. Teachers College Press.

Feuerstein, R., Feuerstein, R. S., & Falik, L. H. (2010). *Beyond smarter: Mediated learning and the brain's capacity for change*. Teachers College Press.

Feuerstein, R., Feuerstein, R. S., Falik, L. H., & Rand, Y. (2006). *The Feuerstein instrumental enrichment program*. ICELP Publications.

Feuerstein, R., & Lewin-Benham, A. (2012). *What learning looks like: Mediated learning in theory and practice, K-6*. Teachers College Press.

Gersten, R., Jordan, N. C., & Flojo, J. R. (2005). Early identification and interventions for students with mathematics difficulties. *Journal of Learning Disabilities, 38*(4), 293–304.

Goddard Blythe, S. (2005a). Releasing educational potential through movement: A summary of individual studies carried out using the INPP test battery and developmental exercise program. *Child Care in Practice, 11*(4), 415–432.

Goddard Blythe, S. (2005b). *Reflexes, learning and behavior: A window into the child's mind: A non-invasive approach to solving learning and behavioral problems*. Fern Ridge Press.

Gray, C. (2000, Winter). Gray's guide to bullying part I: The basics. *The Morning News, 12*(4), 243–247.

Gross, S., & Stevens, T. (2005). Mediation and assessment of a young and low functioning child: An initial session. In O. Tan & A. Seng (Eds.), *Enhancing cognitive functions: Applications across contexts*. McGraw Hill.

Holmes, J., & Gathercole, S. (2009). Working memory deficits can be overcome: Impacts of training and medication on working memory in children with ADHD. *Applied Cognitive Psychology, 24*, 827–836.

Holmes, J., Gathercole, S., Alloway, T., Hilton, T., Place, M., & Elliott, J. (2014). Children with low working memory and children with ADHD: Same or different? *Frontiers in Human Neuroscience, 8*(976). https://doi.org/10.3389/fnhum.2014.00976

Jaeggi, S., Buschkuehl, M., Jonides, J., & Perring, W. (2008). Improving fluid intelligence with training on working memory. *Proceedings National Academy of Science, 105*, 6829–6833.

Jaeggi, S., Buschkuehl, M., Shah, P., & Jonides, J. (2014). The role of individual differences in cognitive training and transfer. *Memory and Cognition, 42*(3), 464–480.

Jaeggi, S. M., Seewer, R., Nirkko, A. C., Eckstein, D., Schroth, G., Groner, R., et al. (2003). Does excessive memory load attenuate activation in the prefrontal cortex? Load-dependent processing in single and dual tasks: Functional magnetic resonance imaging study. *NeuroImage, 19*(2), 210–225.

Johnson, K. (2015). *Maintaining brains everyday. Pyramid of potential*. Author.

Joundry, P., & Joundry, R. (2009). *Sound therapy: Music to recharge your brain*. Success Stream Books.

Joundry, R. (2004). *Why aren't I learning? Listening is the key to overcoming learning difficulties*. Sound Therapy International Pty Ltd.

Kaplan, M., & Kreiger, S. (1990). Improving inattention and reading in inattentive children through MLE: A pilot study. *International Journal of Cognitive Education and Learning, 1*(3), 185–192.

Kaufman, A. S., & Kaufman, N. L. (2004). *Kaufman brief intelligence test* (2nd ed.). Pearson.

Kaufman, P., Chen, X., Choy, S. P., Ruddy, S. A., Miller, A. K., & Fleury, K. K. et al. (2000). *Indicators of school crime and safety, 2000*. (NCES 2000-017/NCJ-184176). US Department of Education.

Kentucky Department of Education. (2019). *2018–2019 Safe Schools Annual Statistical Report*. Frankfort, KY July 15, 2020 from the World Wide Web: https://education.ky.gov/school/sdfs/Documents/2018-19%20Safe%20Schools%20Annual%20Statistical%20Report.pdf

Kozulin, A., Lebeer, J., Madella-Noja, A., Gonzalez, F., Jeffrey, I., Rosenthal, N., & Koslowsky, M. (2010). Cognitive modifiability of children with developmental disabilities: A multicenter study using Feuerstein's instrumental enrichment –basic program. *Research in Developmental Disabilities, 31*(2), 551–559.

Kuo, C., Huang, Y., & Yeh, Y. (2018). Let's play cards: Multi-component cognitive training with social engagement enhances executive control in older adults. *Frontiers in Psychology, 9*. https://doi.org/10.3389/fpsyg.2018.02482

Maguin, E., & Loeber, R. (1996). Academic performance and delinquency. In M. Tonry (Ed.), *Crime and justice: A review of research* (Vol. 20, pp. 145–264). University of Chicago Press.

Martin, D. (2001). Paradigm assessment and treatment for children with autistic features. *ICELP News, 1*(1), 12. http://ictaweb.org/51-2/.

Melby-Lervag, M., & Hulme, C. (2013). Is working memory training effective? A meta-analytic review. *Developmental Psychology, 49*(2), 270–291.

Mentis, M., Dunn-Bernstein, M., Mentis, M., & Skuy, M. (2009). *Bridging learning: Unlocking cognitive potential in and out of the classroom*. Corwin.

Meltzer, L. (2007). *Executive function in education: From theory to practice*. The Guilford Press.

Moffitt, T. E., Arseneault, L., Belsky, D., Dickson, N., Hancox, R. J., & Harrington, H. (2020). A gradient of childhood self-control predicts health, wealth, and public safety. *Proc National Academy Science U.S.A., 108*, 2693–2698.

National Center for Education Statistics. (2020). *Special education July 30*. World Wide Web: https://nces.ed.gov/programs/coe/indicator_cgg.asp

Novick, J., Bunting, M., Dougherty, M., & Engle, R. (2020). *Cognitive and working memory training: Perspectives from psychology, neuroscience, and human development*. Oxford University Press.

Peng, P., Barnes, M., Namkung, J., & Sun, C. (2016). A meta-analysis of mathematics and working memory: Moderating effects of working memory domain, type of mathematics skill, and sample characteristics. *Journal of Educational Psychology, 108*(4), 455–473.

Porges, S. W., & Dand, D. (2018). *Clinical applications of the polyvagal theory: The emergence of polyvagal-informed therapies*. W.W. Norton and Company.

Purvis, K. (2007). *The connected child*. McGraw-Hill.

Raghubar, K., Barnes, M., & Hecht, S. (2010). Working memory and mathematics: A review of developmental, individual difference, and cognitive approaches. *Learning and Individual Differences, 20*, 110–122.

Reichenbe, L. M. (2014). *DSM-5 essentials: The savvy clinicians guide to the changes in criteria.* John Wiley and Sons.

Reuhkala, M. (2001). Mathematical skills in ninth-graders: Relationship with visuo-spatial abilities and working Memory. *Educational Psychology, 21*(4), 387–399.

Rodney, L. W., Rodney, H. E., Crafter, B., & Mupier, R. M. (1999). Variables contributing to grade retention among African American adolescent males. *Journal of Educational Research., 92*, 185–190.

Roth, M., & Szamoskozi, S. (2001). *Activating cognitive functions of children living in an impoverished environment: A Romanian perspective.* Project Inside.

Sanches, P. (1994). The study of instrumental enrichment as a tool for improving language proficiency. *Teaching Thinking and Problem Solving, 13*(3).

Scott, T. M., Nelson, C. M., & Liaupsin, C. J. (2001). Effective instruction: The forgotten component in preventing school violence. *Education & Treatment of Children, 24*, 309–322.

Strobach, T., & Karbach, J. (2021). *Cognitive training: An overview of features and applications.* Springer.

Stroop, J. R. (1935). Studies of interference in serial verbal reactions. *Journal of Experimental Psychology, 18*, 643–662. http://psychclassics.yorku.ca/Stroop/

Tan, O. S., & Seng, S. H. A. (2008). *Cognitive modifiability in learning and assessment: International perspectives.* Cengage Learning.

United States Department of Education, Office of Civil Rights. (2018). (August 1, 2020) 2015–2016 Civil rights data collection: School climate and safety. *World Wide Web.* https://www2.ed.gov/about/offices/list/ocr/docs/school-climate-and-safety.pdf

United States Department of Education, Office of Civil Rights. (2020). (February 25, 2021) 2017–2018 Civil rights data collection: The use of restraint and seclusion on children with disabilities in KK-12 schools. *World Wide Web.* https://www2.ed.gov/about/offices/list/ocr/docs/restraint-and-seclusion.pdf?utm_content=&utm_medium=email&utm_name=&utm_source=govdelivery&utm_term=.

U.S. Department of Education. (2020, August 1). IDEA Section 618 Data Products: Static Tables. *World Wide Web.* https://www2.ed.gov/programs/osepidea/618-data/static-tables/index.html

von Bastian, C., & Oberauer, K. (2013). Distinct transfer effects of training different facets of working memory capacity. *Journal of Memory and Language, 69*, 36–58.

Warmbold-Brann, K. L., Burns, M. K., Preast, J. L., Taylor, C., & Aguilar, L. N. (2017). Meta-analysis of the effects of academic intervention and modifications on student behavior outcomes. *School Psychology Quarterly, 32*(3), 291–305.

Witt, J. C., VanDerHeyden, A. M., & Gilbertson, D. (2004). Troubleshooting behavioral interventions: A systematic process for finding and eliminating problems. *School Psychology Review, 33*, 363–383.

Chapter 24
Character Education Update: Building a Buffer Against School Violence

Thomas W. Miller

Introduction

One's emerging character is based on the moral values and principles which an individual embraces as the guidelines they choose to form their conscience. Moral principles aid an individual in determining what is right and wrong or good and bad behavior. Moral development for human beings throughout their lives is the cornerstone of character development. Therefore, the moral development of an individual yields what we have come to realize as their "character." Character is a developmental process and, for the purposes of this chapter, as an update to the original chapter in the first edition, it is seen as a dynamic process associated with a child's growth and maturity.

The moral fabric of one's emerging personality from infancy through adulthood is based on the individual's ability to understand, shape, and accept respect for self and others based on their education and the interface with the laws of the society in which they live. One's schooling experiences from preschool through their college and university years aid in shaping a significant part of this concept of character development. McGrath et al. (2021) has addressed character education with the development of a specific prototype. In this model, character development is viewed as a branch of one's personal development and includes several key values. Moral

---

Parts of this chapter published previously in: Miller (2019). Used with permission.

T. W. Miller (✉)
Department of Psychiatry, College of Medicine, Department of Gerontology, College of Public Health, University of Kentucky, Lexington, KY, USA

Institute for Collaboration on Health, Intervention, and Policy, University of Connecticut, Storrs, CT, USA
e-mail: tom.miller@uconn.edu

© The Author(s), under exclusive license to Springer Nature Switzerland AG 2023
T. W. Miller (ed.), *School Violence and Primary Prevention*,
https://doi.org/10.1007/978-3-031-13134-9_24

development is the foundation of a person's character. The emerging human being must observe and learn moral responsibility. McGrath et al. (2021) places character as the focus of one's personal psycho-social development based on earlier works of others (Althof & Berkowitz 2006). McGrath et al. (2021) examined more carefully exactly what character education meant to experts on character education in the field. The reader is encouraged to examine his detailed prototypical analysis of what the experts generated.

In approaching and understanding character development, one must recognize that no one is born with character but rather this concept refers to the process of developing a conscience that leads to moral attitudes and behavior by an individual. The process of which we speak is based on learning moral concepts, right from wrong, based on the culture and traditions in which one lives. It includes but is not limited to the inculcation of parental standards, family guidance, religious values, and the influence of peers and social attitudes that one adopts in the course of child, adolescent, and adult personality development. This learning process involves learning the culture, law and social values that influence one's behavior. Each individual is guided by the acceptance of specific rules and guidelines learned during this process and one's ability to gain a general understanding of what is good versus what is evil, what is right and what is wrong, which leads to one's ability to behave appropriately in the society in which one lives. In so doing, the person must develop their own standards and apply them voluntarily, thoughtfully, and self-critically in the behaviors that they adopt in life. This results in the development of a conscience, which for the emerging person is an inward voice of knowledge, experiences and educational guidelines that serves as a decision-making component of the human personality.

Within the school setting, educational scientists and practitioners have recognized that the decision-making process the individual is exposed to in school plays an influential role in character development. More specifically, the classroom climate created by the teacher at each grade level aids in character-building and the potential to expect favorable results realized in acceptable student behavior (Bennett, 1991; Murphy, 1998). Most educators agree that character education programs create a socially healthy environment in the school setting as realized when more than 90 percent of Americans value the inclusion of character education to be a critical part of the curriculum for elementary through high school level education in the United States (Matera, 2001).

Foundation of Character Building

The moral values that an individual adopts during their childhood, adolescence and adult developmental stages form their useable guidelines for individual and group decisions. Those adopted moral values are based on the cultural norms under which they are raised. Among those cultural norms are the spiritual and religious values to which they have been exposed, taught, and learnt through both formal and informal educational experiences. Correlated with this process are the ethical issues that have been offered to them as examples of making appropriate decisions that emerge with age as the personality of the individual. Ethical thinking throughout this process of decision-making becomes the way we translate and transition our thinking into socially appropriate behaviors that are an acceptable part of this character developmental process for the maturing personality. When this occurs, we have the foundation for realizing the development of the "conscientious person," a person with emotional health and social well-being. As our children age, the community accepts a greater role through teachers, neighbors, friends, and peers. Moral development involves the formation of a system of one's beliefs, values, attitudes, and behaviors that emerge as the basis for decision-making and creating a conscience as to who we are as human beings (Miller, 2019).

Understanding the Contributions of Kohlberg and Piaget in Character Development

Perhaps two of the most recognized theoreticians and scientists who contributed to our understanding of how moral development emerges in one's life are Swiss psychologist Jean Piaget, who focused on cognitive development, and Professor Lawrence Kohlberg (University of Chicago and Harvard University), who is credited with the scientific study of moral development. Kohlberg (1987) is an American psychologist who built upon the work of Piaget in understanding cognitive reasoning as to how a human being matures in the society in which they live (Miller, 2019). Through his social learning theory, Kohlberg generated a model involving the stages of moral development that produce a conscience that addresses the decision-making in ethical behavior. The reader is encouraged to examine in more detail the research of these two contributors to the science of character development of individuals throughout the life span. The morality of an individual is also based on his or her childhood experiences. Parents have an immense effect on their children's values. What parents teach their children in the home and family environment is crucial to their development of moral character in childhood, adolescence, and adulthood. Another factor in determining one's moral character is the extent to which they have been introduced to a spiritual or religious lifestyle. The foundations of most religions of the world have their basis in moral development and ethical behavior of their membership. A religious or spiritual basis offers several motivational factors that assist in guiding the development of moral character. The belief in a supernatural being also provides a source of guidance to the person who adopts a religion in forming their personality in much the same way the various social virtues associated with most religions advocate for service, trust, honesty and nonviolence. These virtues provide a source for creating the needed qualities we recognize as associated with character development. Therefore, it seems reasonable to expect that a person who has a foundation in spirituality or religion has an added ingredient in character formation.

In examining the components of moral development and the resulting moral standards that provide the guidelines for conscientious thinking, it is essential that the child develop moral self-awareness of how she/he relates to others as witnessed by the child's emotional understanding of how others respond to the child in social situations. So critical to developing this moral self-awareness is the role of empathy and sensitivity to others in social situations. A child's moral growth begins in infancy, but it is when the child begins to socialize with others that conscientious thought begins to lead to socially acceptable behavior. For most it first shows itself for the child in preschool, transitioning through elementary and secondary school experiences and realizing the necessary and essential challenges of life with respect to ethical behavior at the college and university levels.

The Interface of Character and Social Violence

Where violence in our society presents itself, character also has a role and function. In these situations, whether they are viewed as bullying, exploitation or abuse, their presence in the personality of the individual is a failure on the part of the system from which the individual perpetrator grew and developed. In these situations, the qualities that are frequently associated with character such as honesty, integrity, faithfulness or loyalty and respectfulness are lacking or have not been realized in this individual's personality. Character development, for the purposes of addressing the concept of violence in schools, is seen as a dynamic process associated with growth and maturity. The moral fabric of one's personality is based on the individual's ability to understand and accept respect for self and others in society. It further requires a willingness to abide by the formal guidelines or laws of the society in which one lives.

Perhaps the foundation of understanding compassion, caring and forgiveness often associated with spiritual values can be found in the nonviolent consideration of Gandhi and others. When one begins to adopt characteristics of non-violence in their character formation, they are adopting a commitment to choosing self-restraint along with compassion and caring for others. Character education programs lay the groundwork for learning how to resolve conflict by causing no harm with a non-violent response.

It is important to recognize that character development is a critical component of one's personal development and includes key values. One's moral development and how it emerges through maturity create a person's character. One's personal character based on the behavior of the individual will have a major impact on society throughout one's life. For a healthy character to develop, the emerging human being must be exposed to effective learning experiences. Home, family, and the school environment are the core learning laboratories for effective prevention interventions in the formation of good character development. Where children lack moral education and opportunities to accept responsibility, these children will fail to develop the moral and ethical sensors for incorporating the values recognized as desirable for the society in which these children live. Educational scientists envision moral education and the character traits associated with it as personal growth as the child matures into adolescence and adulthood.

This learning process for character development involves learning the culture, the law and the social values that influence one's behavior. Each individual is guided by the acceptance of specific rules and guidelines learned during this process and must then understand, interpret, and integrate such learning into one's personality. This process formulates one's ability to behave appropriately for the society in which one lives. In doing so, children must develop their own choice in standards, thereby creating a conscience that allows effective decision-making when confronted with ethical and moral issues in their life. The favorable effects that character education can provide offer both the individual student and the student peers improved communication and skills development (Bennett, 1991).

Redesigning Character Education

Trends in shaping character education in our schools have demonstrated that Americans are undergoing a moral transformation driven by the changing mores, values, and ethical standards of our global society. Mores today seem compromised in our political world. In our culture, individuals tend to distinguish between rules that are conventional and those that are convenient. They identify moral issues as those having to do with one's personal welfare and physical harm such as running a stop sign, going through red lights, shoving in line, verbal abuse, and assaulting others. There are examples of psychological harm with such behaviors as bullying, hurting another's feelings, ridiculing, name calling and targeting one's personal self-worth (Miller, 2019). There appears to be a wider distribution of American consciences across the stages of moral development which results in a broader spectrum of ethical and moral thinking and behavior. What is clearly evident is moral development plays an important role in our twenty-first-century society, our shifts in how we behave, our social interactions with others, and our growth and development as a global community. Such shifts in thinking and behavior are shaping the relationships that we have with others in our society today and reflect the changes in our ethical and moral standards of behavior in today's world (Miller, 2019).

The Center for Character and Social Responsibility at Boston University Wheelock College of Education & Human Development is an excellent resource on character development for further consideration and understanding of the issues that we face in this twenty-first-century environment (Center for Character and Social Responsibility, 2014).

In considering the transitions character education has gone through over the past two decades, it is essential to recognize that we are now a global society linked by the latest in social media and scientific technology. It becomes increasingly clear that growth in understanding character development must take a broader perspective to capture the necessary and essential cultural and international perspectives on this topic. Another useful resource is *Character Education: a Bibliography of Recent Research, Reports and Resources*, a literature review primarily aimed at school leaders on approaches to the effective leadership, planning, and delivery of character education that was published by the National Foundation for Education Research (Taylor, 2017).

Character Building and Prevention

Character education has been a valued partner in prevention-based strategies. Prevention education is seen as a key component in addressing school violence. Three hundred and three fourth-grade students in 9 of the 11 elementary schools in a predominantly rural community were provided with a specialized program of character education as a prevention tool to reduce the potential for deviant behavior. Students in three schools were in the no-treatment control condition. Students in the remaining six schools received a school-based and curriculum-driven character education program. These six schools were divided into two conditions. Two of the schools were in the curriculum-only condition, while in the other four schools the students were randomly selected to be in one of three groups: a protocol-driven summer academic (6 weeks' duration) and experiential education/program group; an embedded control group; and a comparison group.

Primary prevention involves the provision of education and training along with efforts to promote school bonding. There are several approaches to addressing school-related violence. Prevention education through character education is considered a critical component of a healthy school environment (U.S. Department of Education, 2002; DeVoe et al., 2002; Edwards & Mullis, 2003). For some time, there has been support for character education in local and state governments, state departments of education, and educational organizations. Successful programs include the process of building community consensus and commitment to helping different religions and cultures realize common values. Several state and federal court decisions refer to the obligation educators have to teach the values upon which democracy and social order depend (Miller et al., 2005).

There are a number of contributing factors in forming one's personality through effective character development. These include parent-child interaction, teacher-child interaction, and socialization experiences with peers (The Ray Center at Drake University, 2019). As Leonard (1997) noted, "character is not everything one learns but refers primarily to [the concepts] a person learns about how he or she should conduct himself or herself or behave in social or interpersonal situations. Part of this shaping of our behavior is based on the need to be seen in a positive way, as moral or virtuous (i.e., as having a good reputation), but another part relates to how people want to see and feel about themselves."

Character building has as a primary characteristic, noted by virtually all theorists and research on this topic, consistency in behavior across time. Character is enduring, not transient like an interest, emotion, or attitude (Leonard, 1997). Character is critical to moral and ethical development. In considering the structure of character development, Benninga and Wynne (1997) documented the record-breaking rates of distress afflicting young Americans and form an essential backdrop for character development. The annual rates of death among 15- to 19-year-old white males by homicide and suicide are at their highest points since national record-keeping began. The rates of out-of-wedlock births among 15- to 19-year-old white females are also at or near their highest points since national record-keeping began. Benninga and Wynne (1997) argue that character educators want children and adolescents to learn to feel a sense of belonging to and responsibility for others. They believe that instability and individual feelings of anxiety and dissatisfaction sometimes result in depression, suicidal ideation, and other forms of disorder.

Educators believe that children need age-appropriate responsibilities, in order to feel socially integrated and respected. They believe that adults with authority should feel comfortable disciplining youngsters who fail to carry out those significant duties. Benninga and Wynne (1997) argue that the responsibility of adults is to critically examine children's and adolescents' social environments and to design and manage school-aged children in those environments that guide them to maturity and into morally responsible adults.

Educators, parents, and healthcare professionals are often involved with several classroom disruptions that teachers face and most are the result of antisocial behaviors. Walker et al. (1996) argue that well-developed antisocial behavior patterns and high levels of aggression evidenced early in a child's life are among the best predictors of delinquent and violent behavior years later. Such behavior patterns negatively affect the child in the school environment and become elaborated and more destructive over time; they poison the school environment and lower the quality of life for students and staff alike (Hawkins & Catalano, 1992; Frey et al., 2000; McMahon et al., 2000). Clayton et al., (1996) provided a model intervention that offers educators a better understanding of the risk and protective factors associated with today's youth and provided a model for prevention intervention strategies that offer critical learning components for students, parents, and teachers for the necessary school-bonding experience.

Processing the Trauma of Violence

Violence in our society seems to be occurring in our everyday lives. Various forms of violence are present in our homes, workplaces, schools, healthcare facilities and communities. Women and children are more often the victims of violence today. As we have come to realize, violence can take several forms as has been realized in the chapters in this volume. Past discussion of bullying, child exploitation and child sexual abuse has focused on adult perpetrators and child victims. However, there is an increased incidence of peer sexual abuse in the school setting involving both males and females. One of the more severe forms is early child sexual abuse among preschool and grade-school peers. This has reached increased prominence because of the exposure and access to websites containing pornographic material.

When young children are exposed to various forms of sexual abuse, it can create for them a number of emotional responses that range from uncertainty or confusion to trauma. Children in such situations who have experienced physical and/or psychological abuse find themselves trying to understand what the abuse means and how they can accommodate it. The Trauma Accommodation Syndrome (Miller & Veltkamp, 1996; Miller, 1998; Miller et al., 2014) provides a clinical understanding of what a child who is sexually abused experiences in adapting to the trauma of the event or events. The Trauma Accommodation Syndrome is based on criteria from the *Diagnostic and Statistical Manual of Mental Disorders, Fifth Edition* (DSM-5) (American Psychiatric Association, 2013), which outlines how individuals who are traumatized through various forms of violence cognitively and emotionally process and adapt to the traumatizing event or events over time. It can be especially helpful to parents, teachers, and others in caring for and supporting the child who has been exposed to sexual abuse (Miller et al., 2002). In applying this model to a child who has experienced sexual abuse, the initial stage is one of the child abuse or victimization itself. This experience is recognized as a stressor for the child and is usually realized as an acute physical and/or psychological event. The victim's response is usually feeling overwhelmed, confused, scared, and intimidated by the event, and the locus of control for the victim is more of external nature. The child victim will often think of the stressful experience and focus on the intimidating act, as well as the physical and emotional pain associated with the perpetrator's violence (Miller & Beane, 2010). This initial stage is followed by stage two, a stage involving more cognitive disorganization and confusion. This stage is marked by a vagueness in understanding both the concept of abuse and the expectations associated with the demands of the perpetrator. The third stage may involve denial and a conscious inhibition wherein an effort is made on the part of the child to actively inhibit thoughts and feelings related to the abuse. A revisiting of the sexual abuse may be experienced as flashbacks to the acute physical and psychological trauma. In order to cope, the child may tend to avoid the psychological trauma associated with the abuse. The victim, therefore, unconsciously denies or minimizes the abuse and/or any efforts to respond to the abusing experience. This may result in isolation, stagnation, and feelings of entrapment, and often results in the victim accommodating to the pain of the violence experienced (Miller et al., 2005). The next stage usually emerges slowly but is one of re-evaluation by the child victim. When this occurs, the child may begin to disclose to a significant other, a parent, a teacher or a trusted friend, specific content related to the sexual abuse. Evidenced at this point in the Trauma Accommodation Syndrome is an understanding on the child victim's part of what has happened and the potential avenues for healing. The final stage is one of acceptance and resolution where the child victim can begin to explore healthier and appropriate lifestyles with respect to sexuality (Miller et al., 2005). Sexual violence in our society is a public health concern and attention along with prevention intervention strategies must be addressed with realistic evidence-based solutions.

Future Directions for Character Education

The character education movement continues to be a valued component in instilling the presence of "good character" as a desirable feature in educating the whole person in the family, the educational system, and the community in which each child lives. Bates (2019) alerted us to the need to be vigilant in recognizing violence in its many forms in the school and community environment as has Herbert (2018). Pattaro (2016) along with Walker et al. (2015) have redefined a new era of character education in theory and in practice emphasizing the emergence of needed character-driven prevention intervention programs to combat violent behavior in our schools. Baehr (2017) and Bartkowski et al. (2019) have examined more carefully the role of a spiritual and religious base for character development in children and adolescents. In their discussion, Bartkowski et al. (2019) cite both the rich benefits along with the potential detrimental effects that religion can play based on their research. Noted for all is the emphasis on resilience, respect and responsibility that schools must take along with parents in providing the essentials for good character development.

The family has traditionally been the child's primary moral educator. Lickona (1993) has noted that "children of marriages that end in divorce and children of single mothers are more likely to be poor, have emotional and behavioral problems, fail to achieve academically, get pregnant, abuse drugs and alcohol, get in trouble with the law, and be sexually and physically abused," resulting in troubled lifestyles. More than ever the character values provided in early development through the family drive the need for moral education that transitions to the character education and values offered in the classroom and school environment. It is a key transitioning that schools have to adopt in teaching the values children, adolescents and young adults need in order to function within the norms of society. The shared responsibility in this transitioning is the provision of ethical values that accompany moral development that is realized through ethical values that sustain human dignity and respect, promote both the best of the individual person as well as the best for all human beings and affirm equality and the rights of all individuals.

Herbert (2018), in his examination of character development and social class, noted that the research results suggest a socioeconomic level of the child impacts the child's development of character traits along with achievement level in the school setting. More specifically, where children were from a lower-social-class background, scores on achievement measures and factors affecting character development showed statistically significant differences as reflected in lower scores in each category than those of child counterparts who represented a middle-class background. While further research is needed to examine this finding, it appears that socioeconomic status, along with family and parental influences, plays a role in children's social development and subsequent character development. Influential in improving the development of character traits and behavior are school experiences in the form of various types of school programs designed for effective verbal and social communication, focusing specifically on social skills training for interaction with peers along with principles of good conduct.

Innovation in Character Development

There are emerging approaches to character education that will likely match the expectation of parents and school-based providers in the face of changing norms and values in our society. There are several contemporary researchers and practitioners who have provided guidance in this area (Bartkowski et al., 2019; Herbert, 2018; Baehr, 2017; Pattaro, 2016; Walker et al., 2015; McGrath et al., 2021; Bates, 2019). For innovation to occur there are emerging themes worth considering that include the following:

- Revisiting current theoretical bases of character development that focus on what represents good character at this time in history. The revisitation process should encompass the cognitive, affective, and behavioral aspects of today's interpretation of morality. A transformation must occur wherein good character is seen as a stage process where the child comes to an understanding of knowing what good behavior is, desiring to adopt good behavior, and translating that into interactions that the child experiences in the school setting (Lickona, 1993).
- The cognitive component of character needs greater attention in a child's recognition and acceptance of a set of moral values accompanied by thoughtful decision-making and moral self-knowledge.
- Character education requires an understanding of the affective and emotional components of moral development. For a child, that emotional element of character development includes empathy and respect for others and it serves as a bridge between making a judgment and choosing an action (Lickona, 1993).
- The emotional component must involve the development of a responsible conscience capable of self-confidence, self-respect, self-control, and self-discipline (Lickona, 1993).

At all levels of education, there are several considerations that can be addressed. For the development of character education, teachers and school personnel are encouraged to assess and consider the following points in the school setting.

- Consider using cross-age grouping and tutorials which offer students an opportunity to think, act and behave responsibly in the school setting. Higher-grade students will benefit by serving as a role model. Younger students will likely benefit on two levels; first, academically and second, learning respect and empathy for others.

- Relate character educational experiences for application in the home, with siblings, immediate family members, and extended family members, and in peer relationships.
- Extend the classroom experience to the community through service projects that will provide student-oriented cooperative activities in the larger community, thereby fostering both responsibility and connection with the students' neighborhood and their larger community.
- Much can be accomplished by utilizing structured learning experiences including reading, writing and verbal rehearsal skills and role-playing to encourage moral and ethical thinking related to specific examples that involve effective communication and behavior.
- Identify at-risk children and provide proven interventions that include a combination of curriculum, parent intervention, and experiential opportunities for students to utilize the skills they learn in the school setting (Miller et al., 2005).
- Offer primary, secondary, and tertiary prevention strategies for at-risk children and adolescents through educational programs that focus on effective family and peer communication, interrupt at-risk behavior, and enhance protective factors available to victims.

The benefits of "character education" can be realized in the school setting when educators use "structured learning experiences" to challenge and inspire their students to conceptualize what character means to them and how it contributes to a respectful climate both in the classroom and the larger community. When students are asked to create an essay that addresses being "character strong," it can inspire a bully-free and socially respectful school environment. The thoughts of students can provide a measure of the moral and ethical growth a student has achieved with an exercise like this. As an example, consider the essay generated by a public school fifth grader when asked to summarize their thoughts on adopting good character and respect for fellow students (see Fig. 24.1). The essay, authored by Hillarie Jeanine Adams when she was a public school fifth grader in an urban school system in 2014, represents a measure of her thoughts on being character strong.

National Institute of Mental Health (NIMH)-supported scientists and others are continuing to conduct research on the effectiveness of strategies that impact the role of character development and school bonding with children and adolescents confronted with violence in schools. Established protocols are examining prevention approaches that address the emotional, social, and academic effects of exposure to violence. In some youth, the researchers examine the role of stress hormones in a child or adolescent's response to traumatic experiences. Also examined are factors that place children at risk for victimization at school and those that protect them. It is particularly important to conduct research to discover which individual, family, school, and community interventions work best for children and adolescents exposed to specific forms of school violence, and to find out whether a well-intended but ill-designed intervention could set youth back by keeping the trauma alive in their minds. Through research, NIMH hopes to gain knowledge to reduce the impact of school violence on children, adolescents, and their families. As has been realized,

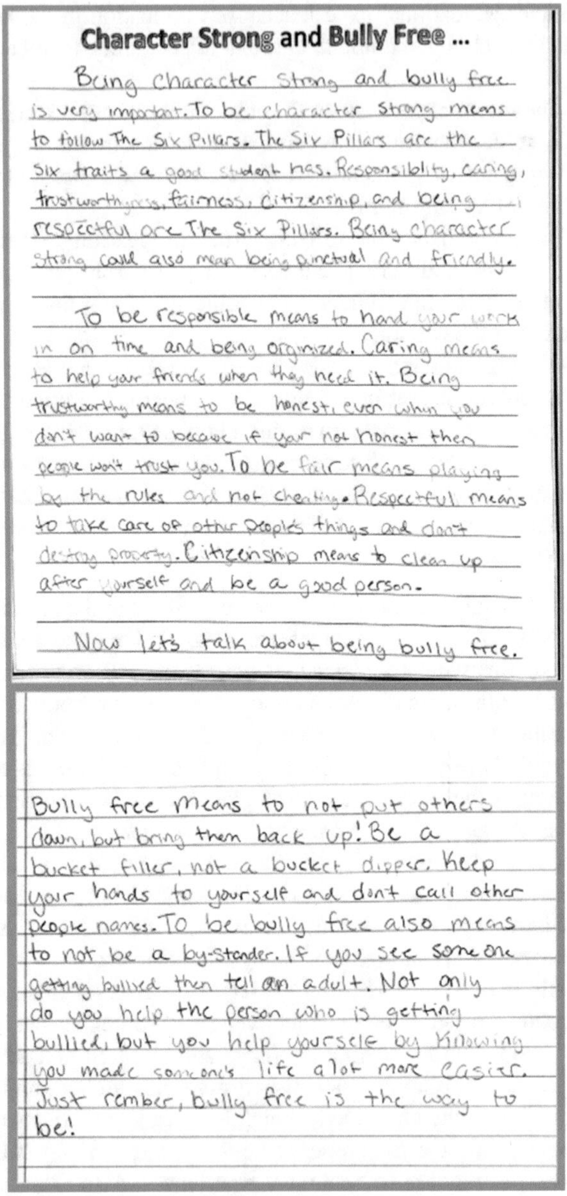

Character Strong and Bully Free ...

Being character strong and bully free is very important. To be character strong means to follow The Six Pillars. The Six Pillars are the six traits a good student has. Responsibility, caring, trustworthiness, fairness, citizenship, and being respectful are The Six Pillars. Being character strong could also mean being punctual and friendly.

To be responsible means to hand your work in on time and being organized. Caring means to help your friends when they need it. Being trustworthy means to be honest, even when you don't want to because if your not honest then people won't trust you. To be fair means playing by the rules and not cheating. Respectful means to take care of other peoples things and don't destroy property. Citizenship means to clean up after yourself and be a good person.

Now let's talk about being bully free.

Bully free means to not put others down, but bring them back up! Be a bucket filler, not a bucket dipper. Keep your hands to yourself and don't call other people names. To be bully free also means to not be a by-stander. If you see someone getting bullied then tell an adult. Not only do you help the person who is getting bullied, but you help yourself by knowing you made someone's life a lot more easier. Just remember, bully free is the way to be!

Fig. 24.1 Character strong and bully-free essay, 5th grade. (Courtesy of Hillarie Jeanine Adams)

there has been a revisiting of the concept of "character" and its integration with character education within the last decade (Bartkowski et al., 2019; Herbert, 2018; Baehr, 2017; Pattaro, 2016; Walker et al., 2015; McGrath et al., 2021; Bates, 2019). This has led to a redefining of what character is for a twenty-first-century school population (McGrath et al., 2021) and subsequent investigations into a reapplication of character education and development for the purposes of generating prevention interventions that are a better fit for today's school environment.

Character education must be seen as both a foundation for psychosocial development and a reemerging discipline in itself. It must be viewed as a school-based process that contributes to the child's personal development with respect to character, moral values, and moral agency. Character education has generated some new directions and emerging trends that reformulate our understanding of how the conscience of today's school population, both for children and adolescents and their public identity, is distinctive from previously held models of socialization and personality development (Bartkowski et al., 2019; McGrath et al., 2021; Bates, 2019). Likewise, the more recent clinical research studies noted in this chapter have provided guidance for teachers and school-based prevention models focused on healthy social communication, attitudes, and values consistent with character growth and development. With the current team of NIMH-supported scientists examining innovative prevention intervention strategies, there is a promise that character education in our schools, colleges and universities will engage more students with the sensitivity, caring, empathy and respect for others that are needed in building a buffer against violence in our educational institutions and larger communities.

Acknowledgments Acknowledged is the guidance and support of our colleagues at the Institute for Collaboration on Health, Intervention and Policy at the University of Connecticut, along with Thomas Holcomb, EdD; Peter McKeown, PhD; Jeanine M. Adams, EdD; Fred Danner, EdD; Janet Saier, M.S.; Jill Livingstone, M.L.S.; Tag Heister, M.L.S.; Kathleen Banner, M.L.S.; and Cathy Martin, M.D., and the Department of Psychiatry at the University of Kentucky, for their contributions to the completion of this chapter.

References

Althof, W., & Berkowitz, M. W. (2006). Moral education and character education: Their relationship and roles in citizenship education. *Journal of Moral Education, 35*(4), 495–518. https://doi.org/10.1080/03057240601012204

American Psychiatric Association (Ed.). (2013). *Diagnostic and statistical manual of mental disorders* (5th ed.). American Psychiatric Association.

Baehr, J. (2017). The varieties of character and some implications for character education. *Journal of Youth Adolescence, 46*, 1153–1161. https://doi.org/10.1007/s10964-017-0654-z

Bartkowski, J., Xiaohe, X., & Bartkowski, S. (2019). Mixed blessing: The beneficial and detrimental effects of religion on child development among third-graders. *Religions, 10*(1), 37. https://doi.org/10.3390/rel10010037

Bates, A. (2019). Character education and the 'priority of recognition'. *Cambridge Journal of Education, 49*(6), 695–710. https://doi.org/10.1080/0305764X.2019.1590529

Bennett, W. (1991). *Moral literacy and the formation of character*. Teachers College.

Center for Character and Social Responsibility. (2014). *Professional development materials*. Available at https://www.bu.edu/ccsr/resources/pd-materials/

DeVoe, J. F., Peter, K., Kaurfam, P., Ruddy, S. A., Miller, A. K., Planty, M., Synder, T. D., Duhart, D. T., & Rand, M. R. (2002). *Indicators of school crime and safety: 2002*. U.S. Department of Education and Justice. NCES 2003-009/NCJ 196753.

Edwards, D., & Mullis, F. (2003). Classroom meeting: Encouraging a climate of cooperation. *Professional School Counseling, 7*, 20–28.

Frey, K., Hirschstein, M., & Guzzo, B. (2000). Preventing aggression by promoting social competence. *Journal of Emotional and Behavioral Disorders, 8*, 102–113.

Hawkins, J. D., & Catalano, R. F. (1992). *Communities that care*. Jossey-Bass Publishers.

Herbert, M. A. (2018). Impact of social stratification and learning on child development and social learning. *International Journal of Pregnancy and Childbirth, 4*(6), 232–236.

Kohlberg, L. (1987). *Child psychology and childhood education: A cognitive-developmental view.* Longman.

Leonard, H. S. (1997). The many faces of character. *Consulting Psychology Journal: Practice and Research, 49*(4), 235–245. https://doi.org/10.1037/1061-4087.49.4.235

Lickona, T. (1993). The return of character education. *Educational Leadership, 51*(3), 6–11. Available at https://www.ascd.org/el/articles/the-return-of-character-education

Matera, D. (2001). *A cry for character*. Prentice Hall Press.

McGrath, R. E., Han, H., Brown, M., & Meindl, P. (2021). What does character education mean to character education experts? A prototype analysis of expert opinions. *Journal of Moral Education*. https://doi.org/10.1080/03057240.2020.1862073

McMahon, S., Washburn, J., Felix, E., Yakin, J., & Children, G. (2000). Violence prevention: Program effects on urban preschool and kindergarten children. *Applied and Preventive Psychology, 9*, 271–281.

Miller, T. W. (1998). *Children of trauma*. International Universities Press Incorporated.

Miller, T. W. (2019). *Moral development is a learning experience*. Health & Wellness Magazine. http://healthandwellnessmagazine.net/moral-development-is-a-learning-experience.html

Miller, T. W., & Beane, A. (2010). Loss of the safety signal in childhood and adolescent trauma. In T. Miller (Ed.), *Handbook of stressful transitions across the lifespan*. Springer. https://doi.org/10.1007/978-1-4419-0748-6_19

Miller, T. W., & Veltkamp, L. J. (1996). *Clinical handbook of child abuse and neglect*. International Universities Press Incorporated. ISSN Number 2035-4983.

Miller, T. W., Veltkamp, L. J., Lane, T., Bilyeu, J., & Elzie, N. (2002). Care pathway guidelines for assessment and counseling for domestic violence. *The Family Journal, 10*(1), 41–48. https://doi.org/10.1177/1066480702101007

Miller, T. W., Kraus, R. F., & Veltkamp, L. J. (2005). Character education as a prevention strategy in school-related violence. *Journal of Primary Prevention, 26*, 455–466. https://doi.org/10.1007/s10935-005-0004-x

Miller, T. W., Williams, D., Nisenbaum, S., & Folman, R. (2014). Trauma resilience and psychological well-being in the 21st century. *American Psychologist, 18*(1), 31–35.

Murphy, M. (1998). *Character education in America's blue ribbon schools*. Scarecrow Press.

Pattaro, C. (2016). Character education: Themes and research. An academic literature review. *Italian Journal of Sociology of Education, 8*(1), 6–30.

Taylor, A. (2017). *Character education: A bibliography of recent research, reports and resources.* NFER. Available at https://nfer.ac.uk/character-education-a-bibliography-of-recent-research-reports-and-resources

The Ray Center at Drake University. (2019). CHARACTER COUNTS! Available at: https://charactercounts.org/

U.S. Department of Education. (2002). *Exemplary and promising safe, disciplined, and drug-free schools*. U.S. Department of Education.

Walker, H. M., Horner, R. H., Sugai, G., Bullis, M., Sprague, J. R., Bricker, D., & Kaufman, M. J. (1996). Integrated approaches to preventing antisocial behavior patterns among school-age children and youth. *Journal of Emotional and Behavioral Disorders, 4*, 194–209.

Walker, D. I., Roberts, M. P., & Kristjánsson, K. (2015). Towards a new era of character education in theory and in practice. *Educational Review, 67*(1), 79–96. https://doi.org/10.1080/00131911.2013.827631

Chapter 25
Building Empathy, Step-by-Step: Prevention Intervention to Promote School Health

Susan K. Reuter

Introduction

Suzy looked deeply into the stranger's eyes and saw something haunting and frightening. It was tender and sad. It was familiar, yet new. It was strong and weak, at the same time. It was hurt. It was tearful. It was real.

IT was a soul.

Suzy, just 9 years old, was surprised to see a little girl in a wheelchair, with clunky braces on her legs and arms. In 1969, seeing anyone in public in a wheelchair was rare, but even more so a child. Girls from 6 to 12 years old from many different towns were gathered for a statewide scout camp.

Suzy noticed a group of older campers starting to huddle up, whisper, and giggle, darting their eyes toward the girl in the wheelchair. Finally, they locked arms and formed a line. They smiled kindly at the girl and marched their human line toward her, singing familiar camp songs. The girl smiled back, apparently thinking they were coming to befriend her. A large crowd of witnesses had now formed.

When the line got within six feet of the wheelchair, the campers suddenly narrowed their eyes, changed their tone, and started singing belittling, hurtful songs at the girl. They chanted "Wheelchair Girl" to her. The whole scene played out to Suzy in slow motion. The girl's hopeful smile dropped and she looked down, trying to avoid the harsh teasing and humiliation. When she finally looked up, Suzy saw into her tearful eyes.

S. K. Reuter (✉)
Step-by-Step, Louisville, KY, USA

© The Author(s), under exclusive license to Springer Nature
Switzerland AG 2023
T. W. Miller (ed.), *School Violence and Primary Prevention*,
https://doi.org/10.1007/978-3-031-13134-9_25

619

Building Empathy

That is when she saw IT... her soul. Suzy's own soul recognized the very delicate soul of the girl in the wheelchair.

The slow-motion moment stopped and everything began swirling for Suzy. She backed up away from the scene as so many realizations and questions flooded her young mind:

- The girl in the wheelchair was a real person who had genuine feelings.
- She must have been brave to come to the camp.
- These older campers deliberately hurt someone. Didn't they know that was wrong?
- What was the girl's name?
- Had she been teased before?
- Why was she in a wheelchair?
- Didn't she have any friends to help her?
- Can someone in a wheelchair have friends?
- Did she have a family that cared about her?
- What was her story?
- *Why was no one going to her to help or comfort her? SOMEONE should go comfort her!*

That last realization was what challenged Suzy and haunted her for years. Deep down she knew someone should help this girl...and why not her? But she did not know how to go comfort and befriend the girl. She was afraid of the older girls. She was afraid of the girl in the wheelchair. She didn't know what to say to someone in a wheelchair. Suzy walked away from the experience with a heavy heart, sad, dejected, and full of regret.

This is MY story! I am Suzy!

If the story ended there, it would have just been a sad tale... one that likely plays out on playgrounds, schools, and neighborhoods everywhere. But this experience planted a seed that germinated in my life and bloomed 40 years later.

I never learned the answers to my questions about the girl in the wheelchair. I never learned her name; however, I will now call her Amy[1] to finally show her the dignity she deserved. I don't know what happened to her after this encounter or how it affected her going forward. I never learned Amy's story.

---

[1] All names and other personal identifiers in the chapter have been changed to protect privacy and confidentiality.

A Step in Learning

What I did learn was that *she had a story*. But all I got to see was the first page. What else could I have learned if only I had gone further into her story? I only knew that I never wanted to see tortured eyes like that again. I certainly never wanted to be the cause of such pain. I would never forget that sight and it was forever etched into my own soul.

At that moment, Amy had become my teacher and I was her unintended student. Even at 9 years old, I realized that this lesson was broader than just Amy. I looked at other people and now wondered what their story was. I yearned to know their stories.

I had no idea how to learn a person's story. But as I grew, I learned to listen and observe. I was labeled a "good listener" by family and friends. In college, nearly every late night, I put my own studying aside to listen to friends looking for someone to hear their heart. I learned and collected real-life stories and perspectives during this time.

Eventually, I went through intensive training to become a crisis intervention volunteer. In this role, I answered phone calls from desperate people seeking someone to hear their story, steer them toward resources, and in some cases "talk them off the cliff." I also counseled people who were brave enough to lose their anonymity to walk into the crisis center. After college, I trained to become a hospice volunteer with an emphasis on bereavement. All these face-to-face interactions allowed me to once again look into the eyes and souls of hurting people. I learned about some very difficult stories.

These collective experiences led me to these conclusions:

- Everyone has a story.
- Stories make people real to us.
- People are strangers to us until we learn their story.
- Stories build understanding and perspective.
- Stories build empathy.
- Stories build compassion.
- Stories build connections.
- Stories build relationships.
- Stories build love.
- You can never assume you know or guess someone's story.
- The outward appearance of people rarely reveals what the internal reality is.
- Everyone's story is sprinkled with both happy and painful experiences… and in some cases, traumatic ones. This is simply the human condition.
- Our stories shape who we are, how we think, how we speak, how we see others, and ultimately how we act and react.
- *Children love stories.*

This last conclusion was another seed that germinated and shaped my own future and purpose for another 20 years.

I would love to claim that these early experiences and training led me to a background in education, research, or psychology. However, I have no credentials in any of those disciplines. Instead, I studied pharmacy at Purdue University and graduated in 1985. I moved to Indianapolis, Indiana, and married my pharmacy school sweetheart, Greg, in 1987. During my career, I practiced pharmacy in a hospital and later, in a nursing home.

Our family grew to include two children, Adrienne and Nate. We moved to Louisville, Kentucky in 2001 when they were in elementary school. I wanted to be involved at their new school and was intrigued by a program called Student Stewardship. The idea was that each grade would identify some way to serve others, make a plan, and then implement it. I was intrigued by the concept, but couldn't understand how it worked and what the purpose was. My children didn't understand it. Other parents I asked couldn't explain it.

I had many questions. What was Stewardship? What was the mission of this program? Was the concept age-appropriate? Were the students truly involved or did the adults do the work? Was the serving hands-on? Did the students understand their involvement? What kind of impact did it have on the students? What impact did it have on those they were serving? Did it truly change hearts?

Apparently, I asked too many questions and didn't get the answers I was seeking. I ended up taking over the committee for the next school year. Over the summer, I dug in to understand it more. My first task was to spend time with the word stewardship to truly embrace it. Eventually, I summarized stewardship as:

Taking responsibility for something or someone under one's care. (Merriam-Webster, 2020)

The school was a Christian school so I also looked up stewardship from a Christian worldview and created this summary:

Taking care of God's creation and everything/everyone in it. (Butler, 1991)

I also found in scripture that, *"The earth is the Lord's, and everything in it, the world, and all who live in it"* (Psalm 24:1 New International Version). Through that, I understood that the Christian's responsibility is to care for the gifts God gives us, such as our talents, families, time, money, health, earth, and people who He puts in our lives.

Previously the Student Stewardship program focused on serving people in our community, but the responsibility for finding ways to serve was on the teachers. That proved to be a challenge for many of them. Some of the projects were well planned and implemented, but many of them were ineffective and confusing for the students.

Since we were new to Louisville, I did not know the people, issues, or initiatives in the community. So for several months, I poured through all possible local sources of community information: the newspaper, local magazines, radio, and the Internet. I paid attention to local TV news features. I clipped print articles and organized them into like categories. What I found was that there were some distinct areas of need in our community that was being addressed by different ministries, agencies, organizations, and groups.

The pile of this information grew to be overwhelming so I made binders for each of the categories. I enlisted my children to help make scrapbooks for each area of need. I realized that I had identified eight distinct areas of need in the community. There were nine grades in the school.

I reflected on the fact that effective education is taught in a stepwise manner, building on a previously acquired knowledge base each year. What if we did the same for Student Stewardship and taught about the different areas of need in a stepwise manner each year, assigning a different community needs to each grade?

This possibility inspired me to make the mission organized and clear. I moved and shifted the scrapbooks around until I had given each grade an age-appropriate scrapbook. I felt that the step-by-step nature would make this program unique, so I named it STEP-by-STEP Student Stewardship©.[2]

I then drew on all my past experiences and remembered the power of stories. What if we taught children about other people through real stories? Would that bring them to life for the students?

I was raised in a home with Christian values. I learned that Jesus, the master storyteller who often taught in parables and stories, had challenged us to *"love our neighbor as ourselves"* (Mark 12:31; Matthew 22:39; John 13:34; John 15:12). It can be natural to love neighbors we know, but how do we love neighbors we do not know? How do we understand neighbors we never met, especially if they look, act, talk, sound, or feel different than us? If we don't understand our neighbors because they are different than us, then how can we love them as ourselves?

We naturally feel most comfortable on our own, with people who are similar to us and have things in common with us. We gravitate to people who are like us and are familiar to us, like the saying: "Birds of a feather flock together."

When we are young, adults teach us about "stranger danger" so we naturally regard people we don't know as potentially harmful to us. So when we meet someone new or someone who is different than us, it is natural that we might respond with feelings of apprehension, uncertainty, suspicion, and even fear.

But Jesus also made it clear through his story of the *Good Samaritan* that our neighbors do not just include the people who live next door (Luke 10:25–37). He taught that our love for neighbor should be as unconditional as God's love for us because every one of our neighbors was also created by God. This instilled inherent dignity in all people.

We also learn that going through the motions of serving is not enough. *"If I give all I possess to the poor and give over my body to hardship that I may boast, but do not have love, I gain nothing."* This is from 1 Corinthians 13 New International Version, the most recognized chapter on love in the Bible. It defines what true love is and what it isn't. It is popular at weddings and is often quoted as *"Love never fails"* or *"Love is patient, love is kind."*

---

[2] Copyright © 2002 Susan K. Reuter. All Rights Reserved.

Without love, there is no heart change. Without heart change, there is no lasting systemic change. So my goal was to ensure that LOVE was a common denominator within the program.

However, the dichotomy of "love your neighbors" and "stranger danger" still perplexed me. I wrestled with this for weeks, until I finally wondered what would happen if we reframed the concept of strangers and called them "neighbors" instead. Would that make them more personal to us?

Would stories of these neighbors change their hearts from ones of apprehension, uncertainty, suspicion, or even fear to hearts of empathy, compassion, understanding, and love? Would this foundational heart change be lasting and inform their perspective in the future?

This caused me to examine the different types of serving. What type of serving was most effective at the different developmental stages of students? Does collecting or donating money or goods change our hearts? Does it really make a difference to our neighbors? My concern was that money would come from the parents' pockets, with no sacrifice on the students' parts. So how could we make serving our neighbors more experiential? How could we put this love into action?

Attentive parents are intentional about exposing their children to different types of activities while they are young: sports, music, dance, arts, travel, etc. They enrich their education with after school lessons, clubs, or activities. They might expose them to different types of foods and flavor profiles. We all want to raise children who are well-rounded. It is one thing to read about a sport or music, but to try our hand at it is a much richer experience. Those hands-on opportunities enrich our lives and make us more confident as we gradually gain skills. Would this same concept work in teaching children about their neighbors? What if we served these neighbors face-to-face, developing meaningful relationships with them?

I reflected back on my own experience of seeing into the soul of a stranger and recognized that that feeling comes when face-to-face with someone. My desire was for the students to get that opportunity. So I called around town, finding places that were safe for our students to serve in person. Stranger danger still exists in this world, so it was important to safely introduce the neighbors to the students. This would require a careful age-appropriate preparation. So I developed a PREPARE… ACT… REFLECT model.

A Three-Step Model

PREPARE would take up most of the time and would include speakers, literature, videos, simulations, research, and games. This old adage applies here: *"Give me six hours to chop down a tree and I will spend the first four sharpening the axe."* ACT would be the culmination of all the preparation. It would entail activities, field trips, and projects to build relationships and serve others. REFLECT would be discussions, reflection, and family follow-up to reinforce the experiences and go deeper with observations, emotions, and opinions.

Could this model also give meaning, purpose, and mission to a child's life from an early age? Could this help to develop character in the children, including commitment, sacrifice, integrity, gratitude, fellowship, and dignity? Could it help them recognize, understand, and embrace their own gifts and talents?

You may have noticed the missing component of evidence-based research in my planning. At least initially, my research was never more sophisticated than learning about the community through print, websites, and media. The program grew organically as we built on a strong foundation and added to it each year. Teachers, parents, and students were surveyed along the way and adjustments were made accordingly.

You may also question the success of the program in other schools, due to the confounding factors of its implementation in a Christian school. Would the program have the same effect in public schools, private schools, or home schools? My aim has never been to prove its success in other settings, but rather to let the program bloom where it was planted. However, it did spread to other Christian schools around the country, but only by word of mouth. It has never been marketed or promoted in any way.

We have not studied the program's impact on school violence. This chapter is included in the primary prevention section of this book because the editor, Dr. Thomas Miller, has been involved in the program for over 10 years as a speaker. He recognized the potential for the program to add value in equipping schools to anticipate problems and address them before they happen. Could helping children become familiar with their neighbors and aware of their needs help them be more accepting of all? Could being a part of something bigger than themselves help a child find purpose, meaning, and value in their own life?

After nearly 20 years, we have observed, listened to feedback, learned, and adapted the program for optimal impact. I am going to share what we learned from each of the components and how you might be able to use small bits of it at your school or with the children in your life. I will also share feedback and reflection from parents, teachers, faculty, and students who have experienced this program.

The consistency and structure of the program have led to a culture of compassion, empathy, and love that has been well received by the schools that have implemented it. There are many school programs available that aim to address social issues, but until there is a heart change, there will not be lasting fruits from these endeavors.

Just like learning music, a sport, or math, building compassion and empathy needs to start young and build on a solid foundation. Let's explore what that looks like through the components of this program.

Overall Structure of STEP-by-STEP Student Stewardship©

The STEP-by-STEP Student Stewardship© program (SBSSS) is multi-layered. The purpose is to introduce students to different neighbors in the community each year so they can:

- Learn about them
- Understand them better
- Develop genuine compassion and empathy for them
- Ultimately meet and serve them in person

The program prepares the students to understand the neighbors they are studying through various in-class modalities and at-home follow-up. The purpose of the preparation is to equip the students with the skills and confidence to meet their neighbors during face-to-face interactions and experiences with them.

Components of Program

The curriculum is vast, but there are many components that can be easily used in any individual classroom, entire school, or at home. As I describe each of the components, I will denote the level of complexity required to implement these symbols:

🕐 = requires *minimal* preparation, time, and resources
🕐🕐 = requires *some* preparation, time, and resources
🕐🕐🕐 = requires a *higher level* of preparation, time, commitment, and resources

Figure 25.1 is an at-a-glance overview of the components we will be covering in this chapter and the level of complexity for each.

A. Stewardship Focus □	M. Global Stories □
B. Stewardship Virtues □□	N. Discussions □
C. Stewardship Curriculum □□□	O. Reflections □
D. Stewardship Parents □□	P. Family Stewardship □
E. Stewardship Friday □□	Q. Games □□ **to** □□□
F. Speakers □□	R. Stewardship Activities □□ **to** □□□
G. Literature □	S. Stewardship Projects □□□
H. Movies / Videos □	T. End-of-Year Wrap Up □
I. Simulation Stations □□□	U. End-of-Year Stewardship Celebration □□
J. Research □□	V. Stewardship Résumé □□
K. Case Studies □□	W. Signature Stewardship Projects □□□
L. Legacy Stories □	X. Stewardship Portfolio □□ Stewardship Graduation □□□

Fig. 25.1 SBSSS components

Stewardship Focus ☉

> SBSSS was such an important part of my younger years. I still remember specific lessons we learned and people we met. I like that we had a different neighbor each year to focus on. I still remember the neighbors for each year. This program prepared me to meet new people when I went to college. I had more confidence and willingness to make friends with people who looked totally different than me or were a different ethnicity, etc. I noticed that my friends weren't like that and would shy away from people they thought were different. – Luke, 24-year-old, reflecting on SBSSS

The Stewardship Focus is the area of need in the community that I originally identified for each grade. We call the people we are learning about "neighbors." We remind the students about the reason for that terminology at the beginning of each school year. We are careful about our phrasing and expect the same from the students. For example, rather than call someone "the homeless man," we say "the neighbor who is homeless" or "the man who is homeless." Just this turn of language helps us to stop and remember they are first a person who happens to be homeless. We also talk about our language when describing others and the students develop a sensitivity around "labeling" people.

After taking into account the age-appropriate aspects of serving each type of neighbor, surveying the teachers, and exploring the learning resources available, I landed on this list for the Stewardship Focus for the program (Table 25.1),

In Kindergarten, the students learn about all eight categories of neighbors, one each month, as a foreshadowing of what they will learn in the following eight grades.

There are other specific neighbors that could be identified and studied, but these were the most striking ones that stood out in our community at the time. The program was written around those particular neighbors. We could have updated this mix as the years progressed, but what we found is that the specific neighbor is not what is important, but the generalization that happens when the students learn about so many different types of people.

We don't have to know every story to know that each person has a story. They learn that ALL people have a story.

Table 25.1 Stewardship Focus per grade

Grade	Stewardship Focus
Kindergarten	Introduction to Stewardship
1st Grade	Neighbors who are in Need
2nd Grade	Neighbors who are Hungry
3rd Grade	Neighbors who are Elderly
4th Grade	Neighbors who are Disabled
5th Grade	Neighbors Living with Illness
6th Grade	Neighbors who are Children in Need
7th Grade	Neighbors who are Homeless/Refugees
8th Grade	Education and Literacy

> I loved the Color Me Healthy game in 2nd grade. I was surprised to hear the stories about the people who were hungry but didn't look like it and the people who weren't hungry but looked disheveled and grumpy. Through SBSSS, I learned that EVERYONE has a story and you can't tell what it is by just looking at them. I now take time to learn about someone instead of making assumptions about them. – Amelia, 8th grade student

Sometimes students are experiencing what is being studied that year. For example, we have had third grade students (Neighbors who are Elderly) who were dealing with a grandparent who was declining in health or function. We have had fourth grade students (Neighbors who are Disabled) with siblings with mental or physical disabilities. We have had fifth grade students (Neighbors Living with Illness) who had a parent or sibling with cancer, diabetes, or cystic fibrosis. We have had sixth grade students (Children in Need) who were adopted or in foster care. We have had seventh grade students (Neighbors who are Homeless) who were homeless.

What we found is that the students felt safe sharing their particular situations with their class. They were met with supportive and understanding reactions from their peers.

> Thank you for letting my daughter share about her diabetes. Since she was diagnosed last year, she has been shy and embarrassed to talk about it with her classmates, thinking they would make fun of her. She was surprised by how supportive they were and they asked her so many questions about it. That gave her the confidence to be open about it. I have noticed that she is more relaxed now that she doesn't have to hide this about herself. It also makes me feel that she is safer if everyone around her knows she is diabetic, in case she has any complications at school or someone's home. – Claire, mom of 5th grade student

What we learned: The neighbors that were chosen for each year were age-appropriate and relatable to the students. Students are able to generalize the concepts for ALL neighbors, even ones we don't study.

Stewardship Virtues ☺☻

> The crumpled $5 bill taught me about dignity of people. When I see neighbors now who look different or messy or dirty, I will remember that they still have value, no matter how they look. I wouldn't want someone to think bad about me by the way I look! – Joel, 3rd grade student

In addition to the Stewardship Focus for each grade, we also introduce character concepts that we call "Stewardship Virtues." Each grade has a Stewardship Virtue that supports their Stewardship Focus and creates a moral framework around the SBSSS experiences (Table 25.2).

We devote 1 month each year to learn about that virtue, but weave the concept into future lessons and discussions. We bring in a "Virtue Speaker" to introduce the concept and to bring it to life. We layer the learning by adding on activities, literature, videos, or role-playing to make the experience more memorable and impactful.

For example, in 5th grade (virtue of integrity), we have a fun role-playing activity called *Integrity Idol©*. The speaker or other adult role-plays as the emcee of a

Table 25.2 Stewardship Virtue per grade

Grade	Stewardship Focus	Stewardship Virtue
Kindergarten	Introduction to Stewardship	Gratitude
1st Grade	Neighbors who are in Need	Sacrifice
2nd Grade	Neighbors who are Hungry	Gifts
3rd Grade	Neighbors who are Elderly	Dignity
4th Grade	Neighbors who are Disabled	Humility
5th Grade	Neighbors Living with Illness	Integrity
6th Grade	Neighbors who are Children in Need	Fellowship
7th Grade	Neighbors who are Homeless/Refugees	Commitment
8th Grade	Education/Literacy	Faith

reality TV show. The students role-play as the studio audience. *Integrity Idol©* is a competition to find the perfect model of integrity. Five boys and five girls role-play as the contestants.

Here is an excerpt of the script for *Integrity Idol©*:

Emcee: Welcome to Integrity Idol, this country's newest reality TV show! We are on the lookout for the person with the greatest character and the most integrity. We have combed the country for the past three months to find the perfect model of integrity. We have narrowed it down to ten contestants who have gone through six highly competitive rounds of cuts already.

Tonight, from these ten people, we will find the new model of integrity! The contestant with the most integrity will be the last one standing! The studio audience will decide who gets to stay and who must go. The winner of Integrity Idol will reign as the man or woman of most character in our country!

The emcee then describes the different dilemmas each of the contestants faced over the months. The audience votes on whether the contestants stay for the next round or leave.

Integrity Idol© is lively, fun, and impactful for the students, but also helps them realize how their own actions affect others, even when no one is watching.

Now every time I am tempted to do something wrong or hurtful, I think of Integrity Idol! Sometimes I pretend that I have a camera crew following me, haha! It is funny, but it helps me see how what I do can help OR hurt someone else! – Karah, 5th grade student

Integrity Idol showed me how much my actions affect other people, even people I don't know. Honestly I don't want to hurt other people! So it was good to see how that can happen. – Joshua, 5th grade student

We also reinforce the virtue concepts for the rest of the school year and challenge the students to practice these virtues so they can become a part of their character as they grow. We call that "Exercise Your Character." Just as we exercise our bodies to get stronger, we can be intentional about exercising our character.

Teachers also are encouraged to use the language of the Stewardship Virtues throughout the year. For example, "Ben, did you treat John with dignity?" or "Make sure you act with integrity and keep your eyes on your own paper."

What we learned: The Virtue Speakers, activities, literature, and discussions are impactful ways to build and practice character.

Stewardship Curriculum ☺☺☺

> I have been involved with SBSSS since it was initiated at my grandkids' school in 2011. I cannot begin to pick any particular lesson as my favorite because they were all tremendous! Many times my grandchildren have referred to one of the lessons, books, or discussions and we can all talk about it together. It has made us closer. It is so well organized and structured. It is so wonderful! – Ben, Stewardship Parent

As the program grew, I realized a written curriculum was necessary to unify the message throughout the entire program and make it easier to implement. The curriculum is now fully laid out and scripted to guide volunteers and teachers with minimal preparation on their part.

Supporting materials for each session always include Curriculum Agenda, Discussion Questions, Reflections, and Family Stewardship. Other supporting materials that may be needed for some months include Activity Plans, Speaker Plans, Project Plans, and Game Plans.

Table 25.3 shows an example of the full in-class curriculum at a glance.

What we learned: The message is unified and scripted throughout the curriculum. It is easy to follow with minimal preparation needed by teachers or volunteers.

Stewardship Parents ☺☺

> As a retired elementary school teacher and administrator, I saw how the students reacted to the lessons that were administered by a parent or grandparent. The teachers have so much responsibility in the classroom so having a neutral, but known adult changed the perception of the lesson for the students. The carryover into the classroom and continuous reference to lessons definitely increases the impact and carryover. Personally, I enjoy continuing the dialog after school with my granddaughter. It is a special thing that she and I have the opportunity to do together. – Caitlin, Stewardship Parent

The program is structured to use volunteers to implement the curriculum. However, teachers can and should be involved at whatever level works for their situation. The majority of the volunteers are parents and have been called Stewardship Parents. However, we have enjoyed having aunts, uncles, friends, seniors, and grandparents involved. To keep things simple, we still call all volunteers Stewardship Parents.

In one of our schools, the parents are typically unavailable or unable to volunteer during the school day. The coordinator of the program reached out to the grandparents of the students and other retired members of their community. This creative

Table 25.3 Example in-class curriculum

Grade	September	October	November	December	January
K Introduction to Stewardship	Intro to Stewardship	Our LIFE is a Blessing	Our HOME is a Blessing	Our FOOD is a Blessing	Speaker: *Our BODY is a Blessing*
1st In Need	Intro Speaker	*Virtue Speaker:* Sacrifice	People NEED Love and Friendship/NH Field Trip Prep	*Christmas for N.H. Buddies/* Gifts of True Love	Shoes for Someone Special Part 1
2nd Hungry	Intro Speaker	What Does it Feel Like to Be Hungry?	BAGS of BLESSINGS	*Virtue Speaker:* Gifts	Stone Soup Trail Mix Snack Packets
3rd Elderly	Intro Speaker	Elderly Stations Memory Box	Pen Pal Huggers	Interesting Facts about Aging	*Virtue Speaker: Dignity Moments with Baxter*
4th Disabled	Intro Speaker.	*Virtue Speaker:* Humility	Disability Stations	Disability Doctors	*Global Story:* Emmanuel's Gift
5th Living with Illness	Intro Speaker	*Speaker:* A Look at Faith & Attitude	Insights about Illness	Legacy Stories	*Speakers:* Diabetes
6th Children in Need	*Intro Speaker*	Recipe for a Well-Balanced Life	*Case Study:* Casey Jackson	*Adoption videos*	*Movie:* Lost & Found Family
7th Homeless/ Refugees	Intro Speaker	THE REALITY GAME Part 2	*Virtue Speaker:* Commitment	Research on Homelessness	*Movie/ Legacy:* The Pursuit of Happyness
8th Education and Literacy	Intro/ Signature Stewardship Project	Every 1 Reads Training	Stewardship Résumé/Project Planning Packet	*Case Study:* Barriers to Literacy & Education	*Case Study:* The Three Little Pigs

Grade	February	March	April	May
K Introduction to Stewardship	Our FAMILY is a Blessing	Our HEALTH is a Blessing	*Virtue Speaker:* Gratitude	End of Year Wrap-up
1st In Need	Shoes for Someone Special Part 2/ Global Stories	People NEED People/Easter Bunny Bags	THE REALITY GAME	End of Year Wrap-up
2nd Hungry	*Global Story:* One Hen	COLOR ME HEALTHY GAME	*Movie:* Kit Kittredge	End of Year Wrap-up
3rd Elderly	*Movie:* A Memory for Tino	Visit with Seniors	THE AGING GAME	End of Year Wrap-up

(continued)

Table 25.3 (continued)

Grade	February	March	April	May
4th Disabled	*Speaker:* Learning Differences	*Legacy Story:* Life Without Limbs	*Movie:* The Front of the Class	End of Year Wrap-up
5th Living with Illness	*Virtue Speaker:* Integrity *INTEGRITY IDOL*	CPR Training/ Cancer Camp Pillowcases	*Movie:* Charlie and Me	End of Year Wrap-up
6th Children in Need	*Speakers:* Foster Care and Adoption	*Legacy Story Global Story*	*Virtue Speaker:* Fellowship	Update Résumé End of Year Wrap-up
7th Homeless/ Refugees	Homeless Chronicles	*Speaker:* Refugee Services/refugee guest	*Movie/Global Story:* God Grew Tired of Us	Update Résumé End of Year Wrap-up
8th Education and Literacy	The Dr. Faith Show Mission Statement	Signature Stewardship Project Presentations	*Movie:* Freedom Writers	Stewardship Graduation Ceremony

solution has made a very vibrant atmosphere for the students. In addition, the volunteers seem pleased to continue every year.

> I have had very few volunteers discontinue their involvement with SBSSS since we started the program at our school in 2011. – Carl, SBSSS Coordinator at an Indiana school

While preparing to write this chapter, I surveyed Stewardship Parents (past and present). I received 30 responses from four schools in four different cities (three states). The years of involvement ranged from three to 18 years, with an average of 10 years. What Carl said earlier is true. When people get involved with the program, the majority stay the course. Some parents stay long after their last child goes on to high school. Stewardship Parents enjoy the experiences, see the fruits of their labor, and make it a priority.

> I used to volunteer for so many things at school, but since I had to go back to work full time, I had to cut everything out… except I will always make time for SBSSS. I work a few extra hours on a different day so I can take off and be there for Stewardship Friday. This program is so valuable and obviously worth my time since I have been involved with it for 7 years now. – Angie, parent of 3

When Stewardship Parents are involved, the students view the curriculum as something outside of their normal routine, which makes it more special.

> The students look forward to the Stewardship Parents, volunteers, and speakers who come in. They seem to pay extra attention to them. The content is so real- life to them and they hang on every word that is spoken by the volunteers. They seem to remember everything they learned, even at the end of the year. The activities, discussions, stories, role-playing, simulations, etc. that the volunteers lead are very impactful. – Patti, 3rd grade teacher

Another benefit of involving Stewardship Parents is that they learn right along with the students. Often times, these adults have not had interactions with many of the neighbors we serve either. It opens their eyes to the needs in the community and the people involved.

> I took a group of students to the soup kitchen. I was so proud of the boys. They were friendly and courteous as they served. I could tell they really appreciated the experience too. I was surprised at how much it opened MY eyes to the plight of the homeless. It made me realize that they are just trying to get along in this life, just like us. We heard some stories of loss, illness, regrettable decisions and actions… but we also heard stories of joy. It made these neighbors more real to ALL of us! Thank you for our awesome Stewardship program! – Maria, parent of a 7th grade student

> I was so touched by the experience at Home of the Innocents. The children we served there were profoundly disabled, but our kids immediately and confidently interacted with them, with no hesitation. They were so well prepared ahead of time through the SBSSS curriculum and previous years of experiences. I was surprised to see that the adult volunteers were less at ease than the children. I am so thankful for these hands-on experiences that transform our kids' hearts! – Kristi, parent of a 4th grade student

What if your school would like to implement parts or all of the program, but doesn't have the support needed to bring in volunteers? The curriculum is set up in a way that teachers could teach it. However, it would be helpful to have a volunteer to help assemble the resources needed for each month.

What we learned: Stewardship Parents make an impactful contribution to the program. They learn valuable lessons along with the students. They often stick with the program once they get involved with it because they believe it is valuable and worth their time.

Stewardship Friday/Stewardship Day ☺☺

> I find that the students are very excited for Stewardship Fridays. ALL of the lessons have a huge impact on them. – Chris, 4th grade teacher

The full curriculum requires an average of 1 hour per month in each of the grades. Schools have found different ways to address the time needed for the monthly curriculum in the classroom. Many schools plan a school-wide Stewardship Friday or Stewardship Day. Most schools have found that the last period on Fridays works well and is less disruptive to the core curriculum. Additionally, there are schools that weave some components of the program creatively into their existing curriculum.

What we learned: It is important to set aside a dedicated time to implement the curriculum, whether it is during the same time for the entire school or broken up by grades or classes. However, schools can implement components of the program as needed.

Speakers ☺☺

> I will never forget the "I GET To" speaker. The lesson was that we GET to do the things we do... we don't HAVE to. It makes a difference in my perspective and attitude when I think about that. I am more thankful and appreciative of the life I have been given and feel it is my duty to use my gifts to help those in need. – Anna, 23-year-old, reflecting on SBSSS

> Speakers really made an impact on students and helped them understand the topic on a deeper level. – Abbie, 4th grade teacher

We start off every school year with an Introduction Speaker for each grade. This is someone with a passion or connection to the Stewardship Focus for the year. Often it is someone from the agency, ministry, or organization we will be serving that year.

Speakers are typically eager to take the time to come and share their area of expertise with the students. Students show their interest through the compelling questions they ask. Our speakers seem happy to come back year after year. In fact, the editor of this book, Dr. Thomas Miller, has been a speaker for one of our schools in Lexington, Kentucky for over 10 years.

We also have speakers throughout the year, as appropriate, to enhance understanding. For example, in fifth grade, we obtain speakers who share their experiences with various medical issues, both patients and professionals.

> My daughter loved hearing about the profession of occupational therapy in 5th grade. The speaker opened up a whole new world for her. Guess what, 15 years later she is now an occupational therapist and loving it! – Joseph, former parent

In sixth grade, we invite a panel of speakers with experience in adoption and foster care.

> My son told me he had a superb speaker in his room today that really touched his heart with a story about the adoption of her son. He came home and wanted to talk about it, which is a rarity so I know it had an impact. He said the Kleenex box had to be passed around the room because there were a lot of tears of joy! – Ann, parent of a 6th grade student

In seventh grade, we bring in refugees to share their unique stories.

> It was so interesting to hear about the refugees coming to Louisville and experiencing electricity and running water for the first time in their lives! I had no idea! It was interesting to find their home on the map and learn about why they left their country. – Blake, 7th grade student

Planning a speaker may take a little time, but the impact is worth it. We are thoughtful about the speakers we choose to talk with the students. Typically, we have the same speakers each year. All the speakers volunteer their time, however, we give them a small gift and a thank-you note signed by all the students in the class.

> I love coming to speak to your students each year! They are so engaged and have such great questions for me. I am always so surprised by their level of awareness and by their compassion and empathy at such a young age. Many shared testimonies that were quite heartfelt and impactful. I can clearly see how well you have prepared them through this program! – Dianne, speaker to 6th grade students

What we learned: Speakers are a memorable and impactful way to enhance the students' knowledge and understanding of their neighbors. Speakers enjoy speaking to our students and sharing their areas of expertise with them.

Literature ⏱

> ALL of the stewardship lessons have had an impact on them! There are three books that we talk about often: (1) Christmas Day in the Morning (Pearl S. Buck): which illustrates the virtue of sacrifice. (2) The Orange Shoes (Trinka Hakes Noble): which shows concepts of sacrifice, resourcefulness, and looking on the bright side. (3) The Teddy Bear (David M. McPhail): which also shows the virtue of sacrifice. – Karen, 1st grade teacher

Relevant literature, both fiction and non-fiction can help us step into the lives of others. Literature helps us know what it feels like to be someone else. In fact, a study confirms that fiction can increase empathy (Johnson, 2012).

We have woven literature, along with rich discussion, reflection, and activities into each of the grades. I spent over 10 years reviewing and cataloging children's literature. There are many titles that we don't have time for in the monthly curriculum but are still valuable. I have a list of those that I call the "Segue Series." These are books that teachers or parents can use between Stewardship Fridays to segue the months.[3]

What we learned: Literature is an effective way to enhance learning about and understanding of our neighbors. It can often be incorporated into the existing curriculum.

Movies/Videos ⏱

> The SBSSS program gives students time to reflect on the circumstances of others. Students realize that although we come from different backgrounds, ethnicity, or cultures, that each person is valuable. Watching and discussing the movie, Freedom Writers, students learn that compassion and understanding for each other brings peace. – Alice, 8th grade teacher

> The Pursuit of Happyness movie was SO good! It was even better that it was a true story. It really helped me see how easy it could be to become homeless. But the dad worked hard and protected his son and made a better life for them. – Cole, 7th grade student

Most grades have a movie that helps to bring their neighbors to life. We have thoughtful discussions before, during, and after the movies. Similar to literature, movies offer endless possibilities. I also curated an extensive list of movies. They can be more difficult to schedule into the school day, so we are creative with timing

---

[3]To download a sample of literature used, visit stepbystepstudentstewardship.mykajabi.com/resources

and scheduling. Sometimes we break up the movies and discuss as we go so students aren't sitting for the entirety of a long movie.

We also have a whole world of online videos available to use in the classroom, but we use these carefully and sparingly throughout the program. There are both movies and videos available for teachers and parents to use in between months in the Segue Series.[4]

> For movie night over the winter, we chose movies in the Segue Series to watch with our daughter who is in 4th grade. We watched Radio one weekend and Shorty the next weekend. We all loved the movies (even our 7th grader) and we had such great discussions about both of the movies. We are going to check out more of them! – Andrea, parent of 4th grader

What we learned: Movies and videos are an effective and engaging tool to increase the students' understanding of their neighbors.

Simulation Stations ☺☺☺

> I have had the privilege of volunteering as a Stewardship Parent since my daughter started Kindergarten. I absolutely love the program and the impact it has had on her. The lessons on disabilities were impactful for her class. The children expressed how they never realized it was so hard to perform a task from a wheelchair or button a shirt with one hand, etc. It opened their eyes to those who have a disability. It was exciting to see the light bulb going off. – Carolyn, 4th grade Stewardship Parent

Hands-on experiences are a valuable way of learning. For a few of the grades, I created simulation stations to help the students "try on" what it might feel like to be in the shoes of someone else.

For third grade, we have the Elderly Stations in which they get to try on different challenges that neighbors who are elderly might face. We suit them up with glasses with limited visibility, gloves with taped fingers, popcorn kernels in their shoes, etc. Then they have scenarios to accomplish with these limitations. These experiences help them to understand what these challenges might feel like.

> The Elderly Stations had a big effect on both of my kids when they were in 3rd grade. They became more compassionate and understanding toward their grandparents. They were actually inquisitive about their grandfather who is in a wheelchair. That made Grandpa feel special to talk about it with them. – Paul, parent of 5th and 6th grade students

In 4th grade, we have the Disability Stations. Once again, we suit up the students with different limitations. Then we give them some real-life scenarios to work through with their disabilities.

> The Disability Stations really helped me understand how someone feels with disabilities, but I only had to do it for an hour and they have to do it their whole life. I can't imagine how

---

[4]To download a sample of movies/videos used, visit stepbystepstudentstewardship.mykajabi.com/resources

hard that is! It helped me understand the children with disabilities we visited at Home of the Innocents. – Lydia, 4th grade student

In fifth grade, we have CPR and emergency training which trains the students to know how to respond in an emergency.

After watching the movie, Charlie and Me, I am so glad to know how to do CPR. You never know when you might need it. It isn't as hard as I thought it would be. – Max, 5th grade student

What we learned: Surveys of students, teachers, Stewardship Parents, and parents have identified the simulation stations as one of the most valuable, hands-on experiences in the program.

Research ☺☺

The research about the neighbors who are elderly really helped our students feel more comfortable when we went on the nursing home field trip a few weeks later. They seemed more accepting of the different things they saw there. Even the staff was surprised at how well our kids related to the residents. What a great perspective to have at such a young age! – Grace, 3rd grade teacher

In some grades, we have used research to help the students learn about issues related to their neighbors. Students usually answer assigned questions ahead of time, then present their findings to the class in creative, fun ways. Here are some examples:

Interesting Facts about Aging: Third graders learn about common issues that their neighbors who are elderly might deal with, such as wrinkled skin, dentures, varicose veins, osteoporosis, gray hair, and cataracts.

Disability Doctors: Fourth grade students learn about conditions that might lead to disabilities such as muscular dystrophy, cerebral palsy, Down Syndrome, blindness, autism, Tourette Syndrome, hearing loss, and dyslexia.

Insights about Illness: Fifth grade students each research a different topic about diseases, illnesses, and conditions they might hear about as they serve neighbors living with illness.

The third, fourth, and fifth grade students then present their findings to their class as if they are the doctor speaking to their patient or caretaker of a patient (role-played by the Stewardship Parents). They wear lab coats and put a stethoscope around their necks. The Stewardship Parents/teachers use props (dolls and puppets) and ask them scripted questions. The students love playing the doctor each year.

What we learned: Research and creative presentations are another layer of understanding the neighbors. Students enjoy role-playing as doctors or experts.

Case Studies ☉☉

> The lesson depicting the three individuals at age 18 and again at age 35 most impacted the students. Because the 8th graders are preparing to enter high school, the lesson causes them to stop and think about how important the decisions are that they make today. The lesson shows the consequences of letting opportunities slip by. – Barbara, 8th grade Stewardship Parent

Case studies are done in sixth and eighth grades. These involve listening to the audio of a story about a girl (Casey Jackson) who finds herself growing up with difficult home life. The students identify all the ways that Casey's parents weren't meeting her basic needs and those of her siblings. They see all the ways Casey tries to work around the deficits of her home life until a school counselor identifies the problem and works to find solutions for Casey.

In 8th grade, the students hear Casey's story again, but this time they explore it from a different angle. They are looking at how Casey's family life led to barriers in literacy and education (family barriers, social barriers, school barriers, and physical barriers).

The following month, they explore the outcome of these issues for Casey. They also hear about two more people and they compare their stories, choices, and outcomes. They hear about these three people at the ages of 18 years old and again at 35 years old.

What we learned: Case studies help students understand their neighbors while also causing them to reflect on their own lives and how the choices they make impact their futures.

Legacy Stories ☉

> Life Without Limbs totally changed my life! I can't believe what Nick can do without arms or legs. He is SO strong and helping other people! It makes me want to do that too. I will never forget this! – Micah, 4th grade student

Legacy stories are about neighbors who have used their own afflictions to bring help, healing, and hope to others. The students learn that circumstances don't need to define who they are. For example, in 4th grade, we learn about Nick Vujicic, the founder of *Life Without Limbs*. He was born without arms and legs but has spoken around the world to give hope to all who hear him.

Then we challenge the students to reflect on their own legacy. Just as we learn about all the neighbors' stories through SBSSS, the students have their own story they are still building. Every year they have the opportunity to reflect on what their story will be, what difference they will make by the end of their lives, and how they will be remembered. They also ask their parents the same question. It is a sobering exercise for everyone and one that is not often discussed but has a big impact on the students every year.

I never thought about my own story before! I want to leave behind a legacy that people will never forget… people will keep doing it. I want to do something that will change the world. It will help others in need. It will start out small then spread big. It will truly change people and their hearts. -Leah, 5th grade student

I want to leave a good legacy that helps our neighbors. I want to show the love I have to make other people happy. I want to teach other people to have good will and to help others. I want my story to be a good one and I want to be known as someone who helps others a lot. – Elisabeth, 5th grade student

What we learned: Students are inspired by the legacy stories. It challenges them to reflect on their own legacy story and how they want to be remembered.

Global Stories ©

The SBSSS program focuses mostly on our local neighbors so we can actually meet them, but we also highlight the fact that our neighbors really extend to the global scale. We use literature and videos to bring these global neighbors and their needs to the students. We also learn about the part of the world these neighbors call home. Here are some examples of global neighbors we meet:

In second grade, we learn about Kojo, in Ghana, West Africa, in the book *One Hen* by Katie Smith Milway. We talk about and illustrate through props the Chinese proverb that says: *Give a man a fish and you feed him for a day. Teach a man to fish and you feed him for a lifetime.* This concept resonates with the students.

In seventh grade, we learn about the Lost Boys of Sudan in the movie, *God Grew Tired of Us.* The students' eyes are opened to the plight of refugees who suffer great persecution in their homeland and how they adjust to life here in the United States.

What we learned: Global stories enlighten the students about neighbors around the world and the conditions they live in.

Discussion ©

During the discussions, the students seem to be more authentic and vulnerable, as if they feel safe expressing themselves in front of their peers. The discussions are fruitful and heartfelt. They ask insightful questions that show us they are growing in their understanding of the dignity of all people. They also seem supportive of other students who are also being vulnerable. It really is so sweet to see this in my students. – Amber, 6th grade teacher

During our discussions, I have seen them make positive comments towards one another when discussing their personal home situations. – Dan, 7th grade teacher

Stewardship Parents/teachers guide discussion for every lesson and experience within SBSSS by using scripted questions designed to create an atmosphere of reflection.[5] These discussions are a time when students can share their opinions, thoughts, questions, and feedback. When students have their own life experiences in a certain area, they often share them with the class in a vulnerable way.

For example, in 6th grade, we invite parents who have adopted or fostered children to speak to the students about their experiences. Sometimes these speakers are parents of a student in that grade. Students often share information that their classmates have never heard before.

> My son was adopted at birth and although he has always known that, he didn't choose to tell his friends. When you asked me to tell our story to the 6th grade students, he didn't want me to at first, but when he heard that two of the other 6th graders were also adopted and going to tell their stories, he changed his mind. It was such a great experience... for ALL of us. His friends were sweet about it and some were even crying at the touching stories. His friends have asked him even more questions later and he has enjoyed being able to talk about it. Since then, it has opened up a lot of meaningful conversations at our house. We love this program and that it has supported us while we learn to support others! – Denise, parent of 6th grade student

What we learned: Discussions are an essential component of the SBSSS experience. Students feel safe to express their thoughts during discussions.

Reflections ⊙

> It helped me understand that all people go through struggles at times, but what matters is how they react to the struggles. – Josiah, 6th grade student Reflection

Every experience within SBSSS is followed by a written Stewardship Reflection.[6] This gives the students a chance to process what they have experienced. It also gives us a chance to see that the students understood the concepts that were presented. Students complete the Stewardship Reflections immediately after the experience, when possible, so their thoughts are fresh in their minds.

What we learned: Reflections help students process their experiences and thoughts. They also help us know the students' level of understanding.

Family Stewardship ⊙

> The Family Stewardship is a great way to take this program outside of the once-a-month lesson. Taking the concepts and asking parents and teachers to apply them in the "real world" is important. – Ron, Stewardship Parent

---

[5] To download a sample Discussion, visit stepbystepstudentstewardship.mykajabi.com/resources
[6] To download a sample Reflection, visit stepbystepstudentstewardship.mykajabi.com/resources

Our family LOVES Family Stewardship! The kids are usually eager to talk about it and having prompts is so helpful. We go through the questions and usually end up going off on some interesting tangent. Family Stewardship has opened up many deep, valuable conversations we would not normally think to have with our kids. Thanks! – Mary and James, parents of 5th and 7th grade students

The Family Stewardship is a brief family preparation and/or follow-up to each Stewardship Friday to enhance the student's understanding and draw from the parents' life experiences.[7] This exercise promotes deep conversations about issues and strengthens family connections. We ask families to spend 5 minutes discussing the questions but we hear from parents that the questions spur rich discussion and they often find themselves in much longer conversations that meander from the original questions. Parents have been thankful to have the conversation prompts that are both meaningful and enjoyable. Since we ask for only a five-minute conversation, parents are not so overwhelmed to add it to their typically hectic schedule. Some families discuss this in the car on the way home or on the way to practices.

What we learned: Family Stewardship promotes family engagement and helps parents feel a part of the SBSSS process. It spurs valuable conversations and draws from parents' unique life experiences.

Games ☺☺ *to* ☺☺☺

The 1st grade Reality Game was when I really saw my kids start to grasp the concept that some have more than others and that some families struggle to provide necessities. – Charlene, 1st grade teacher

I think the discussion/activities around homelessness and The Reality Game Part 2 was very eye opening to the kids. The game showed them how difficult life can be when you are an adult with bills to pay and other pressures of life. – David, Stewardship Parent

Most of the grades have a game that involves the hands-on practice of the concepts they are learning, discussing, and experiencing that year.[8] These games are as follows:

1st Grade: The Reality Game©
2nd Grade: Color Me Healthy Game©
3rd Grade: The Aging Game©
5th Grade: Integrity Idol©
6th Grade: Recipe for a Well-Balanced Life©
7th Grade: The Reality Game Part 2©
8th Grade: The Dr. Faith Show©

---

[7] To download a sample Family Stewardship, visit stepbystepstudentstewardship.mykajabi.com/resources

[8] To obtain games, visit stepbystepstudentstewardship.mykajabi.com/resources

What we learned: The games are unique, involved, engaging, and memorable. They help the students to feel the challenges, obstacles, and hardships that their neighbors might face.

Stewardship Activities ☹☺ to ☹☺☺

> The 1st grade NEEDS vs. WANTS activity is something that seems to stick and is an ongoing theme for my students. We talk about it throughout the whole year. – Lindsey, 1st grade teacher

> My students refer back to the shoe collection project when we recap our school year! The difference is that it was made personal and caused them to think of those receiving the shoes, rather than just collecting cast off shoes. We LOVE the "Shoes for Someone Special" lesson! – Katie, 1st grade teacher

Stewardship Activities are hands-on but not face-to-face ways of serving others remotely. An example is a school-wide food collection (led by the second grade students) for the food bank during the Thanksgiving season. It is called BAGS OF BLESSINGS.

While a food collection may not be a unique activity for a school, we do it in an intentional way to help the students realize that not everyone has the luxury of a stocked refrigerator and pantry. There is a video story that everyone watches followed by announcements every morning to encourage the students to think about their own blessings. To make it more personal, the students write fun, friendly messages of encouragement on the cans and boxes they donate. They are asked to picture the person receiving the food and anticipate how special they might feel to find a little handwritten note.

> BAGS of BLESSINGS made me realize that there is a real person with real feelings receiving this food. It also made me so grateful for what I have. I hope they like our little love notes! – Alex, 6th grade student

Stewardship Activities are used to enhance the relationship with our neighbors. For example, in third grade, students are assigned a pen pal from a local nursing home. They visit their pen pals during a field trip mid-school year. As a Stewardship Activity, they make a Pen Pal Hugger for their pen pals before they go. Pen Pal Huggers are fleece shawls to keep them warm in the winter. The shawls are unique because we specifically designed them for someone in a wheelchair or a bed. It would be easier to make blankets, but the nursing home told us that blankets don't keep their upper body as warm and often fall off of their lap or get caught up in the wheels. We discuss this with the students and we point out to them that it is important to listen to our neighbors' needs, versus assuming we know what their needs are.

What we learned: Stewardship Activities are a special hands-on way to enhance our relationships with our neighbors. They also offer opportunities to learn what our neighbors really need versus what we assume they need.

Stewardship Projects ☉☉☉

> During our outings at nursing homes, interactions with children with disabilities, serving at the soup kitchen – students made an effort to make friends and interact through conversations. This is an incredible life skill for children of any age *and* all adults. I noticed some of the adults were uncomfortable in some of these situations. That is an incredible thing to learn at such a young age! – Sarah, Stewardship Parent

> I was proud of our 1st graders when we visited their preschool buddies at Neighborhood House. Our kids seemed so mature and comfortable watching out for and taking care of their little buddies. They were very prepared for this and it made them feel so big and grown up! – Marilyn, 1st grade Stewardship Parent

> I met this one girl and she was excited about her wind chime she had worked so hard on. I complimented it and right away she offered it to me, one of her most favored possessions, to me! This girl had almost nothing. It really touched my heart. Those are the moments that make Stewardship so special. – Zoe, 6th grade student

Stewardship Projects are truly the culmination and hallmark of the SBSSS experience. They are also the most complex to plan. Stewardship Projects are face-to-face interactions with the neighbors. Sometimes they happen during school hours as a field trip or a few students are taken off-site during lunchtime by parents. Also, Stewardship Projects happen after school with several parents driving students to locations around town.

Stewardship Projects require creativity and thinking outside of the box to create, especially when involving children as young as 6 years old. We have developed relationships with organizations and groups around town that have been invaluable to us. There are typical protocols to follow that are important for privacy, security, and safety. But all these steps are worth it to develop personal and memorable moments for these students and relationships with the neighbors.

Table 25.4 shows an example of possible Stewardship Projects by grade.

What we learned: The in-class preparation throughout the school year culminates in the creative Stewardship Projects in which students meet their neighbors. Stewardship Projects are complex to plan but worth the effort.

End-of-Year Wrap-Up ☉

> The things we learn during Stewardship Friday are so memorable. I think it is because it is all so real! I like learning the stories and perspective about other people's lives. It helps me to understand people better. – Jamison 6th grade

During the last session of the school year, each grade spends time reflecting on what they learned throughout the year. They discuss what things surprised them, helped them grow, and the important take-aways. The Stewardship Parents and teachers are always encouraged by the retention of these lessons, discussions, and experiences from so many months earlier.

As they discuss, the Stewardship Parents take notes about the students' memories to make a script for their End-of-Year Stewardship Celebration.

What we learned: The preparations and experiences are memorable and the students retain the information from throughout the year.

End-of-Year Stewardship Celebration ☉☉

> It's fun to see what everyone else did this year and to realize that we are a part of something bigger than just our own grade. It makes me proud of my school. Also, it helps me know what we will be doing the next year. The video shows how much everyone does! – Cecelia 7th grade

The End-of-Year Stewardship Celebration is a whole school assembly in which representatives from each grade spend a few minutes telling the rest of the school what their grade learned that year. They are encouraged to share by using props, signs, or other visuals. This helps the students see that collectively, the whole school is showing love to neighbors of many kinds.

At the end of the celebration, we show a video (with music) that compiles the photos of experiences from the year. The students enjoy seeing themselves and their classmates in photos as they reminisce about the year of SBSSS.

What we learned: The celebration helps the students realize how much has been accomplished school-wide through the collective efforts of each grade.

Stewardship Résumé ☉☉

> It is amazing to see everything listed on paper. I can't believe how much I have done over these years and how many neighbors we met. It makes me feel like I can accomplish anything in the future! – Micah, 8th grade student

> I used my Stewardship Résumé to start a lawn mowing business. People were impressed when I showed it to them. They hired me right away! – Sean, 8th grade student

> I got a college scholarship using my Stewardship Résumé! They were impressed by how much I knew about our community. It really is incredible how much we were exposed to when we were so young. – Lynne, 22-year-old

Beginning in 6th grade, the students start to create their Stewardship Résumés.[9] This is a compilation of all of their experiences with the different neighbors. They are surprised by how much they have done. At the same time, they learn what a

---

[9]To download a sample Stewardship Résumé, visit stepbystepstudentstewardship.mykajabi.com/resources

Table 25.4 Example Stewardship Projects per grade

Grade	Stewardship Projects
1st Neighbors In Need	Community Center Preschool Buddies Project and Field Trip
2nd Neighbors who are Hungry	Help Sort and Distribute Food at the Food Pantry Serve at the Soup Kitchen
3rd Neighbors who are Elderly	Nursing Home Field Trip and Visit with Pen Pals Visit with the Seniors at School/Memory Boxes
4th Neighbors who are Disabled	Serve at School for Physical Disabilities Special Athletes Basketball Tournament and Interviews Serve at Residential Home for Children with Disabilities
5th Neighbors Living with Illness	Serve Dinners at a Club for Neighbors with Cancer Field Trip to the Children's Hospital
6th Neighbors who are Children in Need	Children's Home Social Outings
7th Neighbors who are Homeless/ Refugees	Serve at the Soup Kitchen Field Trip to the Homeless Shelter
8th Education and Literacy	Story Time and Activities at the After School Club Homework Help at the Children's Home After School Club Library Help

résumé is, how to write one, and how they are used. They are encouraged to add to it in the future.

What we learned: The students enjoy the process of looking back on their gradual accomplishments over 9 years. They feel "grown up" to create a resume and use it to help them in the future.

Signature Stewardship Projects ☺☺☺

> We had one student who started a Mission Collection drive at his high school to help different organizations around the world. Another student chose to spend summers at a camp for disabled children because of the experience gained through SBSSS. – Alma, 8th grade teacher

> Students in 8th grade begin to develop empathy and respect for one another. The Signature Stewardship Project is an opportunity for each student to discern his or her own talents, realize that they can make a difference, and begin to see serving as a part of their everyday life. An added benefit is that it builds confidence and purpose in the child! – Robert, 8th grade Stewardship Parent

Eighth grade students are given the opportunity to create their own Signature Stewardship Project. This is a project they develop, informed by the neighbors they have met, the stewardship experiences over the years, their interests, and their personal gifts and talents. Each year in SBSSS, students have been studying the "trees," but this project helps them see the entire "forest." The creation of the project is broken down into small tasks every month so they can practice time management.

They also begin to define their own personal vision and mission statements. This helps them reflect on their own unique story, who they want to be, what their legacy will be, and what their purpose is. We encourage them to dream big.

> I was surprised that I really loved working with kids who are disabled. Now I want to find a career in that. That makes me SO excited! – Anthony, 8th grade

Later in the school year, they present their Signature Stewardship Projects to a team of adults. The adults give them feedback and ideas to move forward. Students are not required to implement their idea, but rather learn how to creatively plan a project. Some students use their projects later in high school when service projects might be required. The projects help them envision how they could be a leader and the steps necessary to do that.

> The Signature Stewardship Projects help students know what it takes to be leaders. Using my daughter as an example, she joined a service fraternity in college, where she worked with others, often leading them, in various ways of serving the community. This type of passion for service stays with the students beyond their involvement in the SBSSS program. – Meg, Stewardship Parent

What we learned: The students learn about their community over their 9 years with the program. They learn what issues and neighbors they identify with most. They also learn about themselves and begin to discover their purpose in life. These discoveries inform the creation of their own Signature Stewardship Project.

Stewardship Portfolio ☺☺*/Stewardship Graduation* ☺☺☺

> She received her Stewardship Portfolio at her 8th grade graduation and she was so excited to look back at her drawings and stories that she did as the follow up activity. It's definitely a keepsake. – Evan, parent of 8th grade student

Over the years, we collect and file the Stewardship Reflections and other creative work in a Stewardship Portfolio for each student. When they graduate from 8th grade, they receive their Stewardship Portfolios during a Stewardship Graduation Ceremony. The students are surprised and touched that we have saved all of that. They reminisce about the experiences they had over the past 9 years. You can see their sense of accomplishment as they thumb through the papers.

The Stewardship Graduation Ceremony is a way to celebrate and reminisce about all they have learned over the past 9 years. We discuss some of their experiences and the impact they had on the students and on the neighbors. We make a video with music and photos from throughout the years. We line up a few inspiring speakers and choose a couple of the student speakers to reflect back on their experiences.

Students leave 8th grade feeling a sense that they have accomplished something important, complete, and worthwhile. They realize that they already know more about their neighbors than many adults do. It gives them the confidence to go out into the world of new neighbors.

What we learned: Students feel a sense of accomplishment and pride, having been a part of SBSSS for up to 9 years. They have fond, vibrant memories of the neighbors they met and feel encouraged to continue to learn about their neighbors and their community.

Conclusion

Now you might be asking the overarching question: Does SBSSS have any effect on school violence? As previously mentioned, preventing school violence was never my aim when developing the program. Since I have no studies or data to support its use for that purpose, I will draw from the only source I have available: statements taken from surveys of the children and adults who have been involved with SBSSS for over 18 years. These results will inform us about the anecdotal outcomes of SBSSS. We will then explore if and how it could be used in other schools.

Before writing this chapter, I sent out an informal survey through e-mail and social media. I quickly received responses from 75 people. I was struck by the fact that the average years of involvement in the program was TEN years! That speaks to the sustainability of the program and the commitment of the people involved. I have summarized the responses to the most relevant question for this discussion: *Could SBSSS help prevent school violence, bullying, or prejudice? If so, how? 100% of students, teachers, faculty, parents, and stewardship parents said "yes."* Below are excerpts of the responses:

Excerpts from 15 Students or Past Students (ages 8 to 24, average of 11 years old, average of 6.5 years of involvement, 4 students are now college graduates):

- *SBSSS informed us and that helps us avoid prejudice.*
- *It helps us have empathy, which is often the solution to these problems.*
- *By exposing us at a young age to neighbors, we learned about acceptance of people who are different than us. That informs our actions in the future.*
- *It taught us that everyone goes through their own battle.*
- *It gave us a different outlook/perspective on life and helped us find our purpose/ meaning.*
- *Being around people who are different gives us an opportunity to learn and eliminate any feelings of self-superiority.*
- *We learned that we can be the light in a world that seems so dark.*
- *It helped us be more comfortable around people others tend to shy away from.*
- *It taught us integrity and to be more thoughtful towards our friends.*
- *Education, exposure, and experiences...ALL helped us understand and empathize with others who are different and to treat everyone with respect and dignity.*

Excerpts from 15 Teachers/Faculty (2 to 18 years of involvement, average of 8 years):

- *They are more aware of social issues and it teaches them about the real world in a way that they can relate to. They hold onto these concepts.*
- *Students are more tolerant and insightful of those not like themselves. They see the bigger picture. They gain something from it in their soul.*
- *SBSSS could and does have an impact on bullying and prejudice. I have seen my classes over the years become more tolerant of others.*
- *I came from a school without SBSSS and the differences are amazing! They learn to respect and value differences in others! Students get that everyone is precious and valuable.*
- *SBSSS is powerful and comprehensive. It makes their whole class closer as a unit.*
- *The lessons pour over into the classroom in calming, thought-provoking ways.*
- *We talk about the various Stewardship lessons when we discuss bullying. So many lessons that we can use in the classroom. This is an excellent program!*
- *I don't have any scientific proof, but I feel my students are more compassionate since the implementation of SBSSS. The kids love Stewardship Friday!*
- *Students and faculty share a common experience and work together to help others. The results show through how the students treat others in their own classrooms and school buildings. Students are nicer to each other.*

Excerpts from 15 Parents (5 to 18 years of involvement, average of 11 years) **and 30 Stewardship Parents** (3 to 18 years of involvement, average of 10 years):

- *They step outside their comfort zone and establish relationships with each other as they work together to help their neighbors. They have more teamwork and camaraderie as they work toward a common goal. It gives them perspective and the ability to relate to others.*
- *Replicating feelings of helplessness/uncertainty have left deep impressions on them.*
- *We don't understand what we don't know and what we don't experience. More knowledge means more compassion, more understanding, and more love.*
- *SBSSS is eye-opening, powerful, impactful, and real-life! They apply the concepts into real-life experiences with real people. Now they are not quick to judge someone.*
- *SBSSS teaches understanding and patience for one another.*
- *Now students listen well to others and are respectful of the opinions of their peers.*
- *They have concern for others and they support each other.*
- *It helps them create good habits for life. They become aware of others' needs.*
- *Gratitude! A grateful heart is a kinder, less prejudiced heart.*

The statements from the surveys suggest that SBSSS benefits both the giver and the receiver. It also appears to improve the health and social environment of the schools.

I thought the project was helpful and exciting and excellent and fun and neat *and it made me feel wonderful and happy and proud and good inside.* – Alice, 1ˢᵗ grade

Alice, just 6 years old, already recognizes what researchers have long observed and studied; helping others makes us feel good. What she doesn't know is that when we help others, there are real changes in the brain that increase happiness (Park et al., 2017). Could this increased happiness also improve school health, wellness, and social environment in other schools?

So the next important question is: Is SBSSS scalable? And if so, in what types of schools? As I have indicated throughout the chapter, there are several components of the program that can be used at any school or home (literature, movies, videos, discussions, reflections, family stewardship, games, and resumés). We have resources on our website that can help you in those areas.[10]

The whole program is also available on the website; however, there are some caveats:

1. This curriculum requires *time* from the classroom (an average of 1 hour per month per grade), so teachers and faculty must be prepared for that.
2. It requires at least one very committed *coordinator* to organize and lead Stewardship Parents and/or teachers, arrange for speakers, and plan projects.
3. The program itself is *budget-friendly*, requiring mainly one-time purchases of supplies, literature, props, etc., a nominal membership fee each year, and funds for buses for field trips.
4. Each grade requires some adult *volunteers*, preferably the same ones each month, who understand how to build the concepts throughout the year. Teachers could teach the program but would still benefit from some volunteer support.
5. The curriculum is written for Christian schools, but the message of love and compassion is a universal one. With some *adapting*, anyone can use the resources, to the degree that works for them.

You might assume that schools in more impoverished areas would be disadvantaged by the aspect of needing volunteers and resources. However, SBSSS is used in schools that vary widely in terms of geography, demographics, and socioeconomic factors. Our school with the least amount of parental involvement and on the lowest socioeconomic scale is one of the most vibrant of all schools using the program.

Their Stewardship "Parents" are made up mostly of grandparents and retired senior volunteers who have time, commitment, and enthusiasm to enrich their community. Through the surveys, I saw that their students highly value this program.

One of the benefits of SBSSS is that it empowers students to rise above fear and circumstances to see the world as a place of possibility and opportunity. Students realize they have value and special gifts that only they can offer.

SBSSS empowers students, especially in scenarios where home life is dysfunctional or unstable. – Kay, Stewardship Parent

---

[10] For all resources, visit stepbystepstudentstewardship.mykajabi.com/resources

I would suggest that students and schools in impoverished areas could benefit even more from the program. It could also be an encouragement to students who might be struggling with some of the very issues we learn about. In addition, it could offer a perspective and moral framework if that is missing in the home.

> Stewardship doesn't just help the less fortunate. It helps everyone… big and small, a steward or a receiver, someone who has a little or a lot. Our stewardship helps everyone. Even our parents and families. – Kevin, 7th grade

How could it be practical to implement in impoverished schools, especially if parental support is minimal? I have a creative model to suggest:

Sponsor-a-School: What if civic, community, senior, or faith-based groups sponsored a school and ran part or all of the curriculum there? Retired teachers would be another valuable group. Volunteers could teach the same grade each year and become experts in that grade. Or they could rise up with the same group of students each year, so they could develop deeper relationships with them.

> SBSSS puts all the lessons of loving your neighbor, doing the right thing, etc., into the practical terms of today's society. *The world would be a better place if every school had SBSSS.* – Mary Jo, Stewardship Parent

Systemic change ultimately happens one person and one family at a time. Families can also use SBSSS at home. There are resources on the website that can help families get started. They can even encourage other families to join them to create an SBSSS network.

> You may think one person can't make a difference, but if you add all of those people up it makes a HUGE difference. If our country and others follow this trend (SBSSS), then the world will be a better place… – Nathaniel, 8th grade student

SBSSS is a remedy for hearts of indifference, apathy, fear, prejudice, and judgment. We do small, but meaningful things over the long course that add up to a lasting heart change. Students learn that EVERYONE has a story! Through the stories of many neighbors, students also find perspective, gratitude, vision, purpose, and meaning as they create their own stories. They begin to discern their own gifts, talents, value, mission, and legacy. Our neighbors benefit now, but also in the future as these students grow up to be more empathetic and informed citizens, advocates, teachers, professionals, influencers, spouses, and parents.

Looking back, what lessons have we learned since the creation of SBSSS in 2002? At the center of everything is the full-circle approach of PREPARE… ACT… REFLECT model. These three layers work in harmony to make SBSSS vibrant, impactful, and valuable. Remember Suzy's story from the beginning of the chapter? My own *negative, regretful* experience at a young age informed the creation of *positive* experiences for SBSSS students. There are three lessons I have learned that would have prepared my heart for the experience I had with Amy, the girl in the wheelchair.

Lessons Learned

1. *PREPARE... this step is foundational.*

If I had been prepared ahead of time with stories about neighbors, researched some of the issues, and experienced hands-on simulations, I would have been more comfortable meeting a child in a wheelchair.

2. *ACT ... this step is transformative.*

If I had already experienced looking into the eyes of a stranger and realized they were a real person with real feelings, I would have been more open to talking with a girl in a wheelchair.

3. *REFLECT... this step pulls it all together.*

If I had been encouraged to reflect on my experience on paper, through discussion with the adults at the camp, and by talking with my parents, it would have given my experience perspective and meaning.

How might my camp story have been different if Suzy, Amy, and the older campers had ALL been exposed to the SBSSS curriculum in school? Perhaps it would have looked like this:

- Amy would have had an opportunity to share her story during Stewardship Friday.
- The older campers would have done the Disability Stations and experienced the difficulties of completing normal daily tasks in a wheelchair. This would have given them understanding and empathy for Amy. They might have included her in their activities.
- Suzy would have already had interactions with children in wheelchairs during fourth grade Stewardship Projects. She would have felt comfortable talking to Amy, rather than fear and apprehension. Suzy would have learned Amy's story, shown love to her neighbor, and made a new friend.

This version of the story would have been a win for all the girls, rather than a humiliating, regrettable situation. However, it was the seed that germinated in Suzy's life and bloomed into STEP-by-STEP Student Stewardship©... so in the end, it was fruitful!

We may be small, but we can make a big difference. – Malea, 5th grade student

References

Butler, T. C. (Ed.). (1991). Entry for 'Stewardship'. *Holman Bible Dictionary*. Available at: https://www.studylight.org/dictionaries/hbd/s/stewardship.html

Johnson, D. R. (2012). Transportation into a story increases empathy, prosocial behavior, and perceptual bias toward fearful expressions. *Personality and Individual Differences, 52*(2), 150–155.

Park, S. Q., Kahnt, T., Dogan, A., Strang, S., Fehr, E., & Tobler, P. N. (2017). A neural link between generosity and happiness. *Nature Communications, 8*, 15964. https://doi.org/10.1038/ncomms15964

Chapter 26
Preventing Compassion Fatigue Among Educators: An Educator Resiliency Study During the COVID-19 Pandemic

Chunyan Yang ⓘ, Jenna E. Greenstein, Sarah Manchanda, Maedah Golshirazi, and Tammy Yabiku

Introduction

The teacher shortage in the United States is vast and growing. According to the report from Learning Policy Institute (Carver-Thomas & Darling-Hammond, 2017), close to 8% of teachers were leaving teaching, with new teachers (<5 years), leaving at rates between 19% and 30%. Teacher shortages affect student motivation (Shen et al., 2015) and student academic success (Sutcher et al., 2019). With the new challenges teachers are facing during the COVID-19 pandemic, it is vital to understand how the COVID-19 pandemic and its subsequent new challenges may influence teachers' wellbeing and the teacher workforce. The psychological reasons for teacher shortage are most often examined through a stress and burnout lens. Researchers showed that stress and burnout may significantly impair the working relationships that the teachers have with their students, the quality of teaching and commitment they are able to display (Kyriacou, 1987), and teacher retention (Christian-Brandt et al., 2020). One of the most important factors influencing teacher stress and burnout is compassion fatigue.

In this chapter, we will discuss theories and empirical studies related to educators' compassion fatigue, particularly in the context of the COVID-19 pandemic and consequent distance learning. We will begin by defining compassion fatigue and reviewing some key demographic and psychological factors associated with educators' compassion fatigue. Grounded in the job demands-resource (JD-R) model, we will then discuss some key empirical findings from the COVID-19 Educator Resilience Project to illustrate how educators perceived online teaching self-efficacy, educators' social and emotional learning (SEL) competencies, and school-connectedness factors concurrently and interactively influence educators'

C. Yang (✉) · J. E. Greenstein · S. Manchanda · M. Golshirazi · T. Yabiku
Graduate School of Education, University of California, Berkeley, Berkeley, CA, USA
e-mail: yangcy@berkeley.edu

© The Author(s), under exclusive license to Springer Nature Switzerland AG 2023
T. W. Miller (ed.), *School Violence and Primary Prevention*,
https://doi.org/10.1007/978-3-031-13134-9_26

compassion fatigue during the unique context of the COVID-19 pandemic and distance learning. This chapter concludes with a discussion of practical recommendations and strategies to promote educators' online teaching self-efficacy, SEL competencies, and healthy connectedness, and to prevent compassion fatigue and racial trauma.

Compassion Fatigue: Definition and Significance

Compassion fatigue was originally defined by Figley (1995) as "the natural consequent behaviors and emotions resulting from knowing about a traumatizing event experienced by a significant other and the stress resulting from wanting to help a traumatized or suffering person" (p. 7). Following this definition, compassion fatigue is often defined as interchangeable with secondary traumatic stress, which is characterized by stress symptoms that result from wanting to help a traumatized or suffering person. However, Stamm (2010) defined compassion fatigue as the negative aspects of individuals' professional quality of life, in contrast to compassion satisfaction, which alludes to the positive aspects of professional quality of life. He identified the two sub-constructs of compassion fatigue, including (1) secondary traumatic stress; and (2) burnout, which is characterized by chronic work-related stress, exhaustion, frustration, and anger. In this chapter, compassion fatigue was conceptualized as one integrated concept including two key negative indicators of educators' psychological wellbeing: burnout and secondary traumatic stress.

Prior research has identified the high rate of secondary traumatic stress and burnout among educators. Borntrager et al. (2012) found that approximately 75% of school personnel in the Northwestern United States were experiencing high levels of compassion fatigue, according to the Secondary Traumatic Stress Scale. The existing research demonstrates that teachers' compassion fatigue, emotional exhaustion, and burnout contribute to negative student behavioral and academic outcomes, such as learning in mathematics (Klusmann et al., 2016), motivation (Shen et al., 2015; Zhang & Sapp, 2008), and school satisfaction and perceived teacher caring (Ramberg et al., 2020). At the classroom level, educators' burnout has also been shown to negatively impact students' school satisfaction, school grades, and perceptions of teacher support (Arens & Morin, 2016). Furthermore, researchers identified the negative impacts of educators' compassion fatigue and burnout on their level of distress (e.g., Hill et al., 2011; Kokkinos, 2007). Christian-Brandt et al. (2020) also found that teachers with lower compassion satisfaction and higher burnout were more likely to report intentions to leave the teaching profession. While the high prevalence rate of compassion fatigue and its significance to student and teacher outcomes have been indicated by previous research, researchers have argued that educators' stress levels varied depending on school-specific features and contexts (Ramberg et al., 2020). Therefore, it is critical that theoretical and empirical studies examine significant factors associated with compassion fatigue, and investigate how such knowledge can help reduce compassion fatigue among educators.

Demographic and Psychological Correlates of Educator Compassion Fatigue

Although the importance of understanding educator compassion fatigue has been recognized by researchers, a comprehensive theoretical conceptualization of educator compassion fatigue is still lacking. However, the Job Demands-Resources (JD-R) theory has provided some important theoretical insights for understanding the demographic and psychological correlates of educator compassion fatigue. According to Job Demands-Resources (JD-R) theory proposed by Bakker and Demerouti (2017), job characteristics were characterized as two distinct categories: job resources and job demands. Job resources buffer occupational wellbeing and performance through motivational processes, while job demands drain occupational wellbeing and performance through health impairment processes. The motivational process posits that job resources could be either extrinsic or intrinsic assets that help people feel more engaged in their work and perform better. On the other hand, the health impairment process is where highly demanding jobs require the individual to exert more energy and effort, which can lead to exhaustion and increased risk for developing health problems. Consistent with this theoretical framework, some important personal and environmental factors have been identified as contributing to educators' compassion fatigue, which is conceptualized as an important negative indicator for the occupational wellbeing of educators. In this section, we discuss some important demographic factors (i.e., age, years of experience, gender, workload, job roles and responsibilities, poverty, and exposure to trauma) and psychological factors (i.e., self-efficacy, perceived teacher autonomy, and social support and school connectedness) that have been found to contribute to educator's compassion fatigue.

Demographic Factors

Age and Years of Experience Researchers have highlighted the role of some individual characteristics (e.g., gender, age, years of experience) in the development of compassion fatigue. A systematic review study showed that older age and more years of work experience are associated with lower levels of burnout (Brewer & Shapard, 2004). Skaalvik and Skaalvik (2015) also stated that although teachers of different ages experienced the same stressors at school, the senior teachers needed increasingly more time to recover from stress. Furthermore, researchers have suggested that age and years of working experience may moderate the association between individual and environmental factors and burnout. For example, in a meta-analysis study, Shoji et al. (2016) suggested that the association between self-efficacy and burnout was stronger among older workers than among younger workers. They also found that the association between burnout and self-efficacy was stronger among participants with more years of work experience than among participants with fewer years of work experience. The authors argued that older workers have protective beliefs about their own ability to handle stressful events and use those protective resources more effectively, which ultimately leads to lower burnout.

Gender There are limited findings regarding the gender differences in educators' compassion fatigue. Researchers have demonstrated that female teachers reported higher emotional exhaustion than male teachers (Skaalvik & Skaalvik, 2011, 2017). Similarly, in a sample of mental health providers in a rural southern state, Sprang and colleagues (2007) found female providers are at a higher risk of suffering from compassion fatigue than male providers.

Poverty and Exposure to Trauma Researchers have suggested that educators who work in high-poverty urban schools and with traumatized children are most vulnerable to developing burnout and compassion fatigue (Abraham-Cook, 2012; Maslach & Schaufeli, 1993; Beaton & Murphy, 1995; Figley, 1995). Students in high-poverty urban schools usually deal with issues related to community violence, child abuse, and poverty (VanBergeijk & Sarmiento, 2006). Considering the high rates of exposure to traumatic events experienced by this population, teachers working in high-poverty schools interact with children who have been traumatized on a regular basis (Abraham-Cook, 2012). In these environments, educators are usually among the first people to address their students' trauma (Chang & Davis, 2009). Researchers showed that the frequency and intensity of one's engagement with traumatized individuals is a strong predictor of compassion fatigue (Adams et al., 2006; Killian, 2008; Meadors et al., 2009). For example, Abraham-Cook (2012) found that teachers in high-poverty urban public schools are particularly vulnerable to developing compassion fatigue, with approximately 90% of the sample scoring within the high-risk range.

Workload Educator's workload is another risk factor associated with compassion fatigue. Workload is a broad concept that has been used to describe a wide range of job-related tasks, from the size and characteristics of one's caseload (or classroom) to the number of job responsibilities they have (Fimian, 1987). Researchers consistently demonstrate that large caseloads and high percentages of traumatized clients are associated with an increased risk of secondary traumatic stress responses (Creamer & Liddle, 2005; Deighton et al., 2007; Sprang et al., 2007). In educational literature, Abraham-Cook (2012) showed that stress related to work demands is a significant predictor of compassion fatigue and burnout.

Job Roles and Responsibilities Certain specific roles and job responsibilities of educators may be more prone to compassion fatigue than others. For example, researchers have suggested that special education teachers are at high risk for developing compassion fatigue. Researchers have identified several factors that impact special education teachers' burnout, including teacher experience, student disability, role conflict, role ambiguity, and administrative support (Brunsting et al., 2014). Many special education teachers often spend their time performing non-instructional tasks (e.g., IEP meetings, paperwork; Vannest & Hagan-Burke, 2010). Moreover, researchers have demonstrated that special education teachers who work with students with emotional disturbance (ED) experienced higher burnout than those working with students with other disabilities (Brunsting et al., 2014). These findings also align with the general education literature, which suggests that challenging student behavior correlates with burnout for general education teachers (Hastings & Brown, 2002).

Self-Efficacy Self-efficacy is defined as "people's judgments of their capabilities to organize and execute courses of action required to attain designated types of performances." (Bandura, 1986, p. 391). Self-efficacy beliefs are constructed from four sources of information, including enactive mastery experiences (also known as "performance accomplishments"), role modeling, verbal persuasion, and physiological and affective states (Bandura, 1997). Bandura (1997) identified four mediation processes, including cognitive, motivational, affective, and selective processes, which explain the mechanism in which self-efficacy beliefs produce their effects. Social cognitive theory assumes that self-efficacy determines various stress-related outcomes (Bandura, 1997) and compassion fatigue is an example of such an outcome. In the context of occupational stress, self-efficacy represents self-perceived competence that one can employ the skills necessary to deal with job demands, and cope with job-related stress and its consequences (Shoji et al., 2016). In the educational realm, research shows that teacher self-efficacy is positively related to work engagement and job satisfaction, and negatively related to burnout. For example, Skaalvik and Skaalvik (2007) found a strong negative association between teacher self-efficacy and teacher burnout. Skaalvik and Skaalvik (2010) also found moderate negative associations between teacher self-efficacy and two traditional dimensions of burnout (i.e., emotional exhaustion and depersonalization). Furthermore, research conducted in the context of teacher burnout and compassion fatigue shows that self-efficacy may operate as a protective factor and prevent negative consequences of strain (Blecharz et al., 2014).

Perceived Autonomy Researchers have suggested that teachers' perceived autonomy is negatively related to burnout and emotional exhaustion (Skaalvik & Skaalvik, 2009, 2010, 2014). According to self-determination theory (SDT), autonomy is one of the fundamental psychological needs that is universally important for psychological wellbeing and motivation (Deci & Ryan, 2000). Autonomy concerns the experience of integration and freedom (Deci & Ryan, 2000). Skaalvik and Skaalvik (2014) argued that teacher autonomy includes freedom to choose goals, teaching methods, and educational strategies that are consonant with the teacher's personal educational beliefs and values. They also stated that some autonomy is necessary for teachers to be able to deal immediately and adequately with stressful and unexpected situations.

Several studies highlighted the association between educators perceived autonomy and compassion fatigue. For example, Skaalvik and Skaalvik (2009) found that perceived teacher autonomy was negatively correlated with all three traditional dimensions of burnout, including emotional exhaustion, depersonalization, and feelings of reduced accomplishment. Skaalvik and Skaalvik (2010) also found that teacher autonomy was negatively related to emotional exhaustion, controlling for workload, student discipline problems, and relations with both colleagues and the school principal.

Social Support and School Connectedness Previous studies have shown that school connectedness perceived by educators were associated with their burnout and secondary traumatic stress, which are key indicators for educators' compassion fatigue and psychological wellbeing in general (i.e., Collie et al., 2012; O'Brennan et al., 2017). Teacher burnout, particularly in the dimensions of workplace stress and emotional exhaustion, was associated with many school contextual factors, such as adequate access to resources, input in decision making, and supportive supervisors (Collie et al., 2012; Greenglass et al., 1996). Also, supportive mentorship was found to function as a preventative factor for secondary traumatic stress among teachers, whereas supervisory or punitive connection with colleagues functioned as a risk factor associated with heightened teacher stress (Caringi et al., 2015).

Furthermore, mutual relationship and connectedness may function as a protective factor in mitigating the negative impact of compassion fatigue on teacher and student outcomes. According to the relational resilience theoretical model, a person's engagement in mutually empathetic and responsive relationships promotes teacher resilience (Jordan, 2003). Relational resilience is defined as resilience that is promoted by the capacity for connection and mutually empathetic, responsive relationships (Jordan, 2003). Relational resilience as it applies to teachers has been defined as a dynamic process between risk and protective factors that produces the outcome of teachers feeling connected while moving beyond the common stressors of the teaching profession (Gu & Day, 2007). There has been a small amount of research that has focused on the role that personal and professional relationships play in teacher resilience (Le Cornu, 2013), and even fewer studies have examined the topic within the context of distance learning caused by the COVID-19 pandemic.

Compassion Fatigue in the Context of COVID-19

As reviewed in the previous section, there has been an increase in research attention in recent years to understand the conceptualization and importance of educators' compassion fatigue and its risk and protective factors. Due to the helping nature of the teaching profession, compassion fatigue affected many teachers prior to the COVID-19 pandemic. However, the pandemic, the subsequent school closure, and the sudden shift to distance learning have drastically changed the nature of compassion fatigue among educators.

Educators were not alone in experiencing increased stress during the pandemic. Pandemic stress was felt by everyone in one way or another, especially in March 2020 when the World Health Organization declared that the COVID-19 outbreak could be characterized as a pandemic (World Health Organization, 2021). People all over the world were forced to shelter in their homes to prevent further spread of the disease, many working professionals transitioned to working remotely, and children were sent home from school, while healthcare professionals and other essential workers continued to work on the frontlines of the pandemic. Though the pandemic was not an easy transition for anyone, educators especially felt a unique increase in compassion fatigue when schools shifted to distance learning.

Educators felt the specific burden of compassion fatigue because in addition to their own troubles (navigating a new system of teaching, financial concerns, caring for their own families, and anxiety about the future of schooling, to name a few), they experienced higher than usual levels of concern for their students (MacIntyre et al., 2020; Sokal et al., 2020). Educator compassion fatigue has been well documented even before the pandemic (e.g., Donahoo et al., 2017; Hoffman et al., 2007; Koenig et al., 2018). Exposure to student adversities and challenges creates feelings of deep empathetic concern, which can lead to secondary traumatic stress and educator burnout. However, the pandemic brought new concerns such as students' access to safe and comfortable shelter and supportive caretakers, students' access to technological devices and internet connections necessary for distance learning, and families' financial difficulties associated with the economic crisis that accompanied the pandemic. Other long-standing issues such as student mental health and wellbeing, student engagement, and student academic achievement continued to run rampant in the distance learning platform. Psychologist Dr. Richard Shadick stated that "we are seeing some of the same psychological effects from teachers as we saw from frontline health care workers" (Teach for America, 2020).

Because educators are the lifeline for students to make it through the pandemic with as minimal long-term academic and psychological repercussions as possible, it is essential that schools and districts understand how to support their educators' wellbeing. Despite the public awareness about the importance of compassion fatigue prevention during the COVID-19 pandemic, we have a minimal empirical and theoretical understanding of what contributes to educators' compassion fatigue and how to prevent and reduce it in the context of the COVID-19 pandemic. Such an understanding is critical for successfully reopening schools and addressing the educator attrition issue during and following the pandemic.

Overview of the COVID-19 Educator Resiliency Project

In response to the above research needs, we conducted the COVID-19 Educator Resiliency Project in the spring of 2020 through a research-practice partnership with a large urban school district in Northern California. One primary goal of the project is to understand educators' experience with compassion fatigue and its contributing factors to the COVID-19 pandemic. The ultimate goal of this research is to provide school districts with practical implications in devising a plan to systematically support educators' wellbeing in the years to come as schools readjust to a new normal.

The COVID-19 Educator Resiliency Project was grounded in the job demands-resources (JD-R) model, in which educators' demographic and psychological characteristics are conceptualized as a potential risk and promotive factors related to job resources or job demands to interactively influence educator's compassion fatigue, which is conceptualized as a negative indicator of educators' wellbeing and occupational quality. Guided by this theoretical framework, we conducted a series of quantitative and qualitative analyses on the survey data collected from both Likert scale and open-ended questions to examine four main research questions:

1. How did educators' compassion fatigue differ by their demographic backgrounds, including gender, race/ethnicity, and years of working experience?
2. How did educators' sense of school connectedness, attempts to connect with different school members, online teaching self-efficacy, and social-emotional learning (SEL) competencies influence their compassion fatigue?
3. What was educators' experience with compassion fatigue during distance learning and the pandemic?
4. How did educators' experience shift in their self-efficacy while teaching online?

Participants and Data Collection Procedure

The data for this research project were collected in the spring of 2020 through a research-practice partnership between the University of California Berkeley and a large urban school district in the Bay Area. Several meetings were held between university researchers and the district's SEL team to plan and prepare the survey that was administered to all educators in the district. The research-practice partnership was implemented with the goal of supporting local districts with adult and student SEL and understanding and promoting educators' resilience and wellbeing. Our survey was designed collaboratively and carefully to fit the unique needs of the district.

The survey was administered to all 4840 educators in the district, and we received responses from 321 educators, yielding a response rate of about 6.5%. Because of the remote nature of data collection, and a lack of incentive, it was difficult to obtain a higher response rate. Our sample of 321 educators was 80% female, 15% male, and 5% not identified or nonbinary. Caucasian educators comprised 56% of the sample, in addition to 12% African American, 14% Hispanic/Latino, 10% Asian, 9% multi-racial, and 3% from other races; 82% of our sample were classroom teachers, 13% were instructional or pupil support professionals, and 5% held other positions at the school. About a quarter of the teachers in our sample (23%) were in their first 5 years working in the field of education. 51% of the sample had worked in education for 6–15 years, 30% for 16–25 years and 18% had worked in education for more than 25 years.

COVID-19 Educator Resiliency Survey

The COVID-19 Educator Resiliency Survey was an online survey that included demographics questions, 4-point Likert scale measures, and qualitative several open-ended questions. In the demographics section, teachers were asked to report their gender, race/ethnicity, occupational position, years of experience in education, and grades taught. The Likert scales (1 = strongly disagree, 2 = somewhat disagree, 3 = somewhat agree, 4 = strongly agree) measured educators' perception of compassion fatigue, online teaching self-efficacy, school connectedness, and their attempts to connect with four types of school members (i.e., students, parents, teachers/staff, and administrators). Their validity and reliability have been supported in previous studies (Yang, 2021; Yang et al., 2021). In the open-ended written responses on the survey, educators had the opportunity to elaborate on their feelings of stress during the pandemic and their main sources of compassion fatigue.

Data Analysis Procedure

Data collected by demographic survey and Likert scales were analyzed using quantitative approach following three steps to examine educators' perceptions of compassion fatigue's demographic differences, the dual roles of "connect" to compassion fatigue, and the interactive influence of online teaching self-efficacy and SEL competencies on compassion fatigue. In the first step, the structural validations of the Online Teaching Self-Efficacy Scale, Compassion Fatigue Scale, and Distance Learning School Connectedness Scale were examined using CFA in Mplus 8.10, and the reliability of these three scales was also examined using SPSS 26. In the second step, descriptive analyses were conducted using SPSS to examine the means and standard deviations of the key continuous variables and their correlations. In the third step, several sequential sets of linear regression models were used to examine the main and moderating effects.

Qualitative data from the open-ended questions were analyzed using a hybrid process of inductive and deductive thematic analysis as modeled by Fereday and Muir-Cochrane (2006). We first developed codes based on the literature on teaching self-efficacy, compassion fatigue, and school connectedness to analyze the raw data. We then engaged in an open coding process and identified patterns that emerged from the raw data and organized these individual codes into four themes: (1) multiple sources of compassion fatigue emerged during distance learning, (2) shifts in teaching self-efficacy and sources of teaching self-efficacy took place, (3) school connectedness impacts teacher wellbeing and self-efficacy, and (4) educators are struggling to maintain wellbeing but attempting to engage in self-care.

Quantitative Research Findings

Demographic Differences of Compassion Fatigue When the main effects of gender, race/ethnicity, and years of working experience on compassion fatigue were examined, we found that educators with longer years of teaching experience also reported significantly lower compassion fatigue levels than educators with shorter teaching experience (Yang et al., 2021). Consistent with this finding, previous studies also found that more experienced or older helping professionals, including psychiatrists, social workers, and therapists, reported lower levels of burnout and higher levels of compassion satisfaction (Boscarino et al., 2004; Craig & Sprang, 2010). However, contradicted findings were found in other studies, where healthcare professionals with more years of experience reported higher level of compassion fatigue than healthcare professionals with fewer years of experience (Potter 2010; Kelly et al., 2015). The mixed findings might be contributed by the different job demands in different professional groups and individuals' abilities to cope with work stress.

We also found that White educators reported significantly higher compassion fatigue than Black educators and marginally significantly higher compassion fatigue than educators with multi-racial/ethnic backgrounds (Yang et al., 2021). It is important to note that the racial/ethnic compositions of the student and teacher population were very diverse in the participating school district of the study. For the student population, there were 43.8% Latino/Hispanic students, 22.9% Black, 12.3% Asian, 11.7% White, and 9.3% other and multi-racial/ethnic students during the 2018–2019 school year. For the educator population, there were 33.8% White educators, 32.5% Black, 17.8% Latino/Hispanic, 13.0% Asian, 2.9% other and multi-racial/ethnic students during the 2018–2019 school year. Based on the racial/ethnic breakdowns of the student and educator populations, White educators and educators with other/multi-racial/ethnic backgrounds were working with the highest percentages of students whose racial/ethnic backgrounds were different from them (e.g., 88.3% of the district student population identified themselves as not being in the "White" racial/ethnic groups, 90.7% of the district student population identified themselves as not being in the "multi-racial/ethnic or other racial/ethnic" group. Thus, it is possible that the racial/ethnic mismatch between educators and students may contribute to the relative higher compassion fatigue found among White educators and educators from other and multi-racial backgrounds.

It is also important to note the fact that the study was conducted in late May and early June 2020 following George Floyd's murder and other murders of Black Americans by police officers. Given this political context, it is also possible that educators with different racial/ethnic backgrounds might have different experiences and reactions in response to the nation-wide reckoning and healing with systemic racism. For example, one White educator's response to the open-ended question about compassion fatigue indicated this potential connection between educators' wellbeing and the political context at that time. The educator wrote: "As I live a very privileged life, [...], I see the act of sheltering in place is a very privileged idea, it assumes you have a safe, loving environment, one that is healthy and can nourish the amount of people living in it. [...] There are many families living in toxic environments, physically, emotionally, and due to an increased exposure to toxic chemicals and pesticides. I fear for their lives and futures and am working to heal my white guilt so I may transform white privilege into action to end white supremacy." (Yang et al., 2021, p.512)

Dual Role of "Connect" on Compassion Fatigue With the controlling of educators' gender, race/ethnicity, and years of teaching in education, educators' increased sense of school connectedness was associated with decreased compassion fatigue. This finding supports the JD-R model by suggesting that school connectedness could function as a job resource that facilitates the motivational process. Thus, it is important to promote educators' school connectedness to improve educators' occupational wellbeing.

As reported in our recently published study (Yang et al., 2021), we also found that educators' attempts to connect with others functioned as both a job resource and a demand to influence compassion fatigue and its specific function varied depending on the type of school members that educators attempted to connect with. For example, educators' attempts to connect with students might function as a "double-edged sword" by not only directly increasing compassion fatigue but also strengthening the preventative influence of school connectedness on compassion fatigue. It is possible that educators who made more frequent attempts to connect with students hold a stronger belief in the importance of school connectedness than those who made less frequent attempts to connect, thereby contributing to the stronger preventative effect of school connectedness on compassion fatigue.

Interactive Influence of Online Teaching Self-Efficacy and SEL Competencies on Compassion Fatigue Controlling for educators' gender, race/ethnicity, and years of teaching in education, online teaching self-efficacy had a negative and significant association with compassion fatigue. Educators' perceived SEL competencies were not significantly associated with educators' compassion fatigue. However, the negative association between online teaching self-efficacy and compassion fatigue was intensified among educators with higher self-reported levels of SEL competencies. This finding indicates that educators with a higher level of SEL competencies were more likely to attune to the preventative influence of online teaching self-efficacy on compassion fatigue than educators with a lower SEL competency level (Yang, 2021). Educators' stronger SEL competencies might be related to higher senses of awareness and empowerment, which are psychological strengths that could promote educators to use their online teaching self-efficacy as a positive source of motivation to combat their negative feelings of burnout and secondary traumatic stress.

Qualitative Research Findings

Overview Based on the thematic analysis on the qualitative responses to the open-ended questions, several themes and subthemes emerged from the codes and they are illustrated in Fig. 26.1. What follows is a summary of findings from the qualitative analysis of the data.

Multiple Sources of Compassion Fatigue During Distance Learning In general, educators reported high levels of compassion fatigue and burnout as a result of distance learning. Based on their responses to the open-ended questions posed in the survey, four sub-themes arose in the coding process as contributing factors to educators' feelings of compassion fatigue: (1) increased job-related demands and responsibilities with limited resources, (2) changing roles and a decrease in job fulfillment, (3) a sense of helplessness in supporting students in need, and (4) concerns about students' physical and mental health wellbeing.

Increased Job-Related Demands A common sentiment expressed among the educators in our sample was no longer finding joy in their job because of the increased demands and responsibilities and the decreased fulfillment of working with students in person. One educator said that they do not enjoy teaching anymore because the "stress of worrying about students and trying, nagging, calling, texting, emailing, Google classroom-ing, Zooming non-stop is exhausting."

In addition to experiencing a higher level of responsibility and greater job demands, teachers also reported a lack of resources and support in meeting these demands. One educator shared that it was "very stressful trying to find ways with little resources to make [students'] learning experiences accessible." Another teacher expressed feelings of burnout linked to "the isolation of trying to solve so many problems for people with such limited resources." These quotes allude to feelings of isolation, exhaustion, and being overworked.

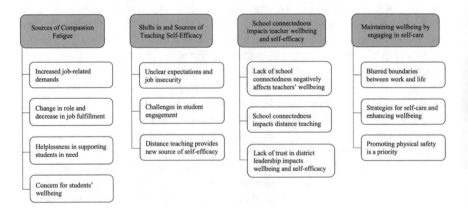

Fig. 26.1 Themes and sub-themes generated from qualitative data analysis

Change in Role and Decrease in Job Fulfillment In many cases, educators described feeling as though their role had changed, and that the responsibilities they had during the pandemic were more emotionally draining than during in-person schooling. One teacher described the frustrations and feelings of being over-whelmed, a common feeling that was reported by educators:

> The combination of childcare responsibility, lack of internet access/computer literacy for students, and the knowledge that almost all of my students' families are unable to pay their rent has given me an overwhelming feeling of "What is the point of all this?" There have been so many nights where I think about my students and cry myself to sleep. It has made me realize that school is about SO MUCH MORE than teaching academics. For me, being away from my students means many of the stresses of teaching, but none of the joy. I've managed to teach for more than a decade in [the district] without burning out or giving up, but this has almost put me over the edge.

Another educator expressed frustration that there are now, "No field trips, no clubs or sports, no parties or celebrations...all the fun and people part of teaching has been stripped away." The new and increased job demands coupled with erasure of some of the greatest sources of joy in teaching have led some educators to feel higher levels of burnout and compassion fatigue.

Helplessness in Supporting Students in Need The helplessness of being unable to support students in need clearly has taken a toll on educators, leading to feelings of burnout and compassion fatigue. The following quote from another teacher further describes the feelings of helplessness that arose during the pandemic:

> This distance learning time has drastically increased my stress levels and has put so many more additional burdens seemingly just on my shoulders. I love my families and checking in with them weekly often makes my day AND feeling like I am the SOLE person support-ing their family's food needs (reminding them of where they can get food, dropping food off at houses), financial needs (passing along fund applications, filling out fund applications on my computer while on the phone with family and a translator), tech support (applying for free internet, talking through how learning programs work, making YouTube videos of how learning programs work), and mental support (hearing family's concerns and needs) is a lot.

Teachers had "so little control over if [their] students were learning or not." Without adequate resources, and with a lack of control over students' lives, teachers felt much higher levels of helplessness and compassion fatigue.

Concern for Students' Wellbeing Teachers' levels of compassion fatigue were also augmented by a greater concern for students' physical and mental wellbeing as a direct result of the pandemic and home learning. For example, a teacher expressed stress about "knowing students who are infected, or work at sites that have reported infections, or have family members that are infected, or are currently self-isolating; and having a mom that was infected; and having students that don't communicate; and having students with extreme economic hardships; and feeling concerned for my physical safety when I go to help the school and students." Never before has there been such a concern for students, families, and teachers themselves catching a deadly disease. Aside from the disease itself, teachers were also worried about students who "experience trauma where they live. Many [...] families were struggling financially, physically, etc., leading [teachers] to worry much more about [their] students and their families."

Shifts in Level of Teaching Self-Efficacy and Sources of Self-Efficacy With the transition to distance learning, educators have worked to quickly adapt in-person instructional strategies and best practices to an online platform with little time and guidance on how to do so successfully. Educators in the district reported a range of feelings of self-efficacy associated with transitioning to distance teaching. The key themes that emerged from educators' reflections on their teaching practice during distance learning were that: (1) educators expressed lower teaching self-efficacy due to unclear expectations from leaders and resulting feelings of job insecurity, (2) challenges in engaging students in distance learning contributed to lower levels of teaching self-efficacy, and (3) distance learning resulted in feelings of empowerment and higher levels of teaching self-efficacy for some teachers.

Unclear Expectations and Job Insecurity Some educators reported heightened levels of anxiety due to the pressure of meeting the district's unclear or unrealistic expectations for successful distance teaching and underlying uncertainty of job security. As one educator shared:

> There was no way I could meet the expectations set forth [by the district]. My stress level was very intense as I just had to kind of pretend. I worried I'd lose my job, something I've never feared as I am very dedicated. It didn't help that a lot of my efforts were for [nothing]. I spent many hours doing district PDs but in the end often realizing they wouldn't work for my students or putting lessons together and having no students show.

Another educator felt stress and lowered teaching self-efficacy primarily due to a lack of reassurance and clarity from the district. This teacher stated:

> How do we know what we are doing has a positive impact on students? This was so overwhelming to implement that my own child's education suffered. So time consuming with little to no feedback from (the district).

During this period of uncertainty around work and safety, educators expressed sentiments that feedback, guidance, and reassurance from the district were necessary in order to maintain feelings of self-efficacy in a high-stress job with rapidly evolving requirements.

Challenges in Student Engagement Many teachers expressed frustration and a lower sense of efficacy in engaging students in distance learning. A core factor that has contributed to lower feelings of self-efficacy in engaging students in distance learning is a lack of control over the learning environment and enactment of pedagogy. One educator reflected that they have felt an "… increase of stress in trying to maintain consistency with students and learning opportunities. [There are] more factors outside of my immediate control that directly impact their own education needs." Another educator reflected that:

> I have never felt more helpless to affect conditions for myself or my students. I grieve for the lost learning, especially for the students who, basically, dropped out. I am stressed that distance learning will continue, making education even more inequitable.

In addition to heightening educators' feelings of compassion fatigue, the change in role linked to online teaching has led to feelings of lower self-efficacy. As one teacher put it:

> Work has become all-encompassing and includes an amplified role as a social worker connecting families to resources. My team has spent hours strategizing how to best engage "unengaged" students and families, but none of our outreach (which has included hand delivering hard copies of assignments, calling, texting, asking what they need, making schedules, making lists of assignments they need to do to pass) has yielded significant results. It feels like putting out a lot of effort into a vacuum. A classroom is so interpersonal that it feels nearly impossible to do this work from a distance.

One specific area of practice that many educators' expressed frustration and low self-efficacy in was engaging students through technology. One educator reflected that the transition to distance teaching "gave me a little more anxiety about getting students to be motivated and involved with distance learning especially when I did hear from a few." Some material and resource constraints contributed to educators' abilities to keep their students motivated to learn during the pandemic as well. For example, an educator shared that a large source of stress was in:

> Changing from teaching a curriculum that is meant for the classroom to figuring out "how to" to do it adequately online. Students, families and teachers are at different places during this pandemic (moving, essential workers, knowing how to help their child use the internet, etc.); nothing about this pandemic is normal.

Another educator identified similar challenges with distance teaching, rooted in competing demands for students' and their families' time and attention during the pandemic:

> It is hard to keep families and students accountable for their learning when there is so many more barriers like technology, internet, family comfort with Zoom or other apps, financial stressors and health stressors.

The limited engagement from students has impacted teachers' feelings of self-efficacy in their practice, as an important source of teaching self-efficacy is feedback from students. As one educator shared:

> It's hard to know if I'm getting through to my students—there is so little useful feedback with this mode of teaching that it often feels like I'm shouting addition[al] strategies into a hole in the ground. There is far less job satisfaction, which makes the stress feel bigger, I guess.

Another teacher reflected on the stress of receiving feedback that indicated their efforts were not enough to meet their students' needs. This educator shared:

> Most of what I hear now is frustration. My students are very young and many have special needs and I am clearly not addressing most of the goals that they have. Am I helpful at all? It is impossible to judge. I do not feel competent at all in what I am doing and that is extremely stressful.

An additional consequence of the lack of student engagement in online instruction is teachers' feelings about the overall quality of their instruction. One educator shared that:

> I feed off being with my students physically. I am struggling teaching online because I cannot gauge whether they are even paying attention and are with me. The rigor of my math lessons has gone down because I could never find the best way for me to teach a lesson. Kids stopped logging into programs like Zearn to help them. They are falling behind and were already behind. This situation is so bad because the academic achievement gap is now even wider and our kids of color are suffering.

For another educator, a combination of challenges in navigating technological platforms, connecting with students and families, and guidance from administrators all came together to contribute to feelings of stress and lowered teaching self-efficacy. This educator stated:

> For me, the greatest stressors were: my lack of technology knowledge and experience, not being able to reach families, families not being responsive to my communication or engaging in the lessons I provided despite constant effort on my part, and lack of support and communication from school administration.

Distance Teaching Provides a New Source of Teaching Self-Efficacy Although many educators reported lower feelings of self-efficacy in their teaching practice, some educators found that teaching online involved developing innovative practices and eventually led to new feelings of efficacy and joy in practice. One teacher stated:

> Adjusting to remote teaching was stressful in that at first, it felt like teaching without the joy, but as I became better at it, I learned a new way to view success with my students. For me, many of my class [student run] routines went out the window when we left school – so distance learning felt very top down. But as I became more used to it, I found ways to continue student routines and student-run routines – which I think has a lot to do with feeling satisfied with a learning experience. Was I stressed about students not learning, families not responding, planning all new assignments – of course, but you carry on. And as you carry on, you become less stressed.

Another educator found the transition to online teaching supportive for developing their practice, saying, "I have been able to learn much more technology, as well as having time to reflect on my teaching practices." Overcoming the initial stress of the transition to distance learning was a source of increase self-efficacy for an educator who reflected:

> Due to the urgency of managing online learning and having to manage a very steep digital learning curve, I now feel that I am able to learn in ways I never imagined. So while the prospect of continuing online learning with a group of students I don't know brings another level of stress, the initial stress of managing online teaching has decreased and been replaced by a feeling of empowerment.

School Connectedness Impacts Teacher Wellbeing and Self-Efficacy As our quantitative results suggested, feelings of school connectedness can greatly impact teachers' wellbeing, both through compassion fatigue and through teaching self-efficacy. Educators' reflections about feeling either connected or disconnected revealed that: (1) a lack of school connectedness negatively affects teachers' well-being, (2) school connectedness, or lack thereof, impacts distance teaching, and (3) a lack of trust in district leadership negatively impacts teachers' emotional wellbeing and teaching self-efficacy.

Lack of School Connectedness Negatively Affects Teachers' Wellbeing Social support appears to boost educators' wellbeing. Unfortunately, however, many educators felt very unsupported in the months following the transition to distance learning. Many teachers cited the isolation and loneliness that accompanied the stay-at-home order in the spring of 2020. One teacher reflected:

> I feel isolated and stressed all the time—sleepless nights, anxiety, doubts and fears pertaining to how to maintain connections with my students and families, despite a strong online presence. I am someone who thrives on interpersonal relationships, in real time and real space, and so I have felt disconnected, lonely, depressed and completely uncertain of the future. There has been no physical contact with anyone since March, and it has affected my social and emotional wellbeing.

Another teacher discussed the lack of community that affected both their emotional wellbeing and occupational efficacy:

> Being at home while being an educator felt isolating. I no longer had the community of other teachers and admin going through the same struggles, validating my own every day. Instead I felt like I was alone in this, attempting to do my best but not doing [anything] that I felt was productive or beneficial for my Kindergarten students and their family. Distance learning took so much away from everyone, and that was clear.

School Connectedness Impacts Distance Learning Some educators in our sample reflected on how feeling connected to other people helped them adapt to distance learning. One educator wrote, "Through the support of my administrator, colleagues, family, and my student's family, distance learning became easier as the days went by." Other teachers discussed how the lack of school connectedness during the pandemic made it extremely difficult to accomplish any tasks to the same degree as they could in person. One educator wrote:

> Online "learning" absolutely cannot replace the benefits of face to face instruction and face to face relationships. Furthermore, online meetings with colleagues feel distant and unproductive. I'm not sure what it is, but I feel a mental block with online meetings that I do not feel about in person meetings. These last few months have been the lowest that I have ever felt as an educator.

Feeling disconnected in the virtual platform clearly impacts educators' emotional wellbeing as well as their feelings of teaching self-efficacy.

In addition to having trouble communicating with colleagues, another educator wrote about challenges with communicating with students: "I need a better way to connect with my students. I tried remind, email, classroom, discord, and personal calls and texts. It was kind of like playing phone tag with 160 at once for 2 months."

Lack of Trust in District Leadership Impacts Wellbeing and Self-Efficacy An important element in developing and maintaining connection is a sense of trust. A common concern among the educators in our sample was the lack of trust in leadership from the district. Educators were largely disappointed and felt neglected by the district's apparent disregard for teachers' health in considering plans to reopen. One teacher wrote:

> Envisioning an elementary school setting operating with social distancing guidelines is like a nightmare. I know it isn't possible and anyone pushing for this prior to a vaccine is not a classroom teacher, does not have a close relative who teaches, and has little regard for the safety of school employees. The stress that I am currently experiencing is due to the unknown about school reopening in August. I'm certain [the district] does not care about my stress level and all decisions will be made through the lens of money, not teacher health and welfare. My life does not matter, neither does the 32 years of service I have provided to the children of [this city].

Another educator wrote about similar frustrations:

> The experience was frustrating beyond belief. First, we're essentially told to create 6 hours of work each day for two weeks. Terrible for both me and the kids. Then, I kept waiting for direction from the district over Spring Break, but I guess (the district) decided to take a week off. I kept waiting and waiting I didn't take the week off so why did the district? Global crises do not allow for holidays. Finally, the district provided help (long after other districts).

Teachers also cited a lack of guidance from the district leadership as a source of stress:

> Stress level has gone way up due to the lack of vision, direction, and communication from leadership. Teachers are expected to "provide support" without specifying what it means, how it's measured, and who is held accountable. It's like screaming at someone to do more and to do better, without providing any real specific or productive feedback.

The educators in our sample largely did not feel supported by the district as a whole, which caused greater stress, frustration, and anxiety.

Importantly, educators also expressed concern that the district was not appropriately supporting their colleagues of color. For example, one educator reported:

> My stress level has remained the same. [The district] continues not to provide needed assistance to veteran staff, students and parents of color, in particular African Americans. Staff and student[s] first, are empty words. Resulting in my continue[d] fight for ALL black and brown students and families, in [this district].

Another teacher noted the interpersonal discrimination within the staff in the district:

> [I have] greater stress due to bullying and both covert and overt racism towards Asian teachers and staff by white admin/instructional coaches. I can handle the technology and lessons just fine. I DO NOT need the racism by support staff who do not have students to teach and are not supportive nor considerate of the time I need to be on-line with my students.

Not only have educators across the district felt unsupported by their administrators and supervisors, but they have also reported that teachers and staff of color are disproportionately disadvantaged because of a lack of district support during distance learning.

Maintaining Wellbeing by Engaging in Self-Care In the midst of a global pandemic, uncertainty about the future, health risks, and changes in educators' living spaces have all contributed to an increased need for self-care in order to maintain emotional and physical wellbeing. Educators in this study touched on three broad themes related to maintaining wellbeing and engaging in self-care: (1) difficulties in enforcing boundaries between work and life outside of work, (2) the importance of having and utilizing strategies of self-care, and (3) the need to prioritize physical safety during the pandemic.

Blurred Boundaries Between Work and Life For many educators in the district, the move to online instruction resulted in significant challenges in setting boundaries between work and life. This blurring of boundaries has had a significant impact on teachers' abilities to maintain their wellbeing and engage in practices that reflect self-care. One educator shared, "My days were always long, but this felt like I was on 24/7. Whether providing feedback to students, troubleshooting the computer, talking to parents. The list goes on." Another teacher added:

> The transition to distance learning largely eliminated that work/life balance that is essential to effectively show up for our students. I found it more difficult to step away from my responsibilities as an educator and check in with my own mental well-being.

These hazy boundaries between work and life have resulted in changes in routines that are detrimental to self-care. As another educator shared:

> Working from home I find it very difficult to distinguish between the work day and the end of the work day (as well as when it starts). I work far later at home than I used to, and my morning routine does not include a "grace period" before I start work.

The increased job demands have had a significant impact on this educator's ability to engage in practices that promote wellbeing:

> My usual outlets for affirmation and joy are no longer available, and the many, daily demands of the job make me not able to manage time, energy, or emotions. I can tell I am reacting in ways that are not typical, but I have no way of really gaining perspective on those reactions. And the demands of the job mean that I don't feel like I have the luxury of slowing down or taking care of myself.

Another teacher reflected on the pressure to be available at all times for students. For this teacher, this pressure is due, at least in part, to the challenges of engaging students in distance learning:

> I feel like I should never turn off work. Because engagement is so low, I feel like I have to be on at all times to maintain the engagement that I do have. One student called me at 10:30pm asking for help and I felt like I had to answer, because she hadn't been engaging in distance learning for over a month and she was finally reaching out.

Although the pressure to support parents and students seemed to peak as the district transitioned to distance learning, for one educator the work demands have already reduced:

> During distance learning, I had parents calling me and texting me from 7am to 10pm, even on the weekends. I understood they had their questions and all but I did find this super stressful to constantly stop whatever I was doing and take care of that. Of course, no one was forcing me to respond right away but I felt it was important to be 100% reachable so families trusted that I was there to help. I suppose I just wasn't expecting that amount of communication and didn't think families would be contacting me so much outside of work hours. These calls and texts calmed down a lot after a few weeks and now my stress level has gone down so much, I feel great.

Making Time for Self-Care Although a common struggle educators expressed during this time of distance learning was in maintaining clear distinctions between work life and personal life, many educators also reflected on the need to prioritize and make time for self-care. Educators reflected on both the importance of carving out time and space in their day for intentional acts of self-care and strategies they find helpful in maintaining their wellbeing. One teacher shared, "I have had to make more of a conscious effort to take care of my social/emotional wellbeing. I have to engage in more self-care, and it is easier for me to get angry and sensitive." Another educator commented on the shift in their self-care practices sparked by the pandemic:

> I have worked to implement self-care and make it a priority in ways that I have not done since ever. The pandemic has made me realize how little I actually implement self-care practices and how rushed they used to be.

Another teacher has brought the focus of self-care both into their own practice but also into their teaching and work with students. This educator wrote:

> I have focused much more on wellness and my own self-care. This has helped me also work with students on wellness and self-care. I want to keep caring for myself and students better, emotionally when I get back to school.

In addition to reflecting on the need for prioritizing self-care activities, some teachers also shared specific practices that have been helpful during this time. One teacher wrote, "Being able to do 'yard duty' in my garden has been my main way of dealing with the huge amount of stress since March 13." For another teacher, the transition to distance learning has led to an increase in self-efficacy in teaching and this educator has been able to engage in intentional practices to promote their wellbeing. This educator shared that:

> I have been able to use tools that I had already developed in order to manage my stress: Al-Anon meetings, exercise, gardening. So I have been able to keep it together. I felt most productive and useful when I had tutoring calls with my students. I was able to work with my lowest students in one-on-one video calls a few times a week. I was so gratified that they advanced their reading more at home than they would have been able to at school.

Self-care practices appear to have a positive and bidirectional impact on teachers' emotional wellbeing and self-efficacy in practice. An outcome of this heightened period of stress seems to be an emphasis on the need to care for oneself and teach students to do the same.

Promoting Physical Safety is a Priority Many educators expressed fears and stress about their physical safety and the physical safety of their students. Because of the imminent risk to physical wellbeing that COVID-19 poses, many educators expressed concerns about the tension between maintaining physical safety and holding onto job security and a steady income stream. One educator expressed their fear of having to choose between work and safety:

> I live in an inter-generational household whose lives will be at high risk if I am told I have to go teach face to face in a classroom full of up to 30+ students. Before all this I made a commitment to stay at my school for 3 years. If I am forced to teach face to face before scientists develop a vaccine or the 2 years it has historically taken COVID viruses to "die" out then I will be forced to find another income stream. I am also concerned that our salaries will be cut WITHOUT the district [or] Dep. of Edu. advocating for rents, car payments, mortgages, etc., be cut by the same amount.

Another educator expressed a similar sentiment, emphasizing the need to protect student and teacher safety during this time:

> I'm worried the schools will open up and people will die. Is one year of education for children worth a student or a teacher LIFE? What's wrong with distance learning, even though younger students can't experience a large amount of growth, isn't accepting a GAP year more prudent than having educators or immune compromised students die?

Another teacher reflected on the need for the district to take adequate steps to ensure safety before reopening:

> I would be extremely stressed if I had to go back into the classrooms before there is an inoculation and useful treatment for COVID. With the risks of being a prep teacher, the concept of going into all the classrooms is simply unacceptable until those conditions have been met.

In educators' written responses on the survey, it is clear that the shift to distance learning was associated with heightened stress for many educators. Stress was correlated with increased demands and shifting expectations. Teachers' changing roles coupled with limited resources and more isolation left teachers feeling high levels of compassion fatigue. Educators have sought to prioritize self-care but struggled to find work life balance. The new roles teachers have taken on have also impacted teachers' self-efficacy in their work. Educators sought guidance from leadership in the district, but the uncertainty of the pandemic and the risks posed left many educators feeling anxious and unsupported. In the next section, we will suggest some evidence-based practices that can reduce compassion fatigue among educators.

Practical Recommendations

Based on the review of existing literature on educators' compassion fatigue and the empirical findings of the COVID-19 Educator Resiliency Project, we made some potential practical recommendations for preventing educators' compassion fatigue and promoting educators' wellbeing in following the sections.

Practical Recommendations for Preventing Compassion Fatigue Among Educators

To prevent or reduce educators' compassion fatigue, it is important to provide professional training and mentoring support to help educators recognize the signs of compassion fatigue and develop personalized self-care practices (Yang et al., 2021). It is also important to assess and monitor educators' top stressors, including their exposure to secondary trauma stress, and then provide needed resources and guidance to help them seek professional help to address these stressors (Yang et al., 2021). In addition to individual-based prevention and intervention, it is equally important for schools to develop initiatives and practices to promote collective compassion and address compassion fatigue as a group. This recommendation has been supported by previous research studies, in which shared social plight has been found to empower individuals to heal as a group and reduces the risks of maladjustment (Brendgen et al., 2013).

Practicing self-compassion has been shown to be related to a decline in occupational stress and symptoms of burnout in educators (Roeser et al., 2013). Research has shown that not only can self-compassion be taught, but that teaching self-compassion can also lead to an increase in wellbeing. These self-compassion techniques can also be long lasting, and how often they are practiced can predict how well they are learned (Neff & Germer, 2012). Following is a list of some self-compassion techniques (Neff & Germer, 2012; Germer & Neff, 2013):

- Practice self-kindness
- Understand that mistakes are a part of the common human experience rather than an oddity occurring in isolation
- Practice mindfulness
- Take time to slow down, study inner thoughts and emotions, and respond with self-compassion when necessary
- Identify core values that bring meaning to your life
- Identify emotions and where they express themselves in the body, and then learn to soothe the emotion with loving-kindness
- Intentionally savor good things in your life and positive qualities about yourself
- Practice formal meditation

Compassion is also something that can be developed collectively, which can be beneficial to a workplace organization. Some examples of collective compassion strategies that can reduce compassion fatigue are as follows (Lilius et al., 2011):

- Share awareness and understanding of a coworker's pain
- Demonstrate empathic concern and shared feelings
- Have a collective response (i.e., collecting donations, help with coworker's work)
- Regularly check up with each other's feelings
- Offer expressions of support
- Establish a buddy system when necessary depending on trauma and need
- Acknowledge each other's successes and celebrate important milestones
- Address problems directly and promptly
- Discuss decisions collectively
- Socialize newcomers

Taking time every day for self-care is also important for an educator's mental and physical health. In fact, practicing self-care strategies can predict vocational strain in educators, teacher quality of life, and compassion fatigue (Alkema et al., 2008; Yang et al., 2009; Yang et al., 2011). Educators must recognize the importance of self-care and make it a priority. As one educator noted, "The kids are only as good as you are. [...] If you are not 100% for them, they are not going to be 100% for you" (Castro et al., 2010). Some examples of individual self-care strategies that educators have found beneficial are listed as follows (Castro et al., 2010; Schussler et al., 2016; Garrick et al., 2017; Yang et al., 2011):

- Exercise regularly
- Get adequate levels of sleep
- Practice relaxation techniques
- Become aware of the process of holding onto stress and how to alleviate it
- Keep a daily log in order to carve out time for self-care
- Participate in fun activities outside of work
- Leave work at the workplace
- Set clear and defined breaks from school
- Invest in social relationships both inside and outside of work

Practical Recommendations for Improving Educators' SEL Competencies

Improving SEL competencies among educators has been found to have significant associations with decreased educator stress and increased job satisfaction (Collie et al., 2012). Findings from the Educator Resilience Project further demonstrated the important role of SEL competencies in the online teaching context and highlighted the importance of improving adult SEL practices and self-care strategies. Ample studies have supported the positive impacts of mindfulness and SEL programs on improving social-emotional skills and awareness, decreasing emotional reactivity, and encouraging self-care among participants (Adimando, 2017; Schussler et al., 2015; Schussler et al., 2019; Taylor et al., 2017). To improve educators' SEL competencies, the following strategies have been used in some of these school-based programs (Adimando, 2017; Schussler et al., 2015):

- Increased awareness of the causes, risk factors, and preventative strategies of compassion fatigue
- Taught participants self-care strategies
- Taught participants how to monitor their compassion fatigue symptoms (learned to administer and score the Professional Quality of Life Scale)
- Taught stress management techniques (i.e., meditation methods, breathing activities)
- Increased awareness of how participants were responding to and physically holding onto their feelings of stress
- Increased awareness of participants' emotions in order to avoid problematic responses
- Taught to take wait time after emotionally stimulating experiences in order to reassess the situation with a calm mind

Schools and districts should utilize strategies such as these in order to help build SEL competencies and awareness of compassion fatigue among educators.

Practical Recommendations for Improving Teaching Self-Efficacy

While teaching is often considered one of the most stressful professions, developing high levels of coping skills and self-efficacy have been shown to relate to decreased burnout in educators with a heightened level of work stress (Herman et al., 2017). During the COVID-19 pandemic, educators have to face an additional myriad of new stressors caused by the demands of navigating online teaching platforms and simultaneously adapting their curriculum to meet the highly rigorous K-12 standards. Consistently, educators in our study expressed decreased teaching self-efficacy as they transitioned to online learning. Thus, it is important to teach educators about how to build self-efficacy and coping skills to manage the increasing demands and stressors during online teaching.

To improve educators' online teaching self-efficacy, it is important to address their basic needs for performing online teaching effectively, especially their needs for technology support and safety. Moreover, it's important to provide professional development for educators to better understand students' learning motivation in the virtual environment. For example, research on the concept of flow in the E-learning environment suggests five key elements for promoting students' flow in the virtual learning environment, which include: (1) congruence between skills and challenges;

(2) both skills and challenges surpass a certain level; (3) sense of control in the virtual environment; (4) focused attention; and (5) feeling of presence. It is important to consider these factors to improve educators' sense of teaching efficacy (Rodríguez-Ardura & Meseguer-Artola, 2017). Some other ways to build teaching self-efficacy are listed as follows (Cardullo et al., 2021; Sehgal et al., 2017; Skaalvik & Skaalvik, 2010):

- Create a safe learning environment by adhering to CDC guidelines
- Provide professional development in online teaching and technology competencies
- Give educators time to explore the online learning platform and experience success prior to focusing on the high stakes of preparing students to meet grade level standards
- Build positive relationships with parents
- Increase feelings of supervisory support (feelings of being cognitively and emotionally supported by the administration) and trust
- Collaborate with other educators

Practical Recommendations for Promoting Healthy School Connectedness

Research has demonstrated that social relationships built with students, coworkers, and administrators are beneficial to teacher by increasing their wellbeing and decreasing compassion fatigue (Aldrup et al., 2018; Greenglass et al., 1996; Hasselquist et al., 2017). Therefore, it is important to promote the development and nourishment of these relationships by positive school climates. However, online teaching was often described as "isolating" (Haber & Mills, 2008; Hawkins et al., 2012) even prior to the global COVID-19 pandemic. Online teaching is also often described as both more stressful and requiring a greater workload than in-person learning (Bolliger & Wasilik, 2009; Haber & Mills, 2008; Lewis & Abdul-Hamid, 2006). Prior to the COVID-19 pandemic, the workload has already been identified as one of the most significant reasons teachers leave the profession (Buchanan, 2010; Smithers & Robinson, 2003). Thus, it is critical to ensure that educators are able to rely on social relationships in order to cope with the increased workload during distance learning, and developing a sense of school connectedness among the school staff is all the more important.

Supporting healthy boundaries and interactions among educators and students is critical for promoting the sense of connectedness among educators and students in schools while minimizing the risk of over-burdening educators, particularly in the social distancing and distance learning context (Institute of Educational Sciences, Pate & Case, 2020; Yang et al., 2021). Some helpful practical recommendations have been provided by researchers (Institute of Educational Sciences, Pate & Case, 2020). For example, "schools could: (1) provide various connection channels to meet the varying needs of different school members; (2) share communication norms for online meetings and interactions; (3) revise and/or create policies and procedures as needed; (4) provide two-way communication opportunities; (5) encourage the use of set working hours and scheduled breaks; and (6) use district and school media channels to share positive stories about the community" (Yang et al., 2021, p. 514). It is also important that administrators (Aldridge & Fraser, 2015; Borup & Stevens, 2016; Hasselquist et al., 2017; Leung & Lee, 2006; Stone & Springer, 2019):

- Develop competent and supportive school leadership
- Create a positive school environment
- Promote a collaborative environment
- Incorporate positive relationship building techniques into professional development
- Provide opportunities for school staff to collaborate and build relationships with each other
- Provide educators and collaboration teams with sufficient time, resources, and training in order to effectively create and modify engaging curriculum to meet distance learning needs

Meanwhile, educators must work to develop relationships with both their colleagues and students. Building positive work relationships with coworkers can allow for educators to (Greenglass et al., 1996):

- Turn to each other during times of high stress at work to boost morale
- Act as a confidante and listen to each other's work-related problems
- Provide practical support (such as help to complete a task) for one another
- Share and discuss best teaching practices

Building positive relationships with students has also been shown to increase teacher wellbeing (Aldrup et al., 2018), and creating a greater teacher presence online has been shown to help alleviate some of the pressures of online teaching (Lewis & Abdul-Hamid, 2006). In fact, online teachers have commonly acknowledged that having more time to spend with students one-on-one was one of their favorite parts of online teaching (Borup & Stevens, 2016). Some strategies that can be used to build positive relationships and create a greater teacher presence are listed here (Rehn et al., 2016; Stone & Springer, 2019):

- Maintain regular and prompt communication with students
- Focus on making lessons interactive and engaging
- Make an effort to use students' names in order to acknowledge all students during each lesson
- Utilize teacher self-disclosure with students in order to get to know students
- Check students regularly for understanding and provide them with informal feedback

Practical Recommendations for Reducing Racial Trauma Among Educators

School connectedness can also play a role in helping bridge the teacher-student racial divide. The race of the teaching population does not often accurately reflect the student population of the school, especially when it comes to teaching students of color. Whereas about half of the student population in the United States are students of color, educators of color only represent about 17% of the teaching workforce (Ingersoll & Merrill, 2017). Meanwhile, racial congruence has been found to be related to teacher job satisfaction. When an educator shares the same race as the majority of the students, and racial composition of the students is at or exceeds 70%, teacher job satisfaction is positively affected (Fairchild et al., 2011). In fact, one study conducted in 2014 by Stearns et al. (2014) and colleagues reported that White educators teaching in a predominately Black classroom were significantly less satisfied with their jobs than White educators teaching in predominantly White classrooms. Interestingly enough, this discrepancy in job satisfaction decreased depending upon the professional community at the school. In schools where educators felt that they were accepted, that administrators effectively communicated with the staff, that the staff had school spirit and a common school mission, and where there was an active teaching-learning community, these relationships among the staff were found to moderate the impact of the teacher-student racial divide (Stearns et al., 2014).

At this time, with the emergence of the COVID-19 pandemic, it is possible that educators are experiencing even more racial distress as they are forced to interact more closely with diverse families due to distance learning. Furthermore, with the emergence of the Black Lives Matter protests and the discrimination and violence experienced by both Asian American and Hispanic students at this time (Ruiz et al., 2020; Tessler et al., 2020), it is very possible that the largely White teaching workforce is being exposed to the racial distress their students and their students' families are experiencing to a greater degree than normal. However, there is little research right now on how that racial discord will or has affected educators. Due to this, it is even more important that teachers rely on their school community in order to address any racial distress they might be exposed to due to distance learning. Some other strategies that might be beneficial for coping with racial trauma are as follows (Truong & Museus, 2012):

- Seek social support from others
- Advocate for peers of color
- Reach out to struggling peers or students to provide them with support
- Partake in activities to provide relief from racism-related stress (i.e., take up a hobby, meditate)
- Reflect on racism and racist encounters
- Speak up when confronted with racism
- Seek out counseling and psychological services

Conclusion

Turnover among educators is remarkably high, with close to 50% of the teaching population leaving the profession within the first 5 years (Ingersoll, 2003). Meanwhile, high levels of burnout have been shown to be related to compassion fatigue, and lower rates of compassion satisfaction have been shown to act as predictors for this turnover in the teaching workforce (Christian-Brandt et al., 2020; Skaalvik & Skaalvik, 2011). Generally, when educators are less weighed down by compassion fatigue, they are better able to provide quality support and education for their students. With the added stressors and traumatic experiences induced by the COVID-19 pandemic, it has become even more necessary to identify and implement strategies to decrease compassion fatigue and stress, and increase wellbeing among educators. In this chapter, based on the findings from the COVID-19 Educator Resiliency Project, we presented quantitative findings about how educator perceived online teaching self-efficacy, educators' social and emotional learning (SEL) competencies, and school connectedness factors concurrently and interactively influence educators' compassion fatigue during the COVID-19 pandemic and distance learning. We also provided qualitative insight on educators' experience with compassion fatigue during distance learning and their individual struggles during distance learning. In addition, we shared practical implications and suggestions for how to reduce compassion fatigue among educators. It is clear that schools must learn from educators' experiences and needs in order to understand how to better support them during difficult times such as this pandemic. Findings from quantitative and qualitative data in this study draw attention to the need for prioritizing educator wellbeing, and offer avenues for future research and policy shifts that prioritize educator wellbeing even in post-pandemic life.

References

Abraham-Cook, S. (2012). *The prevalence and correlates of compassion fatigue, compassion satisfaction, and burnout among teachers working in high-poverty urban public schools.*

Adams, R. E., Boscarino, J. A., & Figley, C. R. (2006). Compassion fatigue and psychological distress among social workers: A validation study. *American Journal of Orthopsychiatry, 76*, 103–108. https://doi.org/10.1037/0002-9432.76.1.103

Adimando, A. (2017). Preventing and alleviating compassion fatigue through self-care: An educational workshop for nurses. *Journal of Holistic Nursing, 36*(4), 304–317. https://doi.org/10.1177/0898010117721581

Aldridge, J. M., & Fraser, B. J. (2015). Teachers' views of their school climate and its relationship with teacher self-efficacy and job satisfaction. *Learning Environments Research, 19*(2), 291–307. https://doi.org/10.1007/s10984-015-9198-x

Aldrup, K., Klusmann, U., Lüdtke, O., Göllner, R., & Trautwein, U. (2018). Student misbehavior and teacher well-being: Testing the mediating role of the teacher-student relationship. *Learning and Instruction, 58*, 126–136. https://doi.org/10.1016/j.learninstruc.2018.05.006

Alkema, K., Linton, J. M., & Davies, R. (2008). A study of the relationship between self-care, compassion satisfaction, compassion fatigue, and burnout among hospice professionals.

Journal of Social Work in End-of-Life & Palliative Care, 4(2), 101–119. https://doi.org/10.1080/15524250802353934

Arens, A. K., & Morin, A. J. (2016). Relations between teachers' emotional exhaustion and students' educational outcomes. *Journal of Educational Psychology, 108*(6), 800. https://doi.org/10.1037/edu0000105

Bakker, A. B., & Demerouti, E. (2017). Job demands–resources theory: Taking stock and looking forward. *Journal of Occupational Health Psychology, 22*(3), 273–285. https://doi.org/10.1037/ocp0000056

Bandura, A. (1986). *Social foundations of thought and action: A social cognitive theory.* Prentice Hall.

Bandura, A. (1997). *Self-efficacy: The exercise of control.* Freeman.

Beaton, R. D., & Murphy, S. A. (1995). Working with people in crisis: Research implications. In C. R. Figley (Ed.), *Compassion fatigue: Coping with secondary stress disorder in those who treat the traumatized* (Vol. 1, pp. 51–81).

Blecharz, J., Luszczynska, A., Scholz, U., Schwarzer, R., Siekanska, M., & Cieslak, R. (2014). Predicting performance and performance satisfaction: The role of mindfulness and beliefs about the ability to deal with social barriers in sport. *Anxiety, Stress, & Coping, 27*, 270–287. https://doi.org/10.1080/10615806.2013.839989

Bolliger, D. U., & Wasilik, O. (2009). Factors influencing faculty satisfaction with online teaching and learning in higher education. *Distance Education, 30*(1), 103–116. https://doi.org/10.1080/01587910902845949

Borntrager, C., Caringi, J. C., van den Pol, R., Crosby, L., O'Connell, K., Trautman, A., & McDonald, M. (2012). Secondary traumatic stress in school personnel. *Advances in School Mental Health Promotion, 5*(1), 38–50. https://doi.org/10.1080/1754730x.2012.664862

Borup, J., & Stevens, M. A. (2016). Factors influencing teacher satisfaction at an online charter school. *Journal of Online Learning Research, 2*(1), 3–22.

Boscarino, J. A., Figley, C. R., & Adams, R. E. (2004). Compassion fatigue following the September 11 terrorist attacks: A study of secondary trauma among New York City social workers. *International Journal of Emergency Mental Health, 6*(2), 57. Retrieved from https://www.ncbi.nlm.nih.gov/pmc/articles/PMC2713725/

Brendgen, M., Vitaro, F., Bukowski, W. M., Dionne, G., Tremblay, R. E., & Boivin, M. (2013). Can friends protect genetically vulnerable children from depression? *Development and Psychopathology, 25*(2), 277–289. https://doi.org/10.1017/S0954579412001058

Brewer, E. W., & Shapard, L. (2004). Employee burnout: A meta-analysis of the relationships between age or years of experience. *Human Resource Development Review, 3*, 102–123. https://doi.org/10.1177/1534484304263335

Brunsting, N. C., Sreckovic, M. A., & Lane, K. L. (2014). Special education teacher burnout: A synthesis of research from 1979 to 2013. *Education and Treatment of Children, 681-711.* https://doi.org/10.1353/etc.2014.0032

Buchanan, J. (2010). May I be excused? Why teachers leave the profession. *Asia Pacific Journal of Education, 30*(2), 199–211. https://doi.org/10.1080/02188791003721952

Cardullo, V., Wang, C.-H., Burton, M., & Dong, J. (2021). K-12 teachers' remote teaching self-efficacy during the pandemic. *Journal of Research in Innovative Teaching & Learning, 4*(1), 32–45. https://doi.org/10.1108/jrit-10-2020-0055

Caringi, J. C., Stanick, C., Trautman, A., Crosby, L., Devlin, M., & Adams, S. (2015). Secondary traumatic stress in public school teachers: Contributing and mitigating factors. *Advances in School Mental Health Promotion, 8*(4), 244–256. https://doi.org/10.1080/1754730X.2015.1080123

Carver-Thomas, D., & Darling-Hammond, L. (2017). *Teacher turnover: Why it matters and what we can do about it.* Learning Policy Institute.

Castro, A. J., Kelly, J., & Shih, M. (2010). Resilience strategies for new teachers in high-needs areas. *Teaching and Teacher Education, 26*(3), 622–629. https://doi.org/10.1016/j.tate.2009.09.010

Chang, M., & Davis, H. A. (2009). Understanding the role of teacher appraisals in shaping the dynamics of their relationships with students: Deconstructing teachers' judgments of disruptive behavior/students. In P. A. Schutz & M. Zemblyas (Eds.), *Advances in teacher emotion research: The impact on teachers' lives.* Springer-Verlag.

Christian-Brandt, A. S., Santacrose, D. E., & Barnett, M. L. (2020). In the trauma-informed care trenches: Teacher compassion satisfaction, secondary traumatic stress, burnout, and intent to leave education within underserved elementary schools. *Child Abuse & Neglect: Part, 3*, 110. https://doi.org/10.1016/j.chiabu.2020.104437

Collie, R. J., Shapka, J. D., & Perry, N. E. (2012). School climate and social-emotional learning: Predicting teacher stress, job satisfaction, and teaching efficacy. *Journal of Educational Psychology, 104*(4), 1189–1204. https://doi.org/10.1037/a0029356

Craig, C. D., & Sprang, G. (2010). Compassion satisfaction, compassion fatigue, and burnout in a national sample of trauma treatment therapists. *Anxiety, Stress, & Coping, 23*(3), 319–339. https://doi.org/10.1080/10615800903085818

Creamer, T. L., & Liddle, B. (2005). Secondary traumatic stress among disaster mental health workers responding to the September 11 attacks. *Journal of Traumatic Stress, 18*(1), 89–96. https://doi.org/10.1002/jts.20008

Deci, E. L., & Ryan, R. M. (2000). The "what" and "why" of goal pursuits: Human needs and the self-determination of behavior. *Psychological Inquiry, 11*, 227–268. https://doi.org/10.1207/s15327965pli1104_01

Deighton, R. M., Gurris, N., & Traue, H. (2007). Factors affecting burnout and compassion fatigue in psychotherapists treating torture survivors: Is the therapist's attitude to working through trauma relevant? *Journal of Traumatic Stress, 20*, 63–75. https://doi.org/10.1002/jts.20180

Donahoo, L. M. S., Siegrist, B., & Garrett-Wright, D. (2017). Addressing compassion fatigue and stress of special education teachers and professional staff using mindfulness and prayer. *The Journal of School Nursing, 34*(6), 442–448. https://doi.org/10.1177/2F1059840517725789

Fairchild, S., Tobias, R., Corcoran, S., Djukic, M., Kovner, C., & Noguera, P. (2011). White and black teachers' job satisfaction. *Urban Education, 47*(1), 170–197. https://doi.org/10.1177/0042085911429582

Fereday, J., & Muir-Cochrane, E. (2006). Demonstrating rigor using thematic analysis: A hybrid approach of inductive and deductive coding and theme development. *International Journal of Qualitative Methods, 5*(1), 80–92. https://doi.org/10.1177/160940690600500107

Figley, C. R. (Ed.). (1995). *Compassion fatigue: Coping with secondary stress disorder in those who treat the traumatized.* Brunner/Mazel.

Fimian, M. J. (1987). The alternate-forms and alpha reliability of the Teacher Stress Inventory. *Psychology in the Schools, 24*, 234–223. https://doi.org/10.1002/1520-6807(198707)24:3%3C234::aid-pits2310240307%3E3.0.co;2-p

Garrick, A., Mak, A. S., Cathcart, S., Winwood, P. C., Bakker, A. B., & Lushington, K. (2017). Non-work time activities predicting teachers' work-related fatigue and engagement: An effort-recovery approach. *Australian Psychologist, 53*(3), 243–252. https://doi.org/10.1111/ap.12290

Germer, C. K., & Neff, K. D. (2013). Self-compassion in clinical practice. *Journal of Clinical Psychology, 69*(8), 856–867. https://doi.org/10.1002/jclp.22021

Greenglass, E., Fiksenbaum, L., & Burke, R. J. (1996). Components of social support, buffering effects and burnout: Implications for psychological functioning. *Anxiety, Stress, and Coping, 9*(3), 185–197. https://doi.org/10.1080/10615809608249401

Gu, Q., & Day, C. (2007). Teachers resilience: A necessary condition for effectiveness. *Teaching and Teacher Education, 23*(8), 1302–1316. https://doi.org/10.1016/j.tate.2006.06.006

Haber, J., & Mills, M. (2008). Perceptions of barriers concerning effective online teaching and policies: Florida community college faculty. *Community College Journal of Research and Practice, 32*(4–6), 266–283. https://doi.org/10.1080/10668920701884505

Hasselquist, L., Herndon, K., & Kitchel, T. (2017). School Culture's influence on beginning agriculture teachers' job satisfaction and teacher self-efficacy. *Journal of Agricultural Education, 58*(1), 267–279. https://doi.org/10.5032/jae.2017.01267

Hastings, R. P., & Brown, T. (2002). Coping strategies and the impact of challenging behaviors on special educators' burnout. *Mental Retardation, 40*(2), 148–156. https://doi.org/10.1352/0047-6765(2002)040<0148:csatio>2.0.co;2

Hawkins, A., Barbour, M. K., & Graham, C. R. (2012). "Everybody is their own island": Teacher disconnection in a virtual school. *The International Review of Research in Open and Distributed Learning, 13*(2), 124. https://doi.org/10.19173/irrodl.v13i2.967

Herman, K. C., Hickmon-Rosa, J., & Reinke, W. M. (2017). Empirically derived profiles of teacher stress, burnout, self-efficacy, and coping and associated student outcomes. *Journal of Positive Behavior Interventions, 20*(2), 90–100. https://doi.org/10.1177/1098300717732066

Hill, H. C., Kapitula, L., & Umland, K. (2011). A validity argument approach to evaluating teacher value-added scores. *American Educational Research Journal, 48*(3), 794–831. https://doi.org/10.3102/0002831210387916

Hoffman, S., Palladino, J. M., & Barnett, J. (2007). Compassion fatigue as a theoretical framework to help understand burnout among special education teachers. *Journal of Ethnographic & Qualitative Research, 2*, 15–22. https://eric.ed.gov/?id=ED558015

Ingersoll, R. (2003). *Is there really a teacher shortage?* Retrieved from https://repository.upenn.edu/gse_pubs/133/

Ingersoll, R., & Merrill, L. (2017). *A quarter century of changes in the elementary and secondary teaching force: From 1987 to 2012.* (Statistical Analysis Report, NCES 2017–092). Washington, DC: U.S. Department of Education, Institute of Educations Sciences, National Center for Education Statistics. Retrieved from https://files.eric.ed.gov/fulltext/ED573526.pdf

Jordan, J. V. (2003). Relational-cultural therapy. In *Handbook of Counseling Women.* Sage.

Kelly, A. M., Gningue, S. M., & Qian, G. (2015). First-year urban mathematics and science middle school teachers: Classroom challenges and reflective solutions. *Education and Urban Society, 47*(2), 132–159. https://doi.org/10.1177/001312451348914

Killian, K. D. (2008). Helping till it hurts? A multimethod study of compassion fatigue, burnout, and self-care in clinicians working with trauma survivors. *Traumatology, 14*, 32–44. https://doi.org/10.1177/1534765608319083

Klusmann, U., Richter, D., & Lüdtke, O. (2016). Teachers' emotional exhaustion is negatively related to students' achievement: Evidence from a large-scale assessment study. *Journal of Educational Psychology, 108*(8), 1193. https://doi.org/10.1037/edu0000125

Koenig, A., Rodger, S., & Specht, J. (2018). Educator burnout and compassion fatigue: A pilot study. *Canadian Journal of School Psychology, 33*(4), 259–278. https://doi.org/10.1177/0829573516685017

Kokkinos, C. M. (2007). Job stressors, personality and burnout in primary school teachers. *British Journal of Educational Psychology, 77*(1), 229–243. https://doi.org/10.1348/000709905X90344

Kyriacou, C. (1987). Teacher stress and burnout: An international review. *Educational Research, 29*(2), 146–152. https://doi.org/10.1080/0013188870290207

Le Cornu, R. (2013). Building early career teacher resilience: The role of relationships. *Australian Journal of Teacher Education, 38*(4), 1. https://doi.org/10.14221/ajte.2013v38n4.4

Leung, D. Y., & Lee, W. W. (2006). Predicting intention to quit among Chinese teachers: Differential predictability of the components of burnout. *Anxiety, Stress & Coping, 19*(2), 129–141. https://doi.org/10.1080/10615800600565476

Lewis, C. C., & Abdul-Hamid, H. (2006). Implementing effective online teaching practices: Voices of exemplary faculty. *Innovative Higher Education, 31*(2), 83–98. https://doi.org/10.1007/s10755-006-9010-z

Lilius, J. M., Worline, M. C., Dutton, J. E., Kanov, J. M., & Maitlis, S. (2011). Understanding compassion capability. *Human Relations, 64*(7), 873–899. https://doi.org/10.1177/0018726710396250

MacIntyre, P. D., Gregersen, T., & Mercer, S. (2020). Language teachers' coping strategies during the Covid-19 conversion to online teaching: Correlations with stress, wellbeing, and negative emotions. *System, 94.* https://doi.org/10.1016/j.system.2020.102352

Maslach, C., & Schaufeli, W. B. (1993). Historical and conceptual development of burnout. In W. B. Schaufeli, C. Maslach, & T. Marek (Eds.), *Professional burnout* (pp. 1–16). Taylor & Francis.

Meadors, P., Lamson, A., Swanso, M., White, M., & Sira, N. (2009). Secondary traumatization in pediatric healthcare providers: Compassion fatigue, burnout, and secondary traumatic stress. *Omega: Journal of Death & Dying, 60*(2), 103–128. https://doi.org/10.2190/om.60.2.a

Neff, K. D., & Germer, C. K. (2012). A pilot study and randomized controlled trial of the mindful self-compassion program. *Journal of Clinical Psychology, 69*(1), 28–44. https://doi.org/10.1002/jclp.21923

O'Brennan, L., Pas, E., & Bradshaw, C. (2017). Multilevel examination of burnout among high school staff: Importance of staff and school factors. *School Psychology Review, 46*(2), 165–176. https://doi.org/10.17105/spr-2015-0019.v46-2

Pate, C. & Case, K. (2020, April 29). *Strategies for districts to support self-care for educators during the COVID-19 pandemic*. [PowerPoint slides]. Institute of Education Sciences. https://mcusercontent.com/a9bab6ebb1d1e641170c090cf/files/67cb8d2c-8ed2-45ba-a9e0-2258e2405db7/Self_Care_for_Educators_Slides_4.29.2020.pdf

Potter, P. (2010). Compassion fatigue and burnout: prevalence among oncology nurses. *Clinical Journal of Oncology Nursing, 14*(5), E56–E62. https://doi.org/10.1188/10.CJON.E56-E62

Ramberg, J., Brolin Låftman, S., Åkerstedt, T., & Modin, B. (2020). Teacher stress and students' school well-being: The case of upper secondary schools in Stockholm. *Scandinavian Journal of Educational Research, 64*(6), 816–830. https://doi.org/10.1080/00313831.2019.1623308

Rehn, N., Maor, D., & McConney, A. (2016). Investigating teacher presence in courses using synchronous videoconferencing. *Distance Education, 37*(3), 302–316. https://doi.org/10.1080/01587919.2016.1232157

Rodríguez-Ardura, I., & Meseguer-Artola, A. (2017). Flow in e-learning: What drives it and why it matters. *British Journal of Educational Technology, 48*(4), 899–915. https://doi.org/10.1111/bjet.12480

Roeser, R. W., Schonert-Reichl, K. A., Jha, A., Cullen, M., Wallace, L., Wilensky, R., et al. (2013). Mindfulness training and reductions in teacher stress and burnout: Results from two randomized, waitlist-control field trials. *Journal of Educational Psychology, 105*(3), 787–804. https://doi.org/10.1037/a0032093

Ruiz, N. G., Horowitz, J. M., & Tamir, C. (2020). *Many black and Asian Americans say they have experienced discrimination amid the COVID-19 outbreak*. Pew Research Center.

Schussler, D. L., Jennings, P. A., Sharp, J. E., & Frank, J. L. (2015). Improving teacher awareness and Well-being through CARE: A qualitative analysis of the underlying mechanisms. *Mindfulness, 7*(1), 130–142. https://doi.org/10.1007/s12671-015-0422-7

Schussler, D. L., Jennings, P. A., Sharp, J. E., & Frank, J. L. (2016). Improving teacher awareness and well-being through CARE: A qualitative analysis of the underlying mechanisms. *Mindfulness, 7*(1), 130–142. https://www.ons.org/cjon/14/5/compassion-fatigue-and-burnout

Schussler, D. L., DeWeese, A., Rasheed, D., DeMauro, A. A., Doyle, S. L., Brown, J. L., et al. (2019). The relationship between adopting mindfulness practice and reperceiving: A qualitative investigation of CARE for teachers. *Mindfulness, 10*(12), 2567–2582. https://doi.org/10.1007/s12671-019-01228-1

Sehgal, P., Nambudiri, R., & Mishra, S. K. (2017). Teacher effectiveness through self-efficacy, collaboration and principal leadership. *International Journal of Educational Management, 31*(4), 505–517. https://doi.org/10.1108/ijem-05-2016-0090

Shen, B., McCaughtry, N., Martin, J., Garn, A., Kulik, N., & Fahlman, M. (2015). The relationship between teacher burnout and student motivation. *British Journal of Educational Psychology, 85*(4), 519–532. https://doi.org/10.1111/bjep.12089

Shoji, K., Cieslak, R., Smoktunowicz, E., Rogala, A., Benight, C. C., & Luszczynska, A. (2016). Associations between job burnout and self-efficacy: A meta-analysis. *Anxiety, Stress, & Coping, 29*(4), 367–386. https://doi.org/10.1080/10615806.2015.1058369

Skaalvik, E. M., & Skaalvik, S. (2007). Dimensions of teacher self-efficacy and relations with strain factors, perceived collective teacher efficacy, and teacher burnout. *Journal of Educational Psychology, 99*, 611–625. https://doi.org/10.1037/0022-0663.99.3.611

Skaalvik, E. M., & Skaalvik, S. (2009). Does school context matter? Relations with teacher burnout and job satisfaction. *Teaching and Teacher Education, 25*(3), 518–524. https://doi.org/10.1016/j.tate.2008.12.006

Skaalvik, E. M., & Skaalvik, S. (2010). Teacher self-efficacy and teacher burnout: A study of relations. *Teaching and Teacher Education, 26*(4), 1059–1069. https://doi.org/10.1016/j.tate.2009.11.001

Skaalvik, E. M., & Skaalvik, S. (2011). Teacher job satisfaction and motivation to leave the teaching profession: Relations with school context, feeling of belonging, and emotional exhaustion. *Teaching and Teacher Education, 27*(6), 1029–1038. https://doi.org/10.1016/j.tate.2011.04.001

Skaalvik, E. M., & Skaalvik, S. (2014). Teacher self-efficacy and perceived autonomy: Relations with teacher engagement, job satisfaction, and emotional exhaustion. *Psychological Reports, 114*(1), 68–77. https://doi.org/10.2466/14.02.pr0.114k14w0

Skaalvik, E. M., & Skaalvik, S. (2015). Job Satisfaction, Stress and Coping Strategies in the Teaching Profession-What Do Teachers Say? *International Education Studies, 8*(3), 181–192. https://dx.doi.org/10.5539/ies.v8n3p181

Skaalvik, E. M., & Skaalvik, S. (2017). Motivated for teaching? Associations with school goal structure, teacher self-efficacy, job satisfaction and emotional exhaustion. *Teaching and Teacher Education, 67*, 152–160. https://doi.org/10.1016/j.tate.2017.06.006

Smithers, A., & Robinson, P. (2003). *Factors affecting teachers' decisions to leave the profession.* Department for Education and Skills.

Sokal, L., Trudel, L. E., & Babb, J. (2020). Canadian teachers' attitudes toward change, efficacy, and burnout during the COVID-19 pandemic. *International Journal of Educational Research Open, 1*. https://doi.org/10.1016/j.ijedro.2020.100016

Sprang, G., Clark, J. J., & Whitt-Woosely, A. (2007). Compassion fatigue, compassion satisfaction, and burnout: Factors impacting a professional's quality of life. *Journal of Loss and Trauma: International Perspectives on Stress & Coping, 12*(3), 259–280. https://doi.org/10.1080/15325020701238093

Stamm, B. H. (2010). *The concise ProQOL manual.* ProQOL.org

Stearns, E., Banerjee, N., Mickelson, R., & Moller, S. (2014). Collective pedagogical teacher culture, teacher–student ethno-racial mismatch, and teacher job satisfaction. *Social Science Research, 45*, 56–72. https://doi.org/10.1016/j.ssresearch.2013.12.011

Stone, C., & Springer, M. (2019). Interactivity, connectedness and 'teacher-presence': Engaging and retaining students online. *Australian Journal of Adult Learning, 59*(2), 146–169.

Sutcher, L., Darling-Hammond, L., & Carver-Thomas, D. (2019). Understanding teacher shortages: An analysis of teacher supply and demand in the United States. *Education Policy Analysis Archives, 27*(35), 1–40. https://doi.org/10.14507/epaa.27.3696

Taylor, R. D., Oberle, E., Durlak, J. A., & Weissberg, R. P. (2017). Promoting positive youth development through school-based social and emotional learning interventions: A meta-analysis of follow-up effects. *Child Development, 88*(4), 1156–1171. https://doi.org/10.1111/cdev.12864

Teach for America. (2020, October 20). *Tackling COVID-19 fatigue as a teacher: How educators can build resilience amid the pandemic.* https://www.teachforamerica.org/stories/tackling-covid-19-fatigue-as-a-teacher

Tessler, H., Choi, M., & Kao, G. (2020). The anxiety of being Asian American: Hate crimes and negative biases during the COVID-19 pandemic. *American Journal of Criminal Justice, 45*, 636–646. https://doi.org/10.1007/s12103-020-09541-5

Truong, K., & Museus, S. (2012). Responding to racism and racial trauma in doctoral study: An inventory for coping and mediating relationships. *Harvard Educational Review, 82*(2), 226–254. https://doi.org/10.17763/haer.82.2.u54154j787323302

VanBergeijk, E., & Sarmiento, T. (2006). The consequences of reporting child maltreatment: Are school personnel at risk for secondary traumatic stress? *Brief Treatment and Crisis Intervention, 6*(1), 79–98. https://doi.org/10.1093/brief-treatment/mhj003

Vannest, K. J., & Hagan-Burke, S. (2010). Teacher time use in special education. *Remedial and Special Education, 31*(2), 126–142. https://doi.org/10.1177/0741932508327459

World Health Organization. (2021). *Timeline: WHO's COVID-19 response.* https://www.who.int/emergencies/diseases/novel-coronavirus-2019/interactive-timeline

Yang, C. (2021). Online teaching self-efficacy, social-emotional learning (SEL) competencies, and compassion fatigue among educators during the COVID-19 pandemic. *School Psychology Review, 50,* 505–518. https://doi.org/10.1080/2372966X.2021.1903815

Yang, C., Manchanda, S., & Greenstein, J. (2021). Educators' online teaching self-efficacy and compassion fatigue during the COVID-19 pandemic: The dual roles of "connect". *School Psychology, 36*(6), 504–515. https://doi.org/10.1037/spq0000475

Yang, X., Ge, C., Hu, B., Chi, T., & Wang, L. (2009). Relationship between quality of life and occupational stress among teachers. *Public Health, 123*(11), 750–755. https://doi.org/10.1016/j.puhe.2009.09.018

Yang, X., Wang, L., Ge, C., Hu, B., & Chi, T. (2011). Factors associated with occupational strain among Chinese teachers: A cross-sectional study. *Public Health, 125*(2), 106–113. https://doi.org/10.1016/j.puhe.2010.10.012

Zhang, Q., & Sapp, D. A. (2008). A burning issue in teaching: The impact of perceived teacher burnout and nonverbal immediacy on student motivation and affective learning. *Journal of Communication Studies, 1*(2) https://digitalcommons.fairfield.edu/english-facultypubs/25/

Chapter 27
Utilizing Effective Bullying Prevention Programs

Allan Beane and Thomas W. Miller

Since a wealth of information regarding the definition and nature of bullying is readily available on the internet, this chapter only briefly reviews the definition and epidemiology of bullying in schools. This is not to minimize the importance of all personnel, students, and parents understanding the nature and destructiveness of bullying and how it is putting students and schools at risk of harm/danger.

Since many schools have failed to adopt systematic and comprehensive school-wide bullying prevention programs (Beane, 2016), the main purpose of this chapter is to review the philosophy, targets, structure, and effective elements and components that should be present in any bullying prevention program adopted by the schools/districts. To provide a framework for discussion, the authors examine The Allan L. Beane Bullying Prevention Program (formerly the Bully Free Program – www.bullyfree.com), developed by Dr. Allan Beane and Linda Beane after the death of their son, who was bullied in middle school and high school. In this chapter, it will be referred to as the BullyingPrevention Program. They have over 20 years of experience helping schools and other agencies prevent and stop bullying. Since the entire program is now available in the form of eBooks and files that can be printed and/or placed on computers, iPads, and other technology in secure locations, it is the most cost-effective and comprehensive bullying prevention program. It includes administrative and classroom-based prevention and intervention strategies. It also includes all of the elements and components that the researcher has

A. Beane
Bully Free Systems, Denton, TX, USA

T. W. Miller (✉)
Department of Psychiatry, College of Medicine, Department of Gerontology, College of Public Health, University of Kentucky, Lexington, KY, USA

Institute for Collaboration on Health, Intervention, and Policy, University of Connecticut, Storrs, CT, USA
e-mail: tom.miller@uconn.edu

© The Author(s), under exclusive license to Springer Nature   687
Switzerland AG 2023
T. W. Miller (ed.), *School Violence and Primary Prevention*,
https://doi.org/10.1007/978-3-031-13134-9_27

recommended for inclusion in an effective bullying prevention program. The program also includes eBooks and files for every student, parent, and all school personnel, including secretaries, maintenance personnel, and cafeteria workers. Some of the program's materials are available in other languages and are being used internationally.

The program even includes a comprehensive training and presentation kit. The kit includes DVDs and/or online for training/educating all school personnel (professional and support), parents, students, bus drivers, school board members, and representatives of the community. The training videos for bus drivers and the manual are available in both English and Spanish.

What Is Bullying?

To establish an effective bullying prevention program, the district/schools must have a clear and complete definition of bullying. Therefore, in 2014, the Centers for Disease Control and Prevention (CDC) and the Department of Education released the first federal uniform definition of bullying for research and surveillance (Gladden et al., 2014). According to the CDC (2017), bullying is unwanted aggressive behavior(s) by another person or groups of people that involves an observed or perceived power imbalance and is repeated multiple times or is highly likely to be repeated. The core elements of this definition include unwanted aggressive behavior; observed or perceived power imbalance; and repetition of behaviors or high likelihood of repetition.

Bullying can be physical, verbal, social/relational, or electronic (cyberbullying). Some bullying can be actions such as harassment, hazing, or assault that may result in criminal charges (Beane, 2017)

National Incidence and Prevalence

The *Youth Risk Behavior Surveillance System (Survey)* started measuring bullying in 2009 in the United States, indicates that the prevalence of bullying has remained approximately 20% since that time (Hall & Chapman, 2018). According to the Stopbullying.gov website, the incidence and prevalence of bullying have not changed much. Between 1 in 4 and 1 in 3 US students say they have been bullied at school. Many fewer have been cyberbullied. Most bullying seems to happen in middle school.

Some studies have found teachers underestimate the incidence of bullying behavior while other studies indicate some teachers are now overestimating the problem (Beane, 2018). Sometimes bullying is ignored by teachers, school administrators, support personnel, and students (Beane, 2017). According to McCann (2018) only four in 100 adults will intervene and only 11 percent of the child's peers might do the same. The other 85 percent will do nothing. Sometimes, they just don't want to get involved, they believe bullying will make the target a stronger person, in the long run, they feel the administration will not significantly back them if they do report it, and sometimes they are just fearful of retaliation from the bullies (Beane, 2017). Some personnel just do not want to be bothered by discipline problems/issues. After one assembly program, Beane (2017) was told, "You are only creating more reasons for students to complain." Rather than seeking solutions within their schools, some principals even suggest that victimized children be transferred to a different school. That appeared to be their quick fix (Beane, 2017).

In some schools, students may be reluctant to inform school personnel about bullying they have witnessed. This is especially true if the one adult designated to receive the reports is a bully or has demonstrated a lack of concern/empathy in the past – non-approachable (Beane, 2016). They are often afraid the adults will blame the target or make the situation worse or put them (the reporter) at risk of being bullied themselves. Unfortunately, some teachers and principals are unsympathetic to pupils who report bullying (Beane, 2016, 2017). Beane (2016) says some students have reported to him that they are given the impression that they have created more work for the adult and that the adult is not pleased to have to deal with the bullying. When adults do not take action, students decide there is no point in the future to report bullying. That also makes them fearful that they may get bullied and that nothing will be done about it.

The Victimizer

According to Miller (1997), children who bully can be high-spirited, active, energetic children. They may be easily bored or envious and/or insecure. They may be jealous of another's academic or sporting success, or of a sibling/new baby. They may have a learning disability, which makes them angry and frustrated; this may also have the opposite effect and make them a target for bullies. They may be angry from the abuse they themselves have suffered (Beane, 2020; Miller, 1997).

The Victim

Children can become victims of bullying for a variety of reasons, but the most prominent cause is that the bully builds his or her self-esteem by hurting others (Miller, 1997). Bullying is rarely caused by the victim. Victim profiles often include children who are gentle, physically weaker than bullies and appear to lack confidence. They are often intelligent, lacking in social skills, and disruptive. They often cannot understand why they have been singled out. According to Beane (2018), the shy, sensitive personality type is often at risk of being bullied. Such individuals tend to take everything to heart and personalize all negative comments. They look and act like easy targets. Bullies will attack to test other potential victims until they find enough victims to satisfy their need to dominate and control others. Even though these characteristics may not initiate direct bullying, bullies often focus on them to maximize their mistreatment. However, bullying occurs because bullies want power and control over their victims and adults allow it either directly or indirectly through the lack of adult supervision and response or through poor supervision (Beane, 2018).

Bullying may result in almost immediate consequences for the victim, especially if their home environment is non-supportive and/or abusive (Beane, 2019, 2020). The victim may experience the following at varying degrees:

- Confusion
- Fear
- Lack of trust
- Loss of confidence
- Lowered self-esteem
- Anxiety
- Avoidance
- Withdrawal from social experience – including school
- Difficulty concentrating
- Poor academic performance (sudden change)
- Development of school phobic responses
- Anger
- Decide to bully siblings
- Sadness/depression
- Feeling trapped
- Loneliness
- Hate
- Rage
- Self-harm or mutilation
- Desire retaliation
- Suicidal ideation

Bullying is traumatic for some victims of bullying, depending on their genetic makeup, resilience, the extent of the bullying, and the during of the bullying (Beane, 2019, 2020; Miller & Beane, 1999; Miller, 1997). It can be more than just mistreatment, it can be abuse, dehumanizing, hate-driven, violent, and traumatic. The trauma may even alter the victim's brain development and functioning, impact their learning, cause behavioral problems, and ignite a cycle of violence (Gunn, 2020). According to Hall & Chapman, 2018) and the Centers for Disease Control and Prevention, 2017), bullying may inflict harm or distress on the targeted person, including physical, social, mental, or educational harm.

Fidelity of Laws and Policies

"Fidelity refers to the extent to which a policy is implemented to address bullying, including policy interventions" (Hall & Chapman, 2018, p. 58). There are several similarities of laws and policies from state to state. However, according to Cornell and Limber (2016, p. 2), even after more than a decade of judicial and legislative actions and a massive increase in scientific research, today's laws and policies are "fragmented and inconsistent."

There is no federal law that specifically applies to bullying. In some cases, when bullying is based on race or ethnicity, color, national origin, sex, disability, or religion, bullying overlaps with harassment and schools are legally obligated to address it.

State laws can drive policies. Every state has an anti-bullying law, but they are not equal. Some contain components that others do not. But all of the state laws are good in that they require schools to have policies, procedures, and some require instruction and training. Even though states require schools to have policies focusing on bullying, little is known about their effectiveness. Hall (2017), reviewed 21 studies and found that anti-bullying policies might be effective at reducing bullying, but only if their content is based on sound theory and evidence.

He also said they have to be implemented with a high level of fidelity. He found that about twice as many educators perceived anti-bullying policies to be effective than those who reported they were ineffective. While several of the studies reviewed showed the presence of quality policies to be associated with lower rates of bullying among students, other studies found no such association. Two of the studies reviewed found lower rates of verbal and physical bullying in schools with high-quality policies. One study found no difference in social/relational bullying.

In fact, another study found higher rates of social/relational bullying in schools with high-quality policies. However, Hall's review consistently found that schools with quality policies protections based on sexual orientation and gender identity were associated with better protection of lesbian, gay, bisexual, transgender, and queer (LGBTQ) students. In fact, these students reported less harassment and more frequent and effective intervention by school personnel. However, the findings were mixed regarding the presence of a policy and how educators responded to bullying of other students, in general.

Unfortunately, Hall (2017) reports that none of the studies reviewed found the schools to precisely implement their anti-bullying policies as intended. So, even though policies are necessary, their mere presence is not sufficient to prevent and stop bullying for all students. Obviously, more research is needed in this area. This is an important message to leaders who feel all they need to prevent bullying are good policies. Beane (2020) reports that some principals have told him they do not need a bullying prevention program because they had a "good discipline plan and good policies" in place. Other schools simply decided on their week-long anti-bullying campaign could be called a program.

Unfortunately, when schools were required by their state to develop anti-bullying policies, some districts/schools only added bullying to their existing harassment policies (Beane, 2016). Therefore, some policies may have some critical anti-bullying components missing, creating some concerns.

The Requirement: "Bullying Prevention Program"

As soon as state laws required or encouraged schools to implement a bullying prevention program, some publishers who had any product related to bullying in any fashion or form rushed to publicize their product to be such a program. This was a disservice to the schools because the "anti-bullying program" was inappropriately and broadly defined (Beane, 2019). Many of these products did not include all of the critical elements and components necessary to effectively change the culture of the school and prevent and stop bullying (Beane, 2019). Some of them only included one or two elements, such as pro-social behaviors and/or empathy with a limited number of lessons on bullying and a limited list of tips for providing good supervision, yet they are publicized as bullying prevention programs. If the product only included a nine-week focus on kindness, it was publicized as a bullying prevention program, and if the program focused on self-esteem, it was publicized as a bullying prevention program. Some schools purchased these products because they were not costly and they were not time-consuming to use. Some schools decided to meet their state's requirement or encouragement to implement a program by searching the web for free materials (i.e., lesson plans, brochures, posters, bracelets) that they could compile and call a "program" (Beane, 2016).

Unfortunately, some schools and districts only focus their bullying prevention efforts main on certain grades. For example, they only focus on the middle school or fifth grade even though bullying starts in preschool, starts becoming more physical around fifth grade, increases in middle school and continues into high school. Other schools rushed to justify they already had a bullying program in place because they addressed some of the areas, such as empathy and self-esteem (Beane, 2020).

As a result of this broad definition of "bullying prevention program," some schools/districts have used a piecemeal approach (Beane, 2016) when the most effective bullying prevention programs are district-wide and school-wide comprehensive programs implemented systematically and consistently at all grade levels (preschool–12th grade). The most effective programs have an array of elements, components, and resources for students, parents, and all personnel. It has to become a way of living in the school at every grade level and involve all personnel, students, and parents in order to change the culture/climate of the school. Therefore, when certain "programs" are adopted by schools/districts that focus on limited grade levels (i.e., K-5) and/or limited implementation timeframes (i.e., 2 weeks, 5 weeks, 9 weeks), it is important that they review their efforts and adopt a comprehensive school-wide bullying prevention program that addresses all of the other grade levels and includes the missing elements and components that will fill the gaps in their efforts.

Selecting an Effective Program

According to Polanin et al. (2012) and Waasdorp et al. (2012), many prevention programs considered effective or evidence-based have been tested in schools with modest results and others have failed to make a difference. It appears that just as "bullying prevention program" has been inappropriately broadly defined by some developers and publishers, so have the terms "evidence-based" and "research-based." It appears that these terms have also become marketing buzzwords. This has been misleading and confusing, as well as a disservice to the schools, especially the targets of bullying and their parents.

Additionally, research regarding the effectiveness of programs can have numerous limitations and should be clearly revealed and not ignored when selecting a program. Unfortunately, school personnel may not read professional journals and may not be aware of the limitations associated with some evidence-based programs. It is also important to recognize that there are good research efforts and poor research efforts associated with evidence-based research efforts. Even good research efforts of good design can be poorly implemented/controlled.

To complicate these issues, even more, is the fact that schools use effective bullying prevention resources and strategies that have not been officially proven effective through a research project in order to be labelled "evidence- or research-based." Even though the schools have seen the benefits and trust the effectiveness of these non-research-based efforts, they are often required to use certain funds only for "evidence-based" or "research-based" resources. It would be a tragedy and a shame if schools were directed away from resources, prevention and intervention strategies that were more effective than those labeled "evidence-based."

So, when required to use funds only for "evidence-based" programs, districts and schools should consider examining the research design, its limitations, as well as the program's effectiveness data in areas such as those listed in Box 27.1 (Beane, 2016; Spurling, 2006).

Box 27.1 Effectiveness Areas

- Initial increase in reports of bullying resulting from awareness training and increased trust.
- Attendance improved.
- Reduced number of students who feel bullies exist at the school and on the school bus.
- Reduced number of students who have been bullied at school and on the school bus.
- Increased number of students who believe they have safe methods/avenues to report bullying at school.
- Increased number of students who trust adults who respond appropriately to reports of bullying.

(continued)

Box 27.1 (continued)

- Increased number of students who feel adults respond appropriately to bullying seen and heard.
- Increased number of students who feel their peers would stand up for them.
- Increased number of students who say adults do a good job supervising students.
- Decreased bullying in identified high-risk areas.
- Decreased number of aggressive occurrences.
- Decreased physical bullying.
- Decreased social/relational bullying.
- Decreased verbal bullying.
- Decreased cyberbullying.
- Decreased number of students who say school personnel bully students.
- Reduced number of suspensions as a result of aggressive behavior.
- Improved dynamics of interpersonal relationships (student/student, student/teacher, teacher/teacher, parent/teacher, parent/parent, and school/community).
- Improved lines of communication between all stakeholders.
- Improved school attendance.
- Improved state test scores.
- Increased students understanding of their role in preventing and stopping bullying.
- Decrease in vandalism.
- Increase in quantity and quality of supervision by adults, especially in high-risk areas.

Gaffney et al. (2019) conducted an extensive systematic and meta-analytical review of the effectiveness of school-based bullying prevention programs. Their meta-analysis included 100 independent evaluations. The results of their study led to recommendations consistent with those listed in Box .

For more information about program effectiveness, visit the following websites.

- Blueprints Program (https://www.blueprintsprograms.org/)
- National Institute of Justice (https://nij.ojp.gov/search/results?keys=bullying)
- What Works Clearinghouse, National Center for Education Evaluation and Regional Assistance, Institute of Education Sciences (https://ies.ed.gov/ncee/wwc/)

The development and implementation of an effective bullying prevention program require an appropriate program philosophy, appropriate program targets, appropriate program elements, appropriate program components, appropriate program implementation plan, and appropriate program training and presentations. The following is a brief discussion of these areas as they relate to the *Bullying Prevention Program.*

Appropriate Program Philosophy

An effective anti-bullying program will also have a program philosophy that reflects the research regarding effective program approaches and components. For example, the philosophy of the *Bullying Prevention Program* states that anti-bullying programs should not only include policies and procedures, but it should include prevention and intervention strategies (administrative, teacher-centered, and student-centered), comprehensive training that includes skill training (not just awareness training), and curricula. The program philosophy should support systematic implementation district-wide (preschool–high school) and school-wide (all grades and involving all stakeholders). The philosophy should express the school's desire to prevent students from becoming victims and bullies, help victims, help bullies change, empower bystanders and educate all stakeholders (school personnel, parents, community representatives, etc.).

The program philosophy should reflect the desire to promote a sense of belonging and acceptance in all students, as well as promote the Golden Rule – treat others the way you want to be treated. It should recognize the fact that bullying is a heart problem and that it is the little things done every day that make a difference in attitudes, thinking, and behavior. It takes time to change hearts.

Therefore, the program philosophy should also encourage a structure that is flexible enough to allow for the creativity of school personnel and the discovery of new effective strategies, activities, and resources while maintaining the integrity of the program.

Appropriate Program Targets

Any effective anti-bullying program should involve all stakeholders. It should impact everyone associated with the district and schools at every grade level (e.g., professional and support personnel, students, parents, and the community). This is important because bullying is not just a school problem; it is also a school system and community problem (Beane, 2019). For example, the *Bullying Prevention Program* targets students in preschool, elementary, middle school (junior high), and high school. Some of the strategies are designed specifically for potential victims, victims, bullies, followers, bystanders, parents, school personnel (professional and support), and community representatives. System-wide, school-wide, classroom, and individual elements and components interrelate throughout the program in order to enhance the impact.

It is unfortunate that because of lack of funding, schools feel forced to focus prevention and intervention on one or two schools where bullying is considered a "bigger" problem. For example, districts often chose to implement a program only in the middle school, when bullying starts in preschool, increases in middle school, and continues through high school (Beane, 2016). If the district is not able to implement a program later in the earlier grades, that could mean that bullying will not be reduced as it could be in the preschool and elementary levels.

Appropriate Program Elements

An effective anti-bullying program will address all the critical elements associated with bullying. The *Bullying Prevention Program* includes all of the critical elements, and more, that correlate to those identified by the CDC and researchers such as Jones et al. (2012), Durlak et al. (2011), Durlak et al. (2010), Kerns and Prinz (2002) and others researchers and agencies.

For example, the *Bullying Prevention Program*:

- Addresses all forms of bullying (e.g., physical, verbal, social, relational, property stolen or damaged, and cyberbullying)
- Utilizes comprehensive research-based strategies and curriculum developmentally tailored to be age appropriate and build on what is learned each year
- Recognizes and allows for the creativity of school personnel and the use of other prevention and intervention strategies and curriculum
- Includes practical teacher-generated lessons and activities that promote acceptance and a sense of belonging, that empower bystanders, and that address all forms of bullying behavior (physical, verbal, social/relational, property stolen or damaged, cyberbullying, etc.)
- Includes a focus on all aspects of bullying
- Addresses anger management, conflict resolution, peer mediation, friendship, information for victims, potential victims, bullies, empowerment of bystanders, parent education, community involvement, etc.
- Empowers school personnel, parents, volunteers, community representatives, and students
- Focuses on process (as opposed to conducting only special events)
- Provides flexibility in delivering the curriculum through classroom meetings, lesson plans, and/or curriculum schedules, yet ensures systematic and consistent implementation – offering options for incorporating the content into the curriculum
- Includes an ongoing effort to promote the Golden Rule – encouraging students and personnel to treat others the way you want to be treated
- Uses a whole school system and school-wide approach
- Includes systematic implementation of prevention and intervention strategies (administrative, teacher-centered, student-centered, and parent-centered) coupled with the curriculum
- Includes procedures for investigating rumors and reports and responding to bullying

- Utilizes a curriculum and strategies that must be age appropriate and address the uniqueness of students, teacher preferences, parent-teacher relationships, school culture, and climate as well as community needs
- Seeks to help all stakeholders (school personnel, students, parents, community representatives, etc.) understand the nature of bullying
- Views student, parent, and community involvement as critical elements
- Harnesses the energy and commitment of students
- Empowers bystanders
- Requires adults to example their beliefs about bullying and seeks to dispel myths about bullying
- Identifies high-risk areas and provides supervision strategies and supportive supervisory strategies (e.g., adding structure to unstructured times and activities, technology)
- Recognizes that both boys and girls bully and is sensitive to the differences in their behavior
- Recognizes that bullies and victims come from all walks of life
- Seeks to create a "telling environment" – all adults must be "safe places" to report bullying
- Does not minimize any forms of bullying behavior and does not classify such behaviors as mild, moderate, and severe – its impact varies too much from one child to another
- Endorses findings that peer mediation and conflict resolution are usually not effective with bullies but should be included for other students.

Appropriate Program Components

The *Bullying Prevention Program* (Beane, 2009) includes the following major components that should be present in any comprehensive anti-bullying program:

- Coordinating committees(s) called the Bullying Prevention Program Team(s)/ Committee(s).
- Mission statement, goals, slogan/motto, and logo are established by the Bullying Prevention Program Team.
- On-going effort to promote acceptance and a sense of belonging in all students by promoting the Golden Rule – treat others the way you want to be treated.
- Anti-bullying policies, procedures, and rules are developed.
- *Response Plans* are developed to allow for immediate and consistent intervention by all adults.
- *Safety Plan for Victims*
- Appropriate progressive negative/reductive consequences and positive consequences, as well as non-punitive/non-blaming approaches.
- A comprehensive bank of research-based and proven prevention and intervention strategies are provided that are:

- System-centered (district-wide and school-wide)
- Child-centered (victim, potential victims, bully, followers, bystanders)
- Peer-centered (empowerment of bystanders)
- Family-centered
- Personnel-centered
- Community-centered

- Bullying prevention training and program implementation training for all school personnel.
- Bully prevention awareness presentation for parents.
- Bully prevention awareness assembly for students.
- Program "kick-off" assembly for students.
- Program "kick-off" meeting for parents, school personnel, and community representatives.
- Serious talks/interviews with victims, bullies, followers, and bystanders.
- Curriculum delivery choices: Classroom Meetings Schedule, Curriculum Schedule, or Lesson Plans.
- Bulletin Boards, Posters, and Banners Schedule.
- Adult involvement that models the Golden Rule – treat others the way you want to be treated.
- Strategies for a Student Involvement and Empowerment Plan.
- Strategies for a Parent Involvement and Education Plan.
- Strategies for a Community Involvement and Education Plan.
- Strategies for identifying high-risk areas.
- Strategies for a Supervision Plan – developed to supervise high-risk areas – supervision.
- Strategies and supportive supervisory strategies (e.g., adding structure) are included.
- Training for supervisors of high-risk areas.
- Strategies for the creation of a "telling environment."
- Strategies for identifying victims, potential victims, bullies, and followers.
- Intervention Plans for potential victims, victims, and bullies.
- Strategies for ongoing communication with stakeholders for maintaining momentum.
- Strategies for communicating leadership's commitment.
- Strategies for creating a "telling environment" – school personnel and parents must become "safe places" to tell.
- On-going review and monitoring of program implementation and effectiveness.
- Staff Focus Meetings, Student Focus Meetings, and Parent Focus Meeting.
- Strategies and tools for evaluating the program.
- Baseline instruments and measurements of the nature and extent of bullying in the setting (e.g., anonymous self-report surveys and/or student focus groups) and follow-up assessments to determine the effectiveness of the interventions – based on reliable survey instruments and other assessment strategies.

Appropriate Program Implementation Plan

The mark of an effective anti-bullying program is the systematic implementation that recommends district-wide and school-wide programming, training, and strategies. Bullying usually starts around age three and continues through high school. If district-wide implementation is not possible, it should be school-wide in as many schools as possible with a plan to implement in all of the schools. The program should also be comprehensive and multifaceted in that it permeates policies, procedures, activities, events, instructional activities, sports events, clubs, bus operations, operating procedures, codes of conduct, discipline policies and procedures, and other areas (Beane, 2016).

Bullying prevention programs usually recommend that schools complete a sequence of program implementation steps. These typically include forming a coordinating committee, surveys/questionnaires, involving teachers and parents, etc. The following steps to implementing the *Bullying Prevention Program* are provided to illustrate a systematic approach (Beane, 2009, pp. 2–3). Some steps can be completed simultaneously through subcommittees and the rest of the steps can be taken, as the team deems appropriate. These steps may be customized to meet the needs of the school system or school(s). However, it is very important not to let planning delay helping students.

Step 1: Establish and train system-wide and/or school-wide Bullying Prevention Program Support Team/ Committee(s) as well as develop the Program Timeline/ Calendar.

Step 2: Provide the Bullying Prevention Awareness Training for school personnel and volunteers.

Step 3: Provide the Bullying Prevention Awareness Assembly for all students.

Step 4: Provide the Bullying Prevention Awareness Session for all parents and the community.

Step 5: Develop the Program Evaluation Plan and determine the status of bullying in the school(s) – collect baseline data.

Step 6: Develop the Bullying Prevention Program's mission statement, goals, slogan/motto, and logo.

Step 7: Develop and implement the Bullying Prevention Program's Administrative Strategies Plan.

Step 8: Identify high-risk locations and high-risk times, as well as develop and implement a Bullying Prevention Supervision Plan.

Step 9: Establish and/or revisit and perhaps revise the bullying prevention policies, rules, discipline rubrics, behavioral expectations in high-risk areas, and response plan(s).

Step 10: Train school personnel, volunteers, and other key individuals to adhere to policies, procedures, discipline rubrics, and response plan(s).

Step 11: Conduct a program kick-off meeting with faculty, staff, volunteers, community representatives, parents, and an assembly program for students to introduce the Bullying Prevention Program and the new policies.

Step 12: Develop and implement the Bullying Prevention Classroom Meeting Schedules, Curriculum Schedules, or Lesson Plans, and Bulletin Boards, Posters, and Banners Schedule as well as provide training for school personnel related to these.

Step 13: Develop and implement a Student Involvement and Empowerment Plan to create a caring and action-oriented community of bystanders.

Step 14: Develop and implement a Parent and Community Involvement and Education Plan.

Step 15: Check the implementation of program plans and strategies.

Step 16: Re-administer survey instrument(s), analyze pre- and post-data and make improvements.

Step 17: Celebrate success and maintain momentum.

Appropriate Program Training and Presentations

Instead of a one-time awareness session, some form of bullying prevention training should occur each school year. All school personnel (professional and supportive) need to be given the training to help them understand the definition and nature of bullying, the rationale for preventing and stopping bullying, and the role they are to play in the school's efforts. They also need training regarding their efforts to provide quality supervision in all areas of the school, especially the high-risk areas. Professional personnel also need additional training to implement prevention and intervention strategies, to add structure to unstructured times, to implement the anti-bullying curriculum, to respond to bullying when it is observed, and to adhere to anti-bullying policies and procedures (including discipline rubrics). It is also important that students hear presentations (assembly programs) and be told what their role will be in the school's campaign against bullying. They are also needed to be trained through lesson plans to be empowered to stop bullying. Their parents also need to be educated about the problem and involved in the campaign.

Providing all of this necessary training and presentations can be expensive and time consuming. That is why the Bullying Prevention Program provides all of the training and presentations online and on DVDs. The program provides the following interactive video training for personnel online and/or DVDs (Beane, 2016): The Definition and Nature of Bullying (2 h), Why Bullying Must Be Prevented and Stopped (1 h), What Schools Must to Prevent and Stop Bullying (2 h), Bullying: A Sampling of Strategies (1 h), How to Respond to Bullying Seen and Heard (2 h), Why Some Targets of Bullying Self-Harm, Retaliate, and/or Commit Suicide (2 h). Personnel can even complete the training at home. Many of these videos can also be used to train school board members (board of directors).

The program also includes two assembly programs online and/or DVD. The videos are: Help Prevent and Stop Bullying – For Grades K-5 (45 min) and Help Prevent and Stop Bullying – For Grades 6–12 (1 h).

The program also includes 6 h of training for school bus drivers and strategies for the prevention of bullying on buses. The bus training videos, handouts, and manual of bullying prevention strategies, forms, etc., are available in English and Spanish.

Parents also need to understand the definition and nature of bullying, the bullying prevention plans of the school, the policies of the school, how they can help their child, and why bullying must be prevented and stopped. Therefore, the *Bullying Prevention Program* provides a presentation online and/or on DVD for parents: Protect Your Child from Bullying (2 h).

Appropriate Program Curriculum/Instruction

To change the school's climate/culture, it makes sense to involve all school personnel in some aspect of the bullying prevention efforts. For example, it is important that most, if not all, the teachers be involved in teaching the curriculum, not just one or two teachers, or just the counselor, or just the school resource officer. Elementary and middle school teachers have been more receptive than high school teachers to teach the lessons (Beane, 2016). However, some high schools teach the *Bullying Prevention Program*'s lessons during their 15-min advisor-advisee times.

It is also important that schools not rely on personnel from outside agencies to visit the schools and teach four or five lessons, as sometimes implemented by some schools. The students need to hear and see all of the teachers demonstrating their commitment to bullying prevention through the instructional process. Therefore, there should be a definite bullying prevention curricula scope and sequence at each grade level (preschool–high school). Additionally, the cyberbullying lesson should also be included in the early elementary grades. The *Bullying Prevention Program* meets this requirement with twenty-plus lesson plans at every level. For example, the following topics (Box 27.2) are covered in a fifth-grade lesson plan book (Beane et al., 2009, 2019):

Box 27.2 Bullying Prevention Lesson Plans (Fifth Grade)
Lesson 1: Are We a Welcoming Class?
Lesson 2: What is Bullying?
Lesson 3: What Does Physical Bullying Look Like?
Lesson 4: What Does Verbal Bullying Look Like?
Lesson 5: What Does "Guarding Your Tongue" Mean?
Lesson 6: What Does Social Bullying Look Like?
Lesson 7: What is Cyberbullying? What Does It Look Like?
Lesson 8: Do You Cyber Bully?
Lesson 9: What Should I Do to Prevent and Stop Cyber Bullying?
Lesson 10: What was My Behavior Like this Past Week?
Lesson 11: Should I Report Bullying?

(continued)

Box 27.2 (continued)

Lesson 12: When and Where Does Bullying Occur in Our School?
Lesson 13: What Should I Do When Someone Tries to Bully Me?
Lesson 14: What Does "Guarding Your Heart" Mean?
Lesson 15: What Should I Do as a Bystander? (Part 1)
Lesson 16: What Should I Do as a Bystander? (Part 2)
Lesson 17: What are Some Myths and Facts about Bullying?
Lesson 18: What is a Classroom Free of Bullying?
Lesson 19: What is a No Bullying Student Pledge?
Lesson 20: Why Do Some Students Bully?
Lesson 21: How was I Bullied this Past Week on School Property?
Lesson 22: What are the Behavioral Expectations in the Bathroom?
Lesson 23: What are the Behavioral Expectations in the Hallway?
Lesson 24: What are the Behavioral Expectations in the Cafeteria?
Lesson 25: Does Bullying Bruise People on the Inside?
Lesson 26: Do Mean Words and Actions Punch Holes in Hearts?
Lesson 27: What is Empathy and Why is it Important?
Lesson 28: How Can We Spread the Golden Rule?
Lesson 29: What Should I Do If I Hurt Someone?
Lesson 30: Would You Rather Be an Onion Person or an Apple Person?
Lesson 31: How Can I Manage My Anger?
Lesson 32: No Bullying Projects: How Do We Go Forward?

Source: Beane et al. (2009, 2019)

Bullying Prevention and Technology

Technology is available that will help schools with some important aspects of their bullying prevention program. For example, the BRIM Software program has features that allow schools to identify more incidents with online and mobile reporting. It also provides pre-screening questions to distinguish actual bullying from other behavior, promotes consistent reporting and investigating processes, and stores incident details including type of bullying, motivation, time of day, demographic information of students, and location of the bullying event. Additionally, this package can help schools identify high-risk areas, and students frequently engaging in bullying. There is also flexibility which allows schools to enter their framework for reporting and investigating bullying and they can enter their preferred interventions that are consistent with their already established district policies and procedures. For more information, visit antibullyingsoftware.com.

Several Apps are also now available. For example, *Know Bullying: Put the Power to Prevent Bullying in Your Hand* is a free app from the Substance Abuse and Mental Health Services Administration. This app includes conversation starters, tips, warning signs, reminders, social media, and a section for educators. For more information, visit https://store.samhsa.gov/apps/knowbullying/.

Another App, *Report Bullying, by No Bullying Schools* can be used to send a confidential report directly to your School Administrators. The app can be used by students, parents, or school personnel. Reports can also be stored in a confidential database that only authorized personnel can see. Individuals can leave their names or remain anonymous, and they can even upload screenshots of cyberbullying. For more information, visit https://apps.apple.com/us/app/report-bullying/id1423232961.

Lessons Learned and Recommendations for Effective Anti-bullying Programs

Bullying occurs in every school and it takes the cooperation of school personnel (professional and support), parents, students, and community representatives to adequately attack bullying. To change the culture of the school, most, if not all, personnel need to demonstrate their commitment to bullying prevention by teaching the lesson plans and responding appropriately to bullying seen, heard, and reported. Bullying prevention cannot be a once-a-month effort, a one-week focus, or a zero-tolerance policy and expulsion are not effective approaches (Espelage et al., 2012). Piece-meal approaches and zero-tolerance policies are not effective.

Preventing and stopping bullying has to become a high priority of the school and it has to become a way of living from preschool through high school. The program should not only teach students pro-social behaviors and promote the Golden Rule but also the consequences for bullying behaviors. Consequences are a fact of life, yet sometimes schools are reluctant to use them and feel like their hands are tied. Innovative, yet acceptable consequences that are effective need to be developed and tested. The selected consequences need to be progressive, in that they progressively become more negative in the mind of the students. Before establishing consequences, research regarding the topic should be considered.

Since some students provoke students to the point of being mistreated, it is important that schools also realize their responsibility to help some victims change, but to also apply consequences to students who mistreat the provocative victim. The Golden Rule does not say, treat others the way you want to be treated if they do not irritate you, or if you like them. Too often, schools blame only the victim.

It is also important for adults to be held accountable for their behavior directed toward students, personnel, and parents. They should model the Golden Rule – treat others the way they want to be treated. They need to demonstrate that it is more than a belief, it is a conviction. It is a belief that controls their attitudes, thoughts, and behavior. Unfortunately, some school personnel bully children and/or bully other adults. They are poor role models and do not model sensitivity, kindness, and empathy.

Summary, Concerns, and Recommendations

Since the *Bullying Prevention Program* is available in the form of eBooks and files, it is the most cost-effective and comprehensive anti-bullying program (preschool through high school) available. When selecting a program, schools are encouraged to focus on programs that include elements and components which correlate to the findings of research on effective anti-bullying programs.

Even though there seems to be a slow-down in the interest of bullying prevention programs among the schools, more and more anti-bullying materials and resources, as well as supportive technology/software solutions are still being developed and published by an array of companies. Even though bullying continues to contribute to school shootings and suicides, those events no longer receive much attention from the media. Regardless of these slowdowns there continues to be a need for research regarding bullying and the development of effective and innovative programs, especially at the preschool level, where bullying tends to start. There is also a need to identify best practices regarding parent involvement and education as an integrated part of any school's bullying prevention program.

The barriers preventing and/or hindering the adoption and implementation of a systematic and comprehensive school-wide bullying prevention program still exist today and have generated several concerns. For example, state laws and school policies need to be revisited, appropriate (comprehensive) training and presentations should be required, and a scope and sequence of curriculum and instruction need to be required and correlated to educational standards and become a greater priority of the leadership of districts and schools. Schools are still being misdirected by inappropriate labeling using terms such as "program" and "evidence-based." State laws need to be revised and there should be clarification regarding the meaning of the term "program." Rather than adopting a comprehensive ongoing program, some districts/schools are still using piece-meal approaches and are convinced that they are using a "bullying prevention program."

Funding is still inadequate for schools to afford comprehensive and long-term bullying prevention programs and to provide quality supervision through personnel and technology in all of the high-risk areas. Finally, research regarding the use of certain counseling/therapy sessions for groups of bullying needs to continue and the results sufficiently communicated to the schools.

When state laws require schools to have bullying prevention training, some school districts responded by offering limited training. After all, state laws may require training but do not specify the amount, content, or delivery method of such training. Therefore, some schools/districts only offered a one-hour awareness session, which is grossly inadequate (Beane, 2016). Also, such training is often only provided for their professional personnel (e.g., teachers, counselors, psychologists, and administrators), even though support staff such as secretaries, maintenance workers, and volunteer supervisors have a role to play in bullying prevention efforts. Comprehensive training can be costly and states have not provided the necessary funds to purchase what is required.

Some of the leaders of the schools still seek to protect the time of their teachers saying they don't have time to teach a scope and sequence of bullying prevention lesson plans. Therefore, they use outside agencies to provide occasional lessons for free or use only the counselor and/or school resource officers to discuss the topic or to teach lessons. Principals feel they must keep teachers focused on state standards and therefore are unable to address bullying as they should, not realizing that a good bullying prevention program will address certain standards and perhaps increase school performance. Other personnel still blame the targets of bullying and their poor home environments and chose to ignore bullying because they do not want to deal with the parents involved (Beane, 2016, 2017).

Additionally, schools/districts do not have adequate funds to provide the quantity of supervision required to keep students safe in high-risk areas, to repair video cameras in those areas or to purchase other supportive supervisory technology. However, sometimes it appears that the lack of supervision is a reflection of "intentional indifference" (Beane, 2019). For example, some schools do not have a formal written supervision plan, and no one has been assigned to monitor and train supervisors to make sure they are doing their job. Beane (2019) has reported that when he visits middle schools and high schools there are several areas of the schools where there are no adults supervising students.

Some schools provide group counseling/therapy for students who bully. Such sessions focus on helping bullies manage their behavior while trying to improve their self-esteem and empathy. According to stopbullying.gov (2017), these programs often have good intentions, but research shows that a student's behavior may get worse. Group members tend to serve as role models for each other, which typically reinforces antisocial or bullying behavior.

Finally, there is sometimes a lack of state and/or district monitoring of the implementation of school bully prevention laws, policies, regulations, and the implementation of "true" anti-bullying programs, which explains why some schools are lacking in their training and programming efforts. Since funds are lacking, state departments should consider making free resources, even commercial ones, available on their websites, to school districts as an optional choice or resources. Unfortunately, some state departments of education have been reluctant to provide such free bullying prevention resources (scope and sequence of lesson plans, reference books for all personnel, books for parents and students). They have been afraid of being viewed as mandating the use of commercial materials (Beane, 2016).

References

Beane, A. L. (2009). *Bullying prevention for schools: A step-by-step guide to implementing a successful anti-bullying program.* Jossey-Bass, Inc.

Beane, A. (2016). *What schools must do to prevent and stop bullying* (Updated). Bully Free Systems, unpublished manuscript.

Beane, A. (2017). *How to respond to bullying seen and heard.* Bully Free Systems (Updated), unpublished manuscript.

Beane, A. (2018). The Definition and Nature of Bullying (Updated). Bully Free Systems, Denton, Texas, unpublished manuscript.

Beane, A. L. (2019). *Antibullying program: The rush to meet the need was a disservice*. Bully Free Systems, unpublished manuscript.

Beane, A. (2020). *Why some victims of bullying self-harm, retaliate, and/or commit suicide* (Updated). Bully Free Systems, unpublished manuscript.

Beane, A. L., Beane, L., & Matlock, P. (2009). *Bullying prevention lesson plans - Fifth GRADE*. Bully Free Systems.

Centers for Disease Control and Prevention. (2017). *Preventing bullying*. Retrieved August 1, 2020, https://www.cde.gov/violenceprevention/pdf/bullying_factsheet508.pdf

Cornell, D. G., & Limber, S. P. (2016). Do U.S. laws go far enough to prevent bullying at school? *American Psychological Association*, 1–8. Retrieved July 19, 2020, https://www.apa.org/monitor/2016/02/ce-corner

Durlak, J. A., Weissberg, R. P., & Pachan, M. (2010). A meta-analysis of after-school programs that seek to promote personal and social skills in children and adolescents. *American Journal of Community Psychology, 45*, 294–309.

Durlak, J. A., Weissberg, R. P., Dymnicki, A. B., Taylor, R. D., & Schellinger, K. B. (2011). The impact of enhancing students' social and emotional learning: A meta-analysis of school-based universal interventions. *Child Development, 82*(1), 405–432.

Espelage, D. L., Green, H. D., & Polanin, J. (2012). Willingness to intervene in bullying episodes among middle school students: Individual and peer-group influences. *Journal of Early Adolescence, 32*(6), 776–801.

Gaffney, H., Farrington, D., & Ttofi, M. (2019). Examining the effectiveness of school-bullying intervention programs globally: A meta-analysis. *International Journal of Bullying Prevention, 1*, 1–42. Retrieved July 11, 2020, https://link.springer.com/article/10.1007/s42380-019-0007-4#citeas

Gladden, R. M., Vivolo-Kantor, A. M., Hamburger, M. E., & Lumpkin, C. D. (2014). *Bullying surveillance among youths: Uniform definitions for public health and recommended data elements*, Version 1.0. National Center for Injury Prevention and Control, Centers for Disease Control and Prevention and US Department of Education. Retrieved August 12, 2020, https://www.cdc.gov/violenceprevention/pdf/bullying-definitions-final-a.pdf

Gunn, J. (2020). This *is a student's brain on trauma*, pp. 1–3. Resilient Educator. Retrieved August 8, 2020, https://resilienteducator.com/classroom-resources/this-is-a-students-brain-on-trauma/

Hall, W. (2017). The effectiveness of policy interventions for school bullying: A systematic review. *Journal of Social Work Research, 8*(1), 45–69.

Hall, W. J., & Chapman, M. V. (2018). Fidelity of implementation of a state anti-bullying policy with a focus on protected social classes. *Journal of School Violence, 17*(1), 58–73. Retrieved August 6, 2020, http://wjhall.web.unc.edu/files/2016/02/Fidelity-of-Implementation-of-a-State-Antibullying-Policy-With-a-Focus-on-Protected-Social-Classes.pdf

Jones, L., Doces, M. Swearer, S., & Collier, A. (2012). *Implementing bullying prevention programs in schools: A how-to-guide* (Draft), page 2. Retrieved August 5, 2020, https://cyber.harvard.edu/sites/cyber.law.harvard.edu/files/ImplementingBullyingPrevention.pdf

Kerns, S. E. U., & Prinz, R. J. (2002). Critical issues in the prevention of violence-related behavior in youth. *Clinical Child and Family Psychology Review, 5*(2), 133–160.

McCann, A. (2018). *States with the biggest bullying problems*. Wallethub. Retrieved August 10, 2020, https://wallethub.com/edu/e/best-worst-states-at-controlling-bullying/9920/

Miller, T. W. (1997). *Children of trauma: Stressful life events and their effects on children and adolescents*. International Universities Press, Inc.

Miller, T., & Beane, A. L. (1999). Clinical impact on child victims of bullying in the schools. *Directions, 9*, 121–129.

National Center for Education Statistics and Bureau of Justice. *Indicator10: Bullying at school and electronic bullying*. Retrieved July 1, 2020., https://nces.ed.gov/programs/crimeindicators/ind_10.asp

Polanin, J., Espelage, D. L., & Pigott, T. D. (2012). A meta-analysis of school-based bullying prevention programs' effects on bystander's intervention behavior. *School Psychology Review, 41*(1), 47–65. Retrieved July 15, 2020, https://www.researchgate.net/publication/235220413

Spurling, R. (2006). *The bully free zone character education program: A study of the impact on five western North Carolina middle schools*. Department of Educational Leadership and Policy Analysis. East Tennessee University.

Stopbullying.gov. (2017). *Misdirections in bullying prevention and interventions*. Retrieved August 10, 2020, https://www.stopbullying.gov/sites/default/files/2017-10/misdirections-in-prevention.pdf

Stopbullying.gov. (2019). *Facts about bullying, definition*. Retrieved June 4, 2020, https://www.stopbullying.gov/bullying/what-is-bullying#types

Waasdorp, T. E., Bradshaw, C. P., & Leaf, P. J. (2012). The impact of School-wide Positive Behavioral Interventions and Supports (SWPBIS) on bullying and peer rejection: A randomized controlled effectiveness trial. *Archives of Pediatrics and Adolescent Medicine, 116*(2), 149–156.

Chapter 28
Empowering Children to Prevent Violence

Nicole Hockley and Mark Barden

Our sons, Dylan and Daniel, were each murdered alongside 18 of their first-grade classmates and six educators at Sandy Hook Elementary School. A lone gunman armed with an AR-15 and hundreds of rounds of ammunition had broken into the school early that morning and opened fire directly into their classrooms before killing himself. Our sweet boys, only 6 and 7 years old, were looking forward to Christmastime with their families and working on holiday decorations at the time.

When we heard the reports of a shooting at our school, we and other parents rushed there to find our children. We searched every child's face, desperately trying to find our boys. We watched while families were reunited with their children that had escaped from the school. When those families left to go home, we were ushered to a backroom at the firehouse located near the school. There we spent hours waiting with other parents, desperate to hear if our loved ones were okay. It was excruciating. Later that afternoon, Gov. Dannel Malloy entered and informed all of us as to what had happened. Twenty-six people were dead. There were no more survivors that would leave the school. Our beautiful boys had been killed.

The sounds of agony filled that room, as hearts were forever ripped to shreds in the most violent way imaginable. Precious parts of our lives were forever gone. The shock and trauma began instantly, affecting all of us in different ways. Even now, almost 10 years later, every day continues to bring new challenges.

Before the shooting, we were both focused on our individual families and careers. Though we didn't know each other before the tragedy, we both chose to live in Newtown, a beautiful and quaint New England community that we thought would be a great environment for our children to grow up. We were both happy. Most of all, we thought we were safe.

N. Hockley (✉) · M. Barden
Sandy Hook Promise, Newtown, CT, USA
e-mail: nicole.hockley@sandyhookpromise.org

T. W. Miller (ed.), *School Violence and Primary Prevention*,
https://doi.org/10.1007/978-3-031-13134-9_28

But we quickly learned that no community, large or small, poor or wealthy, suburban or urban, is immune to school violence. Nationwide, parents who have been unfortunate enough to join this club of having their children murdered in a school shooting have one thing in common – we never thought it would happen to us.

It can, it does, and if we don't do anything to help address the violence in our schools today, it will only continue. Prior to when the pandemic struck there were already indications that gun violence was on the rise. And while the majority of crime decreased as the pandemic gripped the nation, gun violence actually increased.

In reaction to the COVID-19 pandemic and the explosion of racial tensions throughout the country during 2020, many children are facing increased social isolation, frustration, anger, and depression. Additionally, educators and healthcare professionals have reported serious concerns of increased risk of youth suicide.

We started Sandy Hook Promise with a mission to end school shootings and create a culture that prevents violence and other harmful acts that hurt children. In the beginning, we thought the murders of our young children would finally force federal lawmakers to adopt gun reforms that can save lives. But despite broad support from the nation across all political ideologies, measures like background checks have failed – and have continued to fail since our children were murdered. While the measure passed the US House of Representatives in 2019, members of the US Senate refused to bring the proposal to the floor for a vote.

We quickly began to realize that if we were going to create real change, we had to go about it in a different way. We had to look at a more upstream preventative approach that would stop the violence before it could happen. A two-generation approach that could empower both youth and adults to learn the signs and how to get help to prevent violence. This way, we are not dependent solely on legislative action or law enforcement for the safety of our communities. We can rely on each other.

Shortly after the shooting, the investigation revealed that there were many warning signs the shooter had shown in the years prior to the tragedy that went unreported. Warning signs that research, including a report from the US Secret Service on school and mass shootings, indicates are precursors of someone who could be at risk of harming themselves or others. If only someone who had seen these signs had spoken up, our children might still be alive today.

Some of the signs the shooter showed included increased social isolation in the months before the attack. Officials reported after their investigation that the shooter and his mother, one of the few people in his life he had contact with, had only talked through email before the shooting – despite living in the same house (Santora, 2013).

He also had a falling out just months before with his only friend, who told authorities that the shooter had a preoccupation with mass shootings (Kim, 2014). Investigators also discovered that the shooter had easy access to weapons, as the gun safe and ammunition were stored in his bedroom (Daly, 2013). Police reports indicate there were signs as early as the fifth grade, including writings that portrayed the murder of young children in graphic detail (Kovner, 2014).

The more we talked to experts, the more we realized that many of these signs were common among school shooters and in other cases of school violence. Despite this shared understanding among experts, there were no programs in place that were teaching students and educators about these signs. There were also no programs in place that could help empower students to speak up to a trusted adult if they did see concerning behavior.

So, we decided to create our own. We developed our *Say Something* program in collaboration with leading violence prevention researchers and educators including Dr. Dewey Cornell, a forensic clinical psychologist and Professor of Education in the Curry School of Education at the University of Virginia; Dr. Reid Meloy, a forensic psychologist who consults on criminal and civil cases throughout the United States and Europe; and Dr. Kathryn Seifert, one of the leading experts in the fields of multi-victim violence, bullying, trauma, and mental health-related violence.

Research in the field of violence prevention has found that often those who look to harm themselves or others communicate their plans or give some type of warning or indication prior to the event (Meloy & O'Toole, 2011; Silver et al., 2018; Vossekuil et al., 2002). The extensive research in the field provided evidence to suggest the importance of identifying, assessing, and intervening to reduce and prevent violence.

Our *Start With Hello* program was developed using extensive research in the field of inclusion, peer relationships, and social isolation, and in collaboration with subject matter experts, educators, community leaders, parents, and students. We also examined studies that showed social isolation and loneliness can have a significant impact on a student's mental and physical health, academic performance, and peer relationships (Ingram & London, 2015; Cacioppo & Hawkley, 2009; CDC, 2015; O'Malley & Amarillas, 2011).

Today, more than 18 million people have participated in Sandy Hook Promise's evidence-informed *Know the Signs* programs including *Start With Hello* and *Say Something* which teach youth and adults how to address social isolation as well as how to identify at-risk behaviors and intervene to get people the help they may need. These early prevention measures are shown by various studies to save lives and foster a more connected and inclusive school culture.

Each program offers 30- to 40-minute student training that can be delivered in a classroom, an assembly, or remotely through digital tools. All resources needed are provided, including an Educator's Guide and toolkits that offer lesson plans, activities, games, and discussion guides to reinforce and expand on the core teachings. Companion parent brochures explain the features and benefits of these programs.

The *Know the Signs* programs are provided at no cost to schools. With so many schools struggling for resources – particularly those in lower-income communities where school violence also tends to be the highest – it is important to us that cost never be a barrier to keeping kids safe. Our programs also align with the Collaborative for Academic, Social, and Emotional Learning (CASEL) standards for Social and Emotional Learning (SEL) including relationship skills, social awareness, responsible decision-making, and self-awareness.

Each element of the *Know the Signs* program works to help empower students to help prevent violence in their own schools and communities. The *Start With Hello* is an age-appropriate program for grades K-12 that addresses bullying and social isolation by teaching youth to empathize with others and create a more inclusive and connected culture. *Start With Hello Elementary*, specifically designed for grades K-5, is a fun and interactive experience with animated characters that bring these key lessons to life through short-form videos, games, and activities. With so much physical isolation today, the need for innovative and virtual offerings to keep children socially connected will become even greater.

Our *Start With Hello* program teaches three main steps:

1. *See Someone Alone*

   Learn to understand social isolation, empathize with those who may feel alone, learn how "healthy alone time" is different, and emphasize the importance of connecting with others.
2. *Reach Out and Help*

   Develop strategies for connecting with others and ways to alleviate anxiety about reaching out.
3. *Start with Hello*

   Apply methods to include others, build lasting relationships and support a connected and inclusive school and community.

It's the students who are often the best eyes and ears when it comes to what's happening in their school and their peers, things that are often missed or simply unknown to adults. That makes them the first line of defense when it comes to identifying warning signs from their friends or classmates. We developed the *Say Something* program to help empower these students to look for warning signs and threats – especially on social media – of someone at-risk of hurting themselves or others and to "say something" to a trusted adult before a tragedy can occur.

In our research to create the *Say Something* program, we repeatedly heard from students that the biggest barrier to speaking up was fear of being seen as a "tattletale" and the related social consequences. That is why, shortly after the Parkland school shooting in 2018, we launched the *Say Something* Anonymous Reporting System. A companion to the core *Say Something* training, the system makes it easy and safe for students to intervene when they see concerning behavior. Students can anonymously submit warning signs or threats they are seeing via a downloadable app, telephone hotline, or website. The tips go into our Crisis Center, the only 24-hours-a-day, 365-days-a-year center dedicated to school-based anonymous reporting on the national level, where tips are often designated as life-safety concerns and interventions are quickly put into place. Trained counselors dialog with the students and alert school district personnel, and/or local law enforcement depending on urgency and level of risk to life. Since its launch, our system has received more than 100,000 tips through our district and statewide partnerships, and over 300 confirmed lives saved including multiple school shooting plots averted, teen suicides prevented, and countless other acts of violence in schools.

Within the *Say Something* program we emphasize three essential steps:

1. *Recognize warning signs and threats*

   Learn to understand what are warning signs or threats of violence and where you are likely to find them.

2. *Act immediately; take it seriously*

Understand strategies to take action and overcome the barriers that may exist to being an "upstander" rather than a "bystander."

3. *Say something to a trusted adult*

Learn how to intervene when you see warning signs and threats by telling a trusted adult and know who those trusted adults are that you can go to for help. Because many schools pivoted to a remote learning during the COVID-19 pandemic, we adapted our programs to additionally provide both virtual live learning events and recorded training sessions that educators and parents can use with their children to augment our in-person offerings. As schools prepared for the 2020–21 school year, we knew from the tips we saw coming into our anonymous reporting system that many students would be facing mental health and wellness concerns. These included an increased level of social isolation, depression, or thoughts of suicide.

And yet, the 2019 US Department of Education School Crime and Safety Report found that only about 51% of public schools provide diagnostic mental health assessments to evaluate students for mental health disorders (Oudekerk, 2019). And only 38% of public schools provide treatment to students for mental health disorders. Schools cited a lack of funding, as well as a lack of trained mental health professionals, in their communities for the disparagement. Seeing this makes our programs, whether provided in schools, homes, or in the community, more important than ever.

Many studies over the years, including a research report released by the US Government Accountability Office, found that the majority of school violence occurs in impoverished neighborhoods (US Government Accountability Office, 2020). And while the violence is more prevalent in districts with limited resources, the fatality rate of school shootings is much higher in more affluent communities, as their research shows.

Schools where more than 75% of students were on free or reduced lunches experienced more than three times as many shootings from 2009 to the 2019 school year (US Government Accountability Office, 2020). And schools that also had a majority of minority students also saw the highest level of school shootings during the same time period. This just underscores the need to ensure that all of our children are protected and safe while attending school, as no community is immune from violence.

Sandy Hook Promise, along with the American Psychological Association and other prominent organizations, supported and applauded the passage of the twenty-first Century Cures Act in 2016 that was crafted, in part, to prioritize early intervention and increased access to mental health services and suicide prevention programs. Obviously, more recent research suggests that much more needs to be done. That is why we continually work with experts to improve our programs and develop new initiatives, to evolve with the present landscape, and to prevent violence before it happens.

To help educators and students maintain these programs throughout the year, we offer SAVE Promise Clubs. These Clubs are student-led organizations that encourage youth to take charge of keeping schools safe by teaching, modeling, and continually reinforcing the key messages of *Start with Hello* and *Say Something*. Each SAVE Promise Club receives tools and resources to plan events, activities, and projects that promote kindness, inclusiveness, and the value of looking out for one another.

We now have over 4000 SAVE Promise Clubs around the country where students become more actively involved in creating a school culture of inclusion. The clubs also provide students with leadership opportunities, and we've learned through experience that providing students with an opportunity to succeed helps to increase their resilience when unforeseen challenges present themselves. Many of these clubs helped to keep students socially connected and created their own virtual activities for their members during the pandemic.

We have heard some incredible stories and seen our programs' success firsthand.

One such intervention that administrators credited with saving countless lives occurred at a charter middle school in the Watts community of Los Angeles, California – a community that's been plagued by violence and was home to the infamous race riots in 1965 that left 34 dead and more than a thousand injured, as well as the Rodney King riots in 1992.

Many students at the school were already numb to violence, as most street corners in the neighborhood were adorned with memorials to the many young lives lost to gun violence. But when several students trained in the *Say Something* program saw a 13-year-old classmate showing significant behavioral shifts and bragging about his plans to attack the school, they knew it was time to act.

The students told a trusted adult with whom they had a strong relationship at the school, who then immediately contacted the authorities. The student was found by police to be in possession of an AR-15, hundreds of rounds of ammunition, a map of the school, and several hit lists of students and staff members that the teenager wanted to "give presents to."

Students and administrators also found handwritten notes throughout the building warning about the threat, but nobody could tell who had written them. It wasn't until students spoke up about what they had heard that administrators and law enforcement sprang into action.

The student exhibited many of the warning signs discussed in the program, including significant behavioral changes, pulling away from his peers, outright bragging to other students about his planned attacks, and becoming increasingly protective of his belongings.

Thanks to the alert students who put their *Say Something* training into practice, an intervention was made, the 13-year-old student is getting needed help and countless innocent lives were saved.

Our anonymous reporting system has also seen a marked increase in the percentage of tips involving students who are considering suicide, especially those who feel particularly isolated from their peers because of increased social distancing efforts during the COVID-19 pandemic. Many of the students were feeling alone with nobody to talk to, some were concerned about their academic success given the circumstances, and still, others had found themselves stuck in abusive homes with no way to get out.

One student called our system's Crisis Center during the height of the pandemic to report they were feeling helpless and considering suicide. The student said they were being emotionally abused, felt alone and that they had no support, especially during quarantine. Not only did the student have a plan, but they also had access to the weapons they were planning to use. The counselor at the crisis center continued to have a dialog with the student until help arrived. The police were immediately sent to the home and determined that the student did, indeed, pose an immediate threat to themselves. As such, on-site mental health support was provided and a school social worker was assigned to follow-up with the family on a regular basis.

While calls like this have become all too common at the Crisis Center, it is also heartening for us to see that students are getting the help they need. It is clear that we need to expand these types of tools and make them available to every student and educator in the country.

Recent data shows that gun violence has become the second leading cause of death for those under 18 years of age, only behind motor vehicle accidents (Cunningham, 2019). More children die each year from gun violence than from drownings and drug overdoses *combined.* And yet as a society, we spend billions of dollars on the war on drugs, sponsor countless drug prevention programs in schools, but provide very few resources for schools to address gun violence and the student's own emotional wellbeing.

Part of what we do at Sandy Hook Promise is to advocate for common-sense state and federal legislation that will expand the availability of these kinds of tools to more students. Our team wrote and passed the federal Students Teachers and Officers Preventing (STOP) School Violence Act in 2018, making federal funding available for violence prevention training for youth. Our state-level SAVE Students Act also mandate suicide and violence prevention training for all middle and high school students.

But these policy proposals also can't exist in a vacuum, tools and resources are required to implement and sustain them. We need community-based programs that provide consistent education and training on the warning signs that our parents, educators, and students need. The solution to gun violence in our schools and communities is a multi-pronged approach that includes legislative changes along with education, student empowerment, and a greater understanding of the problem at hand. That is our theory of change.

In November 2019, the US Secret Service released "Protecting America's Schools: A U.S. Secret Service Analysis of Targeted School Violence." The research report examines 41 attacks against K-12 schools in the United States from 2008 to 2017 and is hailed as the most comprehensive report on school shootings in decades, delving not only into the incidents themselves but the background of the shooters.

The researchers found that *every* attacker ($n = 41$, 100%) had engaged in some type of concerning behavior prior to the attack (US Secret Service NTAC, 2019). In all but two of the cases, those behaviors were exhibited in a school setting. These behaviors include a history of being bullied, past thoughts of suicide, increased social isolation, depression, and interest in violent topics. The warning signs can also be as obvious as direct threats by the attacker or bringing a gun to school. In most cases ($n = 28$, 80%), these behaviors caused concern among those who knew the attackers (US Secret Service NTAC, 2019). However, these behaviors often go unreported, and too often with tragic consequences.

The study concluded, in part, that the best ways to prevent school shootings include creating a safe school environment built on a culture of respect and emotional support for students, while also empowering students to share their concerns by teaching them the warning signs. The report also suggested an anonymous reporting system that students could use to share their concerns through a smartphone app, as well as training for students, educators, and law enforcement. The report also stressed early intervention is key.

"The threshold for intervention should be low, so that schools can identify students in distress before their behavior escalates to the level of eliciting concerns about safety," the report states (US Secret Service NTAC, 2019). Put simply, to end school shootings, we all must "know the signs" and "say something." And we are on a mission to do just that.

Bibliography

Cacioppo, J. T., & Hawkley, L. C. (2009). Perceived social isolation and cognition. *Trends in Cognitive Sciences, 13*(10), 447–454. https://doi.org/10.1016/j.tics.2009.06.005

Cunningham, R. (2019, August 19). The facts on children and teens killed by guns. *The Trace.* https://www.thetrace.org/2019/08/children-teens-gun-deaths-data/. Accessed 18 Feb 2022.

Daly, M. (2013, March 28). New details are released about contents of the Lanza House. *The Daily Beast.* https://www.thedailybeast.com/new-details-are-released-about-contents-of-the-lanza-house?ref=scroll. Accessed 18 Feb 2022.

Ingram, D., & London, R. (2015). The health consequences of social isolation "It Hurts More Than You Think." *Beyond Differences.* https://www.beyonddifferences.org/wp-content/uploads/2019/04/consequences_of_social_isolation_2015-2016.pdf

Kim, S. (2014, November 21). 5 disturbing things we learned today about Sandy hook shooter. *ABC News.* https://abcnews.go.com/US/disturbing-things-learned-today-sandy-hook-shooter-adam/story?id=27087140. Accessed 18 Feb 2022.

Kovner, J. (2014 November 25). A chilling look into Adam Lanza's World. *Hartford Courant.* https://www.courant.com/news/connecticut/hc-xpm-2013-11-25-hc-sandy-hook-report-lanza-20131125-story.html. Accessed 18 Feb 2022.

Meloy, J. & O'Toole, M. (2011). The concept of leakage in threat assessment. https://doi.org/10.1002/bsl.986.

O'Malley, M., & Amarillas, A. (2011). *Opportunities for meaningful participation* (California safe and supportive schools what works brief, no. 3). California Department of Education. http://californias3.wested.org/tools/3

Oudekerk, B. (2019). Indicators of school crime and safety: 2019. *NCES* 2020063. https://nces.ed.gov/pubsearch/pubsinfo.asp?pubid=2020063

Santora, M. (2013, November 25). Chilling look at Newtown killer, but no 'why'. *New York Times.* https://www.nytimes.com/2013/11/26/nyregion/sandy-hook-shooting-investigation-ends-with-motive-still-unknown.html. Accessed 18 Feb 2022.

Silver, J., Simons, A., & Craun, S. (2018). *A study of the pre-attack behaviors of active shooters in the United States between 2000 – 2013*. https://www.fbi.gov/file-repository/pre-attack-behaviors-of-active-shooters-in-us-2000-2013.pdf/view

U.S. Centers for Disease Control and Prevention (CDC). (2015). *Understanding youth violence*. https://sa1s3.patientpop.com/assets/docs/66045.pdf

U.S. Government Accountability Office. (2020). K-12 education: Characteristics of school shootings. *GAO-20-455*. https://www.gao.gov/products/gao-20-455

U.S. Secret Service National Threat Assessment Center (NTAC), U.S. Department of Homeland Security. (2019). *Protecting America's schools: A U.S. secret service analysis of targeted school violence.*   https://www.secretservice.gov/sites/default/files/2020-04/Protecting_Americas_Schools.pdf

Vossekuil, B., Fein, R., Reddy, M., Borum, R., & Modzeleski, W. (2002). *The final report and findings of the "safe school initiative": Implications for the prevention of school attacks in the United States*. https://www.govinfo.gov/app/details/ERIC-ED466024

Chapter 29
School Violence: Lessons Learned and New Directions

Thomas W. Miller

Introduction

School violence and efforts to address the most current prevention interventions were the goal of the first edition on this topic (Miller, 2008). It provided the foundation for broadening the scope of the new edition to address the necessary dimensions that required our attention over the past nearly two decades.

In Chap. 1, Dr. Thomas W. Miller writes about the lessons learned by conceptualizing school violence in its many forms. Examined in this chapter are the definition, scope, risk factors, intervention strategies, prevention goals, and public health initiatives aimed at the prevention of school-related violence. Recognizing the increase in community-based violence, efforts to reduce and prevent such violence have necessitated the need for greater community awareness of the character and nature of violence in our schools. Essential are innovative prevention programs that involve the community, families, and children that foster resilience and transformational thinking that results in improved relations with peers. Intervention programs, which provide children who are struggling to cope with the challenges that they face at home and in school, must address prevention efforts aimed at reducing the occurrence of violence and developing respect for all members of our schools and communities.

In Chap. 2, William P. French, MD, professor at the University of Washington, Department of Psychiatry and Behavioral Sciences, addresses the need to understand the neurobiology of violence and victimization. Dr. French provides a

T. W. Miller (✉)
Department of Psychiatry, College of Medicine; Department of Gerontology, College of Public Health, University of Kentucky, Lexington, KY, USA

Institute for Collaboration on Health, Intervention, and Policy, University of Connecticut, Storrs, CT, USA
e-mail: tom.miller@uconn.edu

© The Author(s), under exclusive license to Springer Nature
Switzerland AG 2023
T. W. Miller (ed.), *School Violence and Primary Prevention*,
https://doi.org/10.1007/978-3-031-13134-9_29

theoretical framework for understanding the neurobiology of violence and victimization, especially as it relates to school violence. Recognizing the progress in neurobiological study designs, imaging techniques, and animal models has led to an expansion in our knowledge and understanding of the neurobiological structures, chemicals, circuits, and systems that regulate the expression of violence and victimization. The lesson learned is that we must understand how our neurobiological functioning interfaces with a host of relational and environmental factors, especially early childhood experiences, which influence the formation and function of these neurobiological systems. The expression of violence and victimization is best viewed within a developmental context beginning with gene expression in the embryo and continuing throughout the lifespan. Examples are offered by the author as is the interaction between gene expression and violence and victimization.

The developmental issues in the prevention of aggression and violence in the school setting are the focus of Chap. 3 by Sara E. Goldstein, Andrew M. Terranova, Sarah C. Savoy, Shaniqua Bradley, Jeanie Park, and Paul Boxer. The reader will find the results from the National Crime Victimization Survey and the Youth Risk Behavior Surveillance System data project. Notable observations reveal that aggressors and victims alike are at increased risk for negative psychosocial ramifications when involved with aggressive behavior and violence. Noted are more effective and reliable methods to prevent aggressive behavior in the school setting. The authors encourage research supportive toward aggression prevention efforts that are developmentally sound and address aspects of social, cognitive, and psychological development in their design and implementation. Prevention efforts are viewed as most effective when they are easily understood by the targeted population, and when they are culturally, socially, and developmentally relevant to this population.

Examining urban school violence within the context of culture and protective factors among youth of color is the focus of Chap. 4 by Candice M. Wallace, R. Davis Dixon, Zina T. McGee, and Linda Malone-Colon through a joint effort between Central Connecticut State University and Hampton University researchers. Citing recent studies of youth behavior and negative situations, the authors found that those settings that frequently possess aggressive or vicious environments promote nervousness, tension, and antagonism for those who witness it. These environments result in increased exposure to violence that is associated with engagement in school- and community-based violence. This chapter provides a review of the literature that supports the importance of protective factors in violence reduction. It further provides suggestions and recommendations for school violence prevention interventions that specifically address urban youth and youth of color.

Professor Christia Spears Brown and her colleagues Sharla D. Biefeld and Michele J. Tam at the University of Kentucky, Department of Psychology, examine gender-related harassment in the school setting in Chap. 5. The authors define and document the prevalence and negative psychosocial outcomes associated with two types of gendered harassment in schools and discuss how schools may contribute to the prevalence of such harassment, and how educators can respond to and prevent gender-related harassment from occurring. They conclude by providing suggestions and recommendations for the next tier of research in this area. The authors note that most youth will experience gendered harassment, specifically sexual harassment and harassment on the basis of sexual orientation, gender identity, and gender expression at some point in their school experience. The lesson learned is that these harassment experiences are related to a host of negative psychological, social, and academic outcomes. Because much of that harassment happens within school settings, it is especially important to understand the role of schools and teachers in preventing, mitigating, or at times exacerbating students' experiences of gendered harassment. In closing out the first part of this volume, the intergenerational experiences of bullying, violence, support, and survival skills are addressed by Dai Williams, who brings an international perspective to this discussion. In Chap. 6, the author explores a range of topics concerning how intergenerational experiences during child development impact thinking and behaviors that lead to bullying in children, adolescence, and adulthood along with the link between bullying and violence. Also offered are practical coping strategies in addressing bullying situations, and issues that educators, professionals, and community leaders should address in recognizing major incidents and emerging threats to school-aged children in the twenty-first century.

In examining some of the factors and forms of school-related violence, the second part of the volume turns to Dorothy L. Espelage, the William C. Friday Professor of Education at the University of North Carolina at Chapel Hill, and her respected colleague Susan M. Swearer, the Willa Cather Professor of Educational Psychology at the University of Nebraska – Lincoln, who provide us with an update on the link between school bullying and related youth violence research toward more effective prevention strategies for the school setting. In Chap. 7, the authors note that bullying is viewed as a subset of aggression and has been an international focus of scholarship for several decades, and has been declared a public health concern globally. In an era of cyberbullying, the authors note that there have been significant advances in our understanding of adolescent bullying although, within the past decade, serious attention has been given to addressing definitional issues in the adolescent bullying literature. An extensive literature review is provided as are directions for further study in understanding the relationship between bullying and youth violence research in providing improved prevention intervention strategies in the schools.

Dr. Miller examines school-related violence during the extended COVID-19 pandemic from the Delta and Omicron variants in Chap. 8. For more than 2 years, schools and families alike have been faced with compromising life situations that have resulted in forms of anxiety and violence. Early studies are provided as are directions for further research in this area. Addressed are issues related to violence in the home; issues related to quarantined situations; some of the stresses of a global pandemic on children, parents, teachers, and community members; and lessons learned during this very difficult timeframe. It has been observed that at-risk children during extended periods of quarantine face numerous issues. Among them are the fact that they may be living in close quarters, with parents who are out of work. In such situations, the potential for a negative impact on their mental health and psycho-social functioning must be considered. These children are vulnerable to periods of maltreatment, child abuse, and neglect. Recommendations for children's

health during such periods are offered as are future research directions and the guidance offered by the World Health Organization.

In Chap. 9, Dr. Annie Farmer examines sexual exploitation, abuse grooming, technology, sextortion, psychological consequences, misconceptions, and the trafficking of school-aged children. Recent decades have witnessed an increase in reporting of the prevalence of predatory behavior through the media resulting in survivors of powerful perpetrators. Social movements such as #MeToo have led many individuals to speak out about their exploitation and abuse experiences. Speaking from her own experience with Jeffrey Epstein and one of his co-conspirators, Dr. Farmer, now a practicing psychologist, provides a rare glimpse of the grooming and the sexual exploitation of young girls and women by a sexual predator.

The presence of relationship and dating violence among school-aged adolescents is the focus of Chap. 10 by Drs. Barbara Burcham, Mackenzie Leachman, and Virginia Luftman. Noting that sexual assault is the most common form of dating violence among adolescents in America, the authors begin with the definition and prevalence data for relationship and dating violence. Noting that more than one million high school students nationwide experience some form of violence from a dating partner each year, this chapter provides the reader with the definition and prevalence of sexual, cyber, and psychological aggression in dating relationships among adolescents. Further addressed is the impact of this form of violence and evidence-based prevention and intervention initiatives that schools can consider for implementation to prevent relationship and dating violence.

The twenty-first century has witnessed an increase in lethal forms of violence in our schools. School shootings have gained the attention of parents, children, law enforcement, legislators, and the community at large. Chapter 11 provides information that may be useful for prevention to educational, medical, and healthcare professionals; law enforcement personnel; and school boards that oversee administratively and provide care and services to school-aged children. Lessons learned to focus on a better understanding of the theoretical considerations involving escape theory, the risk and protective factors for school violence, analyses of case studies, and discussion of school shootings with fatal injuries involving others. Identifying at-risk and high-risk students is essential as a part of the prevention of school violence. The clinical lessons raise an awareness in understanding children who are at risk for committing lethal acts of violence in the school setting and that are also examined. Offered are suggestions and recommendations, including recommendations provided by the National School Safety Center (2006) for school personnel, and steps to be taken in creating a safer school environment free of violence in its many forms.

Continuing with forms of school violence, Chap. 12 examines boundary violations within the school setting and beyond. Boundary violations along with harassment and exploitation have increased with the presence of cyber links in the school setting where numerous venues through current technology have created concerns about student-teacher relationships. Examined are the values that have emerged in the twenty-first century along with what is being offered with respect to ethics and moral education, boundaries in the school setting, cyber-harassment, abuse, exploitation, character building, moral development, school health service learning, and community standards for ethical and moral decision-making. The lessons learned from this chapter focus on the recognition and response to the issues related to sexual boundary violations by persons in educational settings. So many instances of boundary violations revolve around sexually related encounters. Recognizing and interrupting the sexual boundary violations and addressing the legal and medical needs of the student are essential. Engaging public policymakers and legislators to assure laws and regulations are in the best interests of the public, children and their families are essential. Establishing policies and procedures that manage and monitor sexual boundary issues in the schools should be a priority for all school systems. Utilizing multidisciplinary professionals within the school system and in the community to address the impact and monitoring of sexual boundary violations and the evaluation of policy and procedures is an important lesson learned. Providing follow-up to established guidelines for monitoring and assessing the effectiveness of current policies and procedures in the schools is crucial if we are to prevent future incidents of boundary violations in and around the school setting.

The various forms range from harassment, bullying to psychological and physical types of school violence graduated to the college and university campus and is considered in the final chapter of Part II. When school violence is considered, grades K-12 is thought of as the primary focus. The college campus must be considered when one considers the spectrum of incidents from bullying and relationship and dating forms of abuse and violence, to various forms of hazing in well-recognized fraternities on campuses nationally. The focus of harassment, abuse, and violence on our college and university campuses is addressed by Drs. Thomas W. Miller and Barbara Burcham in Chap. 13. Recognizing that the college campus is a living laboratory for late adolescents and young adults and their emotional and social development, the authors provide a review of the literature along with current issues and trends faced by students, educators, and college administrators in addressing violence in its several forms on the college campus.

The third part of this volume examines the key personnel involved in addressing school violence. Educational administrators, department heads, and superintendents and their role in addressing school violence are the focus of Chap. 14 by Matthew D. Thompson, Ed.D., a superintendent of schools himself. Recognizing that our schools and districts are a microcosm of the society and community in which we live, all of the issues that exist around us are found in our schools. These issues include and are not limited to race, sexuality, bullying, stress, and the mental health needs of developing students. Examples of some of these issues faced by superintendents along with prevention intervention strategies are explored.

In considering the issue of school safety, we turn to Christopher S. Barrier, a Director of School Safety and Law Enforcement who examines the role of law enforcement in twenty-first-century schools in Chap. 15. The role of law enforcement in school violence prevention has grown and developed over the past decades to where relationship-building is critical toward success with violence prevention in the schools. Officer Barrier examines the role of the school resource officer in the school setting to reduce violent incidents in schools. The author examines a historical overview of the function that law enforcement has played over time and how that role within the schools has evolved into the modern school environment. Policing juveniles in schools has grown into a much more intentional method, supported by education and experience that are conducive to a better learning climate and culture for students. This chapter discusses, from the law enforcement practitioner's point of view, approaches that have been used nationally and which have yielded favorable results in the reduction of violent incidents in the school setting.

Understanding the climate and dynamics of the classroom, the authors of Chap. 16 focus on the teacher and the socialization process among students. Jina Yoon, Chunyan Yang, and Marie L. Tanaka address the role of teachers in addressing peer victimization. Offered are effective teacher training and professional development that should also emphasize enhancing teachers' skills in improving school's bullying reporting systems and facilitating confidential discourse among victimized students to help them process their negative experiences, develop a more objective perception of social context, and empower them to seek social support. Moreover, considering the key roles that teachers play in school and existing anti-bullying programs, of particular importance is a consideration of how training programs and professional development opportunities may enhance teachers' knowledge, skills, and ability to effectively manage classroom-related issues with student behavior.

When critical incidents occur and there is a need for those beyond the school system and network, we turn to two well-respected psychiatrists for understanding the mental health approach in responding to school violence. In Chap. 17, Dr. Praveen R. Kambam at the University of California, Los Angeles, and Dr. Elissa P. Benedek of the University of Michigan examine the role of the physician and psychiatrist in school violence. Addressed in this chapter are the impact on and healing process of all those affected in the school and larger community. Often examined is the "cause" of a school shooting, primarily focusing on either violent media content, clinical mental illness, or access to guns. The psychiatrist may be called upon to address misconceptions regarding a predictive "school shooter profile" and risk probability of mass school shootings, contextualizing them in overall school homicides, societal gun violence, and the like. The clinician accepting interview requests should be familiar with research in these areas and avoid oversimplifying factors that may lead an individual to commit a mass school shooting. Drs. Kambam and Benedek provide case examples and discuss the multifaceted role of the emergency room psychiatrist in addressing the aftermath of an incident involving school shootings and the resulting trauma experienced by victims, survivors, and their families.

Finally, this part of the volume concludes with Chap. 18, in which Drs. Amy L. Murphy and Brian Van Brunt focus on the lessons learned in understanding the dynamics that affect the balance and coordination necessary in addressing classroom disruption. Crisis escalation in the classroom creates a disruption to the teaching environment and increases the potential for violence in the educational setting. The importance of safe classroom climates and the adoption of programs to decrease the escalation of the crisis in the classroom remains a priority for K-12 and postsecondary educational institutions. This chapter details a three-tiered approach to preventing classroom disruptive or dangerous behaviors, reducing the escalation of the behaviors if they do occur, and having a community-based, systemic approach to reduce future risk. The first tier of this approach is setting up the classroom environment with a focus on mutual respect, clear expectations about behaviors, and how frustrations are expected to be handled. The second tier ensures that today's teachers have advanced skills in crisis de-escalation in order to offer timely, appropriate, and effective intervention for the disruptive or dangerous students. The third tier encourages teachers to see their role as a part of a systemic, coordinated crisis and violence prevention response and report to centralized threat assessment or behavioral intervention teams.

The final part of this volume provides an introduction to the prevention interventions that may be beneficial in reducing the incidents and prevalence of school-related violence. Susan Logan, an epidemiologist, brings a public health perspective to reducing firearm violence-related mortality in Connecticut youth. Recognizing that violence takes many forms, and affects individuals of all ages, genders, and socio-demographics, the author addresses interpersonal violence as well as self-directed violence in Chap. 19. Interpersonal violence is a contributor to mental and neurological disorders and poor general health. It also leads to externalizing behavior problems, such as "acting out", and subsequent perpetration of violence. The lesson learned is that the far-reaching impact of violence on both victims and perpetrators extends across the lifespan. The public health approach must involve epidemiologists, sociologists, and behavioral scientists who have been using field-specific scientific methodologies to study violence and injury and its impact on our society.

Recognizing that various forms of school violence can be traumatizing, Professor Ginny Sprang, Director of the University of Kentucky Center on Trauma and Children, examines trauma-informed care as a framework for reducing and managing trauma and violence in the school. Chapter 20 addresses the impact on students who are suffering from the effects of trauma and may experience alterations in their thinking, mood, or patterns of reactivity that may contribute to or compound academic difficulties. This chapter also provides a framework for how trauma-informed care can create a culture of safety that can decrease violence in our schools. Drawing on emerging data from trauma systems transformation projects and the empirical literature, the chapter explores the tenets and assumptions of trauma-informed care and proposes intervention and data strategies for integration of trauma-informed care into a multi-tiered system of support model providing essential elements of a data-driven, trauma-informed approach to reducing trauma and violence in schools. Case examples are provided to illustrate these concepts and offer insight into a prevention intervention with clinical application.

The Alberti Center for Bullying Abuse Prevention at the University at Buffalo, The State University of New York, has been an extraordinary source for prevention intervention research and applied efforts. *Bullying as a Form of Abuse: Conceptualization and Prevention* (Chap. 21) by Amanda B. Nickerson, Amanda Breese, and Jean M. Alberti clarifies for the reader that bullying is characterized as repeated, unwanted aggressive behavior involving an imbalance of power, and can have devastating consequences that parallel those of other forms of abuse. Their chapter provides a historical context for bullying as a recognized problem and offers a theoretical understanding of bullying as a learned behavior that is reinforced within the larger social context, including learning and social cognition; social capital, power, and dominance; and social-ecological theories. Prevention interventions targeted toward youth who are at risk for or are already involved in bullying as a perpetrator or targets are carefully examined.

In an effort to broaden our perspective on prevention strategies, Brian Simmons examines mindfulness strategies for primary prevention in Chap. 22. The author has pioneered the use of mindfulness as a classroom teacher for many years and later implemented it to significantly lower school violence as the head of the discipline at a public high school for inner-city kids in Manhattan, New York City. Mindfulness is a form of meditation that focuses on being intensely aware of thoughts and feelings in the moment. Mindfulness is a powerful tool for teachers and students as it helps to provide clarity and context to complex feelings which ultimately allows for better decisions and healthier relationships in the school setting that might otherwise turn to school violence. From the inner-city schools of New York City and Los Angeles to quaint suburbs and sprawling cities across America, mindfulness is increasingly becoming an educational strategy aimed at improved self-awareness. Its use for scheduled inner reflection time, meditation classes, wellness assemblies, after-school stress reduction programs, and schoolwide mindfulness breaks are becoming the norm in many schools and helpful prevention intervention.

Cognitive training may be a missing component in preventing school violence. Dr. Carol T. Brown addresses this important area under study in Chap. 23. In considering the lessons learned, this chapter provides a very practical and realistic approach to examining the needs of children who are easily distracted; experience poor self-regulation; are inattentive, disorganized, impulsive, and easily frustrated; and face numerous cognitive challenges which negatively impact a student's success in school. Cognitive deficits lead to academic failure, which is a significant predictor of students who will exhibit inattentive, aggressive, and disruptive behavior in the classroom. Dr. Brown provides very detailed interventions that include a specific cognitive training curriculum developed through equipping these children with strategies that aid in managing thinking and behavior. Such models of cognitive training can empower victims of school violence by developing the cognitive abilities that will equip them in navigating possible encounters with bullies and other perpetrators at the elementary, secondary, and college levels.

Character education is revisited in Chap. 24 as a follow-up to the presentation of this subject in the first edition. The benefits of character education in schools at all levels may serve as a buffer against many of the forms of school-related violence. Dr. Miller examines the use of character education from a developmental perspective in this chapter, noting that the use of character education provides the foundation for being able to differentiate right from wrong according to the norms of society. Character education from grades K through 12 can aid in shaping an awareness for moral and ethical thinking and behavior as the individual matures. Offered is an understanding of the foundation of building character in our society along with the necessary tools to create a greater sensitivity on the student's part to understanding morality in our contemporary society. With an understating of what is right and wrong, comes the basis for making ethically responsible decisions in adolescence and adulthood. With character education, and as one matures, the foundation of moral thought and behavior may provide an essential buffer against many forms of school violence when conscientious decisions are required.

In understanding the dynamics of the victim-victimizer relationship, creating empathic understanding in students can be a valuable tool. Building empathy is the focus of the "Step-by-Step" prevention intervention and is carefully examined by Susan Reuter, the developer of this prevention intervention, in Chap. 25. The author explores one's perceptions of first encountering a child with a disability. The influence of bystanders is also examined. Through the Step-by-Step program, the author reveals a systematic approach to developing empathy and understanding in children toward peers with a disability.

In Chap. 26, Chunyan Yang, Jenna E. Greenstein, Sarah Manchanda, Maedah Golshirazi, and Tammy Yabiku at the University of California, Berkley discuss efforts to address the prevention of compassion fatigue among educators, especially during the time of a global-wide pandemic.

In *Utilizing Effective Bullying Prevention Programs*, Drs. Allan Beane and Thomas W. Miller provide a review of the necessary and essential components of an effective bullying prevention program. Recognizing that other chapters in this volume have provided considerable information regarding the definition and nature of bullying, in Chap. 27, the authors briefly review the definition and epidemiology of bullying in schools. Since many schools have failed to adopt systematic and comprehensive schoolwide bullying prevention programs, the main purpose of this chapter is to review the philosophy, targets, structure, and effective elements and components that should be present in an effective bullying prevention program.

This part (IV) on prevention interventions recognizes the role of children and their parents in reducing and preventing all forms of asocial behavior and school-related violence. *Empowering Children to Prevent Violence* is the work of Nicole Hockley and Mark Barden, parents and co-founders of Sandy Hook Promise. From a parent's perspective, Chap. 28 provides a pathway to helping children who are victims of school-related violence with the skills and confidence to address a variety of forms that such violence takes. As parents of a murdered child, Nicole and Mark offer a glimpse into the pain and suffering of losing a child to gun violence in the school setting. Losing their children who were murdered alongside 18 of their first-grade classmates and six educators at Sandy Hook Elementary School in Newtown, Connecticut in 2012 has led them to create a meaningful program that educates and empowers children to develop the competencies and skills to address such situations, noting that in their situation, it was a lone gunman armed with an AR-15 and hundreds of rounds of ammunition that opened fire directly into the school's classrooms before killing himself. Their contribution to this volume provides a parent's perspective and the necessary advocacy to provide a pathway toward the prevention of future occurrences of all forms of gun violence in our schools and communities.

Sandy Hook Promise demonstrates a mission to end school shootings and create a culture that prevents violence globally.

The domain of school violence is an ever-evolving challenge for children, parents, educators, school administrators, law enforcement, and our larger communities. Several educators, clinicians, and researchers (Danese et al., 2020; Domenico et al., 2020; Gardner et al., 2019; Center on the Developing Child at Harvard University 2016; McLaughlin et al., 2019) have addressed some new lessons learned and future directions to consider as we enter the third decade of our twenty-first century. With the guidance provided by these professionals in the field and several of the contributors to this volume, numerous public and private organizations and governmental agencies (UNICEF, 2020; Alliance for Child Protection in Humanitarian Action, 2020; World Health Organization, 2020) have been cited in these chapters to provide the futuristic thinking and new directions that are necessary to formulate the models of management we need to consider in addressing school-related violence. These are essential resources for ongoing research that can shape the prevention interventions necessary to accomplish our goals of prevention for our children and the climate of our schools.

We continue to be called upon to seek better solutions to all forms of school violence for the sake of our children. The contributors to this volume are commended for bringing to the forefront of this topic a broad spectrum of necessary and essential strategies that should assist in providing guidance as we continue to venture into global efforts to find the prevention interventions that will provide the tool kit for all who seek to resolve violence in our schools and colleges.

References

Center on the Developing Child at Harvard University. (2016). *Building core capabilities for life: The science behind the skills adults need to succeed in parenting and in the workplace.* Available at: www.developingchild.harvard.edu

Danese, A., Smith, P., Chitsabesan, P., & Dubicka, B. (2020). Child and adolescent mental health amidst emergencies and disasters. *The British Journal of Psychiatry, 216*, 159–162.

Domenico, L. D., Pullano, G., Colizza, V., et al. (2020). Impact of lockdown on Covid-19 epidemic in Ile-France and possible exit strategies. *BMC Medicine, 18*, 240–247.

Gardner, M. J., Thomas, H. J., & Erskine, H. E. (2019). The association between five forms of child maltreatment and depressive and anxiety disorders: A systematic review and meta-analysis. *Child Abuse & Neglect, 96*, 104082. https://doi.org/10.1016/j.chiabu.2019.104082

McLaughlin, K. A., Weissman, D., & Bitrán, D. (2019). Childhood adversity and neural development: A systematic review. *Annual Review of Developmental Psychology, 1*, 277–312. https://doi.org/10.1146/annurev-devpsych-121318-084950

Miller, T. W. (2008). *School violence and primary prevention.* Springer Publications. Available at: https://www.springer.com/us/book/9780387756608?msclkid=42099f69d5f51de0 ed64c164d46d2299&utm_source=bing&utm_medium=cpc&utm_campaign=Springer. com%20%7C%20US%20%7C%20Research%20%7C%20Commercial%20%7C%20 PLA&utm_term=4584070140123879&utm_content=All%20eBooks#otherversion=9781441925992

National School Safety Center. (2006). *Guidelines for a safe school environment*. Task Force on School Violence. Available at: http://www.schoolsafety.us/

The Alliance for Child Protection in Humanitarian Action. (2020). *Technical note: Protection of children during the coronavirus pandemic*. Retrieved from https://alliancecpha.org/en/COVD19

UNICEF. (2020). *COVID-19: Children at heightened risk of abuse, neglect, exploitation and violence amidst intensifying containment measures*. Available at: https://www.unicef.org/press-releases/covid-19-children

World Health Organization. (2020) *Monitoring children's development and primary care services*. Available at: https://www.who.int/publications/i/item/monitoring-children-s-development-in-primary-care-services

Index

Printed in the United States
by Baker & Taylor Publisher Services